Atlas of Dermatopathology
Synopsis and Atlas of Lever's Histopathology of the Skin

FOURTH EDITION

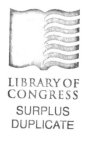

David E. Elder, MB, ChB, FRCPA

Professor of Pathology and Laboratory Medicine
Hospital of the University of Pennsylvania
Philadelphia, Pennsylvania

Rosalie Elenitsas, MD

Professor of Dermatology
Hospital of the University of Pennsylvania
Philadelphia, Pennsylvania

Adam I. Rubin, MD

Associate Professor of Dermatology
Hospital of the University of Pennsylvania
Philadelphia, Pennsylvania

Michael Ioffreda, MD

Associate Professor of Dermatology and Pathology
Penn State Milton S. Hershey Medical Center
Hershey, Pennsylvania

Jeffrey Miller, MD

Professor of Dermatology
Penn State Milton S. Hershey Medical Center
Hershey, Pennsylvania

O. Fred Miller III, MD

Emeritus Director, Department of Dermatology
Geisinger Medical Center
Danville, Pennsylvania

Sook Jung Yun, MD, PhD

Professor of Dermatology
Chonnam National University Medical School
Gwangju, Korea

FOURTH EDITION

Atlas of Dermatopathology
Synopsis and Atlas of
Lever's Histopathology of the Skin

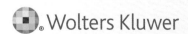 Wolters Kluwer

Philadelphia • Baltimore • New York • London
Buenos Aires • Hong Kong • Sydney • Tokyo

Acquisitions Editor: Nicole Dernoski
Development Editor: Ariel S. Winter
Editorial Coordinator: Anthony Gonzalez
Editorial Assistant: Maribeth Wood
Marketing Manager: Phyllis Hitner
Production Project Manager: Catherine Ott
Design Coordinator: Joseph Clark
Manufacturing Coordinator: Beth Welsh
Prepress Vendor: Aptara, Inc.

Fourth edition

9 8 7 6 5 4 3 2 1

Printed in China

Library of Congress Cataloging-in-Publication Data
Names: Elder, David E., author.
Title: Atlas of dermatopathology : synopsis and atlas of Lever's histopathology of the skin / David E. Elder, Rosalie Elenitsas, Adam I. Rubin, Michael Ioffreda, Jeffrey Miller, O. Fred Miller III, Sook Jung Yun.
Description: Fourth edition. | Philadelphia : Wolters Kluwer, 2021. | Preceded by Atlas and synopsis of Lever's histopathology of the skin / David E. Elder ... [et al.]. 3rd ed. c2013. | Includes bibliographical references and index. | Summary: "In this new edition, as in its predecessors, we have extensively updated the text, based on review of the recent literature, and also on material from the latest (11th) edition of Lever's Histopathology of the Skin. We have added more extensive discussion of several diseases that were either not covered or only briefly mentioned with little or no elaboration in the earlier editions, and have added current references to the literature. We have added multiple new images including clinical images of conditions that were not formerly illustrated. These are original digital images of high quality. As in the last edition, the histopathologic images have been prepared from digital slides and the quality is state of the art, especially noticeable in the low-power images. These images are to be provided online for the reader's convenience. We have continued the use of arrows and labels on the photomicrographs, adapted from the style used in Sara Edward's excellent book Essential Dermatopathology. In addition, we have continued the practice of using tables to summarize the most salient diagnostic features of potential "look-alike" diseases"— Provided by publisher.
Identifiers: LCCN 2020000391 | ISBN 9781975124632 (paperback) | ISBN 9781975124632 (epub)
Subjects: MESH: Skin Diseases—pathology | Skin Diseases—diagnosis | Skin—pathology | Atlas
Classification: LCC RL71 | NLM WR 17 | DDC 616.5—dc23
LC record available at https://lccn.loc.gov/2020000391

CCS0420

BRIEF CONTENTS

In this book, diseases are classified not by the usual pathophysiologic classification but according to a pattern classification, more fully discussed in the Introduction on page xxiii.

In this pattern classification, the diseases are classified first as to their location in the skin, then according to morphologic patterns that may present in those particular locations, and then according to the cell types involved. Generally speaking, these classifiers can be thought of as low-power, medium-power, and high-power microscopic features.

There are eight specified locations, which are assigned Roman numerals I through VIII, as follows below.

I. Disorders Mostly Limited to the Epidermis and Stratum Corneum
II. Localized Superficial Epidermal or Melanocytic Proliferations
III. Disorders of the Superficial Cutaneous Reactive Unit
IV. Acantholytic, Vesicular, and Pustular Disorders
V. Perivascular, Diffuse, and Granulomatous Infiltrates of the Reticular Dermis
VI. Tumors and Cysts of the Dermis and Subcutis
VII. Inflammatory and Other Disorders of Skin Appendages
VIII. Disorders of the Subcutis

Some of these "locations" also combine patterns where these have particularly broad significance. For example, "II. Localized Superficial Epidermal or Melanocytic Proliferations," "IV. Acantholytic, Vesicular, and Pustular Disorders," "V. Perivascular, Diffuse, and Granulomatous Infiltrates of the Reticular Dermis" are all terms that combine a location and one or more patterns, namely proliferations of cells to form plaques or superficial nodules (II), separation of epidermal cells either from each other or from the underlying dermis to form spaces termed vesicles, bullae, or pustules (IV), granulomas which are collections of epithelioid histiocytes (V) or tumors which are mass lesions formed by neoplastic cells (VI), and so on. In this book, it is assumed that basic pathologic processes like suppuration, granulomatous inflammation, and neoplasia can be recognized by the reader.

When looking at a microscopic slide of an unknown disorder using this book, the first approach is to determine what part of the skin is primarily involved in that process. Next, the relevant sections of the book can be scanned in an effort to identify the predominant pattern of the abnormality. This can be done by scanning the table of contents,

or by scanning the images in order to find ones that look similar to the image under the microscope. This process may seem difficult at first, however this pattern recognition method has the potential to lead quite rapidly to the section that contains the disease in question.

In these roman numeral–designated sections, the various patterns that may occur in the various locations are designated by capital letters, A, B, C, … These patterns differ from one location to another. For example, within the very important group of inflammatory disorders of the superficial cutaneous reactive unit, the patterns include reactions involving the epidermis such as *spongiosis* which is a basic pattern of the very common eczematous disorders; reactions involving these highly reactive superficial vessels such as *perivascular lymphocytic inflammation*, which is common in many diseases; reactions at the dermal–epidermal interface such as *vacuolar* or *lichenoid* patterns, and changes in the interstitium such as *sclerosis* to name a few. All of these patterns have their own associations which are redundant and not specific. For example, a lichenoid pattern, discussed in section IIIF can be shared by lichen planus (its prototypic disorder), a lichenoid drug reaction, a lichenoid actinic keratosis, and other conditions. As is often the case in dermatopathology, the term "lichenoid" is not intuitive histologically but is derived from the clinical appearance of the lesion, that is, resembling certain plant-like organisms known as lichens.

The third level of classification is by cell type, designated by Arabic numerals 1, 2, 3, … The cell types in question in the same superficial inflammatory disorders discussed above include among others lymphocytes only (e.g., lichen planus which is section IIIF1), lymphocytes with eosinophils (e.g., lichenoid drug eruption IIIF2a), lymphocytes with plasma cells (e.g., syphilis IIIF2b), or in other patterns the cytologic choices might include neutrophils predominating (e.g., Sweet syndrome VC2), eosinophils predominating (e.g., Wells syndrome VC6), and so on. Neoplasms also often have quite specific cytology. The addition of the cytologic classifier to the location and pattern classifiers can often lead to a very narrow differential diagnosis or even a specific diagnosis. Use of the classification follows in order of the attributes, as outlined in Table 1.

TABLE 1. Method of Slide Evaluation

I. **Location of process (e.g., epidermis and superficial dermis)**
   A. **Determine pattern (e.g., Lichenoid inflammation)**
      1. **Determine cell type(s)—e.g., lymphocytes only**

In the example given in Table 1, the findings would be consistent with lichen planus. Even if a specific diagnosis cannot be made, it is always useful to generate a differential diagnosis which can be correlated with the clinical impressions, often leading to a specific diagnosis based on clinicopathologic correlation. In this book, conditions that may be considered in the differential diagnosis are listed at the end of each section, and these lists may serve as the basis for writing a pathology report that considers, as completely as possible, the range of possibilities for any given case.

We have found in practice that trainees who use this system can develop more comprehensive differential diagnoses as they preview cases for sign out with their teachers. Similarly, experienced dermatopathologists can use the book to ensure that their differential diagnostic considerations are complete, and also to illustrate to their trainees the range of lesions that can have morphology similar to that which is visualized under the microscope. We hope and expect that using these principles will increase the value of the signout process as a learning experience, and ultimately may make itself redundant as the patterns become ingrained into the experience of the learner, who may then begin to recognize diseases like lichen planus, lupus profundus, bullous pemphigoid, superficial spreading melanoma, and so on in a flash of recognition or "gestalt," similar to the manner in which old friends can be rapidly picked out of a crowd of otherwise generally similar human beings. When this stage is reached, our work can be considered to be done and a lifetime of continued learning, useful productivity, and fun, will follow.

DETAILED CONTENTS

I   Disorders Mostly Limited to the Epidermis and Stratum Corneum   1

II   Localized Superficial Epidermal or Melanocytic Proliferations   17

III Disorders of the Superficial Cutaneous Reactive Unit   77

IV Acantholytic, Vesicular, and Pustular Disorders   165

V   Perivascular, Diffuse, and Granulomatous Infiltrates of the Reticular Dermis   217

VI   Tumors and Cysts of the Dermis and Subcutis   323

VIII Disorders of the Subcutis   511

PREFACE

In this new edition, as in its predecessors, we have extensively updated the text, based on review of the recent literature, and also on material from the latest (11th) edition of *Lever's Histopathology of the Skin*. We have added more extensive discussion of several diseases that were either not covered or only briefly mentioned with little or no elaboration in the earlier editions, and have added current references to the literature. We have added multiple new images including clinical images of conditions that were not formerly illustrated. These are original digital images of high quality. As in the last edition, the histopathologic images have been prepared from digital slides and the quality is state of the art, especially noticeable in the low-power images. These images are to be provided online for the reader's convenience.

We have continued the use of arrows and labels on the photomicrographs, adapted from the style used in Sara Edward's excellent book *Essential Dermatopathology*. In addition, we have continued the practice of using tables to summarize the most salient diagnostic features of potential "look-alike" diseases.

As in the past, we acknowledge our gratitude to authors of all of the present and past editions of Lever, and these individuals are listed in the acknowledgments.

As in the previous editions, we emphasize that this book is not intended to be a comprehensive discussion of all of the details of the clinical and histologic features of skin disease. Nevertheless, we have found it to be a useful addition to our armamentarium of reference and teaching dermatopathology texts, particularly as an aid to the understanding of cutaneous reaction patterns and the development of differential diagnosis on the part of trainees, as well as more experienced observers. We hope that our readership will also find this work of value in their practices and in their educational activities.

David E. Elder
Philadelphia
November, 2019

As defined by its title, this volume has been planned and executed as a synopsis and atlas of *Lever's Histopathology of the Skin*. The histopathology of the skin, or dermatopathology, is an important subspecialty discipline of both dermatology and pathology, sharing the language and concepts of each of these major specialties. Comprehensive texts of dermatopathology are typically large and ponderous (both in literary style and in physical weight). These heavy texts serve as excellent references to the literature and provide comprehensive descriptions of a majority of the known classified diseases. However, the knowledge they contain is excessive, in many cases, for readers who may be studying for a nonspecialty board examination, or certainly for residents in the early period of learning their discipline. A more synoptic text can fill this gap by providing information that is selected to provide a framework for future learning, as well as a first step toward the development of basic diagnostic skills in the subject.

The synopsis presented in this book has been literally derived and shortened from the original text published as the eighth edition of *Lever's Histopathology of the Skin* in 1997. Accordingly, we as editors acknowledge a debt of gratitude to the contributors to that edition, who are listed in the Acknowledgments of this book. In a few instances, we have used photomicrographs that were contributed by others to the eighth edition, and in these cases we have specifically acknowledged the contributor in the figure legends. Most of the color photomicrographs in this volume have been painstakingly prepared, to ensure consistency, by Michael Ioffreda. The case material used for these photomicrographs has been taken almost exclusively from cases seen by the Penn Cutaneous Pathology Section of the Department of Dermatology at the Hospital of the University of Pennsylvania, selected by Bernett Johnson,[*] Rosalie Elenitsas, and Michael Ioffreda.[**] Some of the material has been taken from the Course in Dermatopathology offered annually under the direction of Dr. Elenitsas and Dr. Johnson. Some additional cases have been identified from the files of the Section of Surgical Pathology at the Hospital of the University of Pennsylvania. Other new material in this volume includes an excellent series of clinical photographs of fine quality derived for the most part from the collections of our father-and-son colleagues, O. Fred Miller and Jeffrey J. Miller. These clinical images, which represent the gross pathology of the diseases, will no doubt be especially useful to those who may not be in regular contact with patients suffering from a large variety of common and uncommon skin diseases.

Traditionally, dermatopathology texts have been organized according to a classification of diseases by a combination of pathophysiologic and clinicopathologic criteria. As discussed in more detail in the Introduction, this approach may serve well as a compendium of multiple disease characteristics, but it does not truly parallel the way in which common reaction patterns may present in histopathologic material. These reaction patterns often appear similar in different diseases, which may therefore be difficult or impossible to distinguish from one another in a histology preparation. As a result, the reader of a traditional text will often have difficulty building a histologic differential diagnosis because the histologic look-alikes are covered in different chapters of the text. In this volume, the subject matter is organized according to the major patterns and cell types that may be involved in the morphologic expression of various disease entities in different levels of the skin and subcutaneous tissues. This organization should facilitate an understanding of the way in which different diseases may induce similar reaction patterns in the skin, and should aid in developing a more comprehensive differential diagnosis for a given case.

In selecting the materials to be covered in this volume, we have attempted to provide at least one important example of essentially all of the possible reaction patterns in the skin. For those diseases considered prototypic of particular reaction patterns, we have provided brief synopses of clinical aspects and histopathology. We have also attempted to illustrate the major entities in the differential diagnosis of the prototypes, usually with an associated text synopsis. In this manner, we have attempted to cover most of the important dermatologic diseases (e.g., those that might be covered in a board review course for dermatology residents) in one or more sections of the book. Of course, the book is not intended to provide coverage as comprehensive or exhaustive as that in the heavy texts.

This book is directed to all students of dermatopathology, including perhaps some medical students, but in particular pathology and dermatology residents and practicing dermatologists and pathologists. In addition, this book could benefit those family practitioners who do skin biopsies and would like to have a better understanding of the pathology reports that they receive from their laboratories. The particular contributions of this book to the educational experience or diagnostic armamentarium of

---

[*]Deceased.
[**]Now at Penn State Milton S. Hershey Medical Center.

its readers should include an appreciation for the relationships between clinical and microscopic morphology of the
common diseases of the skin, and for the manner in which
different diseases may present with similar reaction patterns and thus simulate one another. This should result in
an enhanced understanding of the process of differential

diagnosis development for unknown skin lesions, and
thus in greater diagnostic accuracy.

David E. Elder
Philadelphia, Pennsylvania
June, 1998

ACKNOWLEDGMENTS

This synopsis has been prepared in part from the eighth through eleventh editions of *Lever's Histopathology of the Skin*. Accordingly, we wish to acknowledge the contributors to those editions for their part in the development of the material that we have presented here in a considerably edited form. If any errors are present in this material, however, it is not attributable to these individuals, but to us.

Among the contributors listed alphabetically below, we wish to acknowledge first and foremost the contributions of the founding author of this text, Walter Lever, MD, and of his spouse and collaborator, Gundula Schaumberg-Lever, MD.

Others to whom we are grateful for assistance in the preparation of this work include many colleagues who have supported our effort, either in the form of helpful discussion, or by the provision of materials used in the book. These include our staff colleagues and the residents and fellows at Penn, Hershey and Geisinger. Several colleagues have graciously provided materials from their collections to complete our work. These colleagues are acknowledged in the text.

We are grateful to Liqat Ali, MD, for invaluable work organizing slides to enable the replacement of most of the images in the third edition with state-of-the-art digital images.

The authors of the previous and present editions of *Lever* are listed below, as a token of our appreciation for their indispensable contributions to those works, and, in many instances, to this.

Edward Abell, MD
Tamer Salah Salama Ahmed, MD
Khadija Aljefri, MB, ChB, MSc, MRCP (UK)
Anne E. Allan, MD
Zsolt Argenyi, MD
Lisa Arkin, MD
Elias Ayli, DO
Johanna Baran, MD
Sarah Barksdale, MD
Raymond Barnhill, MD
Trevor W. Beer, MB, ChB, MRCPath, FRCPA
Martin Black, MD
Heather A. Brandling-Bennett, MD
Thomas Brenn, MD
Walter Burgdorf, MD
Klaus Busam, MD
Sonya Toussaint Caire, MD
Eduardo Calonje, MD
Casey A. Carlos, MD, PhD
Edward Chan, MD
Lianjun Chen, MD, PhD
Emily Y. Chu, MD, PhD
Wallace H. Clark, Jr., MD
Lisa Cohen, MD
Felix Contreras, MD
Jacinto Convit, MD
A. Neil Crowson, MD
Joseph Del Priore, MD
Molly Dyrson, MD
David E. Elder, MB, ChB, FRCPA
Rosalie Elenitsas, MD
Lori A. Erickson, MD

Flavia Fedeles, MD, MS
Robert J. Friedman, MD
Maxwell A. Fung, MD
Earl J. Glusac, MD
Thomas D. Griffin, MD
Eckart Haneke, MD
Terence J. Harrist, MD
John L.M. Hawk, MD
Peter J. Heenan, MB, BS, FRCPath, FRCPA
Edward R. Heilman, MD
Kim M. Hiatt, MD
Molly Hinshaw, MD
Paul Honig, MD
Thomas D. Horn, MD
Mei-Yu Hsu, MD, PhD
Stephanie Hu, MD
Matthew P. Hughes, MD
Michael D. Ioffreda, MD
Christine Jaworsky, MD
Bernett L. Johnson, Jr., MD
Waine C. Johnson, MD
Jacqueline M. Junkins-Hopkins
Hideko Kamino, MD
Gary R. Kantor, MD
J. S. Kattampalli, BMBS, FRCPA
Nigel Kirkham, MD, FRCPath
Walter Klein, MD
Christine J. Ko, MD
Carrie L. Kovarik, MD
Alvaro C. Laga, MD
Min H. Lam, MD
Philip LeBoit, MD
Lara Wine Lee, MD, PhD

Walter Lever, MD
Christine G. Lian, MD
B. Jack Longley, MD
Sebastian Lucas, FRCPath
Cynthia Magro, MD
John C. Maize, MD
John C. Maize, Jr., MD
Timothy McCalmont, MD
N. Scott McNutt, MD
John Metcalf, MD
Martin C. Mihm, Jr., MD
Michael K. Miller, MD
Danny A. Milner, Jr., MD, MSc, FCAP
Michael E. Ming, MD, MSCE
Narciss Mobini, MD
Abelardo Moreno, MD
Elizabeth A. Morgan, MD
George F. Murphy, MD
Narayan S. Naik, MD
Carlos H. Nousari, MD
Roberto A. Novoa, MD
Donna M. Pelowski, MD
Neal Penneys, MD, PhD
Victor G. Prieto, MD, PhD
Donald R. Pulitzer, MD
Bruce D. Ragsdale, MD
Jonathan S. Ralston, MD
Richard J. Reed, MD
Luis Requena, MD
Leslie Robinson-Bostom, MD
Misha Rosenbach, MD
Adam I. Rubin, MD
Brian Schapiro, MB, ChB
Gundula Schaumberg-Lever, MD

Roland Schwarting, MD
Philip O. Scumpia, MD
Klaus Sellheyer, MD
John T. Seykora, MD
Philip E. Shapiro, MD
Debra Skopicki, MD

Neil Smith, MD
Richard L. Spielvogel, MD
Campbell L. Stewart, MD
Elsa Velasquez, MD
James Y. Wang, MD, MBA
Edward Wilson Jones, FRCP, FRCPath

Harry Winfield, MD
Hong Wu, MD, PhD
Xiaowei Xu, MD, PhD
Albert C. Yan, MD
Sook Jung Yun, MD, PhD
Bernhard Zelger, MD

In this work, it is our goal to provide the reader with an expanded introduction to the concept of diagnosis of cutaneous disease by pattern analysis. This concept was developed by others in a body of work stretching back more than 30 years, and was adapted by us in an introductory form in Chapter 5 of the last four editions of *Lever's Histopathology of the Skin*.

As we stated in those chapters, the diagnosis of disease concerns the ability to classify disorders into categories that predict clinically important attributes such as prognosis, or response to therapy. This permits appropriate interventions to be planned for particular patients. A complete understanding of this process would involve mastery of the stages of disease, the mechanisms of changes in morphology over time, and the molecular, cellular, gross clinical, and epidemiologic reasons for the differences among diseases. However, in practice, many diseases are successfully diagnosed using only a few of their distinguishing features or "diagnostic attributes."

As there are hundreds of diseases, each having potentially scores of diagnostic attributes, it is evident that an efficient strategy must be employed to enable diagnoses to be considered, dismissed, or retained for further consideration. Observation of an experienced dermatopathologist reveals a rapidity of accurate diagnosis that precludes the simultaneous consideration of more than a few variables. The process of diagnosis by an experienced observer is quite different from that employed by the novice, and is based on the rapid recognition of combinations or patterns of criteria (1,2). Just as the recognition of an old friend occurs by a process that does not require the serial enumeration of particular facial features, this process of pattern recognition occurs almost instantly, and is based on broad parameters that do not, at least initially, require detailed evaluation.

In clinical medicine, patterns may present as combinations of symptoms and signs, or even of laboratory values, but in dermatopathology, the most predictive diagnostic patterns are recognized through the scanning lens of the microscope, or even before microscopy, as the observer holds the slide up to the light, to evaluate its profile and distribution of colors. Occasionally, a specific diagnosis can be made during this initial stage of pattern recognition, by a process of "gestalt" or instant recognition, but this should be tempered with a subsequent moment of healthy analytical scrutiny. More often, the scanning magnification pattern suggests a small list of possible diagnoses, a "differential diagnosis." Then, features that are more readily recognized at higher magnification may be employed to differentiate among the possibilities. Put in the language of science, the scanning magnification pattern suggests a series of hypotheses, which are then tested by additional observations. The tests may be observations made at higher magnification, the results of special studies such as immunohistochemistry, or external findings such as the clinical appearance of the patient, or the results of laboratory investigations. For example, a broad plaque-like configuration of small blue dots near the dermal–epidermal junction could represent a lichenoid dermatitis, or a lichenoid actinic keratosis. At higher magnification, the blue dots are confirmed to be lymphocytes, and one might seek evidence of parakeratosis, atypical keratinocytes, and plasma cells in the lesion, a combination which would rule out lichen planus and establish a diagnosis of actinic keratosis.

Most diagnoses in dermatopathology are established either by the "gestalt" method, or by the process of hypothesis generation and testing (differential diagnosis and investigation) just described, but in either case the basis of the methods is the identification of simple patterns recognizable with the scanning lens that suggest a manageably short list of differential diagnostic considerations. This pattern recognition method was first developed in a series of lectures given in Boston by the late Wallace H. Clark (3), and has been refined since for inflammatory skin disease by Ackerman (4), for inflammatory and neoplastic skin disease by Mihm (5), and by Murphy (6). These authors have published texts based more or less extensively on the pattern classification. More recently, Ko and Barr have provided a very well–illustrated work that demonstrates dermatopathologic reaction patterns conducive to "diagnosis by first impression," also incorporating the concepts of pattern recognition (7).

In the various editions of *Lever's Histopathology of the Skin*, on which this present Synopsis and Atlas is based (8), the classification of diseases was organized upon traditional lines, in which diseases were discussed on the basis of pathogenesis (mechanisms) or etiology as well as upon reaction patterns. This classification, in our opinion, has the significant advantage of placing disorders such as infections in a common relationship to one another, facilitating the description of their many common attributes. From a histopathologic point of view, however, the novice must learn that some infections, such as syphilis, can resemble disorders as disparate as psoriasis, as lichen planus, as a cutaneous lymphoma, or as a granulomatous dermatitis.

Because there are a limited number of reaction patterns in the skin, morphologic simulants of disparate disease processes are common in the skin, as elsewhere. For this reason, classification methods based on patterns and those based on pathogenesis are only loosely compatible with each other. An observer who is studying an unknown case has available only the morphologic patterns under consideration. Not until the diagnosis is known can the pathogenesis of the disease be well understood. Thus, it is difficult to use a book based on a pathogenic classification as a guide to the diagnosis of an unknown case. To partially circumvent this problem, this book presents a pattern-based classification of cutaneous pathology based on location in the skin, on reaction patterns, and where applicable on cell type. The classification has been based on original lecture notes prepared by the late Wallace H. Clark, Jr., MD in 1965 (with permission), and on the published works cited above, especially that of Hood, Kwan, Mihm, and Horn (5). This book is also closely linked with the "big" Lever (8), and could in fact be used as a morphology-based index to that larger volume.

The classification is presented first in tabular form and is redundant, in that a particular disease entity may appear in several positions in the table, because of the morphologic heterogeneity of disease processes, which are often based on evolutionary or involutional morphologic changes as a disease waxes and wanes. Within each morphologic category, one or more disorders considered to be "prototypic" of that category are described and illustrated. For example, lichen planus is the "prototypic" lichenoid dermatitis. The "prototypic" member of each category is emphasized in the detailed descriptions, because such entities constitute the descriptive standard in a given category, and they are also the standard against which other entities are evaluated. For example, drug eruptions may adopt any of a number of morphologies as reflected by their appearance in the lichenoid category but also in the psoriasiform, perivascular, and bullous categories as well as elsewhere. A "naked" epithelioid cell granuloma may suggest sarcoidosis, the prototypic epithelioid cell granuloma, while the presence of lymphocytes and necrosis in addition to granulomas might suggest tuberculosis, plasma cells might suggest syphilis, and neuritis might suggest leprosy.

After discussion of the prototypic entity in each category, a list of differential diagnostic possibilities is presented. The order of presentation of particular entities in any given position in this list reflects the authors' opinion of the relative frequency of the entities in the list, as encountered in a typical dermatopathology practice. For example, lichenoid drug eruption is likely to be more common than lichen planus in most hospital-based practices. Some of these differential diagnostic possibilities are discussed in more detail because of their importance as diseases in their own right. For example, Spitz nevi are discussed in the section that also contains nodular melanoma, keratoacanthomas are discussed along with squamous cell carcinomas, and so on.

The classification tables may be used as the basis of an algorithmic approach to differential diagnosis, or as a guide to the descriptions in other books, including the VIIIth to XIth editions of *Lever's Histopathology of the Skin*, from which this book has been summarized. For example, a lichenoid dermatitis comprised of lymphocytes, could represent lichen planus, graft-versus-host disease, or mycosis fungoides, patch/plaque stage, whose descriptions are to be found in Chapters 7, 9, and 31 of the "Big Lever," respectively, but are discussed here in juxtaposition in section IIIF1. Terms such as "psoriasiform" and "lichenoid" are defined briefly in this book, and illustrated extensively, so that the reader may review more specific criteria for the distinctions among morphologic simulants. This system of hypothesis generating and testing should lead not only to more efficiency in the evaluation and diagnosis of an unknown case, but should also facilitate the development of pattern recognition skills as more subtle diagnostic clues are absorbed into the diagnostic repertoire to allow for "tempered gestalt" diagnosis in an increasing percentage of cases.

This book is intended as a guide to differential diagnosis but should not be construed as an infallible diagnostic tool. Diagnosis should be based not only on the diagnostic considerations presented here, but also on those discussed elsewhere in the literature, all considered in a clinical and epidemiologic context appropriate to the individual patient.

References

1. Sackett DL, Haynes RB, Guyatt GH, et al. *Clinical Epidemiology. A Basic Science for Clinical Medicine*. 2nd ed. Boston: Little Brown; 1991.
2. Foucar E. Chapter 1: Diagnostic decision-making in surgical pathology. In: Weidner N, ed. *The Difficult Diagnosis in Surgical Pathology*. Philadelphia, PA: W.B. Saunders; 1996.
3. Reed RJ, Clark WH Jr. Pathophysiologic reactions of the skin. In: Fitzpatrick TB, ed. *Dermatology in General Medicine*. New York: McGraw-Hill; 1971; 192–216.
4. Ackerman AB. *Histologic Diagnosis of Inflammatory Skin Diseases. A Method by Pattern Analysis*. Philadelphia, PA: Lea & Febiger; 1978.
5. Hood AF, Kwan TH, Mihm MC, et al. *Primer of Dermatopathology*. Boston, Toronto and London: Little, Brown & Company; 1993.
6. Murphy GF. *Dermatopathology*. Philadelphia, PA: Saunders; 1995.
7. Ko CJ, Barr RJ. *Dermatopathology: Diagnosis by First Impression*. 3rd ed. Oxford, UK, Ames Iowa: John Wiley & Sons, Inc.; 2011.
8. Elder DE, Elenitsas R, Rosenbach M, et al., Eds. *Lever's Histopathology of the Skin*. 11th ed. Philadelphia, PA: Wolters Kluwer; 2015.

Disorders Mostly Limited to the Epidermis and Stratum Corneum

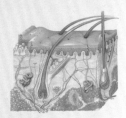

The stratum corneum is usually arranged in a delicate mesh-like or "basket-weave" pattern. It may be shed (exfoliated), or thickened (hyperkeratosis) with or without retention of nuclei (parakeratosis or orthokeratosis, respectively). The granular layer may be normal, increased (hypergranulosis) or reduced (hypogranulosis). Usually, alterations in the stratum corneum result from inflammatory or neoplastic changes that affect the whole epidermis and, more often than not, the superficial dermis. Only a few conditions, mentioned in this section, show pathology mostly or entirely limited to the stratum corneum.

In this Atlas, the cutaneous diseases are listed in morphologic categories based on their location in the skin, their architectural patterns, and their cytology. The lists of diseases in each morphologic category serve as a differential diagnosis for unknown disorders that present with the attributes of that category. The diseases are listed in rough order of their expected frequency in an "average" dermatopathology practice. Representative disorders in each category are briefly described and illustrated. More detailed discussions of most of these and the other lesions in the lists can be found in the parent volume, *Lever's Histopathology of the Skin*.

IA HYPERKERATOSIS WITH HYPOGRANULOSIS

The stratum corneum is thickened, and the granular cell layer is absent or thinned.

IA1 No Inflammation

The dermis contains only the normal scattered perivascular lymphocytes, and there is no epidermal spongiosis or exocytosis. More than 40 genes can cause hereditary ichthyosis, and whole-exome sequencing appears an effective tool in disclosing the molecular cause of individual examples (1). *Ichthyosis vulgaris* (IV) is the prototype.

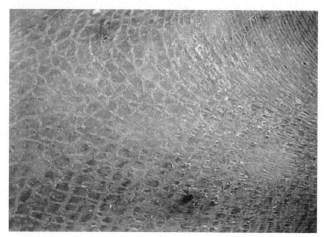

Clin. Fig. IA1

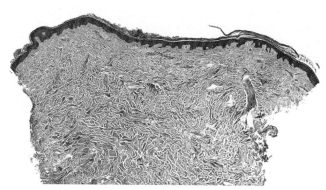

Fig. IA1.a

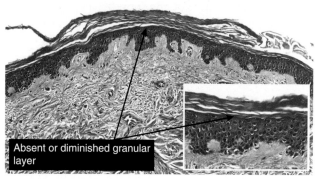

Absent or diminished granular layer

Fig. IA1.b

Clin. Fig. IA1. *Ichthyosis vulgaris: (Autosomal dominant).* Non-inflammatory, fish-like scales are clinically evident on the thigh in a middle-aged male with a strong family history of ichthyosis vulgaris.

Fig. IA1.a. *Ichthyosis vulgaris, low power.* At this power, the epidermis appears normal, except for thickening of the stratum corneum. The dermis is normal.

Fig. IA1.b. *Ichthyosis vulgaris, high power.* The stratum corneum contains no parakeratotic nuclei, constituting orthokeratosis. The granular layer is diminished or, as here, completely absent (*arrow* shows the region of the normal granular layer).

Ichthyosis Vulgaris

CLINICAL SUMMARY. Ichthyosis includes a number of subtypes from congenital severe forms, such as harlequin ichthyosis, to mild noncongenital forms, such as IV, which is a common disorder that is usually first manifest in childhood and is inherited in an autosomal dominant fashion (Table I.1). Filaggrin gene mutations in IV cause keratohyalin granule deficiency, leading to hyperkeratosis and also to loss of barrier function, and increased susceptibility to atopic dermatitis (2,3). The skin shows scales that on the extensor surfaces of the extremities are large and adherent, resembling fish scales, and elsewhere are small. The flexural creases are spared.

HISTOPATHOLOGY. The characteristic finding is the association of moderate compact hyperkeratosis with loss of the normal "basket-weave" pattern of the keratin and a thin or absent granular layer. The hyperkeratosis often extends into the hair follicles, resulting in large keratotic follicular plugs. The dermis is normal.

TABLE I.1. Three Prototypes of Ichthyosis (1)

Disease (Severity)	Molecule	Locus of Disorder	Pattern
IV (mild)	Filaggrin	Keratohyalin (KH) granules	Hyperkeratosis (HK) without KH granules
XLI (moderate)	Steroid Sulfatase	Cornified cell envelope	HK with normal KH granules
HI (severe)	ABCA12	Intercellular lipid transport	HK with abnormal lamellar granules

IV, ichthyosis vulgaris; HI, harlequin ichthyosis; XLI, X-linked ichthyosis.

IB	**HYPERKERATOSIS WITH NORMAL OR HYPERGRANULOSIS**

The stratum corneum is thickened, the granular cell layer is normal or thickened, and the dermis shows only sparse perivascular lymphocytes. There is no epidermal spongiosis or exocytosis.

1. No Inflammation
2. Scant Inflammation

IB1 | No Inflammation

There is hyperkeratosis and the upper dermis contains only sparse perivascular lymphocytes.

X-Linked Ichthyosis

CLINICAL SUMMARY. X-linked ichthyosis is recessively inherited, about 90% caused by gene deletion leading to steroid sulfatase deficiency which results in impaired hydrolysis of cholesterol sulfate leading to accumulation of cholesterol-3 sulfate in the epidermis (1,4). It is only rarely present at birth.

Although female heterozygotes are frequently affected, males have a more severe form of the disorder. The thickness of the adherent scales increases during childhood. In contrast to IV, the flexural creases may be involved.

HISTOPATHOLOGY. There is hyperkeratosis. The granular layer is normal or slightly thickened but not thinned as in dominant IV. The epidermis may be slightly thickened.

Epidermolytic Hyperkeratosis

CLINICAL SUMMARY. This rather striking histologic reaction pattern is also known as *granular degeneration of the epidermis*. It is seen in some linear epidermal nevi and

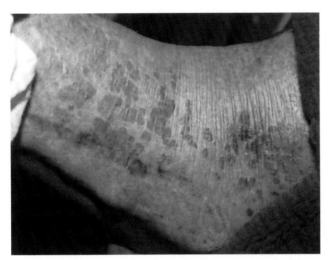

Clin. Fig. IB1.a

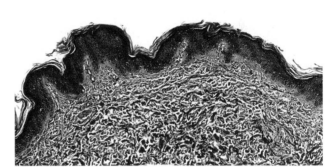

Fig. IB1.a

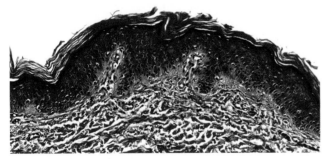

Fig. IB1.b

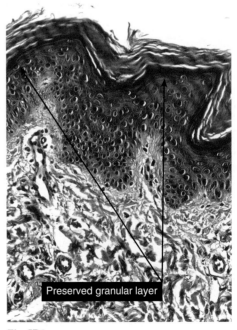

Preserved granular layer

Fig. IB1.c

Clin. Fig. IB1.a. *X-linked ichthyosis.* Large "dirty" scales on the ankle are characteristic.

Fig. IB1.a. *X-linked ichthyosis.* At scanning power, the epidermis appears normal, except for uniform thickening of the stratum corneum.

Fig. IB1.b. *X-linked ichthyosis, medium power.* The thickened stratum corneum contains no parakeratotic nuclei, constituting orthokeratosis.

Fig. IB1.c. *X-linked ichthyosis, high power.* A granular layer is present, visible as a *thin blue line* in the upper epidermis (*arrow*).

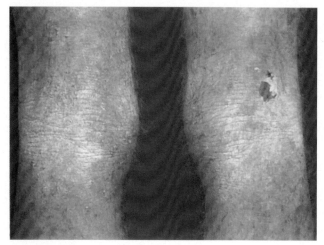

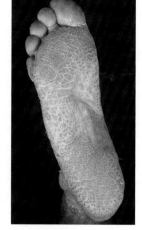

Clin. Fig. IB1.b   **Clin. Fig. IB1.c**

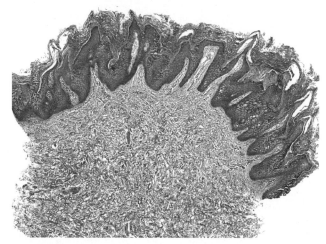

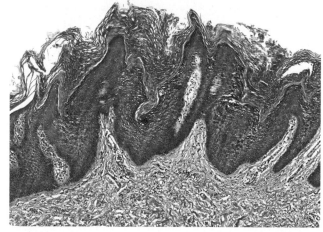

Fig. IB1.d   **Fig. IB1.e**

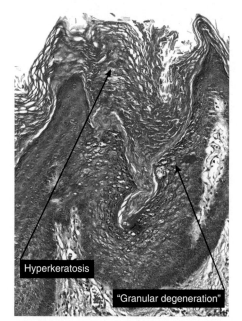

Hyperkeratosis

"Granular degeneration"

Fig. IB1.f

Clin. Fig. IB1.b. *Epidermolytic hyperkeratosis in bullous congenital ichthyosiform erythroderma:* (a). Popliteal flexures are involved with keratotic, almost verrucous, malodorous scale. Erosions appear in sites of bullae.

Clin. Fig. IB1.c. *Bullous congenital ichthyosiform erythroderma.* The sole of the same patient's foot shows characteristic symptomatic yellow keratoderma. The patient's son shares this autosomal dominant condition.

Fig. IB1.d. *Epidermolytic hyperkeratosis, low power.* The epidermis is thickened and there is papillomatosis (these changes are not usually seen in focal acantholytic dyskeratoses). There is compact hyperkeratosis in the stratum corneum.

Fig. IB1.e. *Epidermolytic hyperkeratosis, medium power.* The epidermis shows vacuolated keratinocytes with large keratohyalin granules. There is compact hyperkeratosis in the stratum corneum.

Fig. IB1.f. *Epidermolytic hyperkeratosis, high power.* There is ortho-keratotic hyperkeratosis. The epidermis shows vacuolated keratinocytes with large keratohyalin granules. The keratohyalin granules are irregular and cell borders are ill-defined (*arrows*).

in bullous congenital ichthyosiform erythroderma. The disease results from mutations in the *K1* and *K10* keratin genes (chromosomes 12 and 17, respectively), which encode the keratins in the suprabasal epidermis. These mutations cause faulty assembly of keratin tonofilaments and impair their insertion into desmosomes. These flaws prevent normal development of the cytoskeleton, resulting in epidermal "lysis" and a tendency to form vesicles (5). Similar changes are also seen as one of several reaction patterns in Grover disease, and the same pattern is perhaps more commonly observed as an incidental finding, when it may be referred to as a form of "focal acantholytic keratosis" (FAK, see section IVC1) (6).

HISTOPATHOLOGY. The salient histologic features are (1) perinuclear vacuolization of the cells in the stratum spinosum and in the stratum granulosum; (2) peripheral to the vacuolization, irregular cellular boundaries; (3) an increased number of irregularly shaped, large keratohyalin granules; and (4) compact hyperkeratosis in the stratum corneum.

Epidermodysplasia Verruciformis

CLINICAL SUMMARY: Epidermodysplasia verruciformis (EV) is a genetic disease characterized by HPV infection with types not seen in otherwise healthy individuals (7). It usually begins in childhood and is characterized by a generalized infection by certain subtypes of HPV (referred to as "EV HPVs"), frequent association with cutaneous carcinomas, and abnormalities of cell-mediated immunity. Two forms of EV are recognized. One is induced by HPV-3 and HPV-10 and characterized by a persistent widespread eruption resembling verruca planae with a tendency toward confluence into plaques. Some of the cases are familial. There is no tendency to malignant transformation in this form. The second form is primarily related to HPV-5. There is often a familial history with an autosomal recessive or X-linked recessive inheritance. In addition to the plane warts, irregularly outlined, slightly scaling macules of various shades of brown, red, and white, tinea versicolor-like lesions, and seborrheic keratosis–like lesions have been noted. Development of Bowen disease

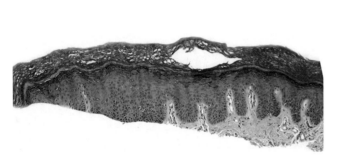

Fig. IB1.g

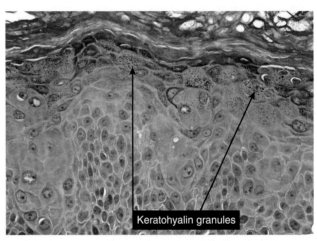

Keratohyalin granules

Fig. IB1.h

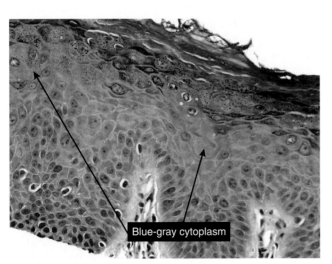

Blue-gray cytoplasm

Fig. IB1.i

Fig. IB1.g. *Epidermodysplasia verruciformis, low power.* Sections show hyperkeratosis, cytoplasmic "blue-gray" change of superficial keratinocytes, and hypergranulosis.

Fig. IB1.h. *Epidermodysplasia verruciformis, medium power.* The superficially located affected keratinocytes are swollen and irregularly shaped. There are a few lymphocytes in the upper dermis.

Fig. IB1.i. *Epidermodysplasia verruciformis, high power.* The nuclei are enlarged, with open chromatin, and there are prominent basophilic keratohyalin granules (*arrow*).

(squamous cell carcinoma *in situ*) within lesions in exposed areas is a common occurrence, and invasive lesions of squamous cell carcinoma are occasionally found. The oncogenic potential is highest for HPV-5 and HPV-8. EV-like lesions can develop in renal transplant patients and in HIV-infected persons. Two known EV susceptibility loci, EV1 and EV2, which belong to the transmembrane channel–like (TMC) gene family, may serve as restriction factors for EV HPVs. In EV individuals, these genes are mutated and malfunctioning, causing a defective cell-mediated immune mechanism against certain types of viruses (8).

HISTOPATHOLOGY. The epidermal changes, although similar to those observed in verruca plana, often differ by being more pronounced and more extensive. Affected keratinocytes are swollen and irregularly shaped. They show abundant, slightly basophilic blue-gray cytoplasm and some contain numerous round, basophilic keratohyalin granules. A few dyskeratotic cells may be seen in the lower part of the epidermis. Although some nuclei appear pyknotic, others appear large, round, and empty owing to marginal distribution of the chromatin. HPV DNA in these lesions is high copy and localized to the upper half of the lesion in cells with cytologic features that included perinuclear halos, blue-gray cytoplasm, and hyper/parakeratosis (9). In immunocompromised patients, EV often lacks the histologic features of verruca planae, a focally thickened granular layer is

a marker for viral detection, and the risk for dysplasia in such lesions is much higher than in EV not associated with acquired immunosuppression. It has been shown that the host response to HPV-5/8 infection in EV includes up regulation of proteins including p16, Ki67, importin-β, exportin-5, Mcl1, and PDL1, and it is suggested that these proteins may serve as biomarkers that can aid in cases that are equivocal on histologic examination (9).

Conditions to consider in the differential diagnosis:

lamellar ichthyosis
X-linked ichthyosis
epidermolytic hyperkeratosis
epidermolytic acanthoma
oculocutaneous tyrosinosis (tyrosinemia)
acanthosis nigricans
large cell acanthoma
verruca plana
EV
hyperkeratosis lenticularis perstans (Flegel disease)

IB2 | Scant Inflammation

There is hyperkeratosis and lymphocytes are minimally increased about the superficial plexus. There may be a few neutrophils in the stratum corneum.

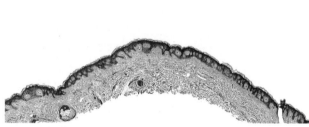

Fig. IB2.a

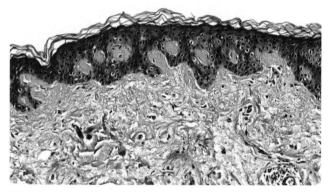

Fig. IB2.b

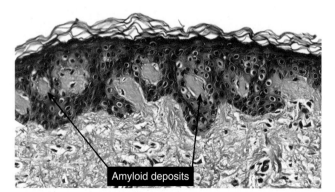

Fig. IB2.c

Fig. IB2.a. *Macular amyloidosis, low power.* At scanning magnification, there is slight hyperkeratosis with minimal inflammation.

Fig. IB2.b. *Macular amyloidosis, medium power.* At this power, the epidermis appears normal, except for slight uniform acanthosis. Subtle deposits of pink amorphous material (amyloid) are seen in dermal papillae.

Fig. IB2.c. *Macular amyloidosis, high power.* There is orthokeratotic hyperkeratosis. The granular layer is normal. There are deposits of amyloid in the dermal papillae (*arrows*).

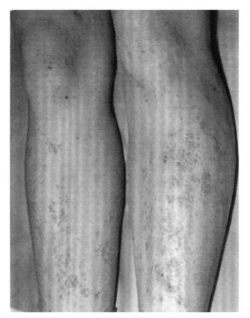

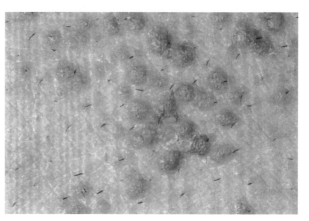

Clin. Fig. IB2.b

Clin. Fig. IB2.a. *Lichen amyloidosis.* Patient presented with pruritic papules on the pretibial areas.

Clin. Fig. IB2.b. *Lichen amyloidosis.* Pigmented discrete papules result from deposition of amyloid derived from keratinocytes.

Clin. Fig. IB2.a

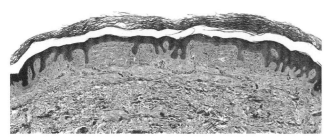

Fig. IB2.d

Fig. IB2.d. *Lichen amyloidosis, low power.* In contrast to macular amyloidosis, lichen amyloidosis reveals irregular acanthosis, papillomatosis, and hyperkeratosis. The papillary dermis is expanded by amorphous eosinophilic material (*arrows*) and there is a mild perivascular inflammatory infiltrate.

Fig. IB2.e. *Lichen amyloidosis, high power.* At higher magnification the amorphous deposits of amyloid are seen in the papillary dermis associated with pigment laden macrophages.

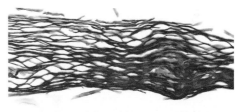

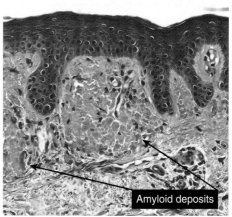

Amyloid deposits

Fig. IB2.e

Lichen Amyloidosis and Macular Amyloidosis

CLINICAL SUMMARY. Lichen amyloidosis and macular amyloidosis are best considered as different manifestations of the same disease process. Lichen amyloidosis is characterized by closely set, discrete, brown-red pruritic often somewhat scaly papules and plaques that are most commonly located on the legs, especially the shins. The plaques often have verrucous surfaces and then resemble hypertrophic lichen planus or lichen simplex chronicus. It is assumed by some that the pruritis leads to damage of keratinocytes by scratching and to subsequent production of amyloid. The amyloid material contains cytokeratins derived from epidermal keratinocytes.

HISTOPATHOLOGY. Lichen and macular amyloidosis show deposits of amyloid that are limited to the papillary dermis. Most of the amyloid is situated within the dermal papillae. Although the deposits usually are smaller in macular amyloidosis than in lichen amyloidosis, differentiation of the two on the basis of the amount of amyloid is not possible. The two conditions actually differ only in the appearance of the epidermis, which is hyperplastic and hyperkeratotic in lichen amyloidosis. Occasionally, the amount of amyloid in macular amyloidosis is so small that it is missed. In such instances, more than one biopsy might be necessary to confirm the diagnosis.

Conditions to consider in the differential diagnosis of this category:

dermatophytosis
lichen amyloidosis and macular amyloidosis

IC HYPERKERATOSIS WITH PARAKERATOSIS

The stratum corneum is thickened, the granular cell layer is reduced, there is parakeratosis. The dermis may show only sparse perivascular lymphocytes, although some of the conditions listed here in other instances may show more substantial inflammation. There is no epidermal spongiosis or exocytosis. Most examples of dermatoses associated with parakeratosis have significant inflammation in the dermis (see Sections IIIA–E). Some neoplastic disorders (e.g., actinic keratoses) present with parakeratosis, usually also associated with epidermal thickening, and inflammation in the dermis (Section IIA).

IC1 Scant or No Inflammation

Lymphocytes are minimally increased about the superficial plexus. There may be a few lymphocytes and/or neutrophils

in the stratum corneum. *Dermatophytosis* is prototypic (10). However, many examples of dermatophytosis have significant inflammation, simulating one or another of the superficial inflammatory dermatoses (see Section III).

Dermatophytosis

CLINICAL SUMMARY. Fungal infections of seven anatomical regions are commonly recognized: tinea capitis (including tinea favosa or favus of the scalp), tinea barbae, tinea faciei, tinea corporis (including tinea imbricata), tinea cruris, tinea of the hands and feet, and tinea unguium. *Tinea corporis* may be caused by any dermatophyte, but by far the most common cause in the United States is *Trichophyton rubrum*, followed by *Microsporum canis* and Trichophyton *mentagrophytes*. In *T. rubrum* infection there are large patches showing central clearing and a polycyclic scaling border, which may be quite narrow and threadlike.

HISTOPATHOLOGY. Fungi may present as filamentous hyphae, arthrospores, yeast forms, or pseudohyphae. Hyphae are threadlike structures that may be septate or nonseptate. Arthrospores are spores formed by fragmentation of septate hyphae at the septum, usually appearing as rounded, boxlike, or short cylindrical forms. Yeasts are single-celled forms that appear as round, elongated, or ovoid bodies; they grow by budding, and their progeny may adhere to each other and form elongated chains called pseudohyphae. If fungi are present in the horny layer, they may be "sandwiched" between two zones of cornified cells, the upper being orthokeratotic and the lower consisting partially

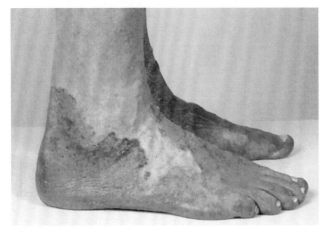

Clin. Fig. IC1.a

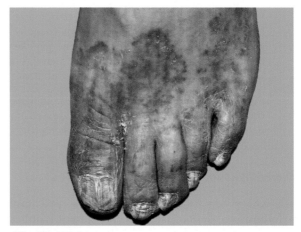

Clin. Fig. IC1.b

Clin. Fig. IC1.a. *Tinea pedis.* A leading edge of scale and erythema in a moccasin distribution characterizes this infection, most commonly caused by the dermatophyte *Trichophyton rubrum*.

Clin. Fig. IC1.b. *Tinea pedis.* Erythema, scale, and dystrophic nail changes consistent with associated onychomycosis.

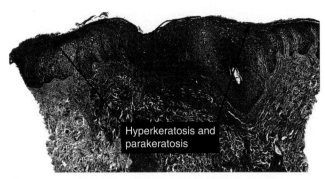

Hyperkeratosis and parakeratosis

Fig. IC1.a

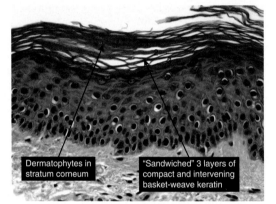

Hyphae

Fig. IC1.b

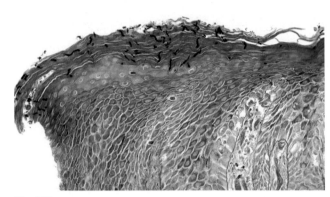

Fig. IC1.c

Dermatophytes in stratum corneum

"Sandwiched" 3 layers of compact and intervening basket-weave keratin

Fig. IC1.d

Fig. IC1.a. *Dermatophytosis, medium power.* At this magnification, the epidermis may appear normal, slightly thickened as here, spongiotic, and/or psoriasiform. There is slight uniform thickening of the stratum corneum.

Fig. IC1.b. *Dermatophytosis, high power.* At high magnification, there is mixed ortho-keratotic hyperkeratosis often "sandwiched" above a layer of parakeratosis, and with focal collections of neutrophils. The granular layer is normal. Hyphal forms may be appreciable even in the H&E section (*arrows*).

Fig. IC1.c. *Dermatophytosis, high power—stain for fungi.* A PAS or a Grocott stain highlights fungal hyphae in the stratum corneum. These are likely to be most numerous in areas away from the collections of neutrophils.

Fig. IC1.d. *"Sandwich sign" in dermatophytosis.* There are alternating layers of "basket-weave" orthokeratosis and compact orthokeratosis; fungal organisms are present in the latter.

of parakeratotic cells. This "sandwich sign" should prompt the performance of a stain for fungi for verification (11). The presence of neutrophils in the stratum corneum is another valuable diagnostic clue. In the absence of demonstrable fungi, the histologic picture of fungal infections of the glabrous skin is not diagnostic. Depending on the degree of reaction of the skin to the presence of fungi, there may be histologic features of an acute, a subacute, or a chronic spongiotic dermatitis.

Granular Parakeratosis

CLINICAL SUMMARY. Granular parakeratosis was initially described as "axillary granular parakeratosis"

because all of the original patients presented with lesions confined to the axillae. Subsequent reports described lesions in inguinal creases, inframammary folds, and other nonintertriginous areas (12). It occurs in both men and women with predominance in the female gender. The characteristic clinical findings are erythematous or hyperpigmented plaques that may be crusted or verrucous. There may be associated pruritus or burning. The total number of lesions is usually small and there are no oral lesions. Because of the clinical presentation, the clinical differential diagnosis usually includes Hailey–Hailey disease, Darier disease, acanthosis nigricans, or contact dermatitis. In the original descriptions, an unusual contact reaction to deodorants was hypothesized, however with

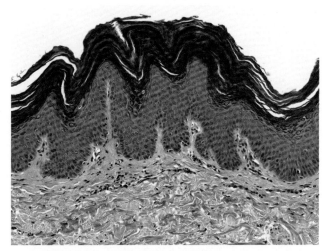

Fig. IC1.e

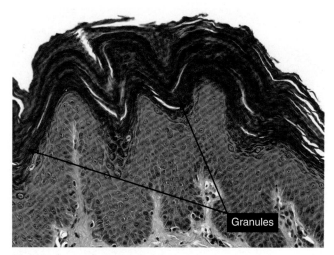

Fig. IC1.f

Fig. IC1.e. *Granular parakeratosis, low power.* There is acanthosis of the epidermis with little to no spongiosis. There is a markedly thickened and compacted stratum corneum. The superficial dermis reveals mild perivascular inflammation.

Fig. IC1.f. *Granular parakeratosis, high power.* The stratum corneum is markedly thickened and compacted. It is basophilic in appearance. Within the thickened stratum corneum, there is retention of the basophilic granules of the granular cell layer (*arrow*).

subsequent reports, this is felt to be less likely. The current hypothesis is that granular parakeratosis is a disorder of keratinization, possibly an abnormality of filaggrin processing.

HISTOPATHOLOGY. The histopathology of granular parakeratosis is distinctive. There is a markedly thickened stratum corneum with parakeratosis and retention of multiple basophilic granules. The epidermis may be normal or slightly thickened. The dermis shows either absent inflammation or either mild perivascular mononuclear cell infiltrate. Except for a rare reported case of granular parakeratosis associated with tinea (13), special stains for fungi are negative.

Conditions to consider in the differential diagnosis of this category:

dermatophytosis
granular parakeratosis
pityriasis rubra pilaris
ichthyosis
seborrheic dermatitis
psoriasiform dermatitis
confluent and reticulated papillomatosis (CARP)
acanthosis nigricans
Dowling–Degos disease
scurvy
vitamin A deficiency

pellagra (niacin deficiency)
Hartnup disease
acrokeratosis neoplastica (Bazex syndrome)
epidermal dysmaturation (cytotoxic chemotherapy variable keratin alterations)
epidermolytic hyperkeratosis
epidermal nevi
porokeratotic eccrine duct nevus
cutaneous horn
oral leukoplakia
leukoplakia of the vulva
syphilis cornee/keratoderma punctatum

ID LOCALIZED OR DIFFUSE HYPERPIGMENTATIONS

Increased melanin pigment is present in basal keratinocytes, without melanocytic proliferation.

1. No Inflammation
2. Scant Inflammation

ID1 No Inflammation

The upper dermis contains only sparse perivascular lymphocytes. *Mucosal melanotic macule (melanosis)* is the prototype (14).

Mucosal Melanotic Macules (Mucosal Lentigines)

CLINICAL SUMMARY. These benign lesions present as a pigmented patch on a mucous membrane. Common locations include the vermilion border of the lip (often the lower lip), the oral cavity, the vulva, and, less often, the penis. The lesions may be synonymously referred to as "mucosal lentigo" or "mucosal melanotic macule." In the common location on the vulva ("vulvar lentigo"), this process may present as a broad, irregular, and asymmetric patch of brown to blue-black hyperpigmentation, resembling a melanoma. The lesions are entirely macular, unlike most invasive melanomas. The so-called "labial lentigo" ("labial melanotic macule"), a hyperpigmented macule of the lip, is uniformly pigmented brown, usually completely macular, and usually less than about 6 mm in diameter. When multiple, these lesions may be associated with hereditary conditions associated with cancer risk, such as Carney complex and Peutz–Jeghers syndrome (15,16).

HISTOPATHOLOGY. At first glance, a biopsy specimen may appear normal. The findings include mild acanthosis without elongation of rete ridges, and hyperpigmentation of basal keratinocytes, recognized in comparison with surrounding epithelium, with scattered melanophages in the dermis. Although melanocytes may be normal in number, in most instances the number is slightly increased. Because of this slight increase in the number of melanocytes, the term "lentiginosis" has been proposed. Although these lesions may simulate melanoma clinically, histologically there is no contiguous melanocytic proliferation and no significant atypia. Occasionally, especially in the penile and vulvar lesions, there are prominent dendrites of melanocytes ramifying among the hyperpigmented keratinocytes. There may be associated mild keratinocytic hyperplasia, and patchy lymphocytes with scattered melanophages in the papillary dermis may account for the heterogeneous blue-black color that may simulate melanoma clinically.

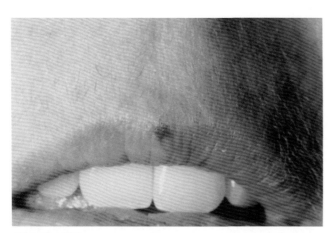

Clin. Fig. ID1.a

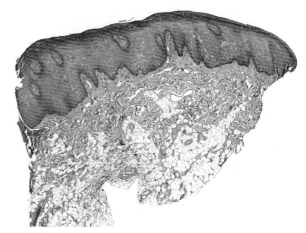

Fig. ID1.a

Clin. Fig. ID1.a. *Labial melanotic macule.* A benign acquired macule with irregular borders and uniform brown pigmentation developed near the vermilion border in a middle-aged female. Melanoma is considered in the differential diagnosis.

Fig. ID1.a. *Labial lentigo, low power.* At this magnification, the epidermis may appear completely normal, unless the difference in melanin pigment content between the lesion and the adjacent skin can be appreciated. Often, however, there is slight acanthosis as in this example. There may be patchy lymphocytes and melanophages in the papillary dermis, or inflammatory cells may be completely absent, as here.

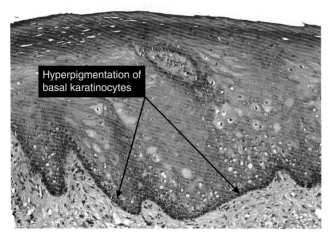

Hyperpigmentation of basal karatinocytes

Fig. ID1.b

Fig. ID1.b. *Labial lentigo, high power.* There is increased brown melanin pigment in basal keratinocytes (*arrows*). Melanocytes may be slightly increased, but there is no contiguous melanocytic proliferation as in nevi and melanomas. A few melanophages are present in the papillary dermis.

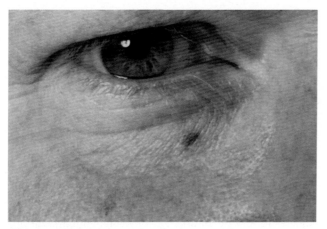

Clin. Fig. ID1.b

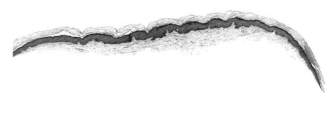

Fig. ID1.c

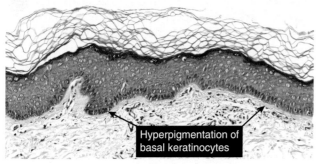

Hyperpigmentation of basal keratinocytes

Fig. ID1.d

Clin. Fig. ID1.b. *Ephelis.* Fair complexioned male has prominent brown macule which darkens in sunlight.

Fig. ID1.c. *Ephelis, low power.* At this magnification, the epidermis may appear completely normal, unless the difference in melanin pigment content between the lesion and the adjacent skin can be appreciated.

Fig. ID1.d. *Ephelis, medium power.* There is increased melanin pigment in basal keratinocytes. Melanocytes are not increased in number.

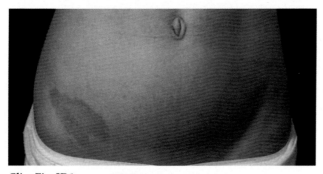

Clin. Fig. ID1.c

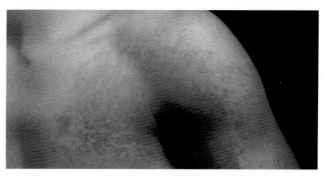

Clin. Fig. ID1.d

Clin. Fig. ID1.c. *Cafe au lait macule.* Evenly tan-colored macules can be seen in normal individuals. Multiple cafe au lait changes raise suspicion for neurofibromatosis.

Clin. Fig. ID1.d. *Becker nevus:* Teenage male acquired an enlarging tan macule with scalloped borders on his shoulder and chest. Hypertrichosis may develop.

Ephelids (Freckles)

CLINICAL SUMMARY. Freckles, or ephelids, are small, brown macules scattered over skin exposed to the sun. Exposure to the sun deepens the pigmentation of freckles, in contrast to lentigo simplex, whose already deep pigment does not change. Freckles, simple lentigines, and solar lentigines are difficult to distinguish from one another clinically (and also overlap histologically), and are considered together in most clinical and epidemiologic studies. Taken together, these lesions constitute a significant risk factor for the development of melanoma (17).

HISTOPATHOLOGY. Freckles have hyperpigmentation of the basal cell layer, but in contrast to lentigo simplex, there is no elongation of the rete ridges and, by definition, no obvious increase in the concentration of melanocytes. In epidermal spreads of freckled skin, the number of dopa-positive melanocytes within the freckles may appear decreased on comparison with the adjacent epidermis. However, the melanocytes that are present may be larger, and they may show more numerous and longer dendritic processes than the melanocytes of the surrounding epidermis.

Conditions to consider in the differential diagnosis:

  simple ephelis
  mucosal melanotic macules
  cafe au lait macule
  actinic lentigo
  pigmented actinic keratosis
  melasma
  Becker nevus
  congenital diffuse melanosis
  reticulated hyperpigmentations
  Addison disease
  alkaptonuric ochronosis
  hemochromatosis

ID2 | Scant Inflammation

Lymphocytes are minimally increased about the superficial plexus. There may be a few lymphocytes and/or neutrophils in the stratum corneum. Melanophages may be present in the papillary dermis. *Pityriasis (tinea) versicolor* is the prototype (18).

Pityriasis (Tinea) Versicolor

CLINICAL SUMMARY. The frequently used term "tinea versicolor" is not accurate since the causative organism, *Malassezia furfur*, is not a dermatophyte. Pityriasis versicolor usually affects the upper trunk, where there are multiple pink to brown papules that may appear hyper- or hypopigmented. On gentle scraping, the surface of the discolored areas is finely scaled.

HISTOPATHOLOGY. In contrast to other fungal infections of the glabrous skin, the horny layer in lesions of pityriasis versicolor contains abundant amounts of fungal elements, which can often be visualized in sections stained with hematoxylin-eosin as faintly basophilic structures. *Malassezia (Pityrosporum)* is present as a combination of both hyphae and spores, often referred to as "spaghetti and meatballs." The inflammatory response in pityriasis versicolor is usually minimal, although there may occasionally be slight hyperkeratosis, slight spongiosis, or a minimal superficial perivascular lymphocytic infiltrate. Although the lesions are pigmented clinically, there is usually no obvious pigment in histologic sections.

Conditions to consider in the differential diagnosis:

  pityriasis (tinea) versicolor
  lichen amyloidosis
  postinflammatory hyperpigmentation (mainly involves
    the upper dermis)
  erythema dyschromicum perstans

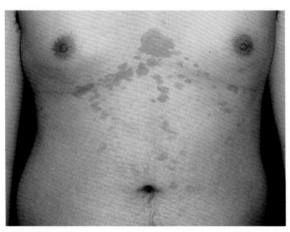

Clin. Fig. ID2

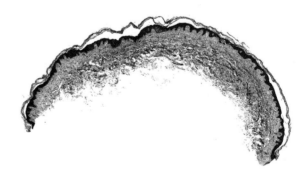

Fig. ID2.a

Clin. Fig. ID2. *Pityriasis versicolor.* Hyperpigmented patches, commonly as here present on the trunk, have "furfuraceous" scale with gentle scraping. KOH examination in this case demonstrated abundant hyphae and spores. The clinical differential diagnosis for this case would include vitiligo.

Fig. ID2.a. *Pityriasis versicolor, low power.* The epidermis may appear completely normal at scanning magnification. There may be a few perivascular lymphocytes in the papillary dermis, or these may be absent. (*continues*)

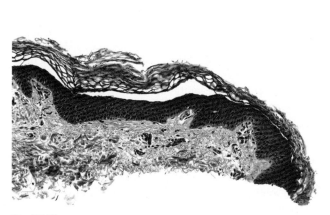

Fig. ID2.b

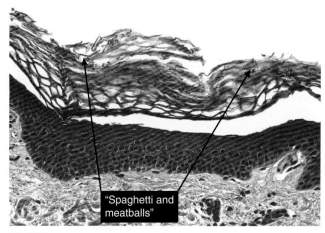

Fig. ID2.c

Fig. ID2.b. *Pityriasis versicolor, medium power.* Upon closer inspection, one can identify a hyperkeratotic stratum corneum, containing organisms.

Fig. ID2.c. *Pityriasis versicolor, high power.* The stratum corneum contains abundant yeasts and hyphae. The classic "spaghetti and meatballs" appearance results.

---

pretibial pigmented patches in diabetes
lichen planus pigmentosus

IE   LOCALIZED OR DIFFUSE HYPOPIGMENTATIONS

Melanin pigment is reduced in basal keratinocytes, with (vitiligo) or without (early stages of chemical depigmentation) a reduction in the number of melanocytes.

IE1   With or Without Slight Inflammation

Lymphocytes may minimally increase about the dermal–epidermal junction, as in the active phase of vitiligo, or may be absent, as in albinism. *Vitiligo* is the prototype (19,20).

Vitiligo

CLINICAL SUMMARY. Vitiligo is an acquired, potentially disfiguring, patchy, total loss of skin pigment. Stable patches often have an irregular border but are sharply demarcated from the surrounding skin. In expanding lesions, there may rarely be a slight rim of erythema at the border and a thin zone of transitory partial depigmentation.

HISTOPATHOLOGY. The central process in vitiligo is the destruction of melanocytes at the dermal–epidermal junction. With immunostains such as Melan-A/Mart-1, well-established lesions of vitiligo are totally devoid of melanocytes. The periphery of expanding lesions that are hypopigmented rather than completely depigmented may have a few melanocytes and some melanin granules in the basal layer. In the outer border of patches of vitiligo, melanocytes are often prominent and demonstrate long dendritic processes filled with melanin granules. Rarely, a superficial perivascular and somewhat lichenoid mononuclear cell infiltrate with vacuolar change is observed at the border of the depigmented areas.

Conditions to consider in the differential diagnosis:

vitiligo
chemical depigmentation
idiopathic guttate hypomelanosis
albinism
tinea versicolor
piebaldism
Chediak–Higashi syndrome
hypopigmented mycosis fungoides

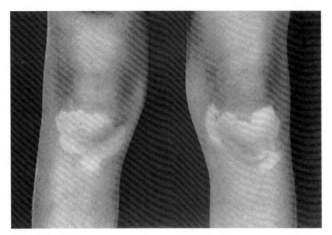

Clin. Fig. IE1

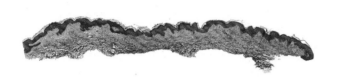

Fig. IE1.a

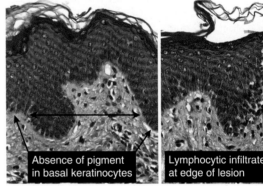

Absence of pigment in basal keratinocytes

Lymphocytic infiltrate at edge of lesion

Fig. IE1.b

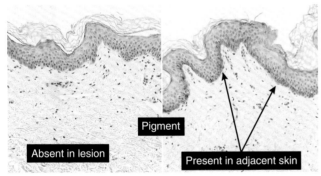

Pigment

Absent in lesion

Present in adjacent skin

Fig. IE1.c

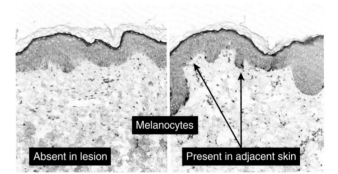

Melanocytes

Absent in lesion

Present in adjacent skin

Fig. IE1.d

Clin. Fig. IE1. *Vitiligo.* Acquired depigmented, well-demarcated patches often appear with striking symmetry.

Fig. IE1.a. *Vitiligo, low power.* The epidermis may appear completely normal at scanning magnification, unless it is appreciated that melanin pigment is reduced compared to surrounding skin.

Fig. IE1.b. *Vitiligo, high power.* At high magnification, in the left panel, a careful search reveals the absence of melanocytes from the basal lamina region. In the right panel, from the periphery of the area of the depigmentation, there is often a subtle lymphocytic infiltrate, as here.

Fig. IE1.c. *Vitiligo, Fontana stain, medium power.* A Fontana stain reveals, in the left panel, the absence of melanin pigment in basal layer keratinocytes, changes typical of vitiligo. In the right panel, from the adjacent skin, there is melanin in the basal layer of the skin, a normal distribution

Fig. IE1.d. *Vitiligo, Melan A stain, medium power.* Similarly, the left panel illustrates a region of vitiligo in which melanocytes are absent, compared to the normal skin in which the distribution of Melan A positive melanocytes (*arrows*) is normal.

References

1. Sitek JC, Kulseth MA, Rypdal KB, et al. Whole-exome sequencing for diagnosis of hereditary ichthyosis. *J Eur Acad Dermatol Venereol* 2018;32(6):1022–1027.
2. Akiyama M, Shimizu H. An update on molecular aspects of the non-syndromic ichthyoses. *Exp Dermatol* 2008;17(5):373–382.
3. McLean WH. Filaggrin failure—from ichthyosis vulgaris to atopic eczema and beyond. *Br J Dermatol* 2016;175(Suppl 2):4–7. Review.
4. Richard G. Molecular genetics of the ichthyoses. *Am J Med Genet C Semin Med Genet* 2004;131C:32–44.
5. Lane EB, McLean WH. Keratins and skin disorders. *J Pathol* 2004;204:355–366.
6. Ackerman AB. Focal acantholytic dyskeratosis. *Arch Dermatol* 1972;106:702–706.
7. Nuovo GJ, Ishag M. The histologic spectrum of epidermodysplasia verruciformis. *Am J Surg Pathol* 2000;24:1400–1406.
8. Dubina M, Goldenberg G. Viral-associated nonmelanoma skin cancers: a review. *Am J Dermatopathol* 2009;31:561–573.
9. Nuovo G, Nicol A, de Andrade CV, et al. New biomarkers of human papillomavirus infection in epidermodysplasia verruciformis. *Ann Diagn Pathol* 2019;40:81–87.
10. Kwon-Chung KJ, Bennett JE. Dermatophytosis. In: Kwon-Chung KJ, Bennett JE, eds. *Medical Mycology*. Philadelphia, PA: Lea & Febiger; 1992:105.
11. Gottlieb GJ, Ackerman AB. The "sandwich sign" of dermatophytosis. *Am J Dermatopathol* 1986;8(4):347–350.
12. Scheinfeld NS, Mones J. Granular parakeratosis: pathologic and clinical correlation of 18 cases of granular parakeratosis. *J Am Acad Dermatol* 2005;52(5):863–867.
13. Resnik KS, Kantor GR, DiLeonardo M. Dermatophyte-related granular parakeratosis. *Am J Dermatopathol* 2004;26(1):70–71.
14. Maize JC. Mucosal melanosis. *Dermatol Clin* 1988;6:283–293.
15. Stratakis CA. Carney complex: a familial lentiginosis predisposing to a variety of tumors. *Rev Endocr Metab Disord* 2016;17(3):367–371.
16. Stratakis CA. Genetics of Peutz-Jeghers syndrome, Carney complex and other familial lentiginoses. *Horm Res* 2000;54(5–6):334–343.
17. Titus-Ernstoff L, Perry AE, Spencer SK, et al. Pigmentary characteristics and moles in relation to melanoma risk. *Int J Cancer* 2005;116:144–149.
18. Galadari I, el Komy M, Mousa A, et al. Tinea versicolor: histologic and ultrastructural investigation of pigmentary changes. *Int J Dermatol* 1992;31:253–256.
19. Zhang XJ, Chen JJ, Liu JB. The genetic concept of vitiligo. *J Dermatol Sci* 2005;39:137–146.
20. Fisher AA. Differential diagnosis of idiopathic vitiligo: Part III. Occupational leukoderma. *Cutis* 1994;53:278–280.

Localized Superficial Epidermal or Melanocytic Proliferations

II

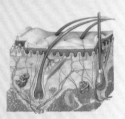

Localized superficial epithelial and melanocytic proliferations may be reactive but are often neoplastic. The epidermis (keratinocytes) may proliferate without extension into the dermis, extend into the dermis and may be squamous or basaloid. Melanocytes within the epidermis may proliferate with or without cytologic atypia (nevi, dysplastic nevi, melanoma *in situ*), in a proliferative epidermis (superficial spreading melanoma [SSM] *in situ*, Spitz nevi) or an atrophic epidermis (lentigo maligna); they can also extend into the dermis as proliferative infiltrates (invasive melanoma with or without vertical growth phase). There may be an associated variably cellular often mixed inflammatory infiltrate, or inflammation may be essentially absent.

IIA — LOCALIZED IRREGULAR THICKENING OF THE EPIDERMIS

Localized irregular epidermal proliferations are usually neoplastic.

1. Localized Epidermal Proliferations
2. Superficial Melanocytic Proliferations

IIA1 | Localized Epidermal Proliferations

The epidermis is thickened secondary to a localized proliferation of keratinocytes (acanthosis). The proliferation can be cytologically atypical, as in squamous cell carcinoma (SCC) *in situ*, or bland, as in eccrine poroma. It may be papillary as in seborrheic keratoses and verrucae, or highly irregular as in pseudoepitheliomatous hyperplasia. Actinic keratosis and SCC are prototypic examples. Clear cell acanthoma may also be included in this category, or may mimic an inflammatory condition.

Actinic Keratosis

CLINICAL SUMMARY. Actinic keratoses (1) are usually seen as multiple lesions in sun-exposed areas of the skin in persons in or past middle life who have fair complexions. Usually, the lesions measure less than 1 cm in diameter. They are erythematous, are often covered by adherent scales, and barely palpable except in their hypertrophic form. Actinic keratoses may be regarded conceptually as local keratinocytic neoplastic proliferations characterized by architectural abnormalities and cytologic atypia, whose histopathology spans a spectrum from mild dysplasia to carcinoma *in situ* (2).

HISTOPATHOLOGY. Five types of actinic keratosis can be recognized histologically: hypertrophic, atrophic, bowenoid, acantholytic, and pigmented. In the *hypertrophic type*, hyperkeratosis is pronounced and is intermingled with areas of parakeratosis. The epidermis is thickened in most areas and shows irregular downward proliferation that is limited to the uppermost dermis and does not represent frank invasion. Keratinocytes in the lower portion of the epidermis have a loss of polarity and thus a disorderly arrangement. Some of these cells have crowding, pleomorphism and atypicality of their nuclei, which appear large, irregular, and hyperchromatic, and some of the cells are dyskeratotic or apoptotic, and there may be increased mitotic activity sometimes with abnormal mitoses. The degree of cytologic atypia and architectural disorder (i.e., dysplasia) can be graded as mild, moderate, or severe and has been correlated with cell cycle marker expression (3). In contrast to the epidermal keratinocytes, the cells of the hair follicles and eccrine ducts that penetrate the epidermis within actinic keratoses retain their normal appearance and keratinize normally, giving rise to the characteristic alternating columns of hyperkeratosis and orthokeratosis.

Atrophic actinic keratoses lack the epidermal proliferation that is strikingly seen in the hypertrophic type; bowenoid keratoses are characterized by high-grade atypia that approaches or achieves full-thickness involvement

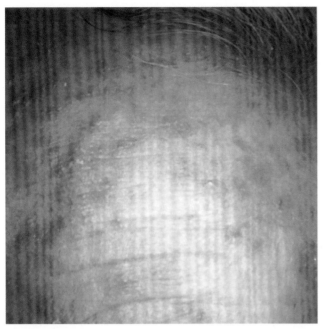

Clin. Fig. IIA1.a

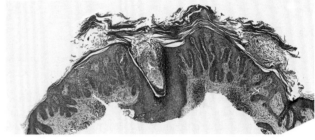

Fig. IIA1.a

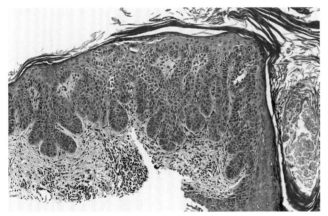

Fig. IIA1.b

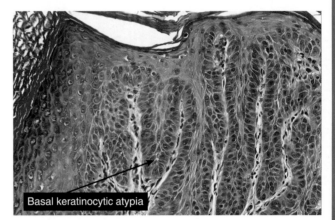

Basal keratinocytic atypia

Fig. IIA1.c

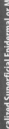

Localized Superficial Epidermal or Melanocytic Proliferations

II

Clin. Fig. IIA1.a. *Actinic keratosis.* Scaly erythematous macules and papules with a "sandpaper" texture appear commonly on face and dorsal hands, areas subject to chronic sun exposure.

Fig. IIA1.a. *Hypertrophic actinic keratosis, low power.* There is hyperkeratosis alternating with parakeratosis, and irregular thickening of the epithelium. In the dermis, there are patchy lymphocytes and plasma cells.

Fig. IIA1.b. *Hypertrophic actinic keratosis, medium power.* The normal epidermal maturation pattern is disturbed, with increased thickness of the basal layer.

Fig. IIA1.c. *Hypertrophic actinic keratosis, high power.* Basal keratinocytes show attributes of dysplasia or *in situ* malignancy—nuclear crowding, enlargement, hyperchromatism and pleomorphism. Note the orthokeratotic column above the hyperplastic follicular infundibulum in the center of the image. (*continues*)

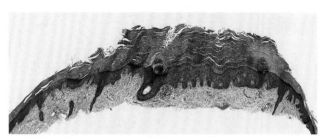

Fig. IIA1.d

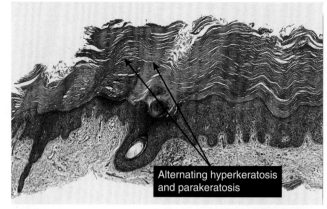

Alternating hyperkeratosis and parakeratosis

Fig. IIA1.e

Fig. IIA1.d. *Actinic keratosis, low power.* This lesion demonstrates striking alternating columns of hyperkeratosis and parakeratosis. The epithelium is irregularly thickened.

Fig. IIA1.e. *Actinic keratosis, low power.* Columns of orthokeratotic keratin extend above the hyperplastic epithelium of skin adnexa (sweat ducts in this instance). Parakeratotic keratin extends above the full-thickness dysplastic epithelium. Atypia is full thickness (bowenoid actinic keratosis/squamous cell carcinoma *in situ*).

(SCC *in situ*); acantholytic keratoses have dyshesion of lesional cells that may simulate a glandular pattern; and pigmented keratoses resemble any of the other forms but contain increased melanin pigment.

In all five types of actinic keratosis, the upper dermis usually shows a fairly dense, often lichenoid or band-like inflammatory infiltrate composed predominantly of lymphoid cells but often also containing plasma cells, which are not seen in lichen planus. The upper dermis usually shows solar or basophilic degeneration.

Eccrine Poroma

CLINICAL SUMMARY. Eccrine poroma (4) is a fairly common solitary tumor, found most commonly on the sole or the sides of the foot, and next in frequency on the hands and fingers, but also in many other areas of the skin, such as the neck, chest, and nose. Eccrine poroma generally arises in middle-aged persons. The tumor has a rather firm consistency, is raised and often slightly pedunculated, is asymptomatic, and usually measures less than 2 cm in diameter. In *eccrine poromatosis*, more than 100 papules are observed on the palms and soles.

HISTOPATHOLOGY. In its typical form, eccrine poroma arises within the lower portion of the epidermis, from where it extends downward into the dermis as tumor masses that often consist of broad, anastomosing bands. The tumor cells are smaller than squamous cells, have a uniform cuboidal appearance and a round, deeply basophilic nucleus, and are connected by intercellular bridges. They show no tendency to keratinize within the tumor,

except on the surface. Although the border between tumor formations and the stroma is sharp, tumor cells located at the periphery have no palisading. The tumor cells may contain significant amounts of glycogen, usually in an uneven distribution. In most but not in all eccrine poromas, narrow ductal lumina and occasionally cystic spaces are found within the tumor, lined by an eosinophilic, PAS-positive, diastase-resistant cuticle similar to that lining the lumina of eccrine sweat ducts and by a single row of luminal cells. There is no severe cytologic atypia, and frequent mitoses would be unusual.

Squamous Cell Carcinoma In Situ and Bowen Disease

CLINICAL SUMMARY. Bowen disease (BD) usually consists of a solitary lesion manifested as a slowly enlarging erythematous patch of sharp but irregular outline, within which there are generally areas of scaling and crusting. It may occur on exposed or on unexposed skin and in pigmented or poorly pigmented skin. It may be caused on exposed skin by exposure to the sun ("Bowenoid actinic keratoses") and on unexposed skin by the ingestion of arsenic. Some cases, especially in immunosuppressed patients and in genital and periungual sites, may be associated with oncogenic viruses including human papilloma virus (HPV) (5), and Merkel cell polyoma virus (6).

HISTOPATHOLOGY. BD (7) is an intraepidermal SCC and may also be referred to as SCC *in situ*. When full-thickness atypia is present in an actinic keratosis, the term SCC *in situ* may also appropriately be applied. The

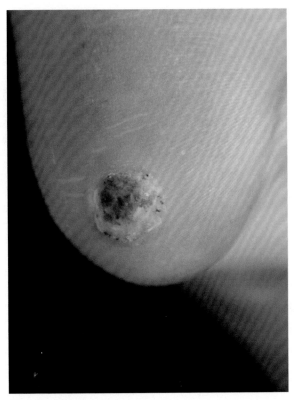

Clin. Fig. IIA1.b

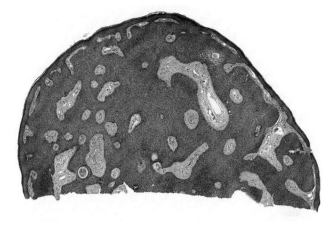

Fig. IIA1.f

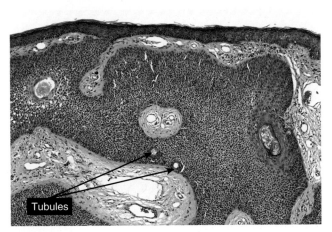

Tubules

Fig. IIA1.g

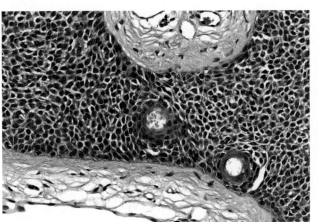

Fig. IIA1.h

Clin. Fig. IIA1.b. *Eccrine poroma.* A pink ulcerated nodular lesion in a characteristic location on the heel in a 52-year-old man.

Fig. IIA1.f. *Eccrine poroma, scanning magnification.* There is a well-defined epidermal proliferation which is sharply circumscribed from the adjacent skin.

Fig. IIA1.g. *Eccrine poroma, high magnification.* At higher magnification this lesion is composed of a uniform, bland-appearing epithelial cells. These lesions are often associated with formation of small ducts.

Fig. IIA1.h. *Eccrine poroma, high magnification.* Ducts at high magnification, lined by an eosinophilic cuticle similar to that of the native eccrine duct.

bowenoid type of actinic keratosis is histologically indistinguishable from BD. As in BD, there is within the epidermis considerable disorder in the arrangement of the nuclei, as well as clumping of nuclei and dyskeratosis. The epidermis is acanthotic and the cells lie in complete disorder, resulting in a "windblown" appearance. Many cells are highly atypical, with large, hyperchromatic nuclei and, frequently, multiple clustered nuclei. In some cases, the atypia is less overt. The horny layer usually is thickened and consists largely of parakeratotic cells with atypical, hyperchromatic nuclei. In contrast to actinic keratoses where the adnexal epithelium is hyperplastic, the infiltrate of atypical cells in BD frequently extends into follicular infundibula and causes replacement of the follicular epithelium by atypical cells down to the entrance of the sebaceous duct. High expression of p16 and Ki-67 or p16 alone are common in BD and can help distinguish it from "microclonal" seborrheic keratosis (8). In a small percentage of cases of Bowen disease (about 3%–5%), an invasive SCC develops.

Bowenoid Papulosis

CLINICAL SUMMARY. As has been reviewed (9), bowenoid papulosis presents as papules and plaques that frequently regress and relapse in vulvar and penile skin. It is best regarded as a form of SCC *in situ* that carries a low risk of progression or transformation to invasive carcinoma. The lesions are contagious and likely transmitted via sexual contact or vertical transmission in the peripartum period. Various high-risk HPV types, including types 16 and 18, have been linked to the disease.

HISTOPATHOLOGY. As in BD, the lesions are characterized by psoriasiform epidermal hyperplasia, hyperkeratosis, and focal parakeratosis. There is full-thickness epidermal dysplasia with crowding of keratinocytes and loss of architecture. The lesional cells are large, with hyperchromatic, pleomorphic nuclei, and demonstrate loss of cellular polarity, and abnormal maturation. Mitoses, some atypical, are often seen and are often suprabasal.

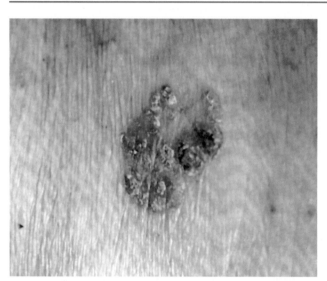

Clin. Fig. IIA1.c

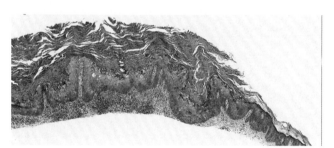

Fig. IIA1.i

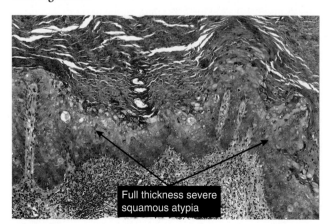

Full thickness severe squamous atypia

Fig. IIA1.j

Clin. Fig. IIA1.c. *Squamous cell carcinoma in situ.* A slightly elevated scaly flesh-colored plaque of long duration. Although Bowen disease is seen commonly on the head and neck, it can arise on sun-protected skin as well. (Photo by William K. Witmer, Department of Dermatology, University of Pennsylvania.)

Fig. IIA1.i. *Squamous cell carcinoma in situ, scanning power.* The epidermis appears irregularly thickened and there is hyperkeratosis. In the dermis, there is a dense inflammatory infiltrate, and solar elastosis.

Fig. IIA1.j. *Squamous cell carcinoma in situ, medium power.* The normal maturation pattern of keratinocytic epithelium is disturbed, imparting a "windblown" look to the neoplastic epithelium. There is a parakeratotic scale.

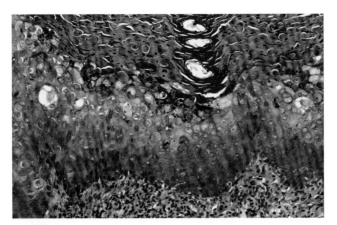

Fig. IIA1.k

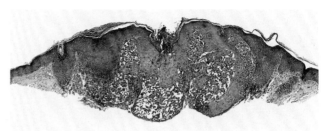

Fig. IIA1.l

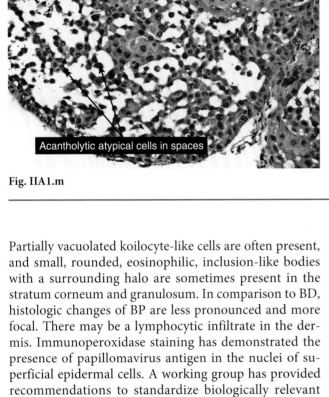

Acantholytic atypical cells in spaces

Fig. IIA1.m

Fig. IIA1.k. *Squamous cell carcinoma in situ, high power.* The lesional cells exhibit nuclear attributes of malignancy—enlargement, hyperchromatism, pleomorphism, and dyskeratosis. The degree of atypia is often less than in this example (see IIA1.o).

Fig. IIA1.l. *Squamous cell carcinoma in situ with acantholysis, low power.* This relatively well circumscribed acanthotic epithelial proliferation shows clear spaces in the mid and lower epidermal layers.

Fig. IIA1.m. *Squamous cell carcinoma in situ with acantholysis, high power.* Acantholysis is seen within the spinous layer. The presence of cytologic atypia is essential in differentiating this lesion from other acantholytic disorders.

Partially vacuolated koilocyte-like cells are often present, and small, rounded, eosinophilic, inclusion-like bodies with a surrounding halo are sometimes present in the stratum corneum and granulosum. In comparison to BD, histologic changes of BP are less pronounced and more focal. There may be a lymphocytic infiltrate in the dermis. Immunoperoxidase staining has demonstrated the presence of papillomavirus antigen in the nuclei of superficial epidermal cells. A working group has provided recommendations to standardize biologically relevant histopathologic terminology and use of biomarkers for HPV-associated squamous intraepithelial lesions and superficially invasive squamous carcinomas across all lower anogenital tract sites. The term "Squamous intraepithelial lesion (SIL)" is recommended, with two grades, high and low. It is stated that, "In the appropriate clinical setting of a patient with small, cutaneous anogenital papules, a note stating that the differential diagnosis includes bowenoid papulosis may be warranted. If the lesion is excised and its small size can be identified, it can be diagnosed as HSIL with an additional designation of bowenoid papulosis in parentheses. Bowenoid papulosis may have a lower risk of progression to cancer than cutaneous HSIL found in larger plaques (BD)" (10).

Clear Cell Squamous Cell Carcinoma In Situ

See Fig. IIA1.q.

Clear Cell Acanthoma

CLINICAL SUMMARY. This not uncommon tumor (11) typically occurs as a solitary lesion on the legs, as a slowly growing, sharply delineated, red nodule or plaque 1 to 2 cm in diameter, covered with a thin crust and exuding some moisture. A collarette is often seen at the periphery. The lesion appears stuck on, like a seborrheic keratosis, and is vascular, like a pyogenic granuloma.

HISTOPATHOLOGY. Within a sharply demarcated area of the epidermis, the epidermal cells, with the exception of those of the basal cell layer, appear strikingly clear and slightly enlarged. Their nuclei appear normal. Staining with the periodic acid–Schiff (PAS) reaction reveals large amounts of glycogen within the cells. The rete ridges are elongated and may be intertwined. The surface is parakeratotic with few or no granular cells. The acrosyringia and acrotrichia within the tumor retain their normal stainability. A conspicuous feature in most lesions is the presence throughout the epidermis of numerous

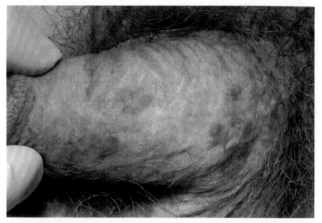

Clin. Fig. IIA1.d

Fig. IIA1.n

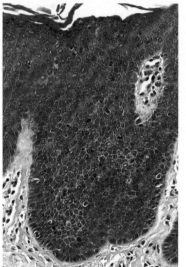

Fig. IIA1.o

Fig. IIA1.p

Clin. Fig. IIA1.d. *Bowenoid papulosis.* A middle aged male presented with a long-standing history of asymptomatic reddish-brown papules.

Fig. IIA1.n. *Bowenoid papulosis, low power.* There is mildly irregular epidermal thickening, and hyperpigmentation.

Fig. IIA1.o. *Bowenoid papulosis, medium power.* Focally, one can identify perinuclear vacuolization similar to what is seen in common condylomata.

Fig. IIA1.p. *Bowenoid papulosis, high power.* In contrast to condyloma acuminatum, bowenoid papulosis reveals nuclear atypia and numerous mitotic figures, and dyskeratotic cells. Bowen disease could be indistinguishable in these fields.

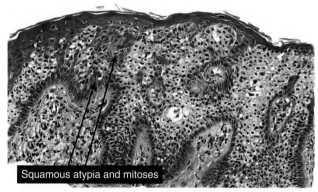

Fig. IIA1.q

Fig. IIA1.q. *Clear cell squamous cell carcinoma in situ, medium power.* In this variant, the atypical keratinocytes show an abundance of clear cytoplasm. Frequently there is sparing of basal layer keratinocytes. Identification of keratinocyte atypia is crucial in distinguishing this lesion from a clear cell acanthoma. Clear cell SCC can overlap morphologically with trichilemmal carcinoma.

neutrophils, many with fragmentation of their nuclei, often forming microabscesses in the parakeratotic horny layer. Slight spongiosis is present between the clear cells. Dilated capillaries are seen in the elongated papillae and often also in the dermis underlying the tumor. In addition, there is a mild to moderately severe lymphoid infiltrate in the dermis. Some clear cell acanthomas appear papillomatous, with the configuration of a seborrheic keratosis.

Conditions to consider in the differential diagnosis:

No Cytologic Atypia
  seborrheic keratosis
  verrucae
  dermatosis papulosa nigra
  stucco keratosis
  large cell acanthoma
  clear cell acanthoma

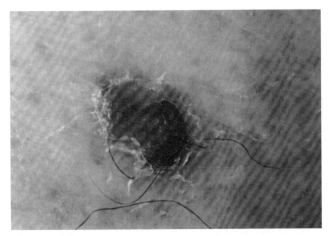

Clin. Fig. IIA1.e

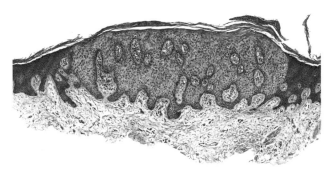

Fig. IIA1.r

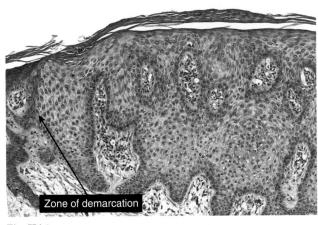

Zone of demarcation

Fig. IIA1.s

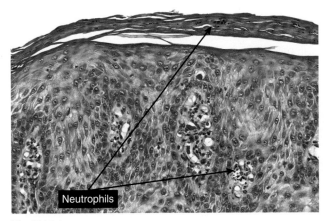

Neutrophils

Fig. IIA1.t

Clin. Fig. IIA1.e. *Clear cell acanthoma.* An elderly male developed an asymptomatic, benign erythematous eroded papule with a collarette of scale on the calf. Differential diagnosis includes amelanotic melanoma, squamous cell carcinoma, and eccrine poroma.

Fig. IIA1.r. *Clear cell acanthoma, scanning power.* There is a zone of epidermal hyperplasia with mild hyperkeratosis. This pale-staining epithelial neoplasm is sharply demarcated from the adjacent normal epidermis.

Fig. IIA1.s. *Clear cell acanthoma, medium power.* The lesion is composed of pale-staining, bland appearing keratinocytes. The cells are pale because of an abundance of glycogen.

Fig. IIA1.t. *Clear cell acanthoma, high power.* Upon close inspection, neutrophils can be seen throughout this lesion; they may also accumulate in the overlying stratum corneum.

epidermal nevi
eccrine poroma
hidroacanthoma simplex
oral white sponge nevus
leukoedema of the oral mucosa
verrucous hyperplasia of oral mucosa (oral florid
　papillomatosis)
With Cytologic Atypia
　actinic keratosis
　arsenical keratosis
　squamous cell carcinoma *in situ*

Bowen disease
erythroplasia of Queyrat
erythroplakia of the oral mucosa
bowenoid papulosis
Paget disease
Pseudoepitheliomatous Hyperplasia
　halogenodermas
　deep fungal infections
　epidermis above granular cell tumor
Spitz nevus
verrucous melanoma

II   Localized Superficial Epidermal or Melanocytic Proliferations

IIA2 | Superficial Melanocytic Proliferations

The epidermis may be thickened (acanthosis) and is associated with a proliferation of single or nested melanocytic cells. The proliferation can be malignant as in SSM or benign as in nevi. These are the prototypes.

Superficial Melanocytic Nevi and Melanomas

CLINICAL SUMMARY. Melanocytic nevi (12,13) vary considerably in their clinical appearance. Five clinical types have been recognized: (1) flat lesions which are for the most part are histologically junctional nevi, and compound nevi which include (2) slightly elevated lesions often with raised centers and flat peripheries many of which are histologically dysplastic nevi, (3) dome-shaped lesions, (4) papillomatous lesions, and (5) pedunculated lesions. The first two types are usually pigmented and are superficial at the histologic level (confined to the epidermis and papillary dermis); the latter three may or may not be pigmented, and may involve the reticular dermis. Most small, flat lesions represent either a lentigo simplex or a junctional nevus; flat lesions or lesions with flat peripheries greater than 5 mm in diameter with irregular indefinite borders and pigment variegation are clinically dysplastic nevi. Dysplastic nevi are most important as simulants and markers of increased risk for melanoma. Although about one-third of melanomas may arise in a dysplastic nevus, dysplastic nevi are vastly more common than melanomas and therefore the risk of progression of any one lesion is very low (14).

Melanomas are neoplastic proliferations of cytologically malignant melanocytes (15). Two major steps or phases of melanoma development can be distinguished. The first is the nontumorigenic or radial growth phase (RGP) which presents clinically as an irregular patch or plaque of variegated pigmentation. Histologically in this step the melanomas may be *in situ* or microinvasive but are nontumorigenic (do not form a mass in the dermis) and nonmitogenic (there are no dermal mitoses). In the next step, the vertical growth phase (VGP), the lesional cells have acquired the capacity for proliferation in the dermis. A clinically evident tumor mass is usually formed (tumorigenic melanoma which may be mitogenic or nonmitogenic), often within the confines of an antecedent RGP constituting a tumor within a plaque. In occasional cases the lesion is nontumorigenic but there are dermal mitoses (mitogenic but nontumorigenic melanoma). Tumorigenic or mitogenic melanomas may have competence for metastasis, while this is extraordinarily rare in the nontumorigenic nonmitogenic RGP melanomas (16). The RGP plaque is seen histologically at the edges of the VGP tumor as a "lateral" or "horizontal" component. Three major clinicopathologic types of cutaneous RGP *in situ* or microinvasive melanoma are recognized: the (1) superficial spreading or pagetoid (discussed in IID2), (2) lentigo maligna (IIB1), and (3)

acral-lentiginous types (IIA2). A fourth type of melanoma is defined by the lack of a discernible adjacent RGP component. This is termed (4) nodular melanoma and is discussed in Section VIB.3. Similar lesions occur in mucosal sites; when a RGP is present it is commonly lentiginous.

In the 2018 WHO melanoma classification (17), the presence of solar elastosis as a marker of cumulative solar damage (CSD) is used to discriminate among melanomas in low versus high CSD skin, and those in skin with no (or incidental) CSD. The genomic landscape of these forms of melanoma vary and taken together with clinical and histologic features, eight patterns or "pathways" to cutaneous and mucosal melanoma have been identified. This classification also includes the benign lesions that share epidemiologic, clinicopathologic, and genomic abnormalities with the various forms of melanoma, and may be potential precursors, risk markers and simulants of these melanomas (see Table II.1).

HISTOPATHOLOGY. Melanocytic nevi are defined and recognized by the presence of nevus cells, which, even though they are melanocytes, differ from ordinary melanocytes by being arranged at least partially in clusters or "nests," by having a tendency toward rounded rather than dendritic cell shape, and by a propensity to retain pigment in their cytoplasm rather than to transfer it to neighboring keratinocytes. Although a histologic subdivision of nevi into junctional, compound, and intradermal nevi is generally accepted, it should be realized that these are

TABLE II.1. Classification of Melanoma (1)

A. Melanomas typically associated with cumulative solar damage (CSD)

Pathway I.	Superficial spreading melanoma/Low-CSD melanoma (SSM)
Pathway II.	Lentigo maligna melanoma/High-CSD melanoma (LMM)
Pathway III.	Desmoplastic melanoma (DM)

B. Melanomas not typically associated with cumulative solar damage (no CSD)

Pathway IV.	Spitz melanomas (SM)
Pathway V.	Acral melanoma (AM)
Pathway VI.	Mucosal melanomas
Pathway VII.	Melanomas arising in congenital nevi (MCN)
Pathway VIII.	Melanomas arising in blue nevi (MBN)
Pathway IX.	Uveal melanoma

C. Nodular melanoma (NM) may occur in all or most of the above pathways

Modified from 2018 WHO Classification.

transitional stages in the "life cycle" of nevi, which start out as junctional nevi and, after having become intradermal nevi, undergo involution, likely through a process of senescence (18).

The lentigo simplex is regarded as an early or evolving form of melanocytic nevus. It has the clinical appearance of a small lenticulate or lens-shaped pigmented spot (hence the term "lentigo"), and is characterized histologically by the presence of single melanocytes arranged in contiguity about elongated rete ridges. The lack of nests at the histologic level distinguishes a lentigo from a nevus. The lentiginous pattern is seen in the common lentiginous junctional nevus, in which nevus cells in nests are present in combination with the "lentiginous pattern" just described. Dysplastic nevi also exhibit a partially lentiginous, but predominantly nested architecture. They are larger (greater than 4 mm in histologic section diameter) and there is cytologic atypia affecting randomly scattered nevus cells, as well as architectural disorder. Individuals with clinically and/or histologically dysplastic nevi are at increased risk of developing melanoma (19–21).

The lentiginous pattern of proliferation is also seen in the "lentiginous" forms of melanoma, in which in contrast to nevi the lesional cells are uniformly atypical, and the pattern is less well organized than in nevi, often with haphazard proliferation of keratinocytes resulting in irregular thickening and thinning of the epidermis. In the most common form of melanoma, the superficial spreading type, the pattern of proliferation is termed "pagetoid" with lesional cells extending singly and in groups up into the keratinocytic epithelium, which as in lentiginous melanomas tends to be irregularly thickened and thinned. Some degree of pagetoid proliferation, often slight, is usually present in the lentiginous melanomas as well, and pagetoid proliferation may also be seen on occasion in benign nevi, especially Spitz nevi (sections IID2 and VIB3), and pigmented spindle cell nevi (see below). The lentiginous, pagetoid and nested patterns, as well as the degree of pigmentation, and the presence of actinic elastosis and also other readily recognizable histologic, clinical and epidemiologic factors, have been linked to the prevalence of mutations of BRAF and NRAS in melanomas, with the canonical BRAFV600E mutation being more likely in the pagetoid melanomas, and NRAS mutations in the lentiginous ones (22); other oncogenes are in the process of categorization, varying among the pathways as seen in Table II.1, and these may potentially be amenable to targeted therapy for metastatic melanoma. Of interest, certain cutaneous syndromes associated with multiple lentigines and cancer risk are also associated with mutations of the RAS/MAPK pathway called RASopathies (23).

Junctional nevi including dysplastic nevi may exhibit an irregularly thickened epidermis but more often they tend to have regularly elongated rete ridges and are discussed in a later section (IIC.1). The pigmented spindle cell nevus of Reed is a lesion that often has a rather irregularly thickened rete pattern, and is discussed here as a prototype. *In situ* or microinvasive melanomas of the superficial spreading and acral-lentiginous types also tend to have an irregularly thickened and thinned epidermis. The former is discussed in the section on pagetoid proliferations (IID.2), while the latter is discussed below.

Pigmented Spindle Cell Nevus

CLINICAL SUMMARY. The pigmented spindle cell nevus (30), first described by Richard Reed, may be regarded as a variant of the classical Spitz nevus. The lesions are usually 3 to 6 mm in diameter, deeply pigmented, and either flat or slightly raised dome-shaped lesions. Most patients are young adults, and the most common location is on the lower extremities. Because of the heavy pigment and the history of sudden appearance, a clinical diagnosis of melanoma is often suspected clinically. The lesions are generally stable after a relatively sudden appearance and a short-lived period of growth. It has been demonstrated that these lesions are driven by oncogenic fusion genes, similar to those in classical Spitz nevi (24).

HISTOPATHOLOGY. The lesion is characterized by its relatively small size and its symmetry, by good circumscription, and by a proliferation of uniform, narrow, elongated, spindle-shaped, often heavily pigmented melanocytes at the dermal–epidermal junction. The epidermis tends to be irregularly thickened, and there is hyperkeratosis often with conspicuous melanin pigment in the stratum corneum. The nests of spindle cells are vertically oriented, and tend to blend with adjacent keratinocytes rather than forming clefts as in Spitz nevi. Kamino bodies may be present as in Spitz nevi. In the papillary dermis, the nevus cells lie in a compact cluster pattern, pushing the connective tissue aside. Involvement of the reticular dermis, common in Spitz nevi, is unusual in pigmented spindle cell nevi. Some lesions may show upward epidermal extension of junctional nests of melanocytes, or of single cells in a "pagetoid scatter pattern." In contrast to SSMs, pigmented spindle cell nevi are smaller, symmetrical, and have sharply demarcated lateral margins. The tumor cells appear strikingly uniform "from side to side." If lesional cells descend into the papillary dermis, they mature along nevus lines in pigmented spindle cell nevi, in contrast to melanomas. Mitoses may be present in the epidermis in either lesion, but are uncommon in the dermis in pigmented spindle cell nevi. Abnormal mitoses are very uncommon indeed.

Acral Melanoma

CLINICAL SUMMARY. Acral lentiginous melanoma (AM) occurs on the hairless skin of the palms and soles and in the ungual and periungual regions, the soles being

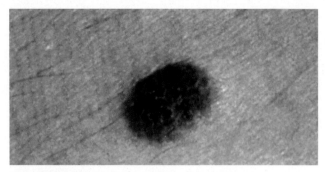

Clin. Fig. IIA2.a

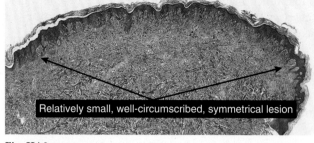

Relatively small, well-circumscribed, symmetrical lesion

Fig. IIA2.a

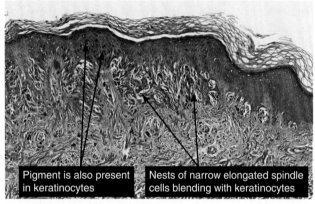

Pigment is also present in keratinocytes

Nests of narrow elongated spindle cells blending with keratinocytes

Fig. IIA2.b

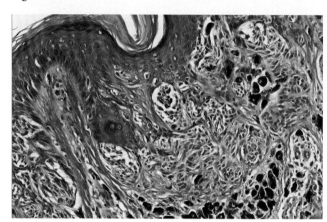

Fig. IIA2.c

Clin. Fig. IIA2.a. *Pigmented spindle cell nevus.* A well circumscribed symmetrical small uniformly pigmented lesion which appeared rapidly on the thigh of a young woman, but then remained stable. The dark blue-black color differs from the pink or tan color of most classic Spitz nevi, and may suggest the possibility of melanoma clinically. (W. Witmer.)

Fig. IIA2.a. *Pigmented spindle cell nevus, low power.* These lesions may be entirely within the epidermis (junctional) or they may be compound. In the latter case, they tend to be confined to the papillary dermis. In this scanning magnification, the lesion is well circumscribed; there is an abundance of brown pigment, both within the thickened epidermal layer and within the superficial dermis.

Fig. IIA2.b. *Pigmented spindle cell nevus, medium power.* At higher magnification this nevus is composed of a proliferation of single and nested uniform melanocytes which contain an abundance of melanin pigment. The nests tend to blend with the surrounding keratinocytes in contrast to the clefting artifact that characterizes classic Spitz nevi.

Fig. IIA2.c. *Pigmented spindle cell nevus, high power.* The melanocytes are spindled in form and frequently oriented perpendicular to the skin surface. The keratinocytes and the stratum corneum also contain an abundance of melanin pigment and there are numerous melanophages in the superficial dermis.

the most common site (25). In groups such as Asians, Hispanics, Polynesians, and blacks, for whom the overall incidence of melanoma is low, most melanomas are of the acral type. However, the absolute incidence of acral melanoma in these groups is similar to that in Caucasians who have a much higher overall incidence of melanoma. In addition, the genetic profile differs from that of the more common superficial spreading type of melanoma, with a relatively low burden of point mutations and with amplification of genes such as Cyclin D and *KIT* (26,27). Mutually exclusive mutations of *BRAF*, *NRAS*, and *KIT* are seen

in a subset of cases, and also kinase fusions have been identified (28). Mutations of *KIT* have been described in 39% of mucosal, 36% of acral, and 28% of melanomas on chronically sun-damaged skin, but not in any (0%) melanomas on skin without chronic sun damage (29). Somatic translocations, copy gains, and missense and promoter mutations, or germline events, involving the telomerase gene *TERT*, were recently described in 41% of patients (30). These considerations suggest that different etiologic factors, likely not involving sunlight, are operative in acral and mucosal compared to other sites, while some of these events may represent examples of melanomas of other pathways occurring in acral sites. Although the survival rate of patients with acral melanomas in most series is poor, this is probably a result of their typically advanced microstage and/or stage at diagnosis.

Clinically, *in situ* or microinvasive AM has uneven pigmentation with an irregular, often indefinite border. The soles of the feet are most commonly involved. If the tumor is situated in the nail matrix, the nail unit may show a longitudinal pigmented band (longitudinal melanonychia), and the pigment may extend onto the nail fold (Hutchinson's sign). Tumorigenic vertical growth may be heralded by the onset of a nodule, with development of ulceration. However, some acral melanomas may be deeply invasive while remaining quite flat, because the thick stratum corneum acts as a barrier to exophytic growth.

HISTOPATHOLOGY. The most common pattern of AM is termed "lentiginous" because the majority of the lesional cells are single and located near the dermal–epidermal junction, especially at the periphery of the lesion. Usually, however, some tumor cells can be found in the upper layers of the epidermis, especially near areas of invasion in the centers of the lesions. The histologic picture differs from that of lentigo maligna, because of irregular acanthosis, the lack of elastosis in the dermis, and the frequently dendritic character of the lesional cells. Early *in situ* or microinvasive lesions may have, especially at the periphery, a deceptively benign histologic picture consisting of an increase in basal melanocytes and hyperpigmentation with only focal atypia of the melanocytes. However, in the centers of the lesions,

uniform, severe cytologic atypia is usually readily evident. There may be a lichenoid lymphocytic infiltrate that may largely obscure the dermal–epidermal junction, and in some cases this may be so dense as to simulate an inflammatory process. In most of the lesions, both spindle-shaped and rounded tumor cells are observed, and, in many cases, pigmented dendritic cells are prominent. Pigmentation is often pronounced, resulting in the presence of melanophages in the upper dermis and of large aggregates of melanin in the broad stratum corneum. As in lentigo maligna, when tumorigenic VGP is present, it is often of the spindle cell type and not uncommonly desmoplastic and/or neurotropic. In other instances, the invasive and tumorigenic cells in the dermis may be deceptively differentiated along nevus lines. Some melanomas in acral skin have a predominantly pagetoid pattern of proliferation and may represent "low CSD" melanomas of the superficial spreading or pagetoid type (31).

Conditions to consider in the differential diagnosis:

junctional nevi
recurrent melanocytic nevi
pigmented spindle cell nevi
junctional and superficial compound Spitz nevi
compound or dermal nevi, papillomatous
junctional or superficial compound dysplastic nevi
in situ or microinvasive melanoma, superficial spreading type
in situ or microinvasive melanoma, acral-lentiginous type

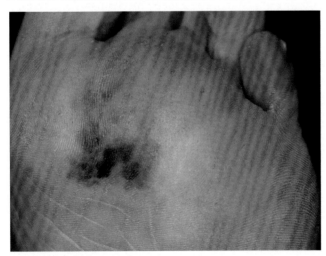

Clin. Fig. IIA2.b

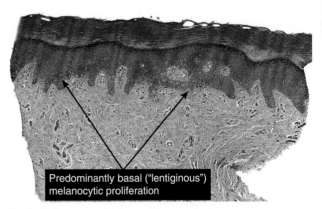

Predominantly basal ("lentiginous") melanocytic proliferation

Fig. IIA2.d

Clin. Fig. IIA2.b. *Acral lentiginous melanoma.* There is an irregular patch of variegated hyperpigmentation in acral skin, including shades of tan, brown, gray-white, red, and blue-black.

Fig. IIA2.d. *Acral lentiginous melanoma, low power.* This punch biopsy of acral skin is from a lesion of the type illustrated above. A thickened stratum corneum is typical of this site. There is a melanocytic proliferation within the epidermis associated with slight inflammation in the superficial dermis.

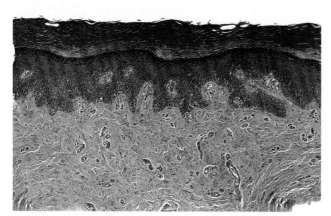

Melanocytic atypia—not always "severe"

Fig. IIA2.e   **Fig. IIA2.f**

Fig. IIA2.e. *Acral lentiginous melanoma, medium power.* Within the epidermis there is a disorganized proliferation of predominantly single but focally clustered heavily pigmented melanocytic cells. Orderly nests are not present in this proliferation. Within the superficial dermis there often may be a lymphocytic infiltrate and numerous melanophages (not prominent here).

Fig. IIA2.f. *Acral lentiginous melanoma, high power.* Higher magnification reveals that the proliferation is almost exclusively of single atypical often dendritic melanocytes mostly in the lower third of the epidermis. This histological appearance is relatively subtle and may be readily missed for example if a specimen is examined only at scanning magnification.

IIB LOCALIZED LESIONS WITH THINNING OF THE EPIDERMIS

A thinned epidermis is characteristic of aged or chronically sun-damaged skin. The epidermis is thinned secondary to diminished number and to decreased size of keratinocytes.

1. With Melanocytic Proliferation
2. Without Melanocytic Proliferation

IIB1 With Melanocytic Proliferation

The epidermis is thinned (atrophic) and there is proliferation of single or small groups of atypical melanocytes, resulting in the localization of melanocytes in contiguity with one another, in the basal layer of the epidermis. *Lentigo maligna* is a prototypic example.

Lentigo Maligna Melanoma, In Situ or Microinvasive (High CSD)

CLINICAL SUMMARY. Lentigo maligna melanoma (LMM) (32), also termed "High CSD melanoma" in the 2018 WHO Classification (33), accounts for about 10%

of all melanomas and typically occurs on the chronically exposed cutaneous surfaces of the elderly, most commonly on the face. The genetic mechanisms of development of these lesions appear to be different from those operating in the more common SSMs, often involving NRAS rather than BRAF (22). The lesion evolves slowly over many years, starting as an unevenly pigmented macule that gradually extends peripherally and may attain a diameter of several centimeters. It has an irregular border and, as long as it remains *in situ* or microinvasive, is not indurated. The color is variegated ranging from light brown to brown, with dark brown, black or gray-white flecks. Fine reticulated lines are usually also present and are helpful in distinguishing the lesions from actinic lentigines.

HISTOPATHOLOGY. Although the earliest stages may be subtle, fully evolved lentigo maligna is characterized by contiguous proliferation of lesional melanocytes, occurring in an atrophic, flattened epidermis. This epidermal architectural pattern is in contrast to SSM, where it is irregularly thickened and thinned, or to actinic lentigines and dysplastic nevi, where there is elongation of the rete. Some lesions, termed "nevoid lentigo maligna," may overlap histologically with dysplastic nevi and are discussed in section IIC. Cytologically, the lesional cells in classic LMM tend to be nevoid to epithelioid and sometimes elongated and spindle-shaped. Their nuclei are atypical, being slightly to moderately, or sometimes more severely enlarged, hyperchromatic, and pleomorphic. This atypia is "uniform" (i.e., present in a majority of the lesional cells), in contrast to dysplastic nevi. Frequently, atypical melanocytes extend along the basal cell layer of hair follicles, often for a considerable distance and frequently extending to the base of a shave biopsy specimen. There is usually some upward pagetoid extension of atypical melanocytes. Although single cells predominate, some nesting of melanocytes in the basal layer may be observed. The atypical melanocytes within the nests usually retain their spindle shape, and they often "hang down" like raindrops from the interface. The upper dermis, which almost always shows severe elastotic solar degeneration, contains numerous melanophages and a rather pronounced, often bandlike, inflammatory infiltrate. Microinvasion may be demonstrable in these areas of dermal inflammation.

Genomically, driver mutations differ in High CSD/LMM from Low CSD/SSM and include loss of function mutations in *NF1* (a tumor suppressor that normally inhibits activation of *RAS*), and usually mutually exclusive gain of function mutations in *BRAF* mutation (other than V600E), *NRAS* (38) and to a lesser extent *KIT* (31).

The differential diagnosis of LMM includes lentiginous junctional nevi and dysplastic nevi, and actinic lentigines. All of these lesions are characterized by lentiginous elongation of rete ridges (section IIC), in contrast to the solar atrophy that characterizes the epidermis in the classic pattern of LMM. Junctional nevi exhibit little or no cytologic atypia, and dysplastic exhibit mild to moderate atypia, in contrast to the uniform moderate to severe atypia that characterizes most examples of LMM. Some examples of lesions thought to be in the general category of LMM have preserved rete ridges, and may have focally bridging nests, usually only in focal areas of a broad proliferation with otherwise more characteristic lentiginous features. These have been termed "nevoid lentigo maligna" or "lentiginous melanoma" and are discussed in Section IIC.

Recurrent ("Persistent") Nevus, Lentiginous Patterns

CLINICAL SUMMARY. First described by Kornen and Ackerman as "pseudomelanoma," this relatively common phenomenon often follows shave biopsy of a nevus (34). Clinically recurrent hyperpigmentation on biopsy may show histologic changes suggestive of melanoma. Recurrence may follow incomplete removal of a nevus, particularly by a shave biopsy or electrodessication, or the nevus may apparently have been completely excised. The pigmentation in recurrent nevi is confined to the region of the scar, and typically presents within a few weeks of the

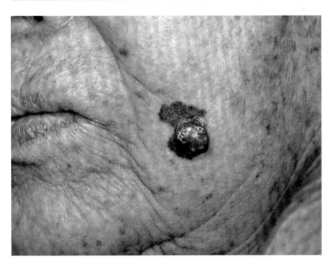

Clin. Fig. IIB1.a

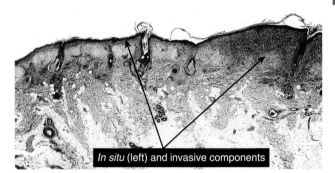

Fig. IIB1.a

Clin. Fig. IIB1.a. *Lentigo maligna melanoma.* An elderly woman had a many year history of an enlarging dark macule on the face, with recent development of a black nodule of tumorigenic vertical growth phase.

Fig. IIB1.a. *Lentigo maligna, low power.* At scanning magnification the lesion is very broad and poorly circumscribed, the epidermis is atrophic and many areas show a flattened rete ridge architecture. This lesion has an invasive and tumorigenic component in the right side of the image.

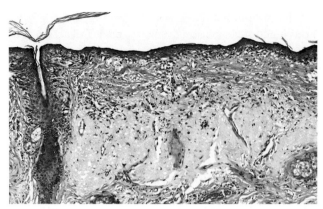

Fig. IIB1.b

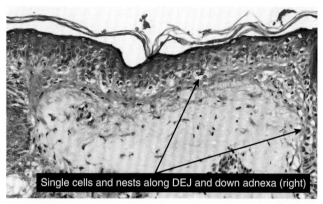

Single cells and nests along DEJ and down adnexa (right)

Fig. IIB1.c

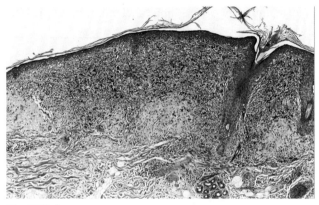

Fig. IIB1.d

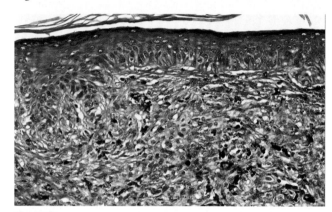

Fig. IIB1.e

Fig. IIB1.b. *Lentigo maligna, medium power.* In the basal cell zone, there is a lentiginous proliferation of predominantly single uniformly atypical melanocytes which focally grow in a confluent or "contiguous" manner. The underlying dermis reveals a broad zone of solar elastosis.

Fig. IIB1.c. *Lentigo maligna, high power.* Higher magnification reveals enlarged, hyperchromatic and irregular nuclei of the majority of the lesional melanocytic cells ("uniform cytologic atypia").

Fig. IIB1.d,e. *Lentigo maligna, medium power.* There is a tumorigenic component comprised of uniformly atypical cells, quite heavily pigmented in this instance.

---

surgical procedure. After this rapid appearance, the pigment is stable. In contrast, recurrent melanoma does not respect the border of the scar, and extends over time into the adjacent skin. Paradoxically, recurrent melanoma occurs more slowly, over months or years, but progresses inexorably.

HISTOPATHOLOGY. Although most recurrent nevi are not cytologically atypical, in a few instances they contain atypical melanocytes, both singly and in nests, arranged mainly along the epidermal–dermal junction, but occasionally also extending into the upper dermis and also into the epidermis in a pagetoid pattern (see IID2) (35). The junctional nests are often composed of pigmented epithelioid melanocytes forming irregular nests possibly the result of their growth within an atrophic epidermal layer that interfaces with scar tissue. Deep remnants of the

nevus may be seen in the reticular dermis beneath the scar (36). A lymphocytic infiltrate with melanophages may be seen in the upper dermis. Nevus cells in the dermis tend to show evidence of maturation, and the Ki-67 proliferation rate is low (37). However, mitotic figures may occasionally be observed. Distinction from melanoma may be difficult without a pertinent history. However, the presence of fibrosis in the upper dermis and often of remnants of a melanocytic nevus beneath the zone of fibrosis, as well as the sharp lateral demarcation, usually make a correct diagnosis possible. This fibrosis need to be distinguished from that seen in partial regression of a melanoma (38). As is true clinically, the recurrent nevus is confined to the epidermis above the scar, while recurrent melanoma may extend into the adjacent epidermis. However, persistent nevus, after a partial biopsy, may also involve skin adjacent to a scar. In this instance, ordinary criteria for the

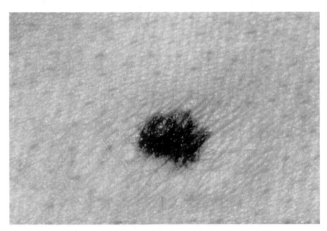

Clin. Fig. IIB1.b

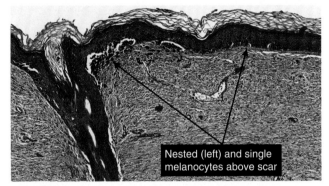

Nested (left) and single melanocytes above scar

Fig. IIB1.g

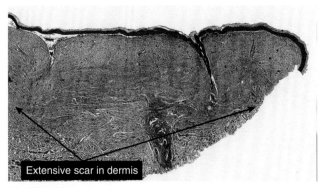

Extensive scar in dermis

Fig. IIB1.f

Clin. Fig. IIB1.b. *Recurrent melanocytic nevus.* Dark brown macule with irregular borders recurred in the surgical site of a previously shave biopsied nevus in a teenaged girl.

Fig. IIB1.f. *Recurrent nevus, lentiginous pattern, low power.* At scanning magnification, one can see a flattened rete ridge architecture, a feature which is a clue to previous trauma or biopsy. There is a proliferation of melanocytes in the epidermis which does not extend beyond the lateral border of the scar.

Fig. IIB1.g. *Recurrent nevus phenomenon, lentiginous pattern, medium power.* At the dermal–epidermal interface there is a lentiginous proliferation of single and nested, heavily pigmented melanocytes which overlie a zone of scar tissue in the superficial dermis. The lesional cells may be large with enlarged nuclei and prominent nucleoli, single cells may be prominent, and there may be cells extending above the dermal–epidermal junction. These features taken together may suggest a lentiginous pattern of melanoma, but the proliferation does not extend beyond the lateral border of the scar, and on review, the original nevus is wholly benign.

distinction between melanomas and nevi apply. In any problematical case in which the diagnosis is in doubt, the original biopsy should be obtained for review.

Superficial Atypical Melanocytic Proliferations of Uncertain Significance (SAMPUS and IAMPUS), Lentiginous Patterns

SAMPUS is a descriptive term that may be applied to lesions that exhibit conflicting or borderline features between melanoma and its benign simulants, such as actinic lentigines with atypia, or dysplastic nevi with focal areas of confluent or continuous basal lentiginous proliferation insufficient for a more definitive diagnosis. A differential diagnosis should always be given, so that appropriate definitive therapy can be planned. Lesions that are entirely intraepidermal may be termed "Intraepidermal melanocytic proliferations of uncertain significance" (IAMPUS"). The term "SAMPUS" is used to reflect the fact that invasion of the dermis, if not accompanied by tumorigenic and/or mitogenic proliferation in the dermis, is not associated with competence for metastasis (9). See also IID2. The differential diagnosis for the lesion illustrated below includes a dysplastic nevus, a "lentiginous nevus of elderly/sun-damaged skin" (39) or an evolving LMM. Because of the locally recurring potential of the latter, complete excision is indicated. Because of the risk marker significance of these diagnoses, the patient should be considered for surveillance, especially if there are other clinically atypical nevi or a family or personal history of melanoma.

Conditions to consider in the differential diagnosis:

melanoma *in situ* (lentigo maligna type)
lentiginous nevus of elderly/sun-damaged skin
recurrent nevus
actinic lentigo (atrophic lesions)

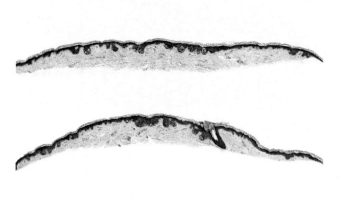

Fig. IIB1.h

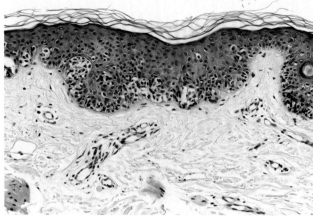

Fig. IIB1.i

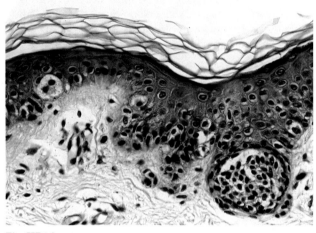

Fig. IIB1.j

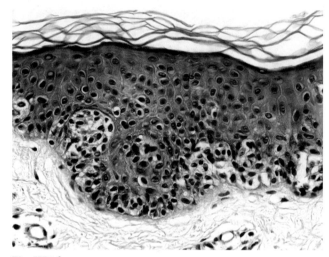

Fig. IIB1.k

Fig. IIB1.h. *SAMPUS, lentiginous pattern.* There is a lentiginous and nested melanocytic proliferation in sun-damaged skin. The rete ridge patterns are incompletely effaced and focally exaggerated.

Fig. IIB1.i. *SAMPUS, lentiginous pattern.* There are increased single cells near the dermal–epidermal junction, with some cells rising above it.

Fig. IIB1.j. *SAMPUS, lentiginous pattern.* Nested and single cells are present, however the basal proliferation is not continuous.

Fig. IIB1.k. *SAMPUS, lentiginous pattern.* In another area there is a suggestion of continuous and focal pagetoid proliferation. Cytologic atypia is moderate, but relatively uniform.

IIB2 | Without Melanocytic Proliferation

The epidermis is thinned without proliferation of keratinocytes or melanocytes. Each melanocyte is separated from the next by several keratinocytes. *Atrophic actinic keratosis* and *porokeratosis* (40) are prototypic examples.

Atrophic Actinic Keratosis

(See also IIA.1.) Atrophic actinic keratoses lack the epidermal proliferation seen in most lesions, especially in the hypertrophic type.

Porokeratosis

CLINICAL SUMMARY. Porokeratosis (41) is characterized by a distinct peripheral keratotic ridge that corresponds histologically to the cornoid lamella. Although five different forms can be distinguished, *disseminated superficial actinic porokeratosis* is by far the most common type. Genomic variations in the mevalonate pathway have been described in various forms of familial and sporadic porokeratosis (42). The lesions often are most pronounced in sun-exposed areas and may be exacerbated by exposure to

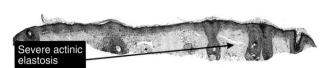

Fig. IIB2.a

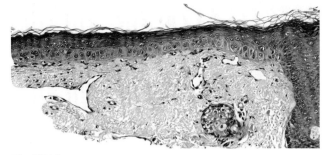

Fig. IIB2.b

Fig. IIB2.a. *Atrophic actinic keratosis, low power.* There is hyperkeratosis with patchy parakeratosis. The underlying epidermis is thin.

Fig. IIB2.b. *Atrophic actinic keratosis, medium power.* There is slight atypia of basal keratinocytes, with patchy to bandlike lymphocytes usually with plasma cells in the papillary dermis (not seen in this example), and actinic elastosis.

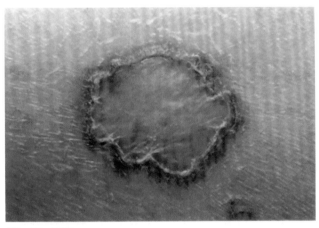

Clin. Fig. IIB2.a

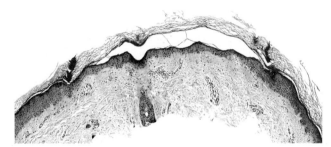

Fig. IIB.2c

Clin. Fig. IIB2.a. *Disseminated superficial actinic porokeratosis.* Illustrated here are two of many oval plaques and papules with slightly raised keratotic rims and atrophic centers that developed on sun exposed legs.

Fig. IIB.2c. *Porokeratosis, low power.* On each end of this shave biopsy specimen there are two cornoid lamellae which can be seen at scanning magnification as discrete foci of parakeratosis. Parakeratotic columns lean toward the center of the lesion.

the sun. They present as small patches surrounded only by a narrow, slightly raised, hyperkeratotic ridge without a distinct furrow.

HISTOPATHOLOGY. The peripheral, raised, hyperkeratotic ridge shows a keratin-filled invagination of the epidermis. In the prototypic *plaque type* of porokeratosis, the invagination extends deeply downward at an angle, the apex of which points away from the central portion of the lesion. In the center of this keratin-filled invagination rises a parakeratotic column, the so-called cornoid lamella, representing the most characteristic feature of porokeratosis of Mibelli. In the epidermis beneath the parakeratotic column, the keratinocytes are irregularly

arranged, and some cells possess an eosinophilic cytoplasm as a result of premature keratinization. Usually no granular layer is found at the site at which the parakeratotic column arises, but elsewhere the keratin-filled invagination of the epidermis has a well-developed granular layer. The histologic changes in disseminated superficial actinic porokeratosis are similar but less pronounced, the central invagination being rather shallow.

Conditions to consider in the differential diagnosis:

atrophic actinic keratosis
porokeratosis
lupus erythematosus

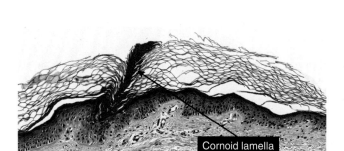

Fig. IIB.2d   **Fig. IIB.2e**

Fig. IIB.2d. *Porokeratosis, medium power.* The cornoid lamella is characterized by a well defined stack of parakeratotic keratin which overlies an invagination of the epidermis. Beneath the parakeratotic column there is focal loss of the granular cell layer and dyskeratosis.

Fig. IIB.2e. *Porokeratosis, high power.* Porokeratosis may be associated with a patchy to bandlike lichenoid mononuclear cell infiltrate in the superficial dermis, though not in this example.

IIC LOCALIZED LESIONS WITH ELONGATED RETE RIDGES

Elongation of the rete ridges without melanocytic proliferation in a localized lesion is termed papillomatosis in which each papilla may be likened to a glove of epidermis covering a finger of stroma. Elongated rete with melanocytic proliferation and predominance of single cells over nests is termed a "lentiginous" pattern. This pattern may be seen in lentiginous junctional and compound nevi, in dysplastic nevi and in the "lentiginous" melanomas. However, in melanomas the epidermal rete pattern is more often irregularly thickened and thinned than regularly elongated.

1. With Melanocytic Proliferation
2. Without Melanocytic Proliferation

IIC1 With Melanocytic Proliferation

The epidermal rete ridges are elongated and within these rete there is melanocytic proliferation. Actinic lentigo, lentigo simplex, lentiginous junctional nevus, and dysplastic nevus are prototypic (43).

Actinic Lentigo

CLINICAL SUMMARY. Lentigines are macular hyperpigmentations in which histologically the number of epidermal melanocytes is increased, but the nests of melanocytes that define nevus cells are not present. In actinic lentigo, which arises most frequently in older adults, there are usually multiple lesions with a predilection to areas of sun exposure. They are relatively large compared to simple lentigines (usually about 5 mm but with some lesions greater than 1 cm), rather asymmetrical, and poorly-circumscribed macules that are variably pigmented in shades of brown usually without black. When the asymmetry and pigmentary variegation are more prominent, biopsy may be necessary to distinguish these lesions from lentigo maligna. Actinic lentigines are the prototypic "freckles" in individuals with severe solar damage; they are important markers of melanoma risk and (like simple ephelids) are associated with polymorphisms of the MC1R gene which has been termed the "freckle gene" and is involved in regulation of melanin synthesis (44). Genomic analysis has identified factors more associated with keratinocytes and matrix cells, rather than melanocytes, which may therefore be only secondarily affected (45).

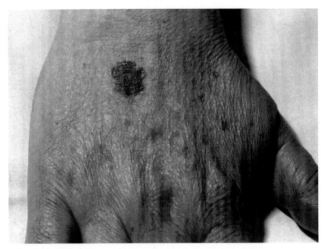

Clin. Fig. IIC1.a

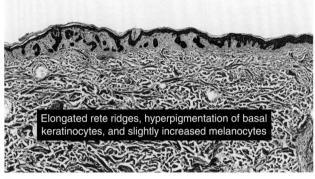

Elongated rete ridges, hyperpigmentation of basal keratinocytes, and slightly increased melanocytes

Fig. IIC1.a

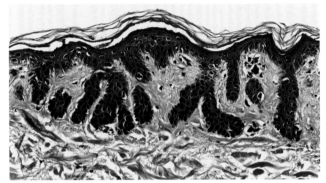

Fig. IIC1.b

Clin. Fig. IIC1.a. *Actinic lentigo.* A 1 cm, rather irregular patch of slightly variegated hyperpigmentation in a background of chronic solar damage.

Fig. IIC1.a. *Actinic lentigo, low power.* At scanning magnification there is uniform elongation of rete ridges with hyperpigmentation. Significant inflammation is not present.

Fig. IIC1.b. *Actinic lentigo, medium power.* Melanocytes are slightly increased in number, but in contrast to lentigo maligna the rete ridges are elongated and there is no contiguous proliferation of uniformly atypical melanocytes.

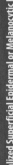

Localized Superficial Epidermal or Melanocytic Proliferations

II

HISTOPATHOLOGY. The findings include, in a relatively large lesion, slight or moderate elongation of the rete ridges, with an obvious increase in the amount of melanin in both the melanocytes and the basal keratinocytes, and often with the presence of melanophages in the upper dermis. In some instances, melanin is also present in the upper layers of the epidermis and stratum corneum. Melanocytes usually appear somewhat increased in number.

Lentigo Simplex

CLINICAL SUMMARY. Lentigines are macular hyperpigmentations in which histologically the number of epidermal melanocytes is increased, but the nests of melanocytes that define nevus cells are not present. In lentigo simplex, which arises most frequently in childhood, there are usually only a few scattered lesions without predilection to areas of sun exposure. They are small (usually 2–3 mm), symmetrical, and well-circumscribed macules that are evenly pigmented but vary individually from brown to black. The definition is a histologic one, and clinically, lentigo simplex is indistinguishable from a junctional nevus.

HISTOPATHOLOGY. The findings include, in a small lesion usually 2 to 3 mm or less in diameter, a slight or moderate elongation of the rete ridges, an increase in the concentration of melanocytes in the basal layer, an increase in the amount of melanin in both the melanocytes and the basal keratinocytes, and the presence of melanophages in the upper dermis. In some instances, melanin is also present in the upper layers of the epidermis and stratum corneum. Because of the existence of these transitional forms, the lentigo simplex is regarded as a form of evolving melanocytic nevus. In a recent study, lentigo simplex lesions lacked the BRAF mutations that characterize most nevi, challenging but not necessarily refuting this presumption (46).

Lentiginous Junctional Nevus

CLINICAL SUMMARY. The term "lentigo" derives from a clinical appearance of a small lenticulate or lens-shaped pigmented spot. The prototype of the lentiginous pattern is seen in the lentigo simplex which is regarded as an early or evolving form of melanocytic nevus. In lesions otherwise clinically characteristic of lentigo simplex, small nests of nevus cells may be present at the epidermal–dermal

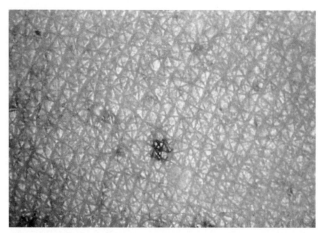

Clin. Fig. IIC1.b

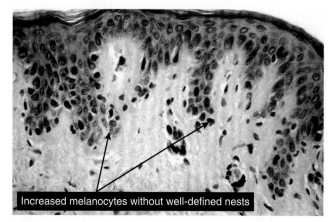

Increased melanocytes without well-defined nests

Fig. IIC1.c

Clin. Fig. IIC1.b. *Lentigo simplex.* A 2–3 mm uniform patch of brown or dark brown to black hyperpigmentation, in normal or sun-damaged skin.

Fig. IIC1.c. *Lentigo simplex, medium power.* In contrast to actinic lentigo, melanocytes are obviously increased at the dermal–epidermal junction and are at least focally contiguous with one another. In contrast to a dysplastic nevus or a lentigo maligna, the lesion is small and there is no significant cytologic atypia.

junction, especially at the lowest pole of rete ridges. These lesions then combine features of a lentigo simplex and a junctional nevus (lentiginous junctional nevus, or "jentigo"). If nevus cells are also present in the dermis but there is a junctional component that extends beyond the dermal component, the term "lentiginous compound nevus" may be used. Lentiginous junctional and compound nevi are typically in the 2- to 4-mm size range and are very common; lesions larger than 5 mm are often dysplastic nevi.

HISTOPATHOLOGY. Although the term "lentigo" is originally of clinical derivation, it has taken on a histologic connotation defined by the presence of single melanocytes arranged in contiguity about elongated rete ridges, as in the lentigo simplex. The lack of nests at the histologic level distinguishes a lentigo from a nevus. In a *lentiginous junctional nevus,* nevus cells lie in well-circumscribed nests either entirely within the lower epidermis or bulging downward into the dermis but still in contact with the epidermis. In addition, varying numbers of diffusely arranged single nevus cells are seen in the lowermost epidermis, especially in the basal cell layer. The rete ridges tend to be uniformly elongated, completing the "lentiginous" pattern. Dysplastic nevi also exhibit a lentiginous architecture, but they are larger (greater than 4 to 5 mm in histologic section) and there is cytologic atypia affecting randomly scattered nevus cells. Lesions smaller than 4 mm that exhibit lentiginous architecture and cytologic atypia are occasionally encountered. These lesions may be diagnosed descriptively (e.g., "lentiginous nevus with atypia"), with a note that additional evaluation of the patient may be indicated to rule out the possibilities of

other clinically atypical nevi, or of a family or personal history of melanoma (47). If these or other risk factors for melanoma are found, then periodic surveillance of the patient may be indicated, depending on the magnitude of the risk as judged clinically.

Nevus Spilus

CLINICAL SUMMARY. The *speckled lentiginous nevus,* or *nevus spilus,* consists of a light brown patch or band present from the time of birth that in childhood becomes dotted with small, dark brown macules. In some apparently related lesions the speckles are papular. These lesions may be syndromic, and familial, and may be associated with neurologic or musculoskeletal abnormalities often ipsilateral to the nevus (48). The melanocytes of nevus spilus have mutations of HRAS (49). The melanocytes in the background patch carry a single mutant allele, which is amplified in the more cellular areas, constituting the speckles. Similar lesions, called nevus spilus–type congenital melanocytic nevi, have large café au lait macules in which there are superimposed lesions that are indistinguishable both clinically and histopathologically from medium/large congenital melanocytic nevi. These differ from nevus spilus in having NRAS rather than HRAS mutations. These lesions can be included in the general category of RASopathies (50).

HISTOPATHOLOGY. The light brown patch or band shows basal hyperpigmentation of keratinocytes similar to a café au lait macule. The speckled areas show junctional nests of nevus cells at the lowest poles of some of the rete ridges and diffuse junctional activity and dermal aggregates of nevus cells, similar to a lentigo simplex.

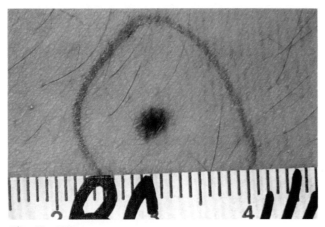

Clin. Fig. IIC1.c

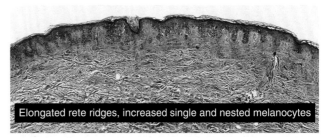

Elongated rete ridges, increased single and nested melanocytes

Fig. IIC1.d

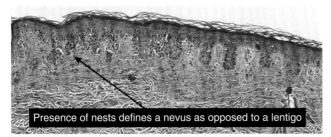

Presence of nests defines a nevus as opposed to a lentigo

Fig. IIC1.e

Clin. Fig. IIC1.c. *Lentiginous junctional nevus.* A 2–5 mm uniform patch of brown or dark brown to black hyperpigmentation.

Fig. IIC1.d. *Lentiginous junctional nevus, low power.* Scanning magnification reveals a small melanocytic lesion confined to the epidermis. There is elongation of rete ridges and a very sparse superficial lymphocytic infiltrate.

Fig. IIC1.e. *Lentiginous junctional nevus, medium power.* Higher magnification reveals a lentiginous proliferation of single and nested melanocytes along the dermal–epidermal junction. The nests are located predominantly at the tips of rete ridges. Atypia of melanocytes is not seen.

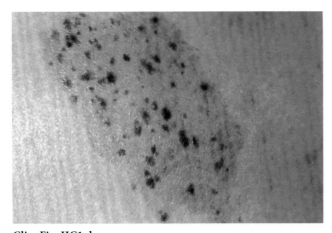

Clin. Fig. IIC1.d

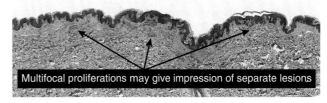

Multifocal proliferations may give impression of separate lesions

Fig. IIC1.f

Clin. Fig. IIC1.d. *Nevus spilus.* This usually congenital lesion presents as a light brown patch in which speckled brown macules appear in childhood.

Fig. IIC1.f. *Nevus spilus, low power.* Scanning magnification may seem to show only a single small melanocytic lesion confined to the epidermis, or to the epidermis and papillary dermis. Depending on the size of the biopsy (which may be submitted to rule out melanoma), there may be more than one of these small lesions. Between the lesions, the epidermis is hyperpigmented, but this may not be apparent histologically unless the normal skin at the edge of the lesion is included for comparison. (*continues*)

II Localized Superficial Epidermal or Melanocytic Proliferations

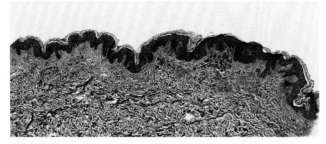

Fig. IIC1.g

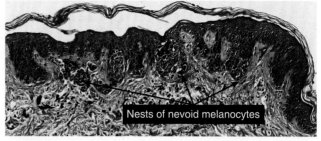

Fig. IIC1.h

Fig. IIC1.g. *Nevus spilus, medium power.* In the focal lesions, there is elongation of rete ridges and a very sparse superficial lymphocytic infiltrate. The appearances are identical to a lentiginous nevus.

Fig. IIC1.h. *Nevus spilus, high power.* Higher magnification reveals a lentiginous proliferation of single and nested melanocytes along the dermal–epidermal junction. Atypia of melanocytes is not seen.

Junctional or Superficial Compound Dysplastic Nevi

CLINICAL SUMMARY. Dysplastic nevi (51) form, clinically and histologically, a continuum extending from a common nevus to an SSM. They may be located anywhere on the body but are most common on the trunk. A clinically dysplastic nevus is defined by (1) the presence of a macular component either as the entire lesion or surrounding a papular center; (2) large size, exceeding 5 mm; (3) irregular or ill-defined "fuzzy" border; and (4) irregular pigmentation within the lesion. Dysplastic nevi are most important as markers of individuals at increased risk for melanoma (14,52); they are also potential precursors of melanoma however most are stable lesions and wholesale excision of them for prevention of melanoma is not recommended. Most dysplastic nevi are excised in order to rule out melanoma histologically. However melanoma risk is related to the degree of histologic atypia in a nevus, being more substantial in moderate to severe dysplasia and negligible in mild dysplasia (14,15). For this reason, the 2018 WHO Classification of Skin Tumours Committee has recommended that lesions formerly called mildy dysplastic should be interpreted as nevi, usually lentiginous junctional or compound nevi. The former moderate dysplasia is characteristized as low-grade dysplasia, and severe dysplasia as high-grade dysplasia (48). Biopsy is most importantly done to rule out melanoma in a clinically concerning lesion, and may also be performed to aid in the assessment of an individual's degree of risk of developing melanoma, and in planning of follow-up schedules.

HISTOPATHOLOGY. *Architectural features* include a "lentiginous" pattern of elongation of the rete ridges with an increase in the number of melanocytes. The latter are arranged as single cells and in nests whose long axes tend

TABLE II.2. Nuclear Features in Different Grades of Dysplasia

Grade (former)	WHO Grade (2017)	Nucleus size compared to resting basal cells	Chromatin	Nuclear size and shape variation	Nucleolus
0 (former mild)	Not a dysplastic nevus	1×	May be hyperchromatic	Minimal	Small or absent
1 (moderate dysplasia[a])	Low-grade dysplasia	1–1.5×	Hyperchromatic or dispersed	Prominent in a minority of cells ("random atypia")	Small or absent
2 (severe dysplasia[a])	High-grade dysplasia	1.5× or more	Hyperchromatic, coarse granular, or peripheral condensation	Prominent in a larger minority of cells	Prominent, often lavender

[a]*Architectural features are required for the diagnosis (see above) and also contribute to the grade of dysplasia. Attributes that indicate a diagnosis of high-grade (severe) dysplasia even when cytologic atypia is low grade include pagetoid scatter above the basal layer (to a lesser degree than in melanoma, usually not above the middle third, and focal i.e. <1 HPF), focal continuous basal proliferation, and intraepidermal mitoses (where more than a rare mitosis and/or any dermal mitosis should raise concern for melanoma).*

Based on Elder DE, Barnhill RL, Bastian BC, et al. Dysplastic naevus. In: Elder DE, Massi D, Scolyer RA, Willemze R, eds. WHO Classification of Melanocytic Tumors. 4th ed. Lyon: IARC; 2018.

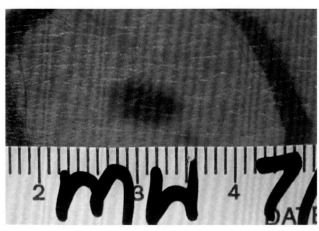

Clin. Fig. IIC1.e

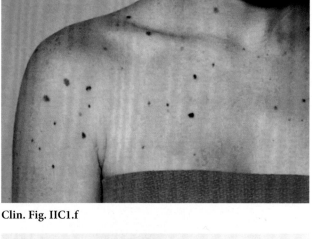

Clin. Fig. IIC1.f

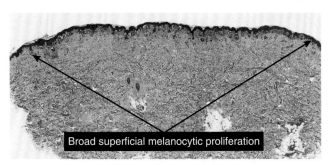

Broad superficial melanocytic proliferation

Fig. IIC1.i

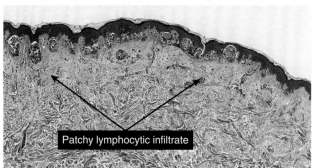

Patchy lymphocytic infiltrate

Fig. IIC1.j

Clin. Fig. IIC1.e. *Dysplastic nevus.* This pigmented lesion fulfills criteria for a dysplastic nevus: (1) macule with indefinite edge; (2) size >5 mm; (3) irregular border; and (4) irregular pigmentation.

Clin. Fig. IIC1.f. *Dysplastic nevi.* This young patient has been followed since childhood. She developed multiple dysplastic nevi around the age of puberty, since this picture was taken she has developed several primary melanomas, all in the curable non-tumorigenic or radial growth phase stage of evolution.

Fig. IIC1.i. *Compound dysplastic nevus, low grade.* At scanning magnification there is a broad compound nevus. Near the center of the lesion the nevus is compound with both an epidermal and dermal component. The "shoulders," at each periphery of the lesion, are composed only of a junctional component.

Fig. IIC1.j. *Compound dysplastic nevus, low grade.* The epidermal rete ridges are uniformly elongated. Nests of melanocytes form "bridges" between these elongated rete. The dermal component of the lesion is at the left of this image, and the junctional component extends to the right, forming the "shoulder." (*continues*)

Localized Superficial Epidermal or Melanocytic Proliferations

II

to lie parallel to the epidermal surface and that tend to form "bridges" between adjacent rete. The melanocytes in the junctional nests are frequently spindle-shaped, but they may be large and epithelioid with abundant cytoplasm containing fine, dusty melanin particles. If the lesion is compound, nests of melanocytes in the papillary dermis have evidence of maturation with descent into the dermis. In these compound dysplastic nevi, the intraepidermal component extends by definition beyond the lateral border of the dermal component, forming a "shoulder" to the lesion histologically, and a "target-like" or "fried-egg" pattern clinically. A patchy lymphocytic infiltrate is present in the rete dermis. "Pagetoid"

extension of melanocytes into the epidermis is absent or slight and is limited to the lowermost layers. *Cytologically*, in addition to the lentiginous melanocytic hyperplasia, melanocytic nuclear atypia is required for the diagnosis, characterized by irregularly shaped, large, hyperchromatic nuclei in more than a few, but nevertheless a minority, of melanocytes. In the WHO classification, nuclear size >1× that of a resting basal keratinocyte is required for a diagnosis of low-grade, and >1.5× for high-grade dysplasia (see Table II.2). Most atypical melanocytes lie singly or in small groups, and the atypia involves only a minority of the lesional cells ("random" cytologic atypia). Focal extension of atypical-appearing

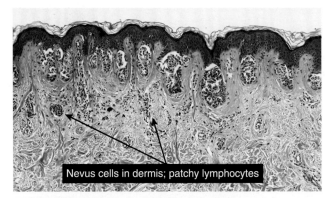

Fig. IIC1.k

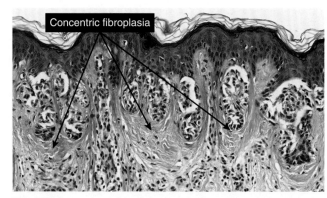

Fig. IIC1.l

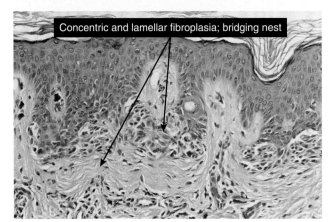

Fig. IIC1.m

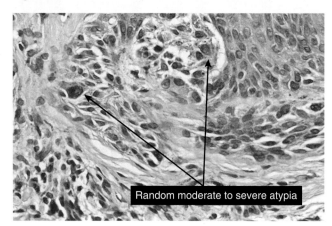

Fig. IIC1.n

Fig. IIC1.k. *Compound dysplastic nevus, low grade.* The intraepidermal component is composed of single and nested melanocytes. The dermis reveals a sparse lymphocytic infiltrate, often with prominent small vessels, and with a sprinkling of melanophages in this example.

Fig. IIC1.l. *Compound dysplastic nevus, low grade.* Beneath the nests of lesional cells, there is lamellar fibroplasia characterized by zones of eosinophilic collagen and spindle cells resembling fibroblasts oriented parallel to the rete epithelium. There are no cells with markedly enlarged nuclei. The dermis reveals a sparse lymphocytic infiltrate, often with prominent small vessels, and with a sprinkling of melanophages.

Fig. IIC1.m. *Compound dysplastic nevus high grade.* In another lesion, at high magnification the majority of the lesional cells are bland in appearance but there are randomly scattered cells which show mild nuclear atypia, characterized by enlargement, irregularity, and hyperchromatism involving a minority of the lesional cell nuclei. Some of the spindle cells in the lamellar fibroplasia contain melanin, suggesting that they are of melanocytic rather than fibroblastic origin.

Fig. IIC1.n. *Compound dysplastic nevus, high grade.* In another field of the same lesion, several of the lesional cell nuclei are markedly enlarged and hyperchromatic. However, the majority of the nuclei are not atypical. This constitutes "random" cytologic atypia. In the dermis, there is eosinophilic concentric and lamellar fibroplasia, in which the collagen contains lamellated spindle cells.

melanocytes into the lower spinous layer may occur, but if this is prominent, transformation into melanoma *in situ* may have occurred.

Nevoid Lentigo Maligna

CLINICAL SUMMARY. This term may be attributed to Kossard who described in 1997 a group of cases of nevoid

melanomas characterized by small cells and a nevoid appearance (53). Rete ridges tend to be preserved, and nesting may be prominent, at least in the centers of these lesions. Similar lesions have been more recently described as "lentiginous melanoma," emphasizing that this is a histologic pattern of melanoma to be distinguished from lentiginous nevus (54). In yet another useful study, 43% of *in situ* lentigo maligna lesions had predominant dysplastic nevus-like features (55). It was concluded that large pigmented lesions on sun-damaged skin and elderly individuals should warrant consideration of an LMM diagnosis even in the setting of dysplastic nevus-like features histologically. Biopsies especially from the centers of the lesions could lead to a mistaken diagnosis of a dysplastic nevus, leading to the possibility of residual melanoma *in situ*, which could persist, recur and progress to a more significant lesion. At least at the periphery, the pattern may be predominantly that of single cells in a continuous distribution along the dermoepidermal junction, more typical of lentigo maligna.

Genomic characteristics have not been studied specifically in this variant of LMM (see also Section IIB1).

Conditions to consider in the differential diagnosis:

lentigo simplex
nevus spilus
lentiginous junctional nevus
junctional nevus
dysplastic nevus
Meyerson nevus
nevoid lentigo maligna
acral-lentiginous melanoma
mucosal-lentiginous melanoma

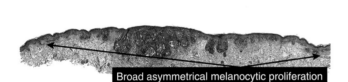

Fig. IIC1.o

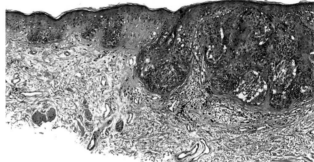

Fig. IIC1.p

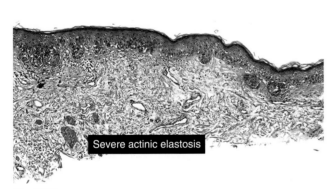

Fig. IIC1.q

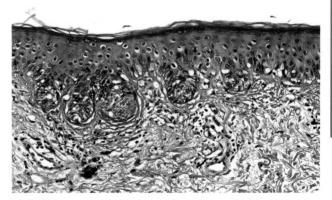

Fig. IIC1.r

Fig. IIC1.o. *Nevoid lentigo maligna, low power.* This lesion is comparatively broad, variably cellular, and is located in skin with moderate to severe actinic elastosis.

Fig. IIC1.p. *Nevoid lentigo maligna, low power.* At the left of this image, the lesion is comprised of small cells, arranged about the tips and sides of elongated rete ridges, without continuous proliferation between the rete at least in all areas. To the right, there is a larger cell type which is uniformly atypical and predominantly nested.

Fig. IIC1.q. *Nevoid lentigo maligna, low power.* At the far periphery of the lesion, to the right of the image, there are two nests which tend to "hang down" from the interface in a "droplet-like" pattern. Elsewhere, similar nests are unevenly scattered along the interface, admixed with some single cells.

Fig. IIC1.r. *Nevoid lentigo maligna, low power.* A high-power view of the periphery of the lesion, demonstrating moderate to severe uniform atypia in the cells within the nests. (*continues*)

Localized Superficial Epidermal or Melanocytic Proliferations

II

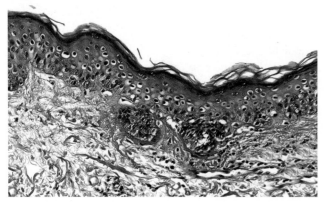

Fig. IIC1.s

Fig. IIC1.s. *Nevoid lentigo maligna, high power.* The nests are somewhat more closely packed, and cytologic atypia is again demonstrated. It might be tempting to consider a field such as this to represent some form of dysplasia, however a cautious approach is appropriate in sun-damaged skin of an elderly subject. The most appropriate diagnosis for this case, in our opinion, is nevoid lentigo maligna (melanoma *in situ*, lentigo maligna type), however alternatively it might be designated as an "intraepidermal atypical melanocytic proliferation of uncertain significance," with a differential diagnosis including *in situ* melanoma, and a recommendation for appropriate management. This lesion was narrowly re-excised but nevertheless recurred locally three years later.

IIC2 | Without Melanocytic Proliferation

The epidermis is thickened (acanthotic). Melanocytes are normal as are keratinocytes. The only change is acanthosis. *Epidermal nevi* are prototypic (56). The differential diagnosis includes *acanthosis nigricans.*

Epidermal Nevus

CLINICAL FEATURES. Epidermal nevi, or verrucous nevi ("nevus verrucosus"), may be either localized or systematized. In the *localized type,* which is present usually but not invariably at birth, only one linear lesion is present, often referred to as *nevus unius lateris.* It consists of closely set, papillomatous, hyperkeratotic papules. In the *systematized type,* papillomatous hyperkeratotic papules often in a linear configuration are present as many lesions. These lesions are often linear in a parallel arrangement, particularly on the trunk. The term *ichthyosis hystrix* is occasionally used, perhaps unnecessarily, for instances of extensive bilateral lesions. Linear epidermal nevi may occasionally be associated with skeletal deformities and central nervous system deficiencies, such as mental retardation, epilepsy, and neural deafness, and, rarely, with basal or SCC. They may also be associated with the distinctive pattern of epidermolytic hyperkeratosis (see also IB1). Various epidermal nevus syndromes exist and have been recently reviewed in terms of their molecular pathogenesis (57).

HISTOPATHOLOGY. Nearly all cases of the localized type of linear epidermal nevus and some cases of the systematized type show the histologic picture of a benign papilloma. One observes considerable hyperkeratosis, papillomatosis, and acanthosis with elongation of the rete ridges resembling seborrheic keratosis, except that the lesions are usually considerably larger. In other instances, papillomatosis may be inconspicuous and orthokeratotic hyperkeratosis may be the major finding.

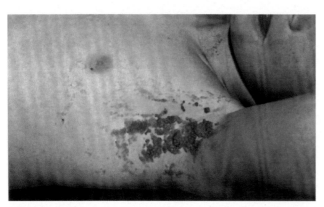

Clin. Fig. IIC2.a

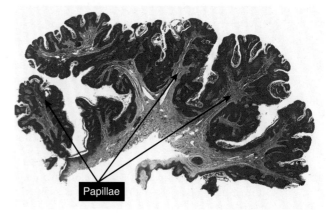

Papillae

Fig. IIC2.a

Clin. Fig. IIC2.a. *Epidermal nevus.* This child had a linear arrangement of brown, warty papules coalescing into plaques. He had no skeletal, ocular or central nervous system involvement.

Fig. IIC2.a. *Epidermal nevus, low power.* At scanning magnification epidermal nevi show papillomatosis and hyperkeratosis. The underlying dermis is essentially unremarkable.

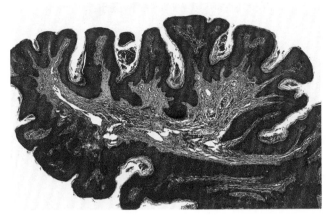

Fig. IIC2.b

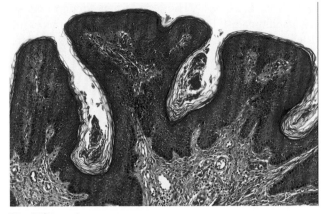

Fig. IIC2.c

Fig. IIC2.b. *Epidermal nevus, medium power.* The epidermis shows varying degrees of acanthosis and papillomatosis with hyperkeratosis. Frequently there is pseudohorn cyst formation resembling a seborrheic keratosis.

Fig. IIC2.c. *Epidermal nevus, high power.* Epidermal maturation is essentially normal. Pigment is variable. The papillary dermis may show fibroplasia with little or no inflammation.

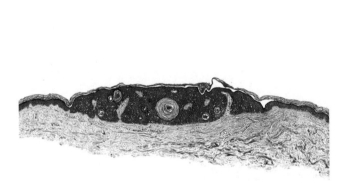

Fig. IIC2.d

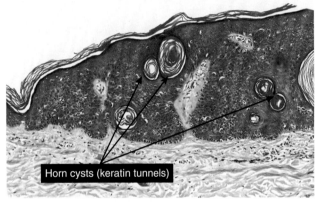

Horn cysts (keratin tunnels)

Fig. IIC2.e

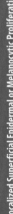

Fig. IIC2.d. *Seborrheic keratosis, low power.* Compared to epidermal nevi, seborrheic keratoses tend to be more sharply circumscribed lesions that lie above the plane of the adjacent epidermal surface.

Fig. IIC2.e. *Seborrheic keratosis, medium power.* Seborrheic keratoses are composed of basaloid cells that show squamous differentiation only near the surface. In an epidermal nevus, the pattern of normal keratinocytic maturation from a single basal layer is more closely maintained (Figures IIC2.b,c).

Seborrheic Keratoses

See also Section IIE2.

Acanthosis Nigricans

CLINICAL SUMMARY. Clinically, acanthosis nigricans presents papillomatous brown patches, predominantly in the intertriginous areas such as the axillae, the neck, and the genital and submammary regions. Syndromes/ associations include: benign inherited, obesity-associated, and syndromic which are often associated with insulin resistance syndromes (58), acral, unilateral, drug-induced, and mixed, and acanthosis nigricans maligna (59). In extensive cases of the malignant type, mucosal surfaces, such as the mouth, the vulva, and the palpebral conjunctivae, may be involved. In the acral type, there is velvety hyperpigmentation of the dorsa of the hands and feet.

HISTOPATHOLOGY. The lesions have hyperkeratosis and papillomatosis but only slight, irregular acanthosis and usually no hyperpigmentation. Thus, the term *acanthosis nigricans* has little histologic justification. In a typical lesion, the dermal papillae project upward as fingerlike projections. The valleys between the papillae show mild to moderate acanthosis and are filled with keratotic material. Horn pseudocysts can occur in some cases. The epidermis at the tips of the papillae and often also on the sides of the protruding papillae appears thinned. Slight hyperpigmentation of the basal layer is demonstrable with silver nitrate staining in some cases but not in others. The brown color

of the lesions is caused more by hyperkeratosis than by melanin.

Conditions to consider in the differential diagnosis:

   epidermal nevi
   psoriasis
   lichen simplex chronicus
   acanthosis nigricans
   actinic lentigo
   confluent and reticulated papillomatosis (CARP)
   seborrheic keratosis

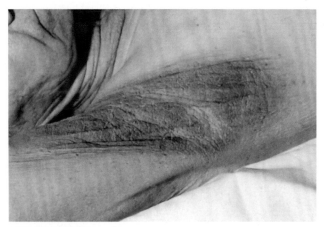

Clin. Fig. IIC2.b

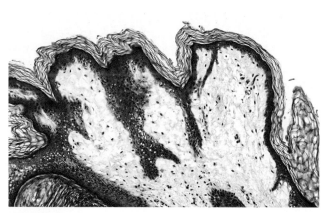

Fig. IIC2.f

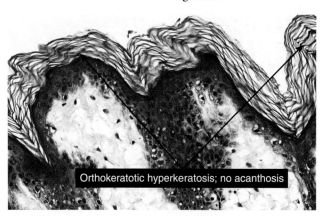

Orthokeratotic hyperkeratosis; no acanthosis

Fig. IIC2.g

Clin. Fig. IIC2.b. *Acanthosis nigricans.* An elderly woman had an explosive development of velvety, hyperpigmented plaques in the intertriginous areas. She had metastatic endometrial carcinoma

Fig. IIC2.f. *Acanthosis nigricans, medium power.* There is papillomatosis with prominent hyperkeratosis which is predominantly orthokeratotic.

Fig. IIC2.g. *Acanthosis nigricans, high power.* In contrast to a seborrheic keratosis, acanthosis nigricans fails to reveal significant acanthosis of the epidermis.

IID | LOCALIZED LESIONS WITH PAGETOID EPITHELIAL PROLIFERATION

A neoplastic proliferation of one cell type distributed as single cells or nests within a benign epithelium is termed "Pagetoid" after Paget disease of the breast (mammary carcinoma cells proliferating in skin of the nipple).

1. Keratinocytic Proliferations
2. Melanocytic Proliferations
3. Glandular Epithelial Proliferations
4. Lymphoid Proliferations

IID1 | Keratinocytic Proliferations

The epidermis has atypical keratinocytes scattered within mature epithelium at all or multiple levels; there is loss of normal maturation. Mitoses are increased and there may be individual cell necrosis. *Pagetoid SCC in situ* is a prototypic example.

Pagetoid Squamous Cell Carcinoma In Situ (Bowen Disease)

(See also IIA1.) An occasional finding in SCC *in situ* (Bowen disease, [BD]) is vacuolization of the cells, especially in the upper portion of the epidermis. Also, in exceptional cases, multiple nests of atypical cells are scattered through a normal epidermis, sometimes with sparing of the basal cell layer.

Clonal Seborrheic Keratosis

In the clonal, or nesting, type of seborrheic keratosis, well-defined nests of cells are located within the epidermis (60). In some instances, the nests resemble foci of basal cell epithelioma, since the nuclei appear small

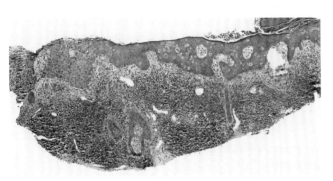

Fig. IID1.a

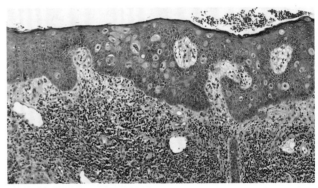

Fig. IID1.b

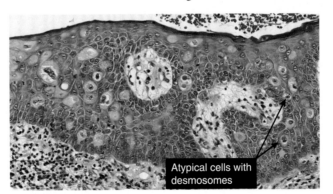

Fig. IID1.c

Fig. IID1.a. *Pagetoid squamous cell carcinoma in situ, low power.* The epidermis is irregularly thickened and thinned, with effaced rete ridges, and a parakeratotic scale-crust. There is a dense bandlike lympho-plasmacytic infiltrate in the dermis.

Fig. IID1.b. *Pagetoid squamous cell carcinoma in situ, medium power.* Large pale cells are present among more compact eosinophilic keratinocytes.

Fig. IID1.c. *Pagetoid squamous cell carcinoma in situ, high power.* At high magnification, a search for desmosomes will usually reveal their presence between the neoplastic cells and their less atypical neighbors, establishing the diagnosis of squamous cell carcinoma *in situ*, and ruling out melanoma and Paget disease.

Localized Superficial Epidermal or Melanocytic Proliferations

II

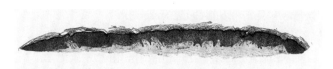

Fig. IID1.d

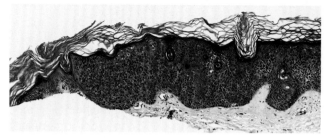

Fig. IID1.e

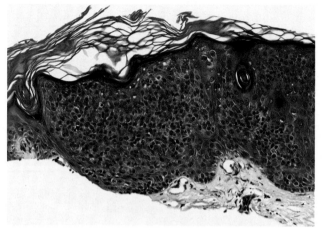

Fig. IID1.f

Fig. IID1.d. *Clonal seborrheic keratosis, low power.* In contrast to a squamous cell carcinoma *in situ*, this lesion shows uniform acanthosis of the epidermis with a predominantly basket-weave stratum corneum.

Fig. IID1.e. *Clonal seborrheic keratosis, medium power.* Within a thickened epidermal layer there are "clones" composed of aggregates of bland appearing epithelial cells clustered within the epidermis.

Fig. IID1.f. *Clonal seborrheic keratosis, medium power.* Lack of features such as cytological atypia, mitotic figures, and an atypical parakeratotic scale help differentiate this lesion from a squamous cell carcinoma *in situ* with a clonal pattern.

and dark-staining and intercellular bridges are seen in only a few areas. In other instances of clonal seborrheic keratosis, the nests are composed of fairly large cells showing distinct intercellular bridges, with the nests separated from one another by strands of cells exhibiting small, dark nuclei. A "microclonal" variant has been described with morphology sometimes challenging to distinguish from pagetoid BD (BD, SCC *in situ*, see IIID1) (8). High expression of p16 and Ki-67 or p16 alone is said to favor the diagnosis of BD over microclonal seborrheic keratosis.

Conditions to consider in the differential diagnosis:

pagetoid squamous cell carcinoma *in situ*
clonal seborrheic keratosis
intraepithelial epithelioma (Borst–Jadassohn)
Paget disease

IID2 Melanocytic Proliferation

Atypical melanocytes are seen at all levels within the otherwise mature but often hyperplastic epidermis. *Melanoma in situ or microinvasive (superficial spreading type)* is prototypic (61,62). Pigmented spindle cell nevus (63) is an important differential.

Melanoma In Situ or Microinvasive, Superficial Spreading Type

CLINICAL SUMMARY. The lesions may occur on exposed skin but are rather more commonly found on intermittently exposed skin and are rare on unexposed skin. The most frequently involved sites are the upper back, especially in men, and the lower legs in women. The lesions are slightly or definitely elevated, with palpable borders and irregular, partly arciform outlines. There is often variation in color that includes not only tan, brown, and black, but also pink, blue, and gray. Gray-white areas may be observed at sites of spontaneous regression. Microinvasion may be clinically inapparent, but the onset of tumorigenic vertical growth is indicated by the development of a papule followed by nodularity and sometimes also ulceration, the latter usually being a late feature.

HISTOPATHOLOGY. *Architectural pattern features* include the large diameter of the lesions, often relatively good circumscription compared to LMM (the last cells at the edge of the lesion are often in a nest), and asymmetry (one half of the lesion does not mirror the other half). The epidermis is irregularly thickened and thinned with distortion of the rete ridge pattern. Rather uniformly rounded, large melanocytes are present near the dermoepidermal junction and usually also scattered in a pagetoid pattern throughout the epidermis. The large cells lie in nests and singly. The nests tend to vary a good deal in size and shape. As previously discussed, the pagetoid and nested patterns in this form of melanoma (and also the relatively prominent pigmentation) tend to be associated with the presence of mutations of the BRAF oncogene (17). Dermal melanophages and a dermal infiltrate are usually present except in some strictly *in situ* lesions. The lymphocytic infiltrate is typically dense and bandlike, especially in invasive lesions. *Cytologically*, the lesional cells are rather uniform and have atypical, hyperchromatic nuclei and abundant cytoplasm containing

varying amounts of melanin that often consists of small, "dusty" particles. This "uniform cytological atypia" is of considerable diagnostic importance and contrasts with the random atypia of dysplastic nevi. Distinction from a dysplastic nevus is based on greater size, asymmetry, and cellularity, the presence of high-level and extensive pagetoid proliferation or of contiguous basilar proliferation of uniformly atypical cells, the presence of moderate to severe and uniform cytologic atypia, and the presence of lesional cell mitoses in some melanomas. Criteria for distinguishing among junctional melanocytic dysplasia versus pagetoid versus lentiginous melanoma *in situ* are presented in Table II.3.

TABLE II.3. Junctional Dysplasia Versus Pagetoid Versus Lentiginous Melanoma *In Situ*

Attribute	Junctional Dysplasia	Pagetoid MIS (SSM-IS)	Lentiginous MIS (LMM-IS)[b]
Melanocytes	Nevoid to epithelioid, small	Epithelioid, large	Nevoid to epithelioid, intermediate
Atypia	Mild to moderate, random	Moderate to severe, uniform	Moderate to severe, uniform
Pagetoid scatter	Minimal	Prominent	Often minimal
Nesting	Predominant	Prominent	Minimal or absent
Pigment	Prominent	Usually prominent	Often minimal/absent
Epidermis	Elongated Rete	Irregular acanthosis	Thinned
Dermal fibrosis[a]	Concentric	Diffuse	Minimal
Lymphocytes[a]	Patchy perivascular	Brisk, bandlike	Patchy to bandlike

[a]*Fibrosis and inflammation may be minimal in some strictly in situ melanomas.*
[b]*"Nevoid lentigo maligna" may have features overlapping with junctional dysplasia.*
IS, in situ; LMM, lentigo maligna melanoma; SSM, superficial spreading melanoma.

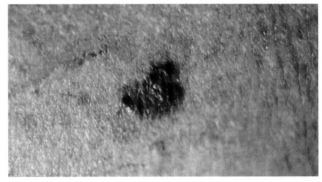

Clin. Fig. IID2.a

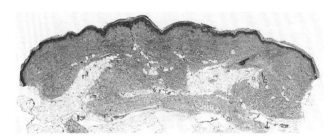

Fig. IID2.a

Clin. Fig. IID2.a. *Melanoma in situ, superficial spreading type.* A slowly enlarging pigmented lesion on the chest of a middle aged male. The asymmetry, irregular notched border, color variegation and size raise suspicion for melanoma.

Fig. IID2.a. *Superficial spreading melanoma in situ, medium power.* There is a broad and poorly circumscribed lesion characterized by an increased number of uniformly enlarged melanocytes in the epidermis. Strictly *in situ* lesions such as this may have little or no dermal inflammation. (*continues*)

II Localized Superficial Epidermal or Melanocytic Proliferations

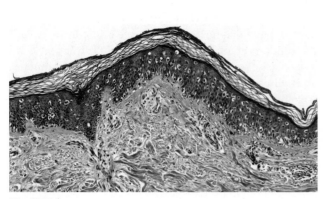

Fig. IID2.b

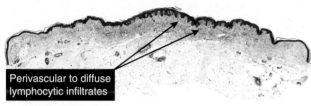

Perivascular to diffuse lymphocytic infiltrates

Fig. IID2.d

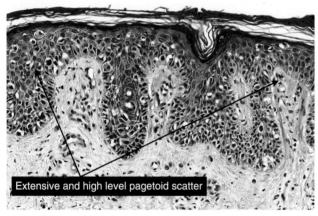

Extensive and high level pagetoid scatter

Fig. IID2.f

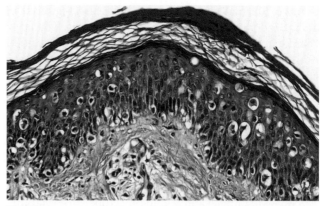

Fig. IID2.c

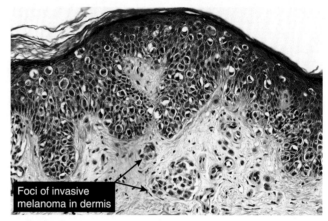

Foci of invasive melanoma in dermis

Fig. IID2.e

Fig. IID2.b. *Superficial spreading melanoma in situ, medium power.* There is extensive pagetoid (or "buckshot") scatter of lesional cells into the epidermis. The cells have a uniform appearance ("uniform cytologic atypia").

Fig. IID2.c. *Superficial spreading melanoma in situ, high power.* Cytologic atypia, characterized here by nuclear enlargement, hyperchromatism, and irregularity, may be moderate, as here, or severe.

Fig. IID2.d. *Superficial spreading melanoma, microinvasive, low power.* The epidermis is irregularly thickened with distortion of the rete ridge pattern. There is a perivascular to diffuse lymphocytic infiltrate in the papillary dermis.

Fig. IID2.e. *Superficial spreading melanoma, microinvasive, medium power.* Enlarged epithelioid melanocytes are scattered in a "pagetoid" or "buckshot scatter" pattern among keratinocytes. A few clusters of lesional cells are seen in the papillary dermis, constituting invasion.

Fig. IID2.f. *Superficial spreading melanoma, microinvasive, high power.* The lesional cells are large, with abundant cytoplasm and, often, finely-divided cytoplasmic melanin pigment. Their nuclei are uniformly enlarged, somewhat hyperchromatic, and have prominent nucleoli.

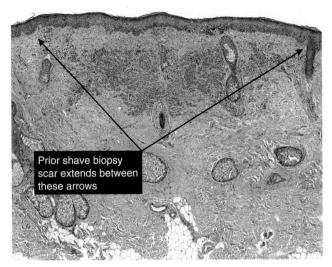

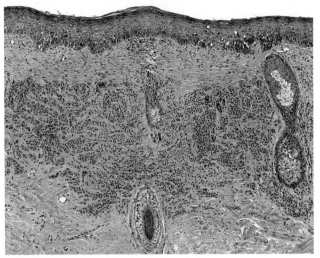

Fig. IID2.g   **Fig. IID2.h**

Fig. IID2.g. *Recurrent nevus phenomenon, lentiginous and pagetoid pattern, low power.* At scanning magnification, one can see a flattened rete ridge architecture, a feature which is a clue to previous trauma or biopsy. There is a proliferation of melanocytes in the epidermis which does not extend beyond the lateral border of the scar.

Fig. IID2.h. *Recurrent nevus phenomenon, lentiginous and pagetoid pattern medium power.* At the dermal–epidermal interface there is a lentiginous and focally pagetoid proliferation of single and nested, heavily pigmented melanocytes, which overlie a zone of scar tissue in the superficial dermis. The lesional cells may be large with enlarged nuclei and prominent nucleoli, single cells may be prominent, and there may be cells extending above the dermal–epidermal junction. These features taken together may suggest melanoma, but the proliferation does not extend beyond the lateral border of scar, and the pre-existing nevus on review is benign.

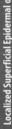

Recurrent Nevus (Pseudomelanoma), Pagetoid Pattern

The atypical proliferation in these lesions may be lentiginous, simulating a lentiginous melanoma as discussed in section IIB1, or pagetoid, simulating SSM.

Junctional Spitz Tumor (Nevus) With Pagetoid Proliferation

Although most Spitz tumors are compound nevi that involve the reticular dermis (discussed in section VIB3), junctional examples are also not uncommonly observed, especially in young children but also occasionally in adults. Some cases are associated with pagetoid proliferation of the lesional cells in the epidermis (64). When this is present, the differential diagnosis of melanoma should always be considered and multiple histologic attributes should be evaluated including size, symmetry, age of the patient, presence of eosinophilic globules (Kamino bodies, depicted in Figure IID2.i) and predominance of nests or single cells. Occasionally in adults, and more commonly in children, pagetoid proliferation of Spitz nevus cells in the epidermis may be seen.

Superficial/Intraepidermal Atypical Melanocytic Proliferations of Uncertain Significance (SAMPUS/IAMPUS), Pagetoid Patterns

SAMPUS is a descriptive term that may be applied to lesions that exhibit conflicting or borderline features between melanoma and its benign simulants, such as pagetoid Spitz nevi, or dysplastic nevi with a few pagetoid cells insufficient for a more definitive diagnosis. A differential diagnosis should always be given, so that appropriate definitive therapy can be planned. See also IIB1. The term "SAMPUS" is used to reflect the fact that invasion of the dermis, if not accompanied by tumorigenic and/or mitogenic proliferation in the dermis, is not associated with competence for metastasis (16).

Conditions to consider in the differential diagnosis:

melanoma *in situ* (superficial spreading type)
pigmented spindle cell nevus
recurrent melanocytic nevus (pseudomelanoma)
certain Spitz nevi with pagetoid proliferation
certain acral nevi with pagetoid proliferation

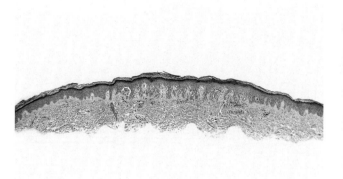

Fig. IID2.i

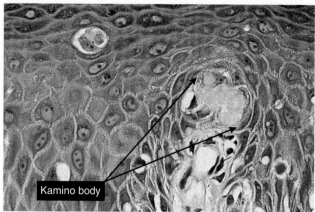

Fig. IID2.j

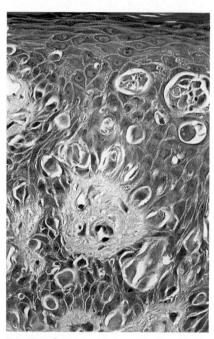

Fig. IID2.k

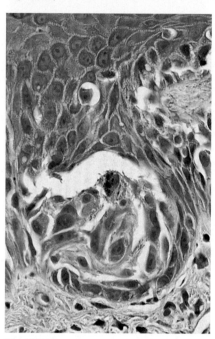

Fig. IID2.l

Fig. IID2.i. *Junctional Spitz nevus, low power.* In contrast to malignant melanoma, this lesion is small and symmetrical.

Fig. IID2.j. *Junctional Spitz nevus, high power.* Pagetoid proliferation of melanocytes is not uncommon in Spitz nevi, especially in young patients. Globoid eosinophilic globules (Kamino bodies) are characteristic of classic Spitz nevi, especially when confluent as here. They may occasionally be seen also in melanomas.

Fig. IID2.k. *Junctional Spitz nevus, high power.* Clefting artifact between the nests of Spitz nevus cells and the adjacent keratinocytes is a characteristic feature.

Fig. IID2.l. *Junctional Spitz nevus, high power.* The Spitz nevus is composed of large nevoid melanocytes with abundant amphophilic cytoplasm and large nuclei with prominent eosinophilic nucleoli.

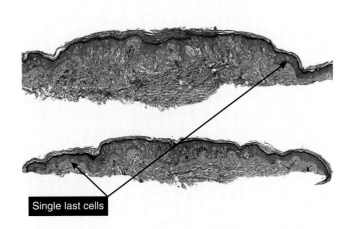

Fig. IID2.m

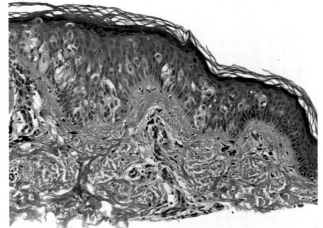

Fig. IID2.n

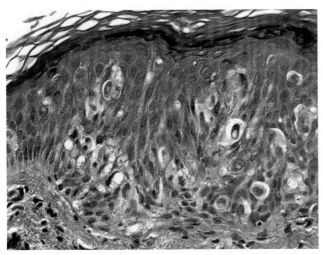

Fig. IID2.o

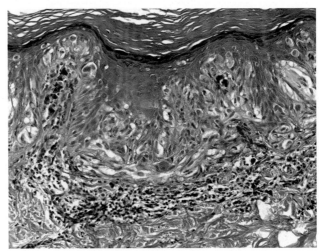

Fig. IID2.p

Fig. IID2.m. *SAMPUS, pagetoid pattern.* This lesion, from the wrist of a 15-year-old girl, is relatively small but not especially well circumscribed or symmetrical at scanning magnification.

Fig. IID2.n. *SAMPUS, pagetoid pattern.* At the periphery of the lesion the last cells are single rather than nested (poor circumscription).

Fig. IID2.o. *SAMPUS, pagetoid pattern.* The lesional cells are large spindle and/or epithelioid cells, with abundant amphophilic cytoplasm, characteristic of the cells of Spitz tumors/nevi. However, there are no Kamino bodies.

Fig. IID2.p. *SAMPUS, pagetoid pattern.* There is pagetoid extension of the lesional cells focally to the stratum corneum, raising the question of melanoma *in situ* (MIS), superficial spreading type. However the differential diagnosis also includes a pagetoid Spitz tumor or even a severely dysplastic nevus. This lesion should be managed taking into consideration the locally recurring potential of MIS and also the risk marker significance of a dysplastic nevus or melanoma. Thus, a re-excision should be considered and the patient's other risk factors should be considered for evaluation of the need for follow-up of her nevi.

Localized Superficial Epidermal or Melanocytic Proliferations

II

IID3 Glandular Epithelial Proliferations

Atypical large clear cells with glandular differentiation (mucin production, lumen formation) proliferate in a normally maturing epidermis. *Paget disease (mammary or extramammary)* is a prototypic example (65,66).

Paget Disease

CLINICAL SUMMARY. The cutaneous lesion in Paget disease of the breast begins either on the nipple or the areola of the breast and extends slowly to the surrounding skin. It is always unilateral and consists of a sharply defined, slightly infiltrated area of erythema showing scaling, oozing, and crusting. There may or may not be ulceration or retraction of the nipple. The cutaneous lesion is nearly always associated with underlying mammary carcinoma. Extramammary Paget disease, which usually occurs in genital skin in either sex, is similar in its clinical appearance, but is not usually associated with an underlying carcinoma.

HISTOPATHOLOGY. In early lesions of Paget disease of the breast, the epidermis usually shows only a few scattered Paget cells. They are large, rounded cells that are devoid of intercellular bridges and contain a large nucleus and ample cytoplasm. The cytoplasm of these cells stains much lighter than that of the adjacent squamous cells. As the number of Paget cells increases, they compress the squamous cells to such an extent that the latter may merely form a network, the meshes of which are filled with Paget cells lying singly and in groups. In particular, one often observes flattened basal cells lying between Paget cells and the underlying dermis. Although Paget cells do not as a rule invade the dermis from the epidermis, they may be seen extending from the epidermis into the epithelium of hair follicles. Criteria to distinguish among Paget disease, and its mimics pagetoid melanoma *in situ* and pagetoid BD have been recently published (67).

Conditions to consider in the differential diagnosis:

Paget disease (mammary or extramammary)
superficial spreading melanoma
pagetoid squamous cell carcinoma *in situ*
pagetoid reticulosis

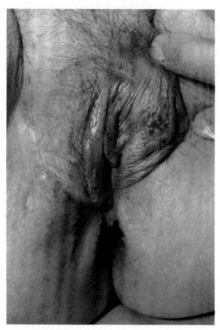

Clin. Fig. IID.3

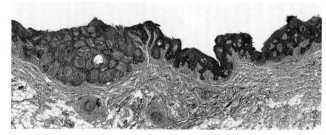

Fig. IID3.a

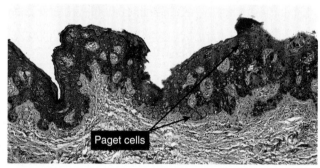

Fig. IID3.b

Clin. Fig. IID.3. *Extramammary Paget's disease.* This elderly female presented with a one-year history of an erythematous plaque with scattered erosions on the left labium majus. Work-up for underlying malignancy was negative.

Fig. IID3.a. *Extramammary Paget's disease, low power.* The epidermis may appear normal or irregularly thickened as here. Even at scanning magnification, large pale cells may be appreciable among otherwise mature keratinocytes.

Fig. IID3.b. *Extramammary Paget disease, medium power.* The large neoplastic cells have pale cytoplasm, sometimes with obvious mucin vacuoles. Their nuclei tend to be enlarged and hyperchromatic, often with prominent nucleoli.

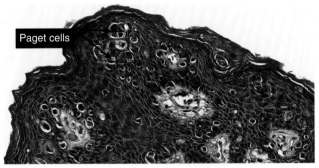

Paget cells

Fig. IID3.c

Fig. IID3.c. *Extramammary Paget disease, medium power.* The stain highlights the glycoprotein constituents of the intracellular mucin contained in the lesional cells, accentuating the "pagetoid pattern" of neoplastic cells scattered among benign epithelial cells. PAS and mucicarmine stains are helpful when the mucin is less obvious than in this H&E section.

IID4 Lymphoid Proliferations

Atypical large clear lymphoid cells proliferate in a normally maturing epidermis.

Pagetoid Reticulosis (Woringer–Kolopp Disease)

Pagetoid reticulosis is a localized variant of mycosis fungoides, characterized by patches and plaques with an intraepidermal proliferation of neoplastic T cells. The atypical cells have medium-sized or large cerebriform nuclei, and usually a CD4-/CD8+ phenotype (68,69).

Conditions to consider in the differential diagnosis:

    pagetoid reticulosis
    localized (Woringer–Kolopp)
    disseminated (Ketron–Goodman)
    Paget disease (mammary or extramammary)
    superficial spreading melanoma
    pagetoid squamous cell carcinoma *in situ*

IIE LOCALIZED PAPILLOMATOUS EPITHELIAL LESIONS

A "papilla" may be likened to a "finger" of stroma with a few blood vessels, collagen fibers, and fibroblasts, covered by a "glove" of epithelium, which may be reactive or neoplastic, benign or malignant.

1. With Viral Cytopathic Effects
2. No Viral Cytopathic Effect

IIE1 With Viral Cytopathic Effects

The epidermis is acanthotic with vacuolated cells (koilocytes), the granular cell layer is usually thickened with enlarged keratohyalin granules, and there is parakeratosis in tall columns overlying the thickened epidermis. Large inclusions are seen in molluscum contagiosum. *Verruca vulgaris* (70) and molluscum contagiosum (71) are prototypic.

Verruca Vulgaris

CLINICAL SUMMARY. Verrucae vulgares are circumscribed, firm, elevated papules with papillomatous ("verrucous") hyperkeratotic surfaces. They occur singly or in groups, most commonly on the dorsal aspects of the fingers and hands. Warts typically regress spontaneously through a combination of cell-mediated and humoral immunity; this may in many cases be accelerated by the topical application of the immune response modifier imiquimod (68).

HISTOPATHOLOGY. Verruca vulgaris is characterized by acanthosis, papillomatosis, and hyperkeratosis. The rete ridges are elongated and, at the periphery of the verruca, are often bent inward so that they appear to point radially toward the center (arborization). The characteristic features that distinguish verruca vulgaris from other papillomas are foci of vacuolated cells located in the upper stratum malpighii and in the granular layer, referred to as koilocytotic cells, vertical tiers of parakeratotic cells, and foci of clumped keratohyalin granules. These three changes are quite pronounced in young verrucae vulgares. The koilocytes possess small, round, deeply basophilic nuclei surrounded by a clear halo and pale-staining cytoplasm. The vertical tiers of parakeratotic cells are often located at the crests of papillomatous elevations of the rete malpighii overlying a focus of vacuolated cells.

Verruca Plana

CLINICAL SUMMARY. Verrucae planae are slightly elevated, flat, smooth papules, which may be hyperpigmented, and affect the face and the dorsa of the hands most commonly. In rare instances, there is extensive involvement, with lesions also on the extremities and trunk. These lesions can be difficult to distinguish clinically from seborrheic keratoses (72).

HISTOPATHOLOGY. Verrucae planae show hyperkeratosis and acanthosis but, unlike verrucae vulgares, have no papillomatosis, only slight elongation of the rete ridges,

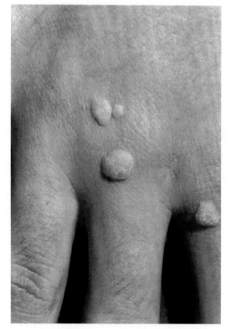

Clin. Fig. IIE1.a

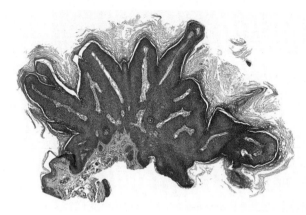

Fig. IIE1.a

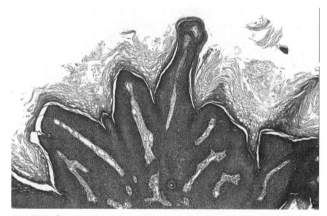

Fig. IIE1.b

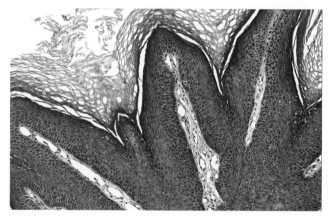

Fig. IIE1.c

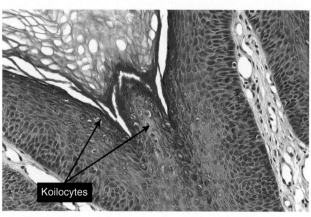

Fig. IIE1.d

Clin. Fig. IIE1.a. *Verruca vulgaris.* Multiple grouped, well circumscribed, flesh colored papules appeared on a child's hand.

Fig. IIE1.a. *Verruca vulgaris, low power.* Elongated rete ridges at the periphery of the lesion often appear to point inward toward the center.

Fig. IIE1.b. *Verruca vulgaris, medium power.* Vertical tiers of parakeratotic cells are often located at the crests of papillomatous elevations of the rete malpighii.

Fig. IIE1.c. *Verruca vulgaris, medium power.* Although no granular cells are seen overlying the papillomatous crests, they are increased in number and size in the intervening valleys and contain heavy, irregular clumps of keratohyalin granules.

Fig. IIE1.d. *Verruca vulgaris, high power.* The virally altered cells, termed koilocytes, possess small, round, deeply basophilic nuclei surrounded by a clear halo and pale-staining cytoplasm.

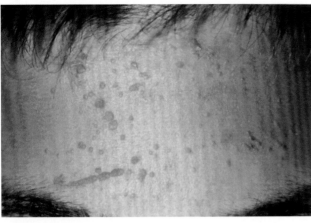

Clin. Fig. IIE1.b

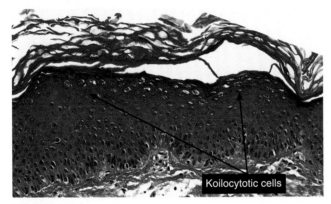

Koilocytotic cells

Fig. IIE1.f

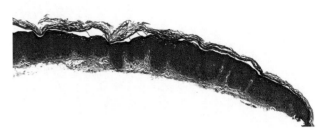

Fig. IIE1.e

Clin. Fig. IIE1.b. *Verruca plana.* Multiple smooth discrete flesh colored papules appeared on a child's forehead. Linear arrangement of papules appear in traumatized areas (Koebnerization).

Fig. IIE1.e. *Verruca plana, low power.* There is irregular acanthosis with a thickened stratum corneum.

Fig. IIE1.f. *Verruca plana, high power.* There is prominent viral cytopathic effect affecting keratinocytes, including vacuolization, enlargement, and nuclear basophilia, with a prominent granular layer.

and no areas of parakeratosis. In the upper stratum malpighii, including the granular layer, there is diffuse vacuolization of the cells, some of which are enlarged to about twice their normal size. The nuclei of the vacuolated cells lie at the centers of the cells, and some of them appear deeply basophilic. The granular layer is uniformly thickened, and the stratum corneum has a pronounced basket-weave appearance resulting from vacuolization of the horny cells. The dermis appears normal.

Deep Palmoplantar Warts (Myrmecia)

CLINICAL SUMMARY. Deep palmoplantar warts can be tender and occasionally swollen and red. Although they may be multiple, they do not coalesce as do mosaic warts, which are verrucae vulgares. Deep palmoplantar warts occur not only on the palms and soles but also on the lateral aspects and tips of the fingers and toes. Unlike superficial, mosaic-type palmoplantar warts, deep palmoplantar warts usually are covered with a thick callus. When the callus is removed with a scalpel, the wart becomes apparent (73).

HISTOPATHOLOGY. Whereas superficial, mosaic-type palmoplantar warts have a histologic appearance

analogous to that of verruca vulgaris and represent HPV-2 or HPV-4, deep palmoplantar warts represent type HPV-1 (74). These lesions, also known as myrmecia ("anthill") or inclusion warts, are characterized by abundant keratohyalin, which differs from normal keratohyalin by being eosinophilic. Starting in the lower epidermis, the cytoplasm of many cells contains numerous eosinophilic granules, which enlarge in the upper stratum malpighii and coalesce to form large, irregularly shaped, homogeneous "inclusion bodies." In addition to the large intracytoplasmic eosinophilic inclusion bodies, some of the cells in the upper stratum spinosum with vacuolated nuclei contain a small intranuclear eosinophilic "inclusion body." It is round and of about the same size as the nucleolus, which, however, is basophilic. Both the intranuclear eosinophilic inclusion body and the basophilic nucleolus disappear as the vacuolated nucleus changes into a smaller, deeply basophilic structure.

Condyloma Acuminatum

CLINICAL SUMMARY. Condylomata acuminata, or anogenital warts, can occur on the penis, on the female genitals, and in the anal region (75). Condylomata of the skin consist of fairly soft, verrucous papules that

II Localized Superficial Epidermal or Melanocytic Proliferations

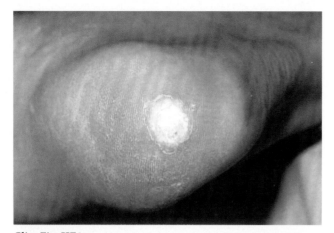

Clin. Fig. IIE1.c

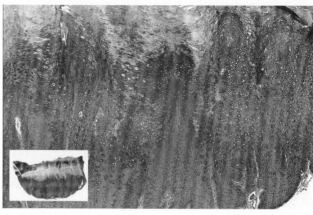

Fig. IIE1.g

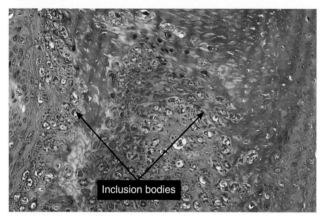

Inclusion bodies

Fig. IIE1.h

Clin. Fig. IIE1.c. *Plantar wart.* A slightly tender rather ill-defined hyperkeratotic nodule on the plantar skin. (Photo by William K. Witmer.)

Fig. IIE1.g. *Deep plantar wart (myrmecia), low power.* There is papillomatosis and thickening of the epidermis with a thickened stratum corneum.

Fig. IIE1.h. *Deep plantar wart (myrmecia), high power.* There are large, irregularly shaped, homogeneous "inclusion bodies" in the cytoplasm of virally affected keratinocytes in the upper stratum spinosum.

occasionally coalesce into cauliflower-like masses. Condylomata are flatter on mucosal surfaces. Diagnostic problems in anal pathology including the significance of dysplastic changes that may occur in condylomas, have been recently reviewed (76). The term "squamous intraepithelial lesion" is favored over "intraepithelial neoplasia." A two tier classification, of "low grade (LSIL)" or "high grade (HSIL)," is favored over a 3- or 4-tier classification (77).

HISTOPATHOLOGY. The stratum corneum is only slightly thickened. Lesions located on mucosal surfaces show parakeratosis. The stratum malpighii shows papillomatosis and considerable acanthosis, with thickening and elongation of the rete ridges. The papillae tended to be rounded rather than more pointed as in verrca vulgaris. Mitotic figures may be present. Usually, invasive SCC can be ruled out because the epithelial cells show an orderly arrangement and the border between the epithelial proliferations and the dermis is sharp. The most characteristic feature, important for the diagnosis, but absent or inconspicuous in many lesions, is the presence of areas in which the epithelial cells show distinct perinuclear vacuolization.

These vacuolated epithelial cells are relatively large and possess hyperchromatic, round nuclei resembling the nuclei seen in the upper portion of the epidermis in verrucae vulgares. It must be kept in mind, however, that vacuolization is a normal occurrence in the upper portions of all mucosal surfaces, so that vacuolization in condylomata acuminata can be regarded as being possibly of viral genesis only if it extends into the deeper portions of the stratum malpighii. Koilocytotic ("raisin") nuclei, double nuclei, and apoptotic keratinocytes may be present but are often less prominent than in uterine cervical lesions. In case of doubt, a descriptive diagnosis should be given. Dysplastic changes, characterized by architectural disorder and cytologic atypia, should be noted and graded, especially in anal lesions. Immunohistochemical studies of p16 may be helpful in this regard (78).

Molluscum Contagiosum

CLINICAL SUMMARY. Molluscum contagiosum, a poxvirus infection (79), occurs most frequently in the pediatric age group and consists of a variable number of small, discrete, waxy, skin-colored, delled, dome-shaped papules,

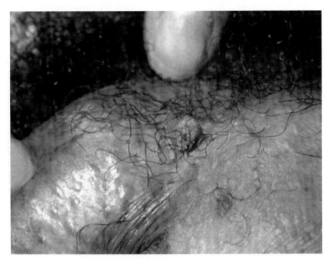

Clin. Fig. IIE1.d

Clin. Fig. IIE1.e

Papillae

Fig. IIE1.i

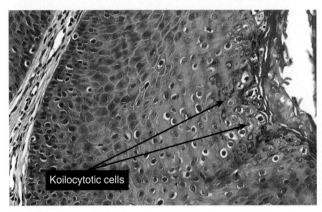

Koilocytotic cells

Fig. IIE1.j

Clin. Fig. IIE1.d. *Condyloma acuminatum.* A pedunculated papilloma at the base of the penis.

Clin. Fig. IIE1.e. *Condyloma acuminatum.* Multiple, papillomas are seen in the anal area of this HIV positive patient.

Fig. IIE1.i. *Condyloma acuminatum, low power.* There is thickening of the epidermis with rounded thickened rete ridges, with little or no thickening of the stratum corneum. There may be focal areas of parakeratosis.

Fig. IIE1.j. *Condyloma acuminatum, high power.* There are koilocytotic changes of virally affected keratinocytes, including hypergranulosis, perinuclear vacuoles, and irregular nuclear membranes.

usually 2 to 4 mm in size. In adults, molluscum contagiosum is primarily a sexually transmitted disease. In immunocompetent patients, the lesions involute spontaneously. During involution, there may be mild inflammation and tenderness. In the setting of immunosuppression, such as in HIV infection, molluscum contagiosum can attain considerable size and be widely disseminated.

HISTOPATHOLOGY. The epidermis is acanthotic, and many epidermal cells contain large, intracytoplasmic inclusion bodies—the so-called molluscum bodies, also known as Henderson–Patterson bodies. These first appear as single, minute, ovoid eosinophilic structures in the lower cells of the stratum malpighii at a level one or two layers above the basal cell layer. As infected cells move toward the surface, the molluscum bodies increase in size and in the upper layers of the epidermis they displace and compress the nucleus so that it appears as a thin crescent at the periphery of the cell. At the level of the granular layer, the staining reaction of the molluscum bodies changes from eosinophilic to basophilic. In the horny layer, the basophilic molluscum bodies lie enmeshed in a network of eosinophilic horny fibers. In the center of the lesion, the stratum corneum ultimately disintegrates, releasing the molluscum bodies, and forming a central crater.

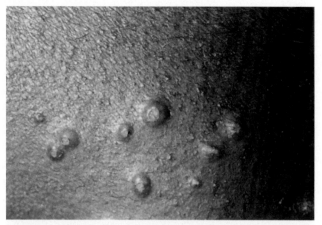

Clin. Fig. IIE1.f

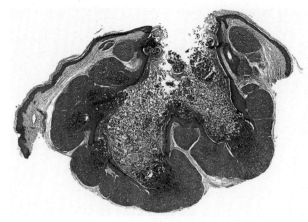

Fig. IIE1.k

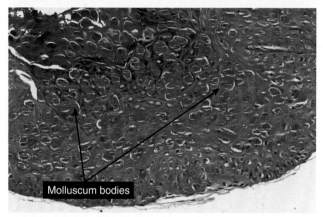

Fig. IIE1.l

Clin. Fig. IIE1.f. *Molluscum contagiosum*. Multiple umbilicated papules in an HIV positive patient contained intracellular inclusions (molluscum bodies) on molluscum prep.

Fig. IIE1.k. *Molluscum contagiosum, low power*. Molluscum contagiosum frequently shows an invagination of hyperplastic epithelium.

Fig. IIE1.l. *Molluscum contagiosum, high power*. The keratinocytes which are infected with this pox virus show large, eosinophilic cytoplasmic inclusions, "molluscum bodies."

Parapox Virus Infections (Milkers' Nodules, Orf)

CLINICAL SUMMARY. Milkers' nodules, orf, and bovine papular stomatitis pox are clinically identical in humans and are induced by indistinguishable parapox viruses. Milkers' nodules are acquired from udders infected with pseudocowpox or paravaccinia (parapox). This disease is called bovine papular stomatitis pox when the source of the infection is calves with oral sores. Orf (ecthyma contagiosum) is acquired from infected sheep or goats with crusted lesions on the lips and in the mouth. After an incubation period of 3 to 7 days, parapox virus infections produce one to three (rarely more) painful lesions measuring 1 to 2 cm in diameter on the fingers, or occasionally elsewhere as a result of autoinoculation. During a period of approximately 6 weeks, they pass through six clinical stages, each lasting about 1 week: (1) the maculopapular stage; (2) the target stage, during which the lesions have red centers, white rings, and red halos; (3) the acute weeping stage; (4) the nodular stage, which shows hard, nontender nodules; (5) the papillomatous stage, in which the nodules have irregular surfaces; and (6) the regressive stage, during which the lesions involute without scarring (80).

HISTOPATHOLOGY. During the maculopapular and target stages, there is vacuolization of cells in the upper third of the stratum malpighii, leading to multilocular vesicles. Eosinophilic inclusion bodies are in the cytoplasm of vacuolated epidermal cells, a distinguishing feature from herpes virus infections. Intranuclear eosinophilic inclusion bodies are also present in some cases. During the target stage, vacuolated epidermal cells with inclusion bodies are only in the surrounding white ring. The epidermis shows elongation of the rete ridges, and the dermis contains many newly formed, dilated capillaries and a mononuclear infiltrate. In the acute weeping stage, the epidermis is necrotic throughout. A massive infiltrate of mononuclear cells extends throughout the dermis. In the later stages, the epidermis shows acanthosis with fingerlike downward projections, and the dermis shows vasodilatation and chronic inflammation, followed by resolution.

Conditions to consider in the differential diagnosis:

verruca vulgaris
orf
condyloma acuminatum
molluscum contagiosum
bowenoid papulosis

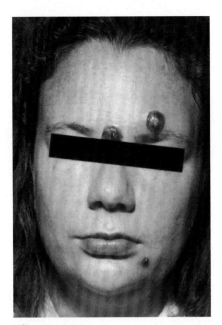

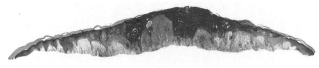

Fig. IIE1.m

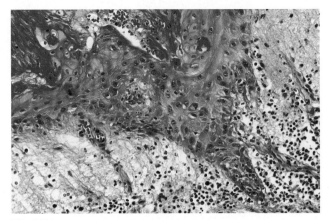

Clin. Fig. IIE1.g   **Fig. IIE1.n**

Clin. Fig. IIE1.g. *Orf.* Multiple, painful erythematous nodules developed gradually in a farmer who fed goats. Examination of goats' mouths by a veterinarian identified the source of the virus.

Fig. IIE1.m. *Orf, low power.* The top of a papillomatous lesion with an overlying scale-crust.

Fig. IIE1.n. *Orf, high power.* The lesional keratinocytes are swollen. Intracytoplasmic eosinophilic inclusions are not readily demonstrated.

IIE2   No Viral Cytopathic Effect

The epidermis proliferates focally. The cells may be basophilic or "basaloid" in type (seborrheic keratoses). There may be increased stratum corneum and elongation of the dermal papillae (squamous papilloma), or there may be basilar keratinocytic atypia (actinic keratosis). *Seborrheic keratosis* (81) is a prototypic example.

Seborrheic Keratosis

CLINICAL SUMMARY. Seborrheic keratoses are very common lesions: sometimes single but often multiple. They occur usually not before middle age, mainly on the trunk and face but also on the extremities, with the exception of the palms and soles. They are sharply demarcated, brownish in color, and slightly raised, so that they often look as if they are stuck on the surface of the skin. Most of them have a verrucous surface, which has a soft, friable consistency. Some, however, have a smooth surface but characteristically show keratotic plugs. Although most lesions measure only a few millimeters in diameter, a lesion may occasionally reach a size of several centimeters. Some may become inflamed. Seborrheic keratoses have been shown to contain mutations of keratinocyte growth factors (45).

HISTOPATHOLOGY. Seven variants may be recognized: irritated, adenoid or reticulated, plane, clonal, melanoacanthoma, inverted follicular keratosis, and benign squamous keratosis (or verrucous keratosis). Often more than one type is found in the same lesion. All have in common hyperkeratosis, acanthosis, and papillomatosis. The acanthosis in most instances is due entirely to upward extension of the tumor. Thus the lower border of the tumor is even and generally lies on a straight line that may be drawn from the normal epidermis at one end of the tumor to the normal epidermis at the other end. Two types of cells are usually seen in the acanthotic epidermis: basaloid cells which resemble the cells found normally in the basal layer of the epidermis tend to predominate over squamous cells.

Dowling–Degos Disease

CLINICAL FEATURES. The patients have multiple pigmented macules of the flexures, usually arranged in a reticular pattern. Less often, there may be more widespread pigmented lesions, dark comedo-like lesions on the neck, and perioral atrophodermic pits or scars (82). Mutations have been detected in keratin 5, and in regulators of the Notch pathway (83). There is overlap with

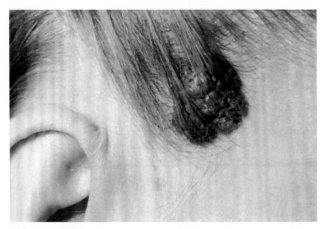

Clin. Fig. IIE2.a

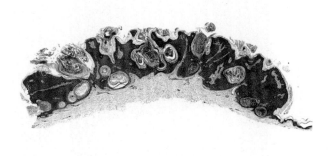

Fig. IIE2.a

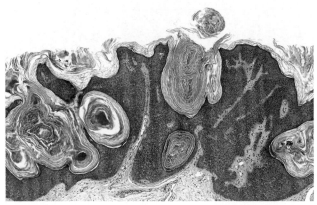

Fig. IIE2.b

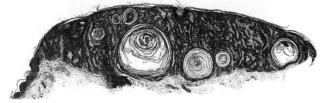

Fig. IIE2.c

Clin. Fig. IIE2.a. *Seborrheic keratosis.* A middle-aged female developed a pigmented "stuck on" papule with a "waxy" feel. Keratin-filled ostia help to distinguish this common lesion. A slightly scaly surface can be accentuated by rubbing or light scratching of the lesion.

Fig. IIE2.a. *Seborrheic keratosis, low power.* The tumor extends upward above a line drawn through the normal epidermis on each side. Pseudohorn cysts (keratin tunnels or horn cysts) containing whorls of keratin are a prominent feature.

Fig. IIE2.b. *Seborrheic keratosis, medium power.* The lesion is composed predominantly of basaloid cells, with squamous differentiation beneath the stratum corneum.

Fig. IIE2.c. *Reticulated seborrheic keratosis, low power.* The lesion is composed of anastomosing cords of cells in a reticulated or "adenoid" pattern, with scattered "horn cysts."

Fig. IIE2.d. *Reticulated seborrheic keratosis, medium power.* The cells in the cords show basaloid and squamous differentiation. In this example, there is moderate melanin pigment in the basaloid cells.

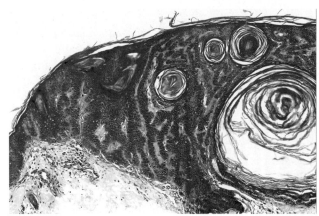

Fig. IIE2.d

Galli–Galli disease, which is now considered to be the same disorder (84).

HISTOPATHOLOGY. The lesions have basaloid epithelial hyperplasia with lacy, hyperpigmented dermal extensions and tiny horn cysts, resembling an adenoid seborrheic keratosis. Acantholysis may be present (80).

Confluent and Reticulated Papillomatosis (Gougerot–Carteaud)

CLINICAL SUMMARY. Confluent and reticulated papillomatosis (CARP) is a condition of unknown cause, originally described in 1927 by Gougerot and Carteaud. The condition presents clinically as collection of

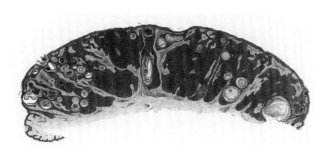

Fig. IIE2.e

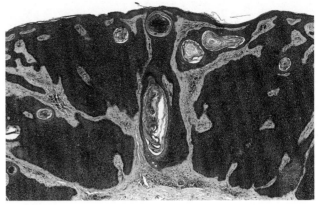

Fig. IIE2.f

Fig. IIE2.e. *Pigmented seborrheic keratosis, low power.* The lesion contains abundant brown melanin pigment, simulating a nodular melanoma clinically.

Fig. IIE2.f. *Pigmented seborrheic keratosis, medium power.* The pigment is located mainly in the basaloid cells. It is produced by melanocytes that populate the lesion.

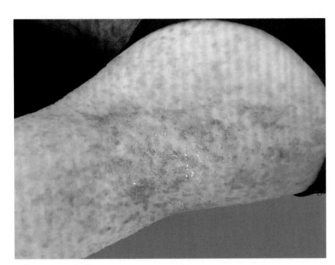

Clin. Fig. IIE2.b

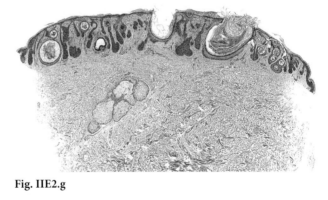

Fig. IIE2.g

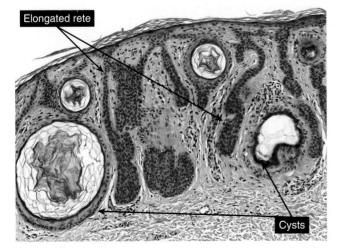

Fig. IIE2.h

Clin. Fig. IIE2.b. *Dowling–Degos disease.* Verrucous and keratotic pigmented rash on the upper thigh of a 49-year-old woman, present for more than 20 years. Also present on neck, axillae, trunk and groin skin. Started as "red raised spots ending up brown in color." (C. Simpson)

Fig. IIE2.g. *Dowling–Degos disease.* Low power, showing hyperkeratosis and elongation of dermal papillae with cysts. (A. Moshiri)

Fig. IIE2.h. *Dowling–Degos disease.* High power of papillae and cysts. (A. Moshiri)

Localized Superficial Epidermal or Melanocytic Proliferations

II

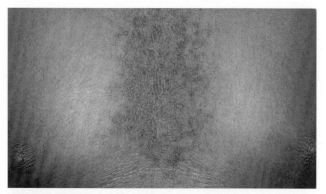

Clin. Fig. IIE2.c

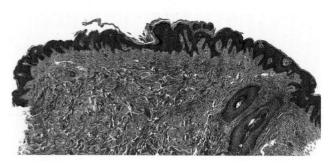

Fig. IIE2.i

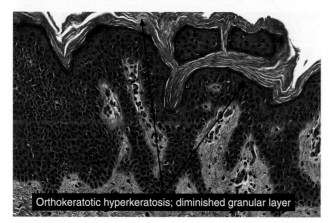

Orthokeratotic hyperkeratosis; diminished granular layer

Fig. IIE2.j

Clin. Fig. IIE2.c. *Confluent and Reticulated Papillomatosis (CARP). Dark brown, reticulated patches are often mistaken for tinea versicolor.*

Fig. IIE2.i. *Low power, showing hyperkeratosis and papillomatosis.*

Fig. IIE2.j. *Hyperkeratosis with a diminished granular layer, with little or no inflammation in the dermis.*

brown-gray hyperkeratotic papules and patches (85). These become confluent centrally and reticulated at the periphery. The initial site is often the mid back with spread to involve the axillae, neck and abdomen. This condition is more common in women of color. Speculation as to the cause varies from an endocrine etiology to that of an organism (yeast—Pityrosporum sp.). The differential diagnosis includes acanthosis nigricans, tinea versicolor, seborrheic keratosis, epidermal nevus, and Naegeli–Franceschetti–Jadassohn syndrome which is a rare autosomal dominant ectodermal dysplasia characterized by the absence of dermatoglyphics, reticulate hyperpigmentation of the skin, hypohidrosis, and heat intolerance, associated with palmoplantar keratoderma, nail dystrophy, and enamel defects (86).

HISTOPATHOLOGY. There is mild papillomatosis, hyperkeratosis, hypogranulosis and an increase of pigment in the basal cell layer. Epidermal pigment is due to an increased number of melanosome granules in the basilar and epidermal keratinocytes. The dermis does not demonstrate significant alteration. Pityrosporum spores may be present in the stratum corneum, but they are few in number.

Verrucous Melanoma

CLINICAL SUMMARY. Occasional examples of nodular melanoma may present with a "warty" or verrucous configuration, with prominent hyperkeratosis. Especially if the lesion is pigmented, the diagnosis is usually obvious, but occasional cases can simulate a wart, or a SCC.

HISTOPATHOLOGY. The keratinocytic epithelium demonstrates papillary hyperplasia and marked hyperkeratosis. Lesional cells in this case are very obvious because of marked hyperpigmentation.

Conditions to consider in the differential diagnosis:

  seborrheic keratosis
  acanthosis nigricans
  confluent and reticulated papillomatosis
  actinic keratosis, hypertrophic
  nonspecific squamous papilloma
  epithelial nevus/epidermal nevus
  hyperkeratosis of the nipple and areola
  verruciform xanthoma
  verrucous melanoma

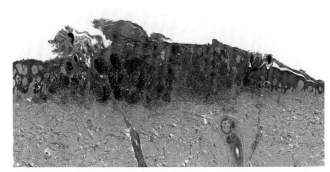

Fig. IIE2.k

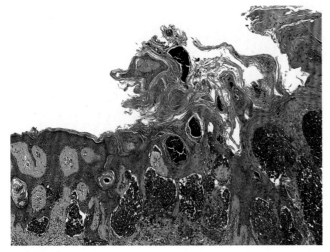

Fig. IIE2.l

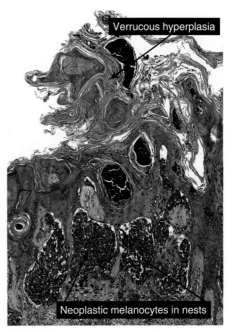

Fig. IIE2.m

Fig. IIE2.k. *A quite large lesion with prominent superficial hyperkeratosis.*

Fig. IIE2.l. *The appearances could resemble a verrucous keratosis of some kind.*

Fig. IIE2.m. *Numerous neoplastic pigmented melanocytes in this case make the diagnosis obvious.*

IIF IRREGULAR PROLIFERATIONS EXTENDING INTO THE SUPERFICIAL DERMIS

Irregular or asymmetrical proliferations of keratinocytes extending into the dermis are usually neoplastic. The differential diagnosis includes reactive pseudoepitheliomatous hyperplasia, which may be seen around chronic ulcers or in association with other inflammatory conditions (refer to VIB1).

1. Squamous Differentiation
2. Basaloid Differentiation

IIF1 Squamous Differentiation

The epidermis is irregularly thickened, the maturation is abnormal and there may be keratinocytic atypia (SCC). The proliferation is often associated with a thick parakeratotic scale. *Superficial SCC* is prototypic (2) (see also VIB1).

Inverted Follicular Keratosis

See Figs. IIF1.d,e.

Conditions to consider in the differential diagnosis:

lichen simplex chronicus
squamous cell carcinoma, superficial
keratoacanthoma
prurigo nodularis
actinic prurigo
inverted follicular keratosis
verrucous carcinoma
  of oral mucosa
  of genitoanal region (giant condyloma of Buschke and
    Lowenstein)
  of plantar skin (epithelioma cuniculatum)
pseudoepitheliomatous hyperplasia
deep fungal infection
halogenoderma
chronic ulcers
granular cell tumor
Spitz nevus
verrucous melanoma

Localized Superficial Epidermal or Melanocytic Proliferations

II

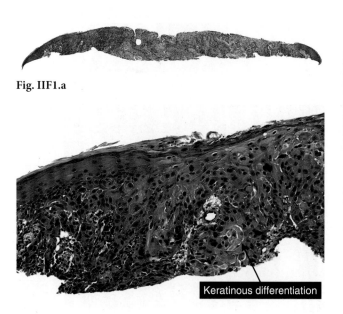

Fig. IIF1.a

Fig. IIF1.b

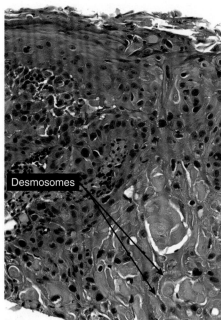

Fig. IIF1.c

Fig. IIF1.a. *Squamous cell carcinoma, invasive, low power.* Arising from the base of the epidermis there are endophytic proliferative lobules of atypical epithelium which are associated with a patchy lymphocytic infiltrate.

Fig. IIF1.b. *Squamous cell carcinoma, invasive, medium power.* The haphazardly oriented lobules are of varying shapes and sizes and show an infiltrative growth pattern within the dermis.

Fig. IIF1.c. *Squamous cell carcinoma, invasive, high power.* At higher magnification there is formation of ill-defined squamous pearls, whorled aggregates of parakeratin within the epithelial islands, and the atypical keratinocytes may show a spectrum of cytologic atypia from mild to severe.

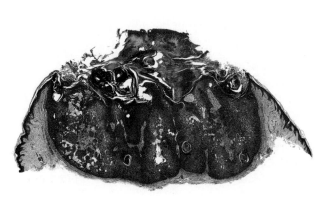

Fig. IIF1.d

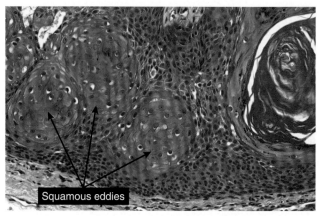

Fig. IIF1.e

Fig. IIF1.d. *Inverted follicular keratosis, low power.* This epithelial neoplasm arises from the epidermis and shows an endophytic lobulated architecture with a symmetrical profile and a regular border. The epithelial proliferation is embedded in a fibrotic stroma and is sharply separated from the adjacent reticular dermal collagen.

Fig. IIF1.e. *Inverted follicular keratosis, high power.* Keratin-filled cystic structures may be seen within the epithelial proliferation, and squamous eddies as depicted here are a characteristic feature of an inverted follicular keratosis.

IIF2 | Basaloid Differentiation

The proliferation is of basal cells from the epidermis, extending into the dermis. The epidermis can be thickened, normal or atrophic. *Basal cell carcinoma* (BCC) is a prototypic example (87).

Basal Cell Carcinoma

CLINICAL SUMMARY. Five clinical types of BCC occur: *Noduloulcerative BCC* begins as a small, waxy nodule that often shows a few small telangiectatic vessels on its surface. The nodule usually increases slowly in size and often undergoes central ulceration surrounded by a pearly, rolled border. This represents the so-called rodent ulcer. *Pigmented BCC* differs from the noduloulcerative type only by the brown pigmentation of the lesion. *Morphea-like or fibrosing BCC* manifests itself as a solitary, flat or slightly depressed, indurated, ill defined, smooth yellowish plaque. This type has a high incidence of local recurrence. *Superficial BCC* consists of one or several erythematous, scaling, centrally atrophic patches that slowly increase in size by peripheral extension and are surrounded, at least in part, by a fine, threadlike, pearly border. The patches usually show small areas of superficial ulceration and crusting. *Fibroepithelioma* presents as a raised, moderately firm, slightly pedunculated reddish nodule resembling a fibroma.

HISTOPATHOLOGY. In the common clinically *noduloulcerative* and histologically *solid* type of BCC, nodular masses of basaloid cells extend into the dermis in relation to a delicate, specialized, somewhat myxoid tumor stroma with a characteristic separation artifact between the two. Cystic spaces may form. The characteristic cells of basal cell carcinoma have a large, oval, or elongated nucleus and relatively little cytoplasm. The nuclei resemble those of epidermal basal cells, but differ by having a larger ratio of nucleus to cytoplasm and by lacking intercellular bridges. Although most BCCs appear well demarcated, some show an infiltrative growth into the reticular dermis. These latter are now widely recognized as a distinct histologic subtype (*infiltrating BCC*).

Superficial BCC shows buds and irregular proliferations of peripherally palisaded basaloid cells attached to the undersurface of the epidermis and penetrating only slightly into the dermis. The overlying epidermis is usually atrophic. Fibroblasts, often in a fairly large number, are arranged around the tumor cell proliferations. In addition, a mild or moderate amount of a nonspecific chronic inflammatory infiltrate is present in the upper dermis.

In *fibroepithelioma of Pinkus*, long, thin, branching, anastomosing strands of BCC are embedded in a fibrous stroma. Many of the strands are connected to the surface epidermis. Here and there, small groups of dark-staining cells showing a palisade arrangement of the peripheral cell layer may be seen along the epithelial strands, like buds on a branch. Usually, the tumor is quite superficial and is well demarcated at its lower border. Fibroepithelioma of Pinkus combines features of the intracanalicular fibroadenoma of the breast, the reticulated type of seborrheic keratosis, and superficial BCC. Most consider the fibroepithelioma of Pinkus to be a variant of a BCC.

MOLECULAR PATHOLOGY. Several tumor suppressor genes and proto-oncogenes have been implicated in the pathogenesis of BCC, including the human homologs of the Drosophila genes patched (PTCH) and smoothened (SMOH), the TP53 tumor suppressor gene, and the RAS proto-oncogene family (88). Patients with PTCH polymorphisms are at increased risk of developing the disease (89). Recent NGS sequencing studies have identified greater than

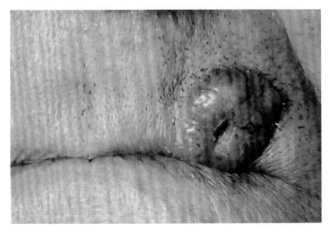

Clin. Fig. IIF2.a

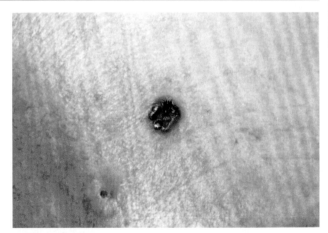

Clin. Fig. IIF2.b

Clin. Fig. IIF2.a. *Nodulo-ulcerative basal cell carcinoma.* The rolled, pearly borders with telangiectases and central ulceration typify basal cell carcinoma, the most common skin malignancy.

Clin. Fig. IIF2.b. *Pigmented basal cell carcinoma.* An elderly man developed a forehead papule with a pigmented rolled border and central concavity. (*continues*)

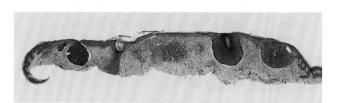

Fig. IIF2.a

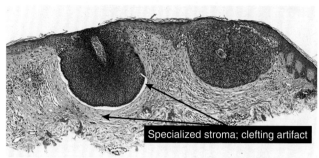

Specialized stroma; clefting artifact

Fig. IIF2.b

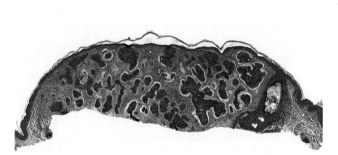

Fig. IIF2.c

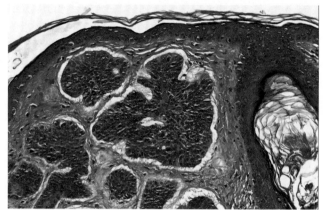

Fig. IIF2.d

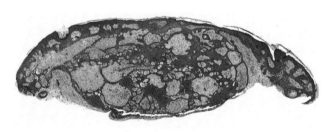

Fig. IIF2.e

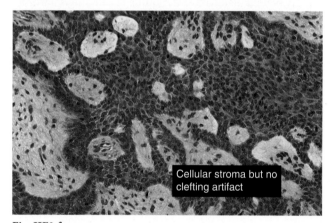

Cellular stroma but no clefting artifact

Fig. IIF2.f

Fig. IIF2.a. *Superficial "multicentric" basal cell carcinoma, low power.* Irregular masses of basophilic cells extend from the epidermis into the dermis.

Fig. IIF2.b. *Superficial "multicentric" basal cell carcinoma, medium power.* The cells at the periphery of the tumor masses are palisaded, and there is a cleft between them and the characteristic delicate collagenous stroma.

Fig. IIF2.c. *Nodular basal cell carcinoma, low power.* Arising from the base of the epithelium there are nodular aggregates of atypical basaloid cells associated with cleft formation.

Fig. IIF2.d. *Nodular basal cell carcinoma, medium power.* Bluish mucinous material is seen in the cleft. The stroma of basal cell carcinomas may be fibrotic, as seen here, or may be loose with an abundance of mucinous material.

Fig. IIF2.e. *Fibroepithelioma of Pinkus, low power.* This variant of basal cell carcinoma shows numerous thin, anastomosing strands of epithelial cells which arise from the base of the epidermis.

Fig. IIF2.f. *Fibroepithelioma of Pinkus, medium power.* These epithelial strands form small basaloid buds with peripheral palisading. The stroma is hypercellular and fibrotic.

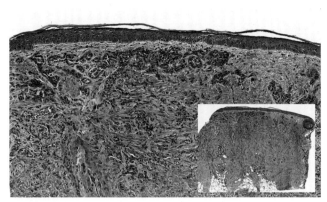

Fig. IIF2.g

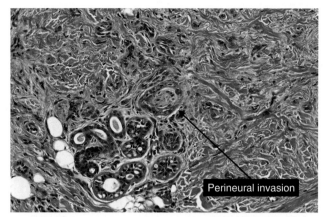

Fig. IIF2.h

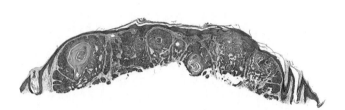

Fig. IIF2.i

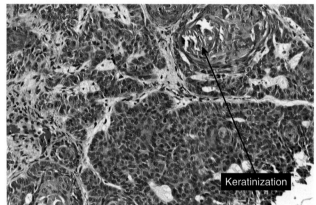

Fig. IIF2.j

Fig. IIF2.g. *Morpheaform basal cell carcinoma, low power (inset), and medium power.* This aggressive variant of basal cell carcinoma is composed of numerous small islands of basal cell carcinoma which generally infiltrate into the reticular dermis.

Fig. IIF2.h. *Morpheaform basal cell carcinoma, high power.* At higher magnification this lesion is composed of very small islands of atypical basaloid cells which are embedded in a fibrotic stroma. There may be perineural involvement, as here.

Fig. IIF2.i. *Keratinizing basal cell carcinoma, low power.* Basal cell carcinoma may show foci of keratinization within the lobules of atypical basaloid cells.

Fig. IIF2.j. *Keratinizing basal cell carcinoma, medium power.* These areas of keratinization may resemble horn cysts or keratin pearls. If a lesion is partially biopsied, this finding may cause confusion between the basal cell carcinoma and squamous cell carcinoma.

previously known complexity of the genomic landscape in BCC, with relevance for targeted therapy strategies (90).

Conditions to consider in the differential diagnosis:

basal cell carcinoma, superficial types

IIG SUPERFICIAL POLYPOID LESIONS

A polyp consists of a "fist" of stroma covered by a "glove" of epithelium. It is to be distinguished from a papilloma, which has elongated papillae.

1. Melanocytic Lesions
2. Spindle Cell and Stromal Lesions

IIG1 Melanocytic Lesions

The polyp contains mature nevus cells in a compound nevus, or atypical melanocytes in a polypoid melanoma. *Polypoid dermal and compound nevi* are prototypic (12). Nevi are benign neoplasms of melanocytes which often have an activating mutation of the oncogene BRAF (or another oncogene such as NRAS), but which undergo a process of maturation and senescence rather than continued proliferation (91).

Localized Superficial Epidermal or Melanocytic Proliferations

II

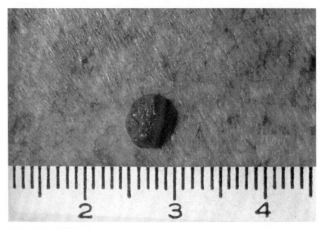

Clin. Fig. IIG1.a

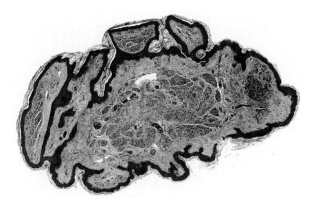

Fig. IIG1.a

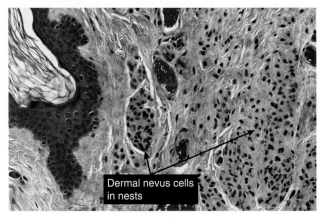

Fig. IIG1.b

Clin. Fig. IIG1.a. *Dermal nevus.* A clinically stable well-circumscribed, symmetrical flesh-colored papule.

Fig. IIG1.a. *Polypoid dermal nevus, low power.* In this tangentially sectioned example, the intradermal location of the dermal nevus cells, and the polypoid character of the lesion, are readily apparent.

Fig. IIG1.b. *Polypoid dermal nevus, medium power.* The polypoid dermal nevus is differentiated from a fibroepithelial polyp or a polypoid neurofibroma by the presence of nevus cells in the dermis, identified by their characteristic cuboidal morphology and nested pattern.

Polypoid Dermal and Compound Nevi

(See also IIA.2.) A compound nevus possesses features of both a junctional and an intradermal nevus. Nevus cell nests are present in the epidermis, as well as in the dermis. Nevus cells in the upper, middle, and lower dermis may present characteristic morphological variations called *types A, B,* and *C,* respectively. Usually, the Type A nevus cells in the upper dermis are cuboidal and show abundant cytoplasm containing varying amounts of melanin granules. Type B cells are distinctly smaller than type A cells, display less cytoplasm and less melanin, and generally lie in well-defined aggregates. Type C nevus cells in the lower dermis tend to resemble fibroblasts or Schwann cells, because they are usually elongated and have spindle-shaped nuclei. Lesions with prominent schwannian differentiation are termed "neurotized." If dermal nevus cells are confined to the papillary dermis, they often retain a discrete, or "pushing" border with the stroma. However, nevus cells that enter the reticular dermis tend to disperse among collagen fiber bundles as single cells or attenuated single files of cells. This pattern of infiltration of the dermis differs from that in melanomas, where groups of cells tend to dissect and displace the collagen bundles in a more "expansive" pattern. Lesions where nevus cells extend into the lower reticular dermis and the subcutaneous fat, or are located within nerves, hair follicles, sweat ducts, and sebaceous glands, may be termed "congenital pattern nevi." Intradermal nevi show essentially no junctional activity. The upper dermis contains nests and cords of nevus cells similar to those described above. Occasional intradermal nevi contain predominantly spindle-shaped schwannian cells embedded in abundant, loosely arranged collagenous tissue. If there are also a few nests of nevus cells, such a lesion may be referred to as aneural nevus however if nests are completely absent the lesion is more likely to be a neurofibroma.

Conditions to consider in the differential diagnosis:

> polypoid dermal and compound nevi
> polypoid melanoma (see also VIB.3)

IIG2 Spindle Cell and Stromal Lesions

The polyp contains stromal cells of types that may be seen in the dermis, including fibroblasts, fat cells, or schwannian cells. *Neurofibroma* is a prototypic example (92).

Neurofibroma

CLINICAL SUMMARY. Extraneural sporadic cutaneous neurofibromas (ESCNs) (the common sporadic neurofibromas) are soft, polypoid, skin-colored or slightly tan, and small (rarely larger than a centimeter in diameter). They usually arise in adulthood. The identification of as many as four, small, cutaneous neurofibromas in a single patient, in the absence of other confirmatory findings, would not qualify as stigmata of neurofibromatosis.

HISTOPATHOLOGY. Most sporadic neurofibromas are faintly eosinophilic, and are circumscribed but not encapsulated: they are extraneural. Thin spindle cells with elongated, wavy nuclei are regularly spaced among thin, wavy collagenous strands. The strands are either closely spaced (homogeneous pattern) or loosely spaced in a clear matrix (loose pattern). The two patterns are often intermixed in a single lesion. Mast cells are often present in the stroma. The regular spacing of adnexa is preserved in cutaneous neurofibromas. Entrapped small nerves occasionally are enlarged and hypercellular. The differentiation from a neurotized nevus may be difficult in routinely stained sections, but distinction may be possible if a few type A or B nevus cells are present in addition to the spindle cells, or with an immunohistochemical stain for myelin basic protein, which is positive only in neurofibromas. Any given neurofibroma could be either sporadic or associated with neurofibromatosis (NF-1), however in a comparative study, neurofibromas in NF-1 were more frequently associated with melanocytic hyperplasia, lentigo simplex-like changes, and diffuse and plexiform neurofibroma patterns (see VIC2) than were the sporadic neurofibromas (93).

Fibroepithelial Polyp

CLINICAL SUMMARY. Fibroepithelial polyps, also called "soft fibromas," "acrochordons" or "cutaneous tags," occur as three types: (1) multiple small, furrowed papules, especially on the neck and in the axillae, generally only 1 to 2 mm long; (2) single or multiple filiform, smooth growths in varying locations, about 2 mm wide and 5 mm

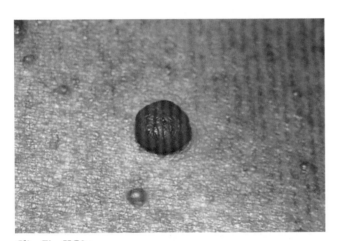

Clin. Fig. IIG2.a

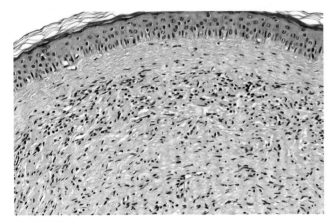

Fig. IIG2.b

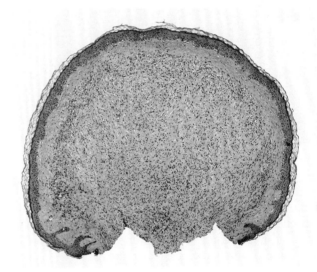

Fig. IIG2.a

Clin. Fig. IIG2.a. *Neurofibroma.* Patient with neurofibromatosis presented with a classical sign—multiple soft flesh colored papules and nodules on the trunk.

Fig. IIG2.a. *Neurofibroma, low power.* At scanning magnification this polypoid lesion shows an essentially normal epidermis. Within the dermis there is a uniformly symmetrical proliferation of spindled cells.

Fig. IIG2.b. *Neurofibroma, medium power.* At higher magnification these small spindled cells are wavy and bland in appearance and they are embedded in an eosinophilic matrix.

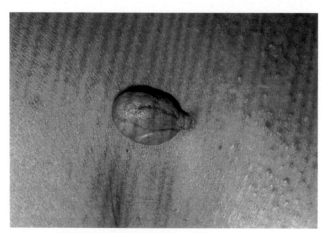

Clin. Fig. IIG2.b

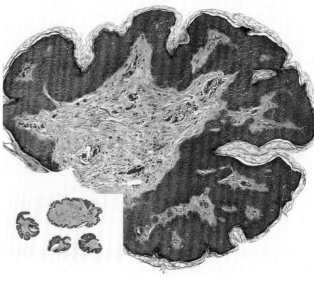

Fig. IIG2.c

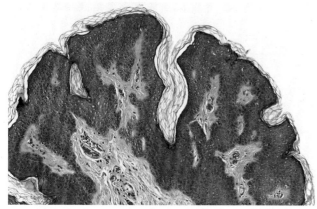

Fig. IIG2.d

Clin. Fig. IIG2.b. *Soft fibroma.* A traumatized pedunculated papule along the bra line.

Fig. IIG2.c. *Fibroepithelial polyp, low power.* At scanning magnification this polypoid lesion may resemble both a nevus and a neurofibroma. However, upon closer inspection, neither nevus cells nor wavy neural cells are seen within the stroma of this lesion.

Fig. IIG2.d. *Fibroepithelial polyp, medium power.* The core of this lesion is composed of well vascularized connective tissue and the lesion is surfaced by slightly acanthotic and papillomatous epithelium. The papillae may be prominent, as here, or may be effaced.

long; and (3) solitary baglike, pedunculated growths, usually about 1 cm in diameter but occasionally much larger, seen most commonly on the lower trunk. There may be associations with diabetes and acromegaly.

HISTOPATHOLOGY. The multiple small furrowed papules usually show papillomatosis, hyperkeratosis, and regular acanthosis and occasionally also horn cysts within their acanthotic epidermis. Thus there is often considerable resemblance to a pedunculated seborrheic keratosis. The common filiform, smooth growths show slight to moderate acanthosis and occasionally mild papillomatosis. The connective tissue stalk is composed of loose collagen fibers and often contains numerous dilated capillaries filled with erythrocytes. Nevus cells are found in many of the filiform growths, indicating that some of them represent involuting melanocytic nevi. The baglike, soft fibromas generally show a flattened epidermis overlying loosely arranged collagen fibers and mature fat cells in the center. In some instances, the dermis is quite thin, so

that the fat cells compose a significant portion of the tumor, which may then be regarded as a lipofibroma.

Conditions to consider in the differential diagnosis:

neurofibroma
neurotized nevus
soft fibroma (fibroepithelial polyp, acrochordon, skin tag)
nevus lipomatosus superficialis

References

1. Sober AJ, Burstein JM. Precursors to skin cancer. *Cancer* 1995;75(2 Suppl):645–650.
2. Davis DA, Donahue JP, Bost JE, et al. The diagnostic concordance of actinic keratosis and squamous cell carcinoma. *J Cutan Pathol* 2005;32(8):546–551.
3. Shin JW, Kim YK, Cho KH. Minichromosome maintenance protein expression according to the grade of atypism in actinic keratosis. *Am J Dermatopathol* 2010;32(8):794–798.

4. Penneys NS, Ackerman AB, Indgin SN, et al. Eccrine poroma. *Br J Dermatol* 1970;82(6):613–615.

5. Gormley RH, Kovarik CL. Dermatologic manifestations of HPV in HIV-infected individuals. *Curr HIV/AIDS Rep* 2009; 6(3):130–138.

6. Kassem A, Technau K, Kurz AK, et al. Merkel cell polyomavirus sequences are frequently detected in nonmelanoma skin cancer of immunosuppressed patients. *Int J Cancer* 2009;125(2):356–361.

7. Callen JP, Headington J. Bowen's and non-Bowen's squamous intraepidermal neoplasia of the skin. *Arch Dermatol* 1980; 116(4):422–426.

8. Bahrani E, Sitthinamsuwan P, McCalmont TH, et al. Ki-67 and p16 Immunostaining differentiates pagetoid Bowen disease from "Microclonal" seborrheic keratosis. *Am J Clin Pathol* 2019;151(6):551–560.

9. Dubina M, Goldenberg G. Viral-associated nonmelanoma skin cancers: a review. *Am J Dermatopathol* 2009;31(6):561–573.

10. Darragh TM, Colgan TJ, Cox JT, et al; Members of LAST Project Work Groups. The Lower Anogenital Squamous Terminology Standardization Project for HPV-Associated Lesions: background and consensus recommendations from the College of American Pathologists and the American Society for Colposcopy and Cervical Pathology. *Arch Pathol Lab Med* 2012;136(10): 1266–1297.

11. Degos R, Civatte J. Clear-cell acanthoma: experience of 8 years. *Br J Dermatol* 1970;83(2):248–254.

12. Elder DE, Clark WH Jr, Elenitsas R, et al. The early and intermediate precursor lesions of tumor progression in the melanocytic system: common acquired nevi and atypical (dysplastic) nevi. *Semin Diagn Pathol* 1993;10(1):18–35.

13. Xu X, Elder DE. A practical approach to selected problematic melanocytic lesions. *Am J Clin Pathol* 2004;121 Suppl:S3–S32.

14. Elder DE. Dysplastic naevi: an update. *Histopathology* 2010; 56(1):112–120.

15. Elder DE. Pathology of melanoma. *Clin Cancer Res* 2006;12(7 Pt2): 2308s–2311s.

16. Gimotty PA, Van BP, Elder DE, et al. Biologic and prognostic significance of dermal Ki67 expression, mitoses, and tumorigenicity in thin invasive cutaneous melanoma. *J Clin Oncol* 2005; 23(31):8048–8056.

17. Elder DE, Barnhill RL, Bastian BC, et al. Melanocytic tumor classification and the pathway concept of melanoma pathogenesis. In: Elder DE, Massi D, Scolyer RA, Willemze R, eds. *WHO Classification of Melanocytic Tumors.* 4th ed. Lyon: IARC; 2018: 62–71.

18. Gray-Schopfer VC, Cheong SC, Chong H, et al. Cellular senescence in naevi and immortalisation in melanoma: a role for p16? *Br J Cancer* 2006;95(4):496–505.

19. Arumi-Uria M, McNutt NS, Finnerty B. Grading of atypia in nevi: correlation with melanoma risk. *Mod Pathol* 2003;16(8): 764–771.

20. Shors AR, Kim S, White E, et al. Dysplastic naevi with moderate to severe histological dysplasia: a risk factor for melanoma. *Br J Dermatol* 2006;155(5):988–993.

21. Hussein MR. Melanocytic dysplastic naevi occupy the middle ground between benign melanocytic naevi and cutaneous malignant melanomas: emerging clues. *J Clin Pathol* 2005;58(5): 453–456.

22. Broekaert SM, Roy R, Okamoto I, et al. Genetic and morphologic features for melanoma classification. *Pigment Cell Melanoma Res* 2010;23(6):763–770.

23. Tajan M, Paccoud R, Branka S, et al. The RASopathy Family: consequences of germline activation of the RAS/MAPK pathway. *Endocr Rev* 2018;39(5):676–700.

24. VandenBoom T, Quan VL, Zhang B, et al. Genomic fusions in pigmented spindle cell nevus of reed. *Am J Surg Pathol* 2018; 42(8):1042–1051.

25. Coleman WP 3rd, Loria PR, Reed RJ, et al. Acral lentiginous melanoma. *Arch Dermatol* 1980;116(7):773–776.

26. Curtin JA, Fridlyand J, Kageshita T, et al. Distinct sets of genetic alterations in melanoma. *N Engl J Med* 2005;353(20):2135–2147.

27. Sauter ER, Yeo UC, Von Stemm A, et al. Cyclin D1 is a candidate oncogene in cutaneous melanoma. *Cancer Res* 2002;62(11): 3200–3206.

28. Niu HT, Zhou QM, Wang F, et al. Identification of anaplastic lymphoma kinase break points and oncogenic mutation profiles in acral/mucosal melanomas. *Pigment Cell Melanoma Res* 2013;26(5):646–653.

29. Curtin JA, Busam K, Pinkel D, et al. Somatic activation of KIT in distinct subtypes of melanoma. *J Clin Oncol* 2006;24(26): 4340–4346.

30. Liang WS, Hendricks W, Kiefer J, et al. Integrated genomic analyses reveal frequent TERT aberrations in acral melanoma. *Genome Res* 2017;27(4):524–532.

31. Yeh I, Jorgenson E, Shen L, et al. Targeted genomic profiling of acral melanoma. *J Natl Cancer Inst* 2019;111(10):1068–1077.

32. Clark WH Jr, Mihm MC Jr. Lentigo maligna and lentigo-maligna melanoma. *Am J Pathol* 1969;55(1):39–67.

33. Elder DE, Bastian BC, Kim J, et al. Lentigo maligna melanoma. In: Elder DE, Massi D, Scolyer RA, Willemze R, eds. *WHO Classification of Melanocytic Tumors.* 4th ed. Lyon: IARC; 2018.

34. Kornberg R, Ackerman AB. Pseudomelanoma. Recurrent melanocytic nevus following partial surgical removal. *Arch Dermatol* 1975;111(12):1588–1590.

35. Haupt HM, Stern JB. Pagetoid melanocytosis: histologic features in benign and malignant lesions. *Am J Surg Pathol* 1995; 19(7):792–797.

36. Park HK, Leonard DD, Arrington JHI, et al. Recurrent melanocytic nevi: clinical and histologic review of 175 cases. *J Am Acad Dermatol* 1987;17(2 Pt 1):285–292.

37. Hoang MP, Prieto VG, Burchette JL, et al. Recurrent melanocytic nevus: a histologic and immunohistochemical evaluation. *J Cutan Pathol* 2001;28(8):400–406.

38. King R, Hayzen BA, Page RN, et al. Recurrent nevus phenomenon: a clinicopathologic study of 357 cases and histologic comparison with melanoma with regression. *Mod Pathol* 2009; 22(5):611–617.

39. Kossard S. Atypical lentiginous junctional naevi of the elderly and melanoma. *Australas J Dermatol* 2002;43(2):93–101.

40. Kaur S, Thami GP, Mohan H, et al. Co-existence of variants of porokeratosis: a case report and a review of the literature. *J Dermatol* 2002;29(5):305–309.

41. Schwarz T, Seiser A, Gschnait F. Disseminated superficial actinic porokeratosis. *J Am Acad Dermatol* 1984;11(4 Pt 2): 724–730.

42. Zhang Z, Li C, Wu F, et al. Genomic variations of the mevalonate pathway in porokeratosis. *Elife* 2015;4:e06322.

43. Elder DE, Elenitsas R, Murphy GF, et al. Benign pigmented lesions and malignant melanoma. In: Elder DE, Elenitsas R, Johnson BL, Murphy GF, eds. *Lever's Histopathology of the Skin.*

Philadelphia, PA: Lippincott Williams & Wilkins; 2005:715–805.

44. Bastiaens M, ter Huurne J, Gruis N, et al. The melanocortin-1-receptor gene is the major freckle gene. *Hum Mol Genet* 2001;10(16):1701–1708.

45. Choi W, Yin L, Smuda C, et al. Molecular and histological characterization of age spots. *Exp Dermatol* 2017;26(3):242–248.

46. Hafner C, Stoehr R, van Oers JM, et al. The absence of BRAF, FGFR3, and PIK3CA mutations differentiates lentigo simplex from melanocytic nevus and solar lentigo. *J Invest Dermatol* 2009;129(11):2730–2735.

47. Elder DE, Barnhill RL, Bastian BC, et al. Dysplastic naevus. In: Elder DE, Massi D, Scolyer RA, Willemze R, eds. *WHO Classification of Melanocytic Tumors*. 4th ed. Lyon: IARC; 2018:82–86.

48. Torchia D, Happle R. Papular nevus spilus syndrome: old and new aspects of a mosaic RASopathy. *Eur J Dermatol* 2019; 29(1):2–5.

49. Sarin KY, McNiff JM, Kwok S, et al. Activating HRAS mutation in nevus spilus. *J Invest Dermatol* 2014;134(6):1766–1768.

50. Kinsler VA, Krengel S, Riviere JB, et al. Next-generation sequencing of nevus spilus-type congenital melanocytic nevus: exquisite genotype-phenotype correlation in mosaic RASopathies. *J Invest Dermatol* 2014;134(10):2658–2660.

51. De Wit PEJ, Van't Hof-Grootenboer B, Ruiter DJ, et al. Validity of the histopathological criteria used for diagnosing dysplastic naevi. *Eur J Cancer* 1993;29A(6):831–839.

52. Tucker MA, Halpern A, Holly EA, et al. Clinically recognized dysplastic nevi. A central risk factor for cutaneous melanoma. *JAMA* 1997;277(18):1439–1444.

53. Kossard S, Wilkinson B. Small cell (naevoid) melanoma: a clinicopathologic study of 131 cases. *Australas J Dermatol* 1997;38 Suppl 1:S54–S58.

54. King R, Page RN, Googe PB, et al. Lentiginous melanoma: a histologic pattern of melanoma to be distinguished from lentiginous nevus. *Mod Pathol* 2005;18(10):1397–1401.

55. Farrahi F, Egbert BM, Swetter SM. Histologic similarities between lentigo maligna and dysplastic nevus: importance of clinicopathologic distinction. *J Cutan Pathol* 2005;32(6):405–412.

56. Su WPD. Histopathologic varieties of epidermal nevus. A study of 160 cases. *Am J Dermatopathol* 1982;4(2):161–170.

57. Happle R. The group of epidermal nevus syndromes Part I. Well defined phenotypes. *J Am Acad Dermatol* 2010;63(1):1–22; quiz 23–24.

58. Cruz PD, Hud JA. Excess insulin binding to insulin-like growth factor receptors: proposed mechanism for acanthosis nigricans. *J Invest Dermatol* 1992;98(6 Suppl):82S–85S.

59. Wilgenbus K, Lentner A, Kuckelkorn R, et al. Further evidence that acanthosis nigricans maligna is linked to enhanced secretion by the tumour of transforming growth factor alpha. *Arch Dermatol Res* 1992;284(5):266–270.

60. Okun MF, Edelstein LM. Clonal seborrheic keratosis. In: Okun MF, Edelstein LM, eds. *Gross and Microscopic Pathology of the Skin*. Vol. 2. Boston: Dermatopathology Foundation Press; 1976:576.

61. Elder DE, Murphy GF. Malignant tumors: melanomas and related lesions. In: Elder DE, Murphy GF, eds. *Melanocytic Tumors of the Skin*. Washington, DC: Armed Forces Institute of Pathology; 1991:103.

62. Duncan LM, Bastian BC, Elder DE, et al. Low CSD Melanoma (Superficial spreading melanoma). In: Elder DE, Massi D, Scolyer RA, Willemze R, eds. *WHO Classification of Melanocytic Tumors*. 4th ed. Lyon: IARC; 2018:76–77.

63. Barnhill RL, Barnhill MA, Berwick M, et al. The histologic spectrum of pigmented spindle cell nevus: a review of 120 cases with emphasis on atypical variants. *Hum Pathol* 1991;22(1):52–58.

64. Busam KJ, Barnhill RL. Pagetoid Spitz nevus. Intraepidermal Spitz tumor with prominent pagetoid spread. *Am J Surg Pathol* 1995;19(9):1061–1067.

65. Raiten K, Paniago-Pereira C, Ackerman AB. Pagetoid Bowen's disease vs. extramammary Paget's disease. *J Dermatol Surg Oncol* 1976;2(1):24–25.

66. Wilkinson EJ, Brown HM. Vulvar Paget disease of urothelial origin: a report of three cases and a proposed classification of vulvar Paget disease. *Hum Pathol* 2002;33(5):549–554.

67. Elbendary A, Xue R, Valdebran M, et al. Diagnostic criteria in intraepithelial pagetoid neoplasms: a histopathologic study and evaluation of select features in Paget disease, Bowen disease, and melanoma in situ. *Am J Dermatopathol* 2017;39(6):419–427.

68. Haghighi B, Smoller BR, LeBoit PE, et al. Pagetoid reticulosis (Woringer-Kolopp disease): an immunophenotypic, molecular, and clinicopathologic study. *Mod Pathol* 2000;13(5):502–510.

69. Cerroni L, Sander CA, Smoller B, et al. Mycosis fungoides. In: Elder DE, Massi D, Scolyer R, eds. *WHO Classification of Skin Tumours*. 4th ed. Lyon: IARC; 2018:226–235.

70. Silverberg NB. Human papillomavirus infections in children. *Curr Opin Pediatr* 2004;16(4):402–409.

71. Smith KJ, Skelton H. Molluscum contagiosum: recent advances in pathogenic mechanisms, and new therapies. *Am J Clin Dermatol* 2002;3(8):535–545.

72. Kim WJ, Lee WK, Song M, et al. Clinical clues for differential diagnosis between verruca plana and verruca plana-like seborrheic keratosis. *J Dermatol* 2015;42(4):373–377.

73. Witchey DJ, Witchey NB, Roth-Kauffman MM, et al. Plantar warts: epidemiology, pathophysiology, and clinical management. *J Am Osteopath Assoc* 2018;118(2):92–105.

74. Laurent R, Kienzler JL, Croissant O, et al. Two anatomoclinical types of warts with plantar localization: specific cytopathogenic effects of papillomavirus. Type I (HPV-1) and type 2 (HPV-2). *Arch Dermatol Res* 1982;274(1-2):101–111.

75. Rock B, Shah KV, Farmer ER. A morphologic, pathologic, and virologic study of anogenital warts in men. *Arch Dermatol* 1992;128(4):495–500.

76. Longacre TA, Kong CS, Welton ML. Diagnostic problems in anal pathology. *Adv Anat Pathol* 2008;15(5):263–278.

77. Wilkinson EJ, Cox JT, Selim MA, et al. Evolution of terminology for human-papillomavirus-infection-related vulvar squamous intraepithelial lesions. *J Low Genit Tract Dis* 2015;19(1):81–87.

78. Albuquerque A, Rios E, Dias CC, et al. p16 immunostaining in histological grading of anal squamous intraepithelial lesions: a systematic review and meta-analysis. *Mod Pathol* 2018;31(7):1026–1035.

79. Forghani B, Oshiro LS, Chan CS, et al. Direct detection of Molluscum contagiosum virus in clinical specimens by in situ hybridization using biotinylated probe. *Mol Cell Probes* 1992; 6(1):67–77.

80. Bergqvist C, Kurban M, Abbas O. Orf virus infection. *Rev Med Virol* 2017;27(4).

81. Sanderson KV. The structure of seborrheic keratoses. *Br J Dermatol* 1968;80(9):588–593.

82. Batycka-Baran A, Baran W, Hryncewicz-Gwozdz A, et al. Dowling-Degos disease: case report and review of the literature. *Dermatology* 2010;220(3):254–258.

83. Basmanav FB, Oprisoreanu AM, Pasternack SM, et al. Mutations in POGLUT1, encoding protein O-glucosyltransferase 1,

cause autosomal-dominant Dowling-Degos disease. *Am J Hum Genet* 2014;94(1):135–143.

84. Wilson NJ, Cole C, Kroboth K, et al. Mutations in POGLUT1 in Galli-Galli/Dowling-Degos disease. *Br J Dermatol* 2017;176(1): 270–274.

85. Jimbow M, Talpash O, Jimbow K. Confluent and reticulated papillomatosis: clinical, light and electron microscopic studies. *Int J Dermatol* 1992;31(7):480–483.

86. Sprecher E, Itin P, Whittock NV, et al. Refined mapping of Naegeli-Franceschetti-Jadassohn syndrome to a 6 cM interval on chromosome 17q11.2-q21 and investigation of candidate genes. *J Invest Dermatol* 2002;119(3):692–698.

87. Rubin AI, Chen EH, Ratner D. Basal-cell carcinoma. *N Engl J Med* 2005;353(21):2262–2269.

88. Reifenberger J, Wolter M, Knobbe CB, et al. Somatic mutations in the PTCH, SMOH, SUFUH and TP53 genes in sporadic basal cell carcinomas. *Br J Dermatol* 2005;152(1):43–51.

89. Strange RC, El-Genidy N, Ramachandran S, et al. Susceptibility to basal cell carcinoma: associations with PTCH polymorphisms. *Ann Hum Genet* 2004;68(Pt 6):536–545.

90. Pellegrini C, Maturo MG, Di Nardo L, et al. Understanding the molecular genetics of basal cell carcinoma. *Int J Mol Sci* 2017; 18(11):E2485.

91. Michaloglou C, Vredeveld LC, Soengas MS, et al. BRAFE600-associated senescence-like cell cycle arrest of human naevi. *Nature* 2005;436(7051):720–724.

92. Requena L, Sangueza OP. Benign neoplasms with neural differentiation: a review. *Am J Dermatopathol* 1995;17(1): 75–96.

93. Ball NJ, Kho GT. Melanocytic nevi are associated with neurofibromas in neurofibromatosis, type I, but not sporadic neurofibromas: a study of 226 cases. *J Cutan Pathol* 2005;32(8): 523–532.

II Localized Superficial Epidermal or Melanocytic Proliferations

Disorders of the Superficial Cutaneous Reactive Unit

III

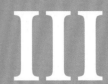

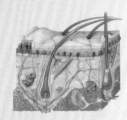

The epidermis, papillary dermis, and superficial capillary–venular plexus react together in many dermatological conditions, and were termed the "superficial cutaneous reactive unit" by Clark. Many dermatoses are associated with infiltrates of lymphocytes with or without other cell types, around the superficial vessels. The epidermis in pathological conditions can be thinned (atrophic), thickened (acanthotic), edematous (spongiotic) and/or infiltrated (exocytosis). The epidermis may proliferate in response to chronic irritation, infection (bacterial, yeast, deep fungal, or viral). The epidermis may proliferate in response to dermatological conditions (psoriasis, atopic dermatitis, prurigo). The papillary dermis and superficial vascular plexus may contain a variety of inflammatory cells, can be edematous, may have increased ground substance (hyaluronic acid), and may be sclerotic or homogenized.

IIIA · SUPERFICIAL PERIVASCULAR DERMATITIS

Many dermatoses are associated with infiltrates of lymphocytes with or without other cell types, around the vessels of the superficial capillary–venular plexus, termed by Clark the "superficial cutaneous reactive unit (SCRU)." The vessel walls may be quite unremarkable, or there may be slight to moderate endothelial swelling. Eosinophilic change ("fibrinoid necrosis") is not seen except in cases of true vasculitis. The term "lymphocytic vasculitis" may encompass some of the conditions mentioned here, but is of debatable validity in the absence of vessel wall damage. The epidermis is variable in its thickness, amount and type of exocytotic cell, and the integrity of the basal cell zone (liquefaction degeneration). In some of the entities listed here, the perivascular infiltrate may in some examples also involve vessels of the mid and deep vessels. These conditions are also listed in Chapter V: Pathology Substantially Involving the Reticular Dermis.

1. Superficial Perivascular Dermatitis, Mostly Lymphocytes
   1a. Superficial Perivascular Dermatitis With Eosinophils
   1b. Superficial Perivascular Dermatitis With Neutrophils
   1c. Superficial Perivascular Dermatitis With Plasma Cells
   1d. Superficial Perivascular Dermatitis, With Extravasated Red Cells
   1e. Superficial Perivascular Dermatitis, Melanophages Prominent
2. Superficial Perivascular Dermatitis, Mast Cells Predominant

IIIA1 · Superficial Perivascular Dermatitis, Mostly Lymphocytes

Viral Exanthem

Lymphocytes are seen about the superficial vascular plexus. Other cell types are rare or absent. Viral exanthems are prototypic (1).

CLINICAL SUMMARY. At least five groups of viruses are well known to affect the skin or the adjoining mucous surfaces: (1) the herpesvirus group, including herpes simplex types 1 and 2 and the varicella-zoster virus, which are DNA-containing organisms that multiply within the nucleus of the host cell; (2) the poxvirus group, including smallpox, milkers' nodules, orf, and molluscum contagiosum, which are DNA-containing agents that multiply within the cytoplasm; (3) the papovavirus group, including the various types of verrucae, which contain DNA and replicate in the nucleus; (4) the picornavirus group, including coxsackievirus group A, causing hand-foot-and-mouth disease, which contain RNA rather than DNA

in their nucleoids; and (5) retroviruses, including human immunodeficiency virus (HIV), the cause of acquired immunodeficiency syndrome (AIDS). Primary HIV infection may be associated with both an exanthem and an enanthem, which are histologically nondescript lymphocytic infiltrates. The array of skin lesions associated with HIV is generally a consequence of eventual immunosuppression. Seborrheic dermatitis, psoriasis, xerosis, and pruritic papular eruptions may be seen in the early stages. As the infection advances and the CD4/CD8 ratio decreases, oral hairy leukoplakia, chronic herpes simplex, recurrent herpes zoster, Kaposi sarcoma, and other opportunistic infections are also common (2). These associations have been reviewed (3).

The prototypic viral rash is the morbilliform rash of measles. Measles virus is a single-stranded RNA virus that belongs to the family Paramyxoviridae. Measles is an epidemic disease with a worldwide distribution. Measles virus is transmitted via respiratory secretions, predominantly as aerosols but also by direct contact. The symptoms usually last for 10 days and resolve without consequence. However, there is an increased risk of more severe diseases, such as severe pneumonitis or encephalitis, in immunocompromised individuals.

HISTOPATHOLOGY. There is no unique histology of HIV infection in the skin. Primary exanthems of HIV show nonspecific lymphocytoid infiltrates with mild epidermal changes, primarily spongiosis (4). Seborrheic dermatitis in patients with AIDS may show nonspecific changes, including spotty keratinocytic necrosis, leukoexocytosis, and plasma cells in a superficial perivascular infiltrate (5). A "papular eruption" may exhibit nonspecific perivascular eosinophils with mild folliculitis, although epithelioid cell granulomas have also been reported (6). An "interface dermatitis" shows, as the name implies, vacuolar alteration of the basal cell layer, scattered necrotic keratinocytes, and a superficial perivascular lymphohistiocytic infiltrate. The vacuolar alteration and number of necrotic keratinocytes tend to be more pronounced than in drug eruptions. Biopsies of AIDS-related eruptions are often nonspecific.

Histopathologic features of the measles exanthem are said to be quite distinctive and are characterized by a combination of multinucleated keratinocytes, and individual and clustered necrotic keratinocytes in the epidermis with pronounced folliculosebaceous as well as acrosyringeal involvement (7). Biopsies from AIDS patients with measles may have necrosis of clusters of keratinocytes in the upper spinous layer and granular layer of the epidermis. Unlike in erythema multiforme the necrosis occurs in the basal layer keratinocytes. Multinucleated keratinocytes may or may not be prominent in the measles biopsy. Cytoplasmic swelling of the keratinocytes in the granular layer may be present even when multinucleated cells are sparse.

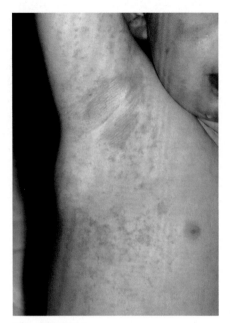

Clin. Fig. IIIA1.a

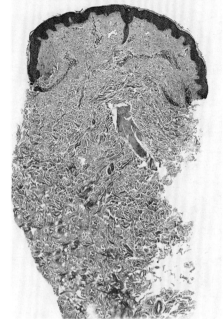

Fig. IIIA1.a

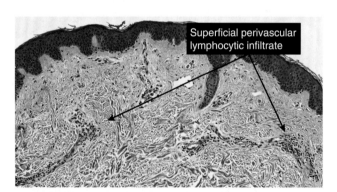

Fig. IIIA1.b

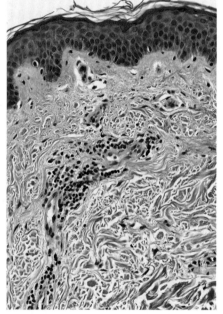

Fig. IIIA1.c

Clin. Fig. IIIA1.a. *Viral exanthem.* Red macules and papules that blanch are characteristic of this unique exanthem called unilateral laterothoracic viral exanthem.

Fig. IIIA1.a. *Morbilliform viral exanthem, low power.* There is an inflammatory infiltrate about dermal vessels in the reticular dermis.

Fig. IIIA1.b. *Morbilliform viral exanthem, medium power.* A thin keratin scale overlies a slightly acanthotic epidermis. There is vascular ectasia in the upper reticular dermis.

Fig. IIIA1.c. *Morbilliform viral exanthem, high power.* A lymphocytic inflammatory infiltrate is seen about the dermal vessels. There are no eosinophils and no plasma cells.

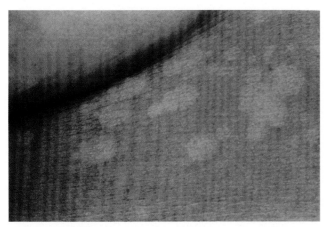

Clin. Fig. IIIA1.b

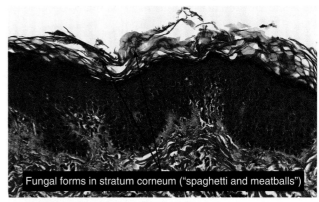

Fungal forms in stratum corneum ("spaghetti and meatballs")

Fig. IIIA1.d

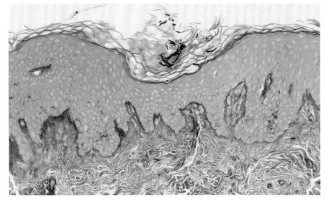

Fig. IIIA1.e

Clin. Fig. IIIA1.b. *Pityriasis versicolor.* Macular areas of hypopigmentation on the upper trunk. On gentle scraping, the surface of the discolored areas shows a fine scale.

Fig. IIIA1.d. *Pityriasis versicolor, medium power.* In the hyperkeratotic stratum corneum there are basophilic staining hyphae and spores. The epidermis is acanthotic with basal layer pigmentation and a sparse lymphocytic infiltrate.

Fig. IIIA1.e. *Pityriasis versicolor, medium power.* A Grocott stain demonstrates the fungal forms in the stratum corneum.

Pityriasis Versicolor

Malassezia furfur is a genus of lipophilic yeast that causes two dermatoses: pityriasis versicolor and Malassezia (Pityrosporum) folliculitis (8). The frequently used term tinea versicolor is not accurate, because Malassezia are not dermatophytes.

CLINICAL SUMMARY. In pityriasis versicolor, multiple round-to-oval pink-to-light-brown patches with fine white scale are seen primarily on the trunk and upper extremities. Gentle scraping of the patches will induce the scale that can be examined for spores and short hyphae. Malassezia (Pityrosporum) folliculitis is a pruritic eruption of 2- to 4-mm acneiform follicular papules and pustules on the trunk and arms of otherwise healthy hosts.

HISTOPATHOLOGY. In contrast to other fungal infections of the glabrous skin, the horny layer in lesions of pityriasis (tinea) versicolor contains abundant fungi, which can often be visualized in sections stained with H&E as faintly basophilic structures. The fungus is present as a combination of both hyphae and spores, creating an appearance often referred to as spaghetti and meatballs. The inflammatory response is usually minimal;

there may occasionally be slight hyperkeratosis, slight spongiosis, or a minimal superficial perivascular lymphocytic infiltrate.

Lupus Erythematosus, Acute

CLINICAL SUMMARY. In acute systemic lupus erythematosus (SLE), the cutaneous manifestations usually appear gradually and may be subtle, so that systemic disease may overshadow the cutaneous manifestations (9). These include erythema lesions, photosensitivity, palmar erythema, periungual telangiectases, diffuse hair loss as a result of telogen effluvium, and urticarial vasculitis or bullous lesions. The erythematous lesions consist of ill-defined red, slightly edematous patches without scaling or atrophy, most commonly on the malar region.

HISTOPATHOLOGY. Early lesions of the erythematous, edematous type may have only mild, nonspecific changes. In well-developed lesions, there is an interface dermatitis with vacuolar degeneration of the basal cell layer in association with edema of the upper dermis and extravasation of erythrocytes. Fibrin deposits in the connective tissue of the skin are often seen in erythematous lesions, appearing as granular, strongly eosinophilic, PAS-positive, diastase-resistant deposits between collagen bundles, in the walls of dermal vessels, in the papillary dermis, or beneath the epidermis in the basement membrane zone. The reticular dermis and subcutaneous fat are often involved. There may be focal mucin deposition associated with a predominantly perivascular and periadnexal lymphocytic infiltrate.

See also IIIH.

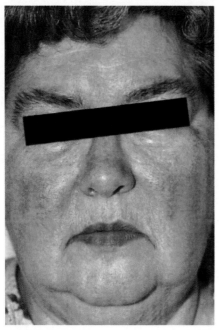

Clin. Fig. IIIA1.c

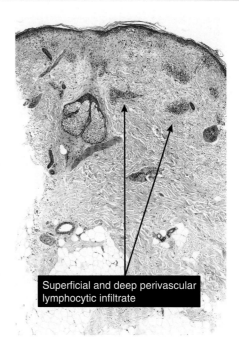

Superficial and deep perivascular lymphocytic infiltrate

Fig. IIIA1.f

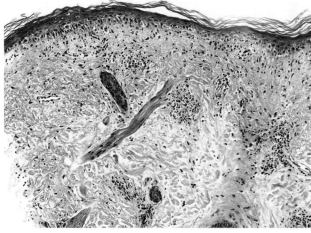

Fig. IIIA1.g

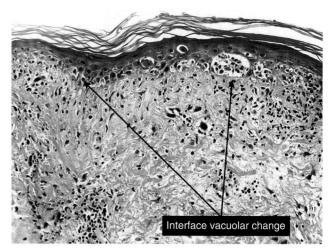

Interface vacuolar change

Fig. IIIA1.h

Clin. Fig. IIIA1.c. *Lupus erythematosus, acute.* A photosensitive female presented with edematous malar erythema—a "butterfly rash." Lack of papules and pustules helps to distinguish lupus from rosacea.

Fig. IIIA1.f. *Lupus erythematosus, acute, low power.* There is hyperkeratosis with a thinned and focally thickened epidermis and vacuolar change at the interface. There is an infiltrate about dermal vessels seen in the reticular dermis.

Fig. IIIA1.g. *Lupus erythematosus, acute, medium power.* Vacuolar change is seen at the dermal–epidermal interface with an overlying hyperkeratotic scale. The inflammatory infiltrate in the dermis is lymphocytic.

Fig. IIIA1.h. *Lupus erythematosus, acute, medium power.* There is prominent vacuolar change at the dermal–epidermal interface. The inflammatory cells are exocytotic to the alternatingly acanthotic and atrophic epidermis.

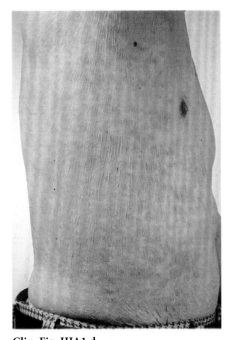

Clin. Fig. IIIA1.d

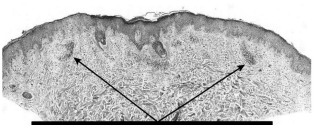

Dense superficial perivascular lymphocytic infiltrate

Fig. IIIA1.i

Clin. Fig. IIIA1.d. *Parapsoriasis.* Brown finely scaled macular fingerlike morphology with atrophy characterizes the benign digitate variant.

Fig. IIIA1.i. *Small plaque parapsoriasis, low power.* There is a focal parakeratotic scale overlying an acanthotic epidermis. In the dermis there is a dense infiltrate about superficial dermal vessels in a localized area.

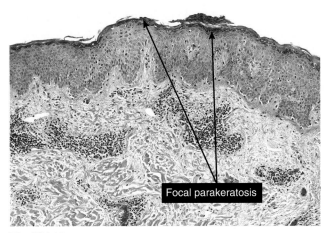

Focal parakeratosis

Fig. IIIA1.j

Fig. IIIA1.j. *Small plaque parapsoriasis, medium power.* A parakeratotic scale overlies an acanthotic epidermis in which there is sparse exocytosis and mild spongiosis. There is a dense inflammatory cell infiltrate about dermal vessels.

Fig. IIIA1.k. *Small plaque parapsoriasis, high power.* There is a dense infiltrate of mononuclear cells about the dermal vessels.

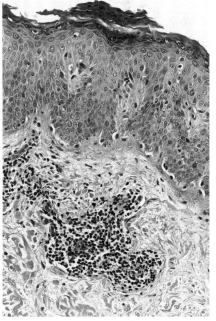

Fig. IIIA1.k

Small Plaque Parapsoriasis (Guttate Parapsoriasis)

Parapsoriasis is a chronic dermatosis whose biologic distinction from early mycosis fungoides (MF), the most frequent form of cutaneous T-cell lymphoma, is still not clearly defined. Two types of parapsoriasis have been delineated: large-plaque parapsoriasis, likely to be related to MF, and small-plaque parapsoriasis, which is generally not considered to be likely to progress to lymphoma (10).
   See also IIID.

Conditions to consider in the differential diagnosis:

   morbilliform viral exanthem
   papular acrodermatitis (Gianotti–Crosti—more often
      spongiotic)
   stasis dermatitis
   pityriasis lichenoides et varioliformis acuta (PLEVA),
      early
   Jessner's lymphocytic infiltrate
   tinea versicolor

candidiasis
superficial gyrate erythemas
lupus erythematosus, acute
mixed connective tissue disease
dermatomyositis
early herpes simplex, zoster
morbilliform drug eruption
cytomegalovirus inclusion disease
polymorphous drug eruption
progressive pigmented purpura
parapsoriasis, small plaque type (digitate dermatosis)
guttate parapsoriasis
Langerhans cell histiocytosis (early lesions)
mucocutaneous lymph node syndrome (Kawasaki disease)
secondary syphilis

IIIA1a Superficial Perivascular Dermatitis With Eosinophils

In addition to lymphocytes, eosinophils are present in varying numbers, with both a perivascular and interstitial distribution. Morbilliform drug eruptions and urticarial reactions are prototypic (11).

Morbilliform Drug Eruption

CLINICAL SUMMARY. Virtually any drug may be associated with a morbilliform eruption; the nonspecific clinical and histologic changes make definitive implication of a specific agent difficult (12). The most common class of medications causing morbilliform eruptions is antibacterial antibiotics. The morbilliform rash consists of fine blanching papules, which appear suddenly, are symmetric, and often are brightly erythematous in Caucasian patients.

HISTOPATHOLOGY. The typical morbilliform drug eruption displays a variable, often sparse, mainly perivascular infiltrate of lymphocytes and eosinophils. Eosinophils may be absent. In a recent study, 82% of 108 cases of drug eruptions (which had been identified in a single institution by pathologic diagnosis supported by chart review) exhibited an inflammatory infiltrate confined to the superficial dermis. Eighty percent exhibited a perivascular and interstitial pattern of dermal infiltrate. The infiltrate was composed of lymphocytes and eosinophils in approximately 29% of cases, lymphocytes and neutrophils in approximately 10% of cases, and lymphocytes, eosinophils, and neutrophils in approximately 21% of cases. Therefore, eosinophils were present in only 50% of cases. Approximately half (53%) of the cases exhibited epidermal–dermal interface (e.g., vacuolar) changes (13). There is a variable degree of urticarial edema (allergic urticarial eruption, see below). Distinction of morbilliform drug eruption from viral exanthem in the absence of eosinophils is generally not possible. More than occasional dyskeratotic epidermal cells should prompt consideration of erythema multiforme and related conditions, for example, toxic epidermal necrolysis (TEN), Stevens–Johnson syndrome, or fixed drug eruption.

Urticaria

CLINICAL SUMMARY. Urticaria is characterized by the presence of transient, recurrent wheals, which are raised, and erythematous areas of edema usually accompanied by itching. When large wheals occur, in which the edema

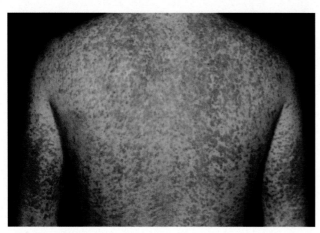
Clin. Fig. IIIA1a.a

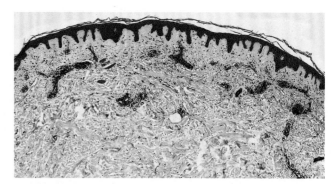
Fig. IIIA1a.a

Clin. Fig. IIIA1a.a. *Morbilliform drug eruption.* A teenage boy abruptly developed a blanchable erythematous maculopapular exanthem with areas of confluence after several days of ampicillin therapy for a sore throat.

Fig. IIIA1a.a. *Morbilliform drug eruption, low power.* The stratum corneum and epidermis are little altered (with time there may develop hyperkeratosis and acanthosis). The dermis shows a dense, perivascular inflammatory infiltrate.

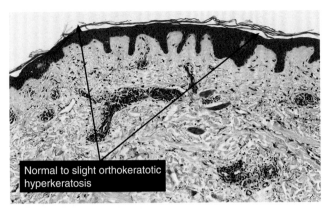

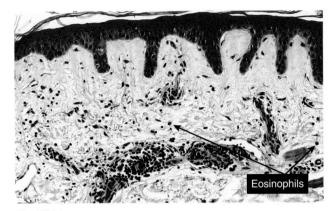

Fig. IIIA1a.b

Fig. IIIA1a.c

Fig. IIIA1a.b. *Morbilliform drug eruption, medium power.* The papillary dermis is edematous with a dense infiltrate about thick-walled dermal vessels.

Fig. IIIA1a.c. *Morbilliform drug eruption, high power.* There is an inflammatory infiltrate about the dermal vessels composed of lymphocytes and eosinophils.

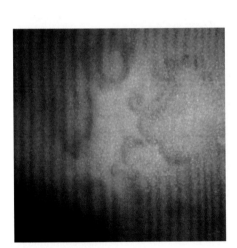

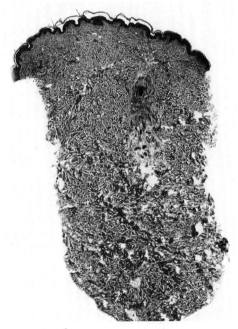

Clin. Fig. IIIA1a.b

Fig. IIIA1a.d

Clin. Fig. IIIA1a.b. *Urticaria.* Large edematous plaques with central clearing and geographic configuration are typical of urticaria.

Fig. IIIA1a.d. *Urticaria, low power.* Sparse superficial perivascular and interstitial inflammatory infiltrate, and separation of collagen bundles by edema fluid.

extends to the subcutaneous tissue, the process is referred to as angioedema (14). Acute episodes of urticaria generally last only several hours. When episodes of urticaria last up to 24 hours and recur over a period of at least 6 weeks, the condition is considered chronic urticaria. Urticaria and angioedema may occur simultaneously, in which case the affliction tends to have a chronic course. In approximately 15% to 25% of patients with urticaria, an eliciting stimulus or underlying predisposing condition can be identified, including soluble antigens in foods, drugs, insect venom, and contact allergens; physical stimuli such as pressure, vibration, solar radiation, cold temperature; occult infections and malignancies; and some hereditary

syndromes. The reaction pattern of urticaria can also be seen in other conditions, notably bullous pemphigoid (9).

HISTOPATHOLOGY. In acute urticaria one observes interstitial dermal edema, dilated venules with endothelial swelling, and a paucity of inflammatory cells. In chronic urticaria interstitial dermal edema and a perivascular and interstitial mixed-cell infiltrate with variable numbers of lymphocytes, eosinophils, and neutrophils are present. In angioedema the edema and infiltrate extend into the subcutaneous tissue. In hereditary angioedema there is subcutaneous and submucosal edema without infiltrating inflammatory cells.

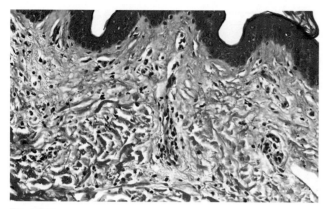

Fig. IIIA1a.e

Fig. IIIA1a.e. *Urticaria, high power.* Interstitial infiltrate of eosinophils, neutrophils, and lymphocytes.

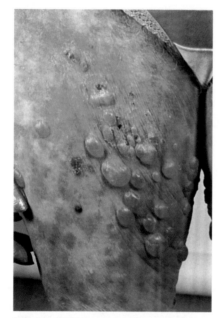

Clin. Fig. IIIA1a.c

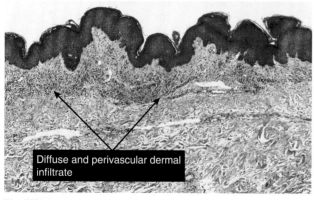

Diffuse and perivascular dermal infiltrate

Fig. IIIA1a.g

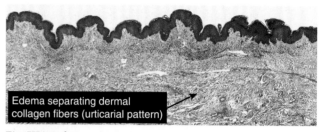

Edema separating dermal collagen fibers (urticarial pattern)

Fig. IIIA1a.f

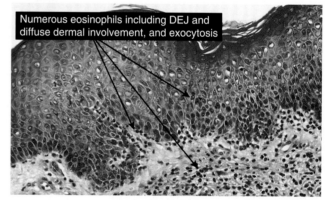

Numerous eosinophils including DEJ and diffuse dermal involvement, and exocytosis

Fig. IIIA1a.h

Clin. Fig. IIIA1a.c. *Bullous pemphigoid, urticarial and bullous phases.* Urticarial plaques on the thigh evolved into tense bullae.

Fig. IIIA1a.f. *Urticarial bullous pemphigoid, low power.* The features seen are those of an orthokeratotic scale overlying an epidermis that is acanthotic. There is edema of the papillary dermis without (in this early lesion) dermal–epidermal separation. A perivascular infiltrate is seen about dermal vessels.

Fig. IIIA1a.g. *Urticarial bullous pemphigoid, medium power.* There is papillary dermal edema with a diffuse as well as perivascular infiltrate of lymphocytes and eosinophils.

Fig. IIIA1a.h. *Urticarial bullous pemphigoid, high power.* The epidermis is acanthotic and spongiotic and in the edematous papillary dermis is an infiltrate of eosinophils and lymphocytes. Several eosinophils are exocytotic to the overlying spongiotic epidermis.

Urticarial Bullous Pemphigoid

Bullous pemphigoid is a subepidermal blistering disorder that commonly presents with a prebullous urticarial phase. See also Sections IVB and IVE.

Conditions to consider in the differential diagnosis:

> arthropod bite reaction
> allergic urticarial reaction (drug)
> bullous pemphigoid, urticarial phase
> urticaria
> erythema toxicum neonatorum
> Well syndrome
> mastocytosis/telangiectasia eruptiva macularis perstans
> angiolymphoid hyperplasia with eosinophilia
> Kimura disease
> Langerhans cell histiocytosis (early lesions)

IIIA1b Superficial Perivascular Dermatitis With Neutrophils

In addition to lymphocytes, neutrophils are present in varying numbers, with both a perivascular and interstitial distribution. *Cellulitis and erysipelas* are prototypic (see also VC.2).

Erysipelas

CLINICAL SUMMARY. Erysipelas, once termed "St. Anthony's fire," is an acute superficial cellulitis of the skin caused by group A streptococci (15). It is characterized by the presence of a well-demarcated, slightly indurated, dusky red area with an advancing, palpable border. In some patients, erysipelas has a tendency to recur periodically in the same areas. In the early antibiotic era, the incidence of erysipelas appeared to be on the decline and most cases occurred on the face. More recently, however, there appears to have been an increase in the incidence, and facial sites are now less common whereas erysipelas of the legs is predominant. Potential complications in patients with poor resistance or after inadequate therapy may include abscess formation, spreading necrosis of the soft tissue, infrequently necrotizing fasciitis, and septicemia. Erysipelas is usually produced by nonnephritogenic and nonrheumatogenic strains of streptococci.

HISTOPATHOLOGY. In the dermis, there are marked edema and dilatation of the lymphatics and capillaries. There is a diffuse infiltrate, composed chiefly of neutrophils, that extends throughout the dermis and occasionally into the subcutaneous fat. It has a loose arrangement around dilated blood and lymph vessels. This pattern may be descriptively termed "cellulitis"; it is not diagnostic of erysipelas specifically, and may be caused by a variety of organisms. In erysipelas, streptococci may be found in the tissue and within lymphatics, in Gram stained sections.

Erysipelas/Cellulitis

See Clin. Fig. IIIA1.b and Figs. IIIA1b.a–c.

Conditions to consider in the differential diagnosis:

> cellulitis
> erysipelas

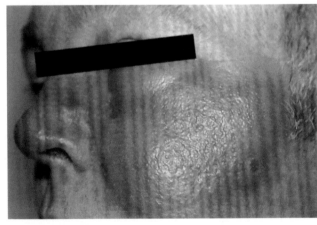

Clin. Fig. IIIA1.b

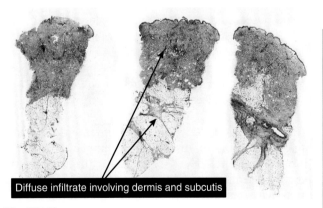

Diffuse infiltrate involving dermis and subcutis

Fig. IIIA1b.a

Clin. Fig. IIIA1.b. *Erysipelas.* A 51-year-old man had fever, chills and an expanding sharply marginated erythematous edematous plaque on the cheek.

Fig. IIIA1b.a. *Cellulitis, low power.* The dermis shows marked edema with separation of collagen bundles and there is a diffuse cellular infiltrate involving the dermis and subcutis. (*continues*)

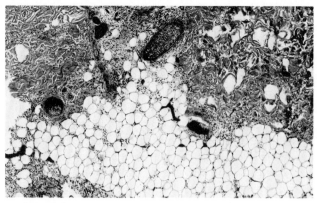

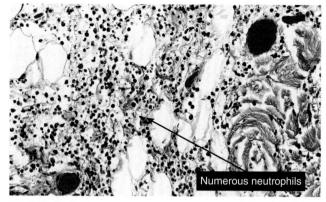

Numerous neutrophils

Fig. IIIA1b.b

Fig. IIIA1b.c

Fig. IIIA1b.b. *Cellulitis, medium power.* There is marked dermal edema and a diffuse infiltrate of lymphocytes and neutrophils as well as fragmented neutrophils.

Fig. IIIA1b.c. *Cellulitis, medium power.* In the dermis and subcutis there is a prominent inflammatory infiltrate, with neutrophils predominating and with histiocytes, lymphocytes and perhaps plasma cells. Bacteria may be demonstrable; however their apparent absence does not rule out sepsis.

IIIA1c Superficial Perivascular Dermatitis With Plasma Cells

Plasma cells are seen about the dermal vessels as well as in the interstitium. They are most often admixed with lymphocytes. *Secondary syphilis* is the prototype.

Secondary Syphilis

CLINICAL SUMMARY. Secondary syphilis (16,17) is typically characterized by a generalized eruption, comprising brown-red macules and papules, papulosquamous lesions resembling guttate psoriasis, and, rarely, pustules. Lesions may be follicular-based, annular, or serpiginous, particularly in recurrent attacks. Other skin signs include alopecia and condylomata lata, the latter comprising broad, raised, gray, confluent papular lesions arising in anogenital areas, pitted hyperkeratotic palmoplantar papules termed "syphilis cornee," and, in rare severe cases, ulcerating lesions that define "lues maligna." Some patients develop mucous patches composed of multiple shallow, painless ulcers.

HISTOPATHOLOGY. The two fundamental pathologic changes in syphilis are (1) swelling and proliferation of endothelial cells and (2) a predominantly perivascular infiltrate composed of lymphoid cells and often plasma cells. In late secondary and tertiary syphilis, there are also granulomatous infiltrates of epithelioid histiocytes and giant cells. Biopsies generally reveal varying degrees of lichenoid inflammation and psoriasiform hyperplasia of the epidermis with variable spongiosis and basilar vacuolar alteration. Exocytosis of lymphocytes, spongiform pustulation, and parakeratosis

also may be observed, with or without intracorneal neutrophilic abscesses. Scattered necrotic keratinocytes may be observed. The dermal changes include variable papillary dermal edema and a perivascular and/or periadnexal infiltrate that usually includes plasma cells and may be lymphocyte predominant, lymphohistiocytic, histiocytic predominant, or frankly granulomatous and that is of greatest intensity in the papillary dermis and extends as loose perivascular aggregates into the reticular dermis. Vascular changes such as endothelial swelling and mural edema accompany the angiocentric infiltrates in about half of the cases. In a review of 106 cases, it was concluded that "combinations of endothelial swelling, interstitial inflammation, irregular acanthosis, and elongated rete ridges should raise the possibility of syphilis, along with the presence of vacuolar interface dermatitis with a lymphocyte in nearly every vacuole and lymphocytes with visible cytoplasm" (18). A silver stain shows the presence of spirochetes in about a third of the cases, mainly within the epidermis and less commonly around the blood vessels of the superficial plexus. Immunohistochemistry, especially when combined with specialized microscopy, results in superior detection rates (19). Lesions of condylomata lata show all of the aforementioned changes observed in macular, papular, and papulosquamous lesions, but more florid epithelial hyperplasia and intraepithelial microabscess formation are observed. Silver or IHC stains show numerous treponemes. In addition to small, sarcoidal granulomata in papular lesions of early secondary syphilis, late secondary syphilis may have extensive lymphoplasmacytic and histiocytic infiltrates resembling nodular tertiary syphilis.

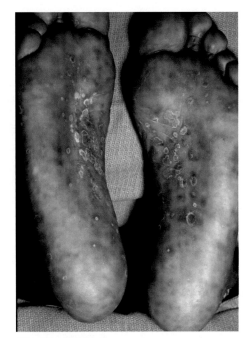

Clin. Fig. IIIA1c.a

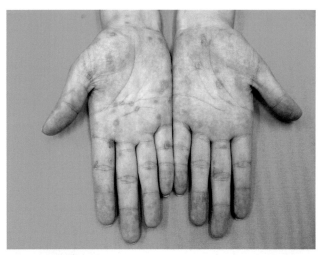

Clin. Fig. IIIA1c.b

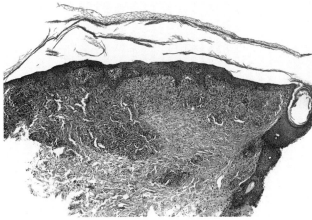

Fig. IIIA1c.a

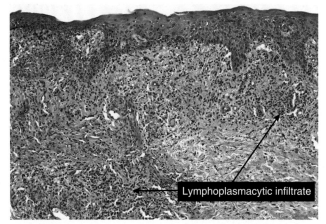

Fig. IIIA1c.b

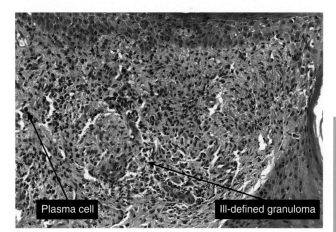

Fig. IIIA1c.c

Clin. Fig. IIIA1c.a. *Secondary syphilis.* Note characteristic scaly brown macules on the soles of the feet.

Clin. Fig. IIIA1c.b. *Secondary syphilis.* Papulosquamous lesions on the palms in an 18-year-old woman.

Fig. IIIA1c.a. *Secondary syphilis, low power.* There is a thin keratin scale overlying an acanthotic epidermis. There is a dense infiltrate at the dermal–epidermal interface and about the superficial dermal vessels.

Fig. IIIA1c.b. *Secondary syphilis, medium power.* There is exocytosis of mononuclear cells into an acanthotic epidermis. The dermis is edematous and there is a dense collection of cells about dermal vessels and in the interstitium.

Fig. IIIA1c.c. *Secondary syphilis, high power.* The inflammatory infiltrate in the dermis is composed of plasma cells, lymphocytes and histiocytes, the latter forming ill-defined granulomas.

Kaposi Sarcoma, Patch Stage

See also VIC5.

Kaposi sarcoma (KS) is a multifocal neoplasm of lymphatic endothelium-derived cells infected with human herpesvirus 8. Whether it qualifies as a true sarcoma is still a matter of debate (20). Four clinical subtypes are distinguished: the classic, the endemic, the epidemic in HIV positive patients, and the iatrogenic subtypes (21). The histologic spectrum of Kaposi disease can be divided into stages roughly corresponding to the clinical type of lesion: early and late macules, plaques, nodules, and aggressive late lesions. In early macules there is usually a patchy, sparse, upper-dermal perivascular infiltrate consisting of lymphocytes and plasma cells. Narrow cords of cells, with evidence of luminal differentiation, are insinuated between collagen bundles. Usually a few dilated irregular or angulated lymphatic-like spaces lined by delicate endothelial cells are also present. Vessels with "jagged" outlines tending to separate collagen bundles are especially characteristic. Normal adnexal structures and pre-existing blood vessels often protrude into newly formed blood vessels, a finding known as the "promontory sign." In late macular lesions there is a more extensive infiltrate of vessels in the dermis, with "jagged" vessels and with cords of thicker-walled vessels similar to those in granulation tissue. At this stage, red blood cell

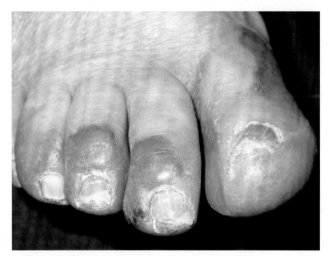

Clin. Fig. IIIA1c.c

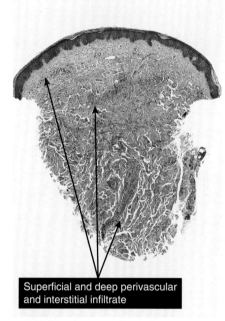

Superficial and deep perivascular and interstitial infiltrate

Fig. IIIA1c.d

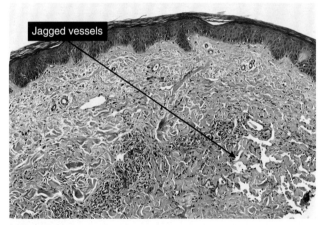

Jagged vessels

Fig. IIIA1c.e

Clin. Fig. IIIA1c.c. *Kaposi sarcoma.* These purplish macules and plaques developed in an elderly Italian male.

Fig. IIIA1c.d. *Kaposi sarcoma, patch stage, medium power.* The epidermis is effaced. In the dermis there is an impression of increased cellularity.

Fig. IIIA1c.e. *Kaposi sarcoma, patch stage, low power.* There is a perivascular and diffuse cellular infiltrate and an increased number of thin-walled blood vessels.

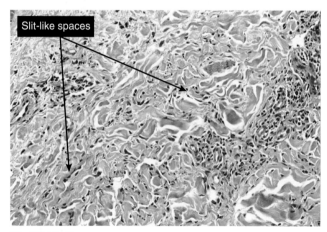

Slit-like spaces

Fig. IIIA1c.f

Fig. IIIA1c.f. *Kaposi sarcoma, patch stage, high power.* There are ill-defined jagged thin-walled vessels with hemorrhage and a mononuclear cell infiltrate. The infiltrate about the dermal vessels includes lymphocytes and plasma cells.

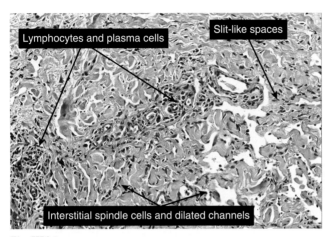

Fig. IIIA1c.g

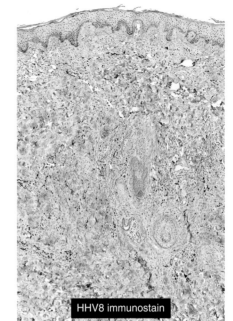

Fig. IIIA1c.h

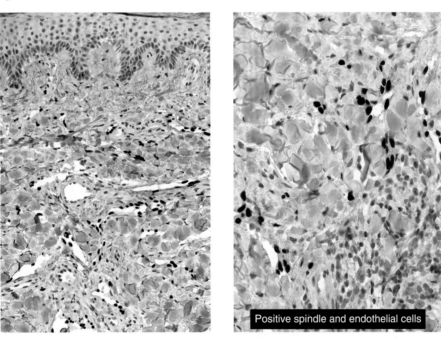

Fig. IIIA1c.i
Fig. IIIA1c.j

Fig. IIIA1c.g. *Kaposi sarcoma, patch stage, high power.* In addition to the jagged vessels, there are spindle cells placed among dermal collagen bundles, with a tendency to form slit-like spaces.

Fig. IIIA1c.h. *Kaposi sarcoma, patch stage, low power.* HHV8 immunostaining in a patch stage lesion shows intranuclear positivity in scattered cells in the reticular dermis.

Fig. IIIA1c.i. *Kaposi sarcoma, patch stage, low power.* The HHV8 positive cells are seen to be lining vascular channels.

Fig. IIIA1c.j. *Kaposi sarcoma, patch stage, low power.* HHV8 positive cells infiltrating among reticular dermis collagen bundles as single cells and as cells lining vascular channels.

III

Disorders of the Superficial Cutaneous Reactive Unit

extravasation and siderophages may be encountered. The presence of slit-like vascular spaces is a characteristic histologic finding. This condition is associated with HHV-8 infection in a susceptible host (see VIC5).

Conditions to consider in the differential diagnosis:

secondary syphilis
arthropod bite reaction
Kaposi sarcoma, nonspecific patch stage
actinic keratoses and Bowen disease
Zoon's plasma cell balanitis circumscripta
erythroplasia of Queyrat

IIIA1d Superficial Perivascular Dermatitis, With Extravasated Red Cells

A perivascular lymphocytic infiltrate is associated with extravasation of lymphocytes, without fibrinoid necrosis of vessels. *Pityriasis rosea* (22,23) and *pityriasis lichenoides et varioliformis acuta* (PLEVA) are prototypic.

Pityriasis Rosea

CLINICAL SUMMARY. Pityriasis rosea (PR) is an acute exanthematous disease associated with the endogenous systemic reactivation of human herpesvirus HHV-6 and/ or HHV-7 (24). It is a self-limited dermatitis lasting from 4 to 7 weeks. It frequently starts with a larger herald patch followed by a disseminated eruption. The lesions, found chiefly on the trunk, neck, and proximal extremities, consist of round-to-oval salmon-colored patches following the lines of cleavage and showing peripherally attached, thin, cigarette-paper–like scales. Several typical and atypical clinical variants have been described including papular, vesicular, urticarial, purpuric, and recurrent forms. Cell-mediated immunity may be involved in the pathogenesis due to the presence of activated helper-inducer T lymphocytes in the epidermal and dermal infiltrate in association with an increased number of Langerhans cells, and the expression of HLA-DR$^+$ antigen on the surface of keratinocytes located around the area of lymphocytic exocytosis (25).

HISTOPATHOLOGY. The patches of the disseminated eruption show a superficial perivascular infiltrate in the dermis that consists predominantly of lymphocytes, with occasional eosinophils and histiocytes. Lymphocytes extend into the epidermis (exocytosis), where there is spongiosis, intracellular edema, mild to moderate acanthosis, areas of decreased or absent granular layer, and focal parakeratosis with or without plasma cells. Intraepidermal spongiotic vesicles and a few necrotic keratinocytes are found in some cases. A common feature is the presence of extravasated erythrocytes in the papillary

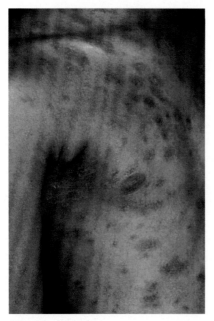

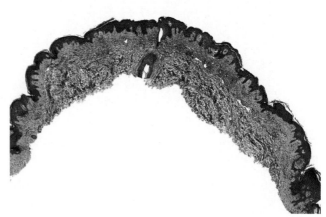

Clin. Fig. IIIA1d.a   Fig. IIIA1d.a

Clin. Fig. IIIA1d.a. *Pityriasis rosea.* Oval brown patches following the lines of cleavage which may show peripheral, thin scales.

Fig. IIIA1d.a. *Pityriasis rosea, low power.* There is an ortho and parakeratotic scale overlying an epidermis that is acanthotic and spongiotic. The papillary dermis is edematous and contains an infiltrate of lymphocytes and red blood cells. This inflammatory infiltrate is seen about dermal vessels.

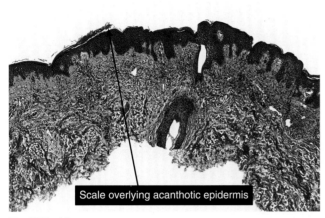

Fig. IIIA1d.b

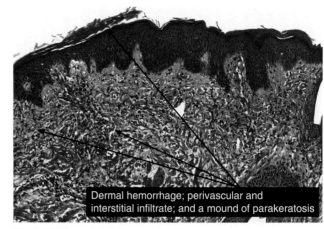

Fig. IIIA1d.c

Fig. IIIA1d.b. *Pityriasis rosea, medium power.* The dermal papillae are widened, edematous and contain an infiltrate of lymphocytes and red blood cells.

Fig. IIIA1d.c. *Pityriasis rosea, high power.* The edematous papillary dermis is hemorrhagic. There may be exocytosis of mononuclear cells as well as red blood cells into the acanthotic, spongiotic epidermis. The ortho and parakeratotic scale forms characteristic small mounds of parakeratosis.

dermis, which sometimes extends into the overlying epidermis. Occasionally, multinucleated keratinocytes in the affected epidermis can be seen. Late lesions from the disseminated eruption are more likely to have a psoriasiform or lichen planus–like appearance and a relatively increased number of eosinophils in the inflammatory infiltrate.

Pityriasis Lichenoides

CLINICAL SUMMARY. Pityriasis lichenoides (PL) is an uncommon cutaneous eruption usually classified in two forms that differ in severity. The milder form, called *pityriasis lichenoides chronica,* is characterized by recurrent crops of brown-red papules 4 to 10 mm in size, mainly on the trunk and extremities, which are covered with a scale and generally involute within 3 to 6 weeks with postinflammatory pigmentary changes. The more severe form, called *pityriasis lichenoides et varioliformis acuta* (PLEVA) or Mucha–Habermann disease, consists of a fairly extensive eruption, present mainly on the trunk and proximal extremities. It is characterized by erythematous papules that develop into papulonecrotic, occasionally hemorrhagic or vesiculopustular lesions that resolve within a few weeks, and can result in scarring. (See also VB2.) Febrile ulceronecrotic Mucha–Habermann disease is a rare very severe variant that can be life-threatening (26). Rarely, PL may evolve into mycosis fungoides. A prolonged clinical course, with development of patches and larger plaques, with prominent lymphocytic nuclear atypia, diminution of apoptotic keratinocytes and of CD7 and CD8 lymphocytes, and presence of clonal T-cell receptor gene rearrangement may be associated with increased risk (27).

HISTOPATHOLOGY. In pityriasis lichenoides chronica, there is a superficial perivascular infiltrate composed of lymphocytes that extend into the epidermis, where there is vacuolar alteration of the basal layer, mild spongiosis, a few necrotic keratinocytes, and confluent parakeratosis. Melanophages and small numbers of extravasated erythrocytes are commonly seen in the papillary dermis. In PLEVA, the more severe form, the perivascular (predominantly lymphocytic) infiltrate is dense in the papillary dermis and extends into the reticular dermis in a wedge-shaped pattern. The infiltrate obscures the dermal–epidermal junction with pronounced vacuolar alteration of the basal layer, marked exocytosis of lymphocytes and erythrocytes, and intercellular and intracellular edema leading to variable degree of epidermal necrosis. Ultimately, erosion or even ulceration may occur. The overlying cornified layer shows parakeratosis and a scaly crust with neutrophils in the more severe cases. Variable degrees of papillary dermal edema, endothelial swelling, and extravasated erythrocytes are seen in the majority of cases. Most of the cells in the inflammatory infiltrate are activated T lymphocytes. There is a predominance of CD8$^+$ (cytotoxic-suppressor) over CD4$^+$ (helper-inducer) T lymphocytes in the infiltrate, and there is expression of HLA-DR on the surrounding keratinocytes, suggesting a direct cytotoxic immune reaction in the pathogenesis of epidermal necrosis. Some studies have suggested that PLEVA is a clonal T-cell disorder (28), although reports of patients with pityriasis lichenoides who have developed cutaneous lymphoma are rare. It is suggested that monoclonal expansion of T cells results most likely from a host immune response to an as yet unidentified antigen, perhaps a viral one (15).

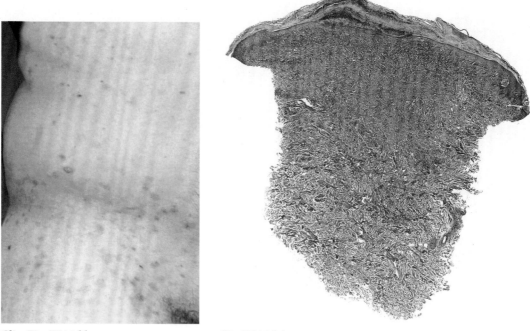

Clin. Fig. IIIA1d.b   **Fig. IIIA1d.d**

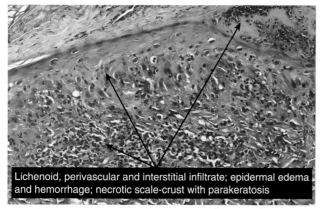

Lichenoid; perivascular and interstitial infiltrate; epidermal edema and hemorrhage; necrotic scale-crust with parakeratosis

Fig. IIIA.1d.e

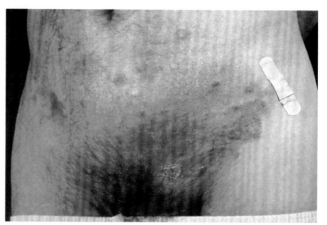

Clin. Fig. IIIA1d.c

Clin. Fig. IIIA1d.b. *Pityriasis lichenoides et varioliformis acuta (PLEVA).* Erythematous papules and papu-lonecrotic lesions developed suddenly on the trunk of a young man.

Fig. IIIA1d.d. *Pityriasis lichenoides et varioliformis acuta (PLEVA), low power.* Lichenoid inflammatory pattern with a superficial and mid dermal perivascular inflammatory infiltrate and a necrotic scale-crust.

Fig. IIIA.1d.e. *Pityriasis lichenoides et varioliformis acuta, medium power.* Closer view reveals lichenoid inflammation with an infiltrate of lymphocytes, extravasated erythrocytes, irregular acanthosis, pallor of the upper layers of the epidermis, spongiosis; and confluent mounds of parakeratosis with plasma cells, neutrophils, and lymphocytes. Necrotic keratinocytes may also be seen in the more acute stages.

Clin. Fig. IIIA1d.c. *Pityriasis lichenoides chronica.* A 29-year-old man gave an 8-month history of asymptomatic dully erythematous macules and papules with light scale on the trunk and extremities.

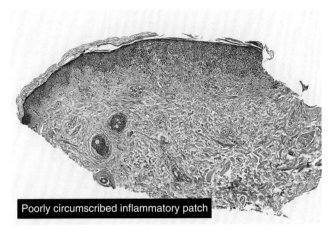

Poorly circumscribed inflammatory patch

Fig. IIIA1d.f

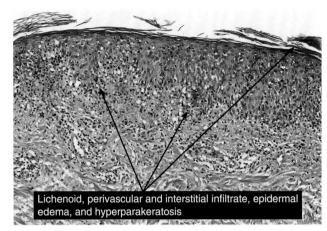

Lichenoid, perivascular and interstitial infiltrate, epidermal edema, and hyperparakeratosis

Fig. IIIA1d.g

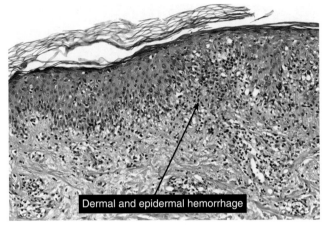

Dermal and epidermal hemorrhage

Fig. IIIA1d.h

Fig. IIIA1d.f. *Pityriasis lichenoides chronica.* A focal lesion characterized by hyperkeratosis and a lichenoid inflammatory infiltrate.

Fig. IIIA1d.g. *Pityriasis lichenoides chronica.* There is hyperkeratosis without the scale-crust or frank necrosis that may be seen in lesions of PLEVA.

Fig. IIIA1d.h. *Pityriasis lichenoides chronica.* There is vacuolar alteration of the basal layer, with mild spongiosis. In addition to lymphocytes, extravasated erythrocytes are present in the papillary dermis and in the epidermis.

Pigmented Purpuric Dermatosis

CLINICAL SUMMARY. Although several variants of pigmented purpuric dermatosis (PPD) have been described, they are all closely related and often cannot be reliably distinguished on clinical or histologic grounds (29). Clinically, the primary lesion consists of discrete puncta often limited to the lower extremities. Gradually, telangiectatic puncta appear as a result of capillary dilatation, and pigmentation as a result of hemosiderin deposits. In some cases, the findings may mimic those of stasis. Not infrequently, clinical signs of inflammation are present, such as erythema, papules, scaling, and lichenification. Several clinical patterns have been distinguished. There are no systemic symptoms related to this disease process. The categorization of PPD as a form of cutaneous lymphoid dyscrasia has been suggested (30).

HISTOPATHOLOGY. The basic process is a lymphocytic perivascular infiltrate limited to the papillary dermis. In some instances, the infiltrate may assume a bandlike or lichenoid pattern, and may involve the reticular dermis in a perivascular distribution. Evidence of vascular damage may be present. The extent of vascular injury is usually mild and insufficient to justify the term "vasculitis,"

commonly consisting only of endothelial cell swelling and dermal hemorrhage. Extravasated red blood cells are usually found in the vicinity of the capillaries. In old lesions, the capillaries often show dilatation of their lumen and proliferation of their endothelium. Extravasated red blood cells may no longer be present, but one frequently finds hemosiderin, in varying amounts. The inflammatory infiltrate is less pronounced than in the early stage.

In a study of 107 cases, five major pathologic patterns were identified: lichenoid (clinically correlating to lichen aureus, a gold-colored papule), perivascular, interface, spongiotic, and granulomatous. Several cases had partial features of mycosis fungoides but none were confirmed (31).

Conditions to consider in the differential diagnosis:

pityriasis rosea
lupus erythematosus, subacute
lupus erythematosus, acute
postinflammatory hyperpigmentation
stasis dermatitis
Kaposi sarcoma, patch stage
pityriasis lichenoides et varioliformis acuta (PLEVA)
pityriasis lichenoides chronica
pigmented purpuric dermatoses (Gougerot–Blum)

III   Disorders of the Superficial Cutaneous Reactive Unit

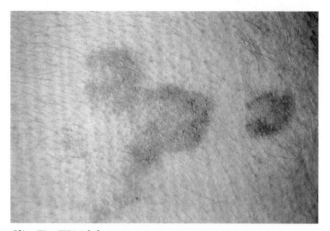

Clin. Fig. IIIA1d.d

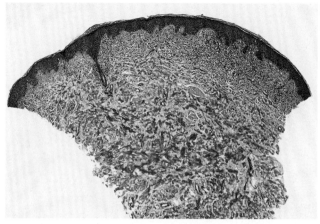

Fig. IIIA1d.i

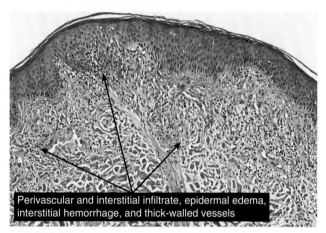

Perivascular and interstitial infiltrate, epidermal edema, interstitial hemorrhage, and thick-walled vessels

Fig. IIIA1d.j

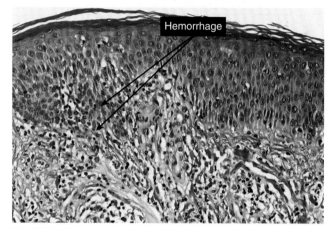

Hemorrhage

Fig. IIIA1d.k

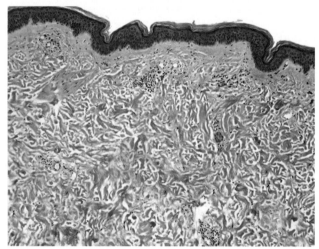

Fig. IIIA1d.l

Clin. Fig. IIIA1d.d. *Pigmented purpuric dermatosis (Gougerot–Blum).* A 15-year-old boy developed asymptomatic nonblanching orange-brown and erythematous lichenoid papules on the lower extremities.

Fig. IIIA1d.i. *Pigmented purpuric dermatosis, low power.* An ortho and parakeratotic scale are present overlying an acanthotic epidermis. There is an inflammatory infiltrate in the papillary dermis.

Fig. IIIA1d.j. *Pigmented purpuric dermatosis, medium power.* The papillary dermis shows hemorrhage and a mononuclear cell infiltrate. There is superficial telangiectasia. Hemorrhage may be seen within the papillary dermis.

Fig. IIIA1d.k. *Pigmented purpuric dermatosis, high power.* The epidermis is acanthotic and shows exocytosis of lymphocytes as well as red blood cells. There is inflammation and hemorrhage in the papillary dermis.

Fig. IIIA1d.l. *Pigmented purpuric dermatosis, low power.* There is a superficial perivascular lymphocytic infiltrate.

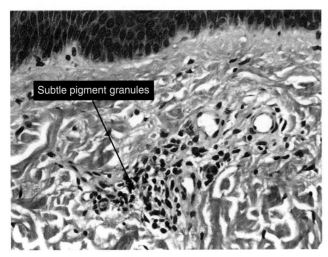

Fig. IIIA1d.m

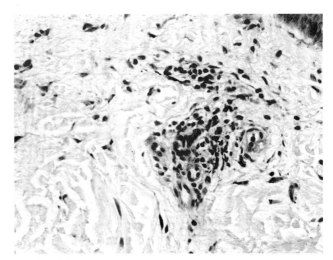

Fig. IIIA1d.n

Fig. IIIA1d.m. *Pigmented purpuric dermatosis, medium power.* Lymphocytes and a few extravasated erythrocytes are present around thick-walled superficial vessels. Faint brown pigment granules can be discerned.

Fig. IIIA1d.n. *Pigmented purpuric dermatosis, high power.* The brown granules stain blue in an iron stain.

IIIA1e Superficial Perivascular Dermatitis, Melanophages Prominent

There is a perivascular infiltrate of lymphocytes, with an admixture of pigment-laden melanophages, indicative of prior damage to the basal layer, and "pigmentary incontinence." Some degree of residual interface damage may also be evident. *Postinflammatory hyperpigmentation* is a prototype (32).

Postinflammatory Hyperpigmentation

CLINICAL SUMMARY. Postinflammatory hyperpigmentation (PIH) may follow any dermatitis that affects the

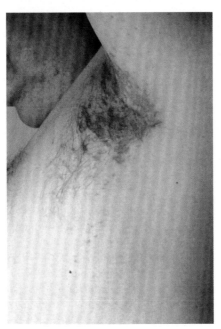

Clin. Fig. IIIA1.e

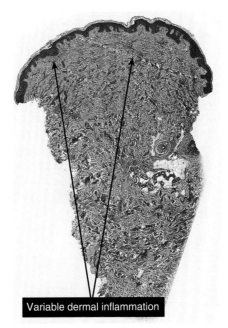

Fig. IIIA1e.a

Clin. Fig. IIIA1.e. *Postinflammatory hyperpigmentation.* A 77-year-old man presented with macular brown changes in sites of previous lichen planus.

Fig. IIIA1e.a. *Postinflammatory hyperpigmentation, low power.* There is an inflammatory infiltrate of lymphocytes and melanophages. *(continues)*

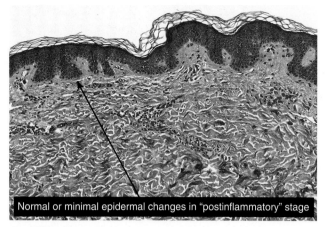

Fig. IIIA1e.b

Normal or minimal epidermal changes in "postinflammatory" stage

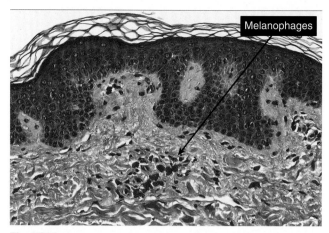

Fig. IIIA1e.c

Melanophages

Fig. IIIA1e.b. *Postinflammatory hyperpigmentation, high power.* In the epidermis there is patchy basal layer pigmentation. In the dermis there are melanophages containing brown pigment granules. About dermal vessels is a mononuclear cell infiltrate.

Fig. IIIA1e.c. *Postinflammatory hyperpigmentation, high power.* The papillary dermis shows melanophage pigmentation with mononuclear cells about the dermal vessels. There is no evidence in this lesion of active inflammation involving the epidermis.

dermal–epidermal junction and results in release of melanin pigment from basal keratinocytes into the dermis. Lichenoid dermatoses such as lichen planus, vacuolar dermatoses such as discoid lupus, or apoptotic/cytotoxic dermatoses such as erythema multiforme or fixed drug eruptions may all result in this reaction pattern. PIH is also a common complication of procedures performed using laser and other light sources (33). Lesions are sometimes biopsied to rule out melanoma. If features diagnostic of a specific underlying dermatosis are lacking in the biopsy, the descriptive diagnosis of PIH may be all that can be made.

HISTOPATHOLOGY. Sections show the phenomena of pigmentary incontinence. Melanin pigment deposited in the dermis is taken up by melanophages. These are large cells with abundant cytoplasm stuffed with pigment and with plump nuclei having open chromatin and sometimes a small nucleolus.

Conditions to consider in the differential diagnosis:

postinflammatory hyperpigmentation
postchemotherapy hyperpigmentation
chlorpromazine pigmentation
amyloidosis

IIIA2 | Superficial Perivascular Dermatitis, Mast Cells Predominant

Mast cells are the main infiltrating cells seen in the dermis. Lymphocytes are also present, and there may be a few eosinophils. *Urticaria pigmentosa* is the example.

Urticaria Pigmentosa

CLINICAL SUMMARY. Urticaria pigmentosa (34) can be divided into four forms: (1) urticaria pigmentosa arising in infancy or early childhood without significant systemic lesions, (2) urticaria pigmentosa arising in adolescence or adult life without significant systemic lesions, (3) systemic mast cell disease, and (4) mast cell leukemia. Five types of cutaneous lesions are seen. The maculopapular type, the most common, consists usually of dozens or even hundreds of small brown lesions that urticate on stroking; a second type exhibits multiple brown nodules or plaques, and, on stroking, shows urtication and occasionally blister formation. A third type, seen almost exclusively in infants, is characterized by a usually solitary, large cutaneous nodule, which on stroking often shows not only urtication but also large bullae. The fourth type, the diffuse erythrodermic type, always starts in early infancy and shows generalized brownish red, soft infiltration of the skin, with urtication on stroking. The fifth type of lesion, telangiectasia macularis eruptiva perstans (TMEP), which usually occurs in adults, consists of an extensive eruption of brownish red macules showing fine telangiectasias, with little or no urtication on stroking. Despite this phenotypic diversity, a mutation of the KIT gene, most commonly D816V, is found in almost all cases and believed to be a driver lesion (35). Although mastocytosis is most typically a benign, self-limited disorder of childhood, up to 30% of adolescent and adult-onset disease represents cutaneous involvement by underlying systemic mastocytosis. CD25 immunoreactivity in a skin infiltrate may be a useful, though not specific, marker for systemic involvement (36).

HISTOPATHOLOGY. In all five types of lesions, the histologic picture shows an infiltrate composed chiefly of mast cells, which are characterized by the presence of metachromatic granules in their cytoplasm. These granules can be visualized with a Giemsa or toluidine blue stain, or with the naphthol AS-D chloroacetate esterase reaction (Leder stain). The lesional cells are also positive with immunostains for KIT and mast cell tryptase (25). In the maculopapular type and in TMEP, the mast cells are limited to the upper third of the dermis and are generally located around capillaries. In some mast cells, the nuclei may be round or oval, but in most, they are spindle shaped. The diagnosis may be missed unless special staining is employed. In cases with multiple nodules or plaques or with a solitary large nodule, the mast cells lie closely packed in tumor-like aggregates and the infiltrate may extend into the subcutaneous fat. In the diffuse, erythrodermic type, there is a dense, band-like infiltrate of mast cells in the upper dermis. Eosinophils may be present in small numbers in all types of urticaria pigmentosa with the exception of TMEP, in which eosinophils are generally absent because of the small numbers of mast cells within the lesions.

Conditions to consider in the differential diagnosis:

urticaria pigmentosa, nodular type
TMEP, adult mast cell disease

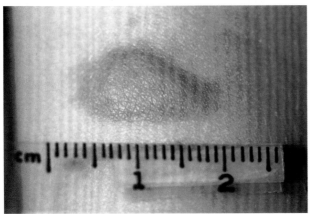

Clin. Fig. IIIA2.a

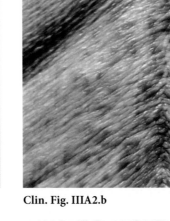

Clin. Fig. IIIA2.b

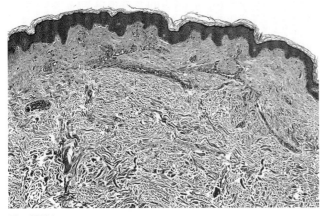

Fig. IIIA2.a

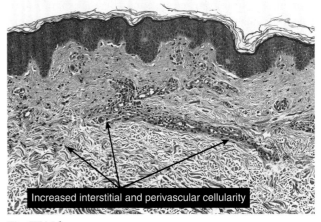

Increased interstitial and perivascular cellularity

Fig. IIIA2.b

Clin. Fig. IIIA2.a. *Urticaria pigmentosa, nodular type.* A 2-year-old boy had a recurrently erythematous and a "swollen" solitary 2 cm yellow brown nodule on the volar forearm.

Clin. Fig. IIIA2.b. *Telangiectasia macularis eruptive perstans.* A 78-year-old woman with 2-year history of telangiectatic erythematous blanching macules on the trunk, neck, and thighs. Darier sign (urtication after stroking) was positive.

Fig. IIIA2.a. *Adult mast cell disease (TMEP), low power.* The epidermis is slightly acanthotic. There is a perivascular infiltrate of mononuclear cells about dermal vessels.

Fig. IIIA2.b. *Adult mast cell disease, medium power.* There is, in the dermis, a diffuse as well as perivascular infiltrate of lymphocytes and mast cells. (*continues*)

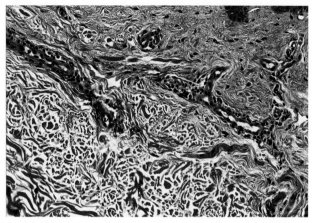

Fig. IIIA2.c   **Fig. IIA2.d**

Fig. IIIA2.c. *Adult mast cell disease, high power.* Mast cells are seen about the thick-walled dermal vessels.

Fig. IIA2.d. *Adult mast cell disease, high power, Giemsa stain.* Large mast cells containing metachromatic granules are seen in the dermis and about dermal vessels.

IIIB SUPERFICIAL DERMATITIS WITH SPONGIOSIS (SPONGIOTIC DERMATITIS)

Spongiotic dermatitis is characterized by intercellular edema in the epidermis (37). In mild or early lesions, the intercellular space is increased with stretching of desmosomes but the integrity of the epithelium is intact. In more severe spongiotic conditions, there is separation of keratinocytes to form spaces (vesicles). For this reason, the spongiotic dermatoses are also listed below in Section IV: Acantholytic, Vesicular and Pustular Disorders (IVB).

    Acute Spongiotic Dermatitis
    Subacute Spongiotic Dermatitis
    Chronic Spongiotic Dermatitis

1. Spongiotic Dermatitis, Lymphocytes Predominant
    1a. Spongiotic Dermatitis, With Eosinophils
    1b. Spongiotic Dermatitis, With Plasma Cells
    1c. Spongiotic Dermatitis, With Neutrophils

Acute Spongiotic Dermatitis

In acute spongiotic dermatitis (38), the stratum corneum is normal in a very early lesion, but there is slight hyperkeratosis in a somewhat later lesion. If the lesion persists, parakeratosis will develop as it evolves further. The epidermal keratinocytes are partially separated by intercellular edema, which stretches the intercellular bridges or desmosomes and renders them more prominent than normal. If the lesion is more severe, the desmosomal attachments rupture, and intercellular spaces appear, usually in the spinous layer, forming spongiotic vesicles. Lymphocytes and occasionally larger Langerhans histiocytes are present in

the spaces and in the edematous epidermis. In addition, there is a loose perivascular infiltrate around the vessels of the superficial capillary-venular plexus.

Subacute Spongiotic Dermatitis

In subacute spongiotic dermatitis, after a spongiotic lesion persists, there is epithelial hyperplasia, which tends to elongate the rete ridges in a pattern that is termed "psoriasiform." Unlike in psoriasis, the suprapapillary plates of keratinocytes are not thinned, indeed they tend to be somewhat thickened. The etiology of the process is made apparent by the presence of spongiotic changes in the epidermis similar to those described above, though vesicle formation is often minimal. A similar perivascular infiltrate is present in the superficial dermis. Because the pattern of subacute spongiotic dermatitis is predominantly psoriasiform, these conditions are also discussed in section IIID, "psoriasiform dermatitis."

Chronic Spongiotic Dermatitis

In chronic spongiotic dermatitis, there is prominent hyperkeratosis and parakeratosis. Spongiosis is usually present but may be quite inconspicuous in a given biopsy. Psoriasiform hyperplasia is prominent and when florid and complex may border on pseudoepitheliomatous hyperplasia (see IIIE). A perivascular lymphocytic infiltrate is present and may include an admixture of histiocytes and even plasma cells, depending on the etiology of the condition. There is often a distinctive pattern of increased collagen fibers arranged vertically between the elongated rete ridges. This papillary dermis sclerosis may be attributable to chronic rubbing or scratching of the lesions, resulting in the condition termed lichen simplex chronicus, which may have as its underlying basis any of the chronic pruritic dermatoses.

The disorders listed below all tend to follow the course listed above, from an acute to a subacute to a chronic spongiotic dermatitis, if the condition persists, and depending on associated factors such as the severity of the condition, the effects of treatment, and the effects of added irritants including the presence of excoriations of chronic rubbing and scratching. The differential diagnosis suggested by a given biopsy specimen may vary to some extent as discussed below, depending for example on the admixture of cell types such as eosinophils or plasma cells, and on the patterns of hyperkeratosis and parakeratosis, of psoriasiform epidermal hyperplasia, and of papillary dermis sclerosis. However, in a given biopsy it is often difficult or impossible to distinguish among the various etiologic categories of spongiotic dermatitis. While a biopsy may be of value to rule out other competing possibilities, such as lymphoma, and may tend to favor one or another of the possibilities listed in the differential diagnosis tables, the exact classification of these disorders usually depends on clinicopathologic correlation.

IIIB1 | Spongiotic Dermatitis, Lymphocytes Predominant

There is marked intercellular edema (spongiosis) within the epidermis. In the dermis, perivascular lymphocytes are predominant. *Nummular dermatitis* is prototypic.

Nummular Dermatitis (Eczema)

CLINICAL SUMMARY. The eruption is characterized by pruritic, coin-shaped (nummular), erythematous, scaly, crusted plaques. The lesions tend to develop on the extensor surfaces of the extremities. Hypersensitivity to haptens such as metals may be involved in the pathogenesis of nummular dermatitis in some patients (39).

HISTOPATHOLOGY. Nummular dermatitis is the prototype of acute and subacute spongiotic dermatitis. There is mild to moderate spongiosis, usually without vesiculation, and a superficial perivascular infiltrate composed of lymphocytes, histiocytes, and occasional eosinophils. The epidermis is moderately acanthotic and parakeratotic. The stratum corneum contains aggregates of coagulated plasma and scattered neutrophils, forming a crust. Mild papillary dermal edema and vascular dilatation may be present.

Meyerson Nevus

CLINICAL SUMMARY. Meyerson nevus is a melanocytic nevus that is associated with an erythematous, eczematous halo that may symmetrically or eccentrically encircle the nevus (40). The lesion may be pruritic and scaly. Spontaneous resolution of the eczema over the course of weeks, without disappearance of the nevus, usually occurs. Meyerson nevi usually occur on the trunk and are more common in males. The simultaneous appearance of a Sutton (halo) nevus and Meyerson nevus has been reported after sunburn, as has the subsequent development of a Sutton nevus and vitiligo 6 months after removal of a Meyerson nevus, but this is not typical. Interferon-alpha therapy has been shown to induce Meyerson nevus (41). Spongiotic inflammation can occur in melanomas as well as nevi. Prominent upward pagetoid scatter and severe atypia can suggest this diagnosis (43).

HISTOPATHOLOGY. The melanocytic nevus may be banal, congenital (42), or dysplastic (43), with superimposed changes of an eczematous dermatitis characterized by epidermal acanthosis and spongiosis which encompass the nevus and the adjacent epidermis (the eczematous halo).

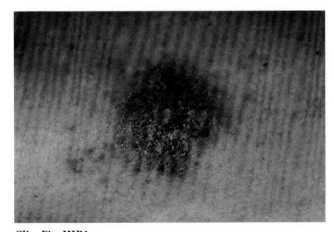

Clin. Fig. IIIB1.a

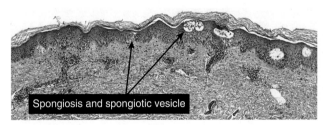

Spongiosis and spongiotic vesicle

Fig. IIIB1.a

Clin. Fig. IIIB1.a. *Nummular eczema.* A crusted, coin-shaped plaque with serous exudate on the extensor surface of the lower-extremity typifies this pruritic, episodic condition.

Fig. IIIB1.a. *Acute spongiotic dermatitis, low power.* In this acute lesion, the stratum corneum retains its basket-weave character, and the epidermis is only slightly acanthotic. In the dermis there is a perivascular mononuclear cell infiltrate. (*continues*)

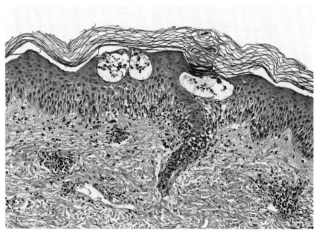

Fig. IIIB1.b

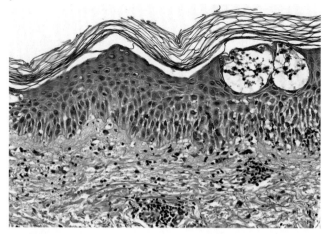

Fig. IIIB1.c

Fig. IIIB1.b. *Acute spongiotic dermatitis, medium power.* The epidermis is slightly acanthotic and markedly spongiotic. The papillary dermis shows an infiltrate of lymphocytes about superficial dermal vessels.

Fig. IIIB1.c. *Acute spongiotic dermatitis, high power.* The epidermal keratinocytes are partially separated by edema (spongiosis), stretching the intercellular desmosomes.

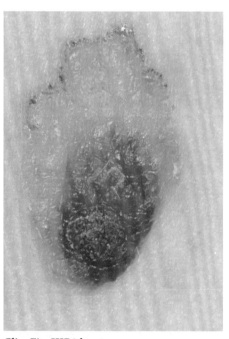

Clin. Fig. IIIB1.b

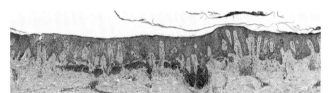

Fig. IIIB1.d

Clin. Fig. IIIB1.b. *Meyerson nevus.* Note the "eczematous" reaction surrounding the atypical nevus.

Fig. IIIB1.d. *Meyerson nevus, low power.* The epidermis is acanthotic, spongiotic, and surmounted by parakeratotic scale with collections of serum.

Spongiotic intraepidermal vesicles and eosinophilic spongiosis may be present. The stratum corneum may show focal parakeratosis with collections of serum. The superficial dermal infiltrate is composed of lymphocytes, histiocytes, and eosinophils. The lymphocytes have been shown to be predominantly CD4+ (helper) T cells, in contrast to the CD8+ (suppressor) T cells that are found in halo nevi.

Conditions to consider in the differential diagnosis:

eczematous dermatitis
atopic dermatitis
allergic contact dermatitis
photoallergic drug eruption
irritant contact dermatitis
nummular eczema

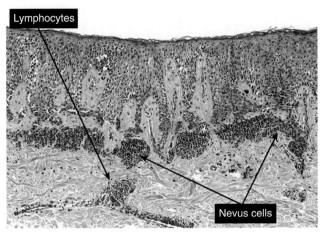

Fig. IIIB1.e

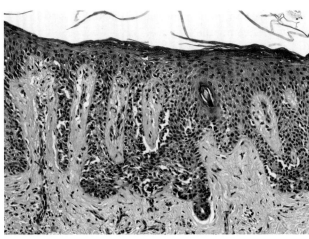

Fig. IIIB1.f

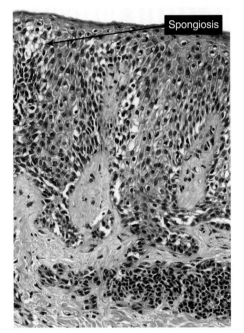

Fig. IIIB1.g

Fig. IIIB1.e. *Meyerson nevus, low power.* A mononuclear cell inflammatory infiltrate is present in the upper dermis, predominantly around vessels. Nevus cells are inconspicuous.

Fig. IIIB1.f. *Meyerson nevus, medium power.* Pigmented nevomelanocytes and melanophages are seen in the dermis on closer inspection. The overlying epidermis shows separation of keratinocytes by intercellular edema.

Fig. IIIB1.g. *Meyerson nevus, high power.* There is intense spongiosis in the epidermis. Nested nevus cells are seen in the dermis.

---

dyshidrotic dermatitis
Meyerson nevus
parapsoriasis, small plaque type (digitate dermatosis)
polymorphous light eruption
lichen striatus
chronic actinic dermatitis (actinic reticuloid)
actinic prurigo, early lesions
"id" reaction
seborrheic dermatitis
stasis dermatitis
erythroderma
miliaria
pityriasis rosea
Sezary syndrome
papular acrodermatitis (Gianotti–Crosti)

IIIB1a   Spongiotic Dermatitis, With Eosinophils

There is marked intercellular edema (spongiosis) within the epidermis. In the dermis, lymphocytes are predominant. Eosinophils can be found in most examples of atopy, and allergic contact dermatitis, and are numerous in incontinentia pigmenti. *Allergic contact dermatitis* is the prototype (39).

Allergic Contact Dermatitis

CLINICAL SUMMARY. The prototype of acute spongiotic dermatitis is allergic contact dermatitis, for example as a reaction to poison ivy exposure. Usually between 24 and 72 hours after exposure to the antigen, the patient develops pruritic, edematous, erythematous papules and plaques and, in some cases, vesicles. Linear papules and vesicles are common in allergic contact dermatitis to poison ivy, reflecting the points of contact between the plant and the skin. Markers of genetic susceptibility to contact allergy are beginning to be identified (44).

HISTOPATHOLOGY. Early lesions are an acute spongiotic dermatitis. If vesicles develop, they may contain clusters of Langerhans cells. Eosinophils may be present in the dermal infiltrate as well as within areas of spongiosis. In patients with continued exposure to the antigen, the biopsy may show a subacute or later a chronic spongiotic

dermatitis, often lichen simplex chronicus due to rubbing. Eosinophilic spongiosis and multinucleate dermal dendritic fibrohistiocytic cells, in the presence of acanthosis, lymphocytic infiltrate, dermal eosinophils, and hyperkeratosis, are particularly suggestive of allergic contact dermatitis compared to other spongiotic dermatoses (39).

Allergic Contact Dermatitis

See Clin. Fig. IIIB1a.a and Figs. IIIB1a.a–c; Clin. Fig. IIIB1a.b and Figs. IIIB1a.d–g.

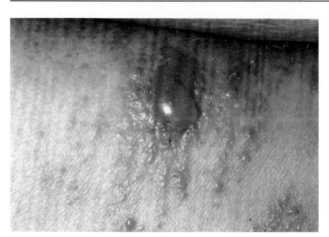

Clin. Fig. IIIB1a.a

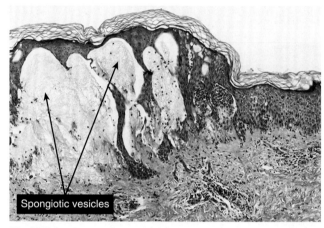

Fig. IIIB1a.a

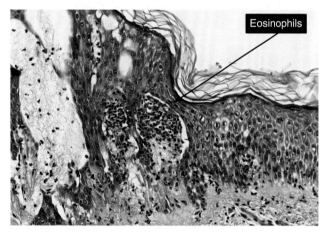

Fig. IIIB1a.b

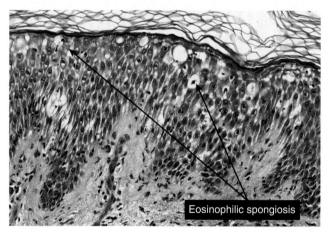

Fig. IIIB1a.c

Clin. Fig. IIIB1a.a. *Allergic contact dermatitis.* Vesicles and bullae developed on volar forearm after application of perfume.

Fig. IIIB1a.a. *Acute allergic contact dermatitis, low power.* The stratum corneum consists of normal basketweave keratin, indicative of an acute disorder that has not had time to elicit alterations in the pattern of keratinization. The epidermis is thickened by spongiosis and exocytosis, with prominent vesicle formation. A dense infiltrate of mononuclear cells is seen about dermal vessels.

Fig. IIIB1a.b. *Acute allergic contact dermatitis, high power.* Tense spongiotic vesicles are formed by the confluence of spongiotic intercellular edema.

Fig. IIIB1a.c. *Acute allergic contact dermatitis, high power.* The epidermis is spongiotic with a diffuse infiltrate of eosinophils (eosinophilic spongiosis).

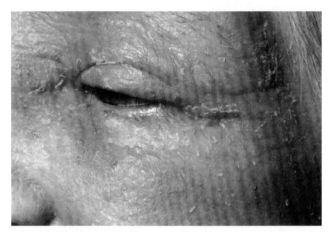

Clin. Fig. IIIB1a.b

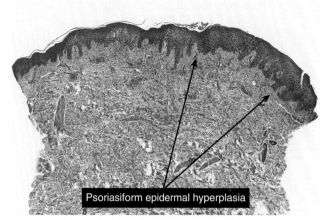

Psoriasiform epidermal hyperplasia

Fig. IIIB1a.d

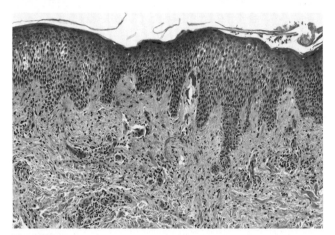

Fig. IIIB1a.e

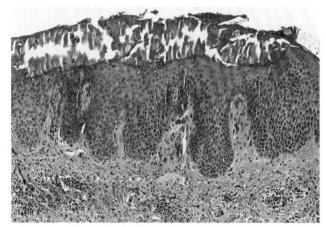

Fig. IIIB1a.f

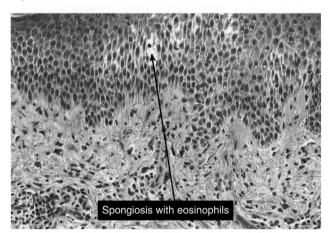

Spongiosis with eosinophils

Fig. IIIB1a.g

Clin. Fig. IIIB1a.b. *Subacute contact dermatitis.* Elderly woman had several month history of pruritic scaly facial erythema and positive fragrance mix patch test.

Fig. IIIB1a.d. *Subacute allergic contact dermatitis, low power.* The stratum corneum is altered by compact orthokeratosis. The epidermis is thickened by mild spongiotic edema, and by moderately prominent psoriasiform hyperplasia (i.e., characterized by elongation of the rete ridges as in psoriasis).

Fig. IIIB1a.e. *Subacute allergic contact dermatitis, medium power.* The epidermis is spongiotic. There is an inflammatory infiltrate in the edematous papillary dermis.

Fig. IIIB1a.f. *Subacute allergic contact dermatitis, medium power.* There is a focal scale-crust in the superficial epidermis, the site of a several day old vesicle. The papillary dermis is edematous and has an infiltrate of lymphocytes and eosinophils diffusely as well as about dermal vessels.

Fig. IIIB1a.g. *Subacute allergic contact dermatitis, high power.* There is a parakeratotic scale overlying a spongiotic epidermis that shows exocytosis of eosinophils. There are numerous eosinophils in the dermal infiltrate.

Conditions to consider in the differential diagnosis:

> spongiotic (eczematous) dermatitis
> atopic dermatitis
> allergic contact dermatitis
> photoallergic drug eruption
> incontinentia pigmenti, vesicular stage
> eczematous nevus (Meyerson nevus)
> erythema gyratum repens
> scabies
> erythema toxicum neonatorum

IIIB1b | Spongiotic Dermatitis, With Plasma Cells

There is marked intercellular edema (spongiosis) within the epidermis. In the dermis, perivascular lymphocytes are predominant, and plasma cells are present. Syphilis is the prototype (see IIIA1c).

Conditions to consider in the differential diagnosis:

> syphilis, primary or secondary lesions
> pinta, primary or secondary lesions
> seborrheic dermatitis in HIV

IIIB1c | Spongiotic Dermatitis, With Neutrophils

There is marked intercellular edema (spongiosis) within the epidermis. Lymphocytes are present in the dermis. There is focal and shoulder parakeratosis, with a few neutrophils in the stratum corneum. *Seborrheic dermatitis* is a prototype (45).

Seborrheic Dermatitis

CLINICAL SUMMARY. Clinically, patients develop erythema and greasy scale on the scalp, paranasal areas, eyebrows, nasolabial folds, and central chest. Rarely, patients with seborrheic dermatitis develop generalized lesions. Patients with HIV infection often have severe, recalcitrant disease (2). In infants, the scalp ("cradle cap"), face, and diaper areas are often involved.

HISTOPATHOLOGY. The histopathologic features are a combination of those observed in psoriasis and spongiotic dermatitis. Mild cases may exhibit only a slight subacute spongiotic dermatitis. The stratum corneum contains focal areas of parakeratosis, with a predilection for the

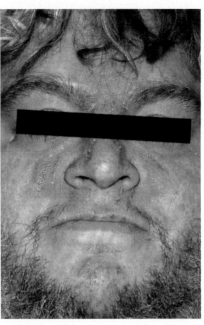

Clin. Fig. IIIB1.c

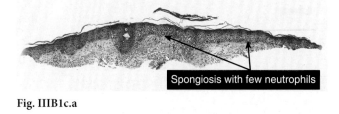

Fig. IIIB1c.a

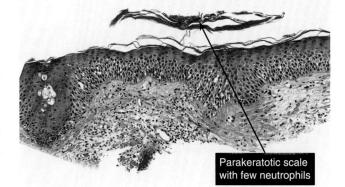

Fig. IIIB1c.b

Clin. Fig. IIIB1.c. *Seborrheic dermatitis.* Greasy erythema involving the nasolabial folds, glabella, medial eyebrows and chin characterize this condition.

Fig. IIIB1c.a. *Seborrheic dermatitis, medium power.* An ortho and parakeratotic scale overlie an acanthotic epidermis that also has spongiosis and exocytosis.

Fig. IIIB1c.b. *Seborrheic dermatitis, high power.* Fragments of polymorphonuclear leukocytes are seen within the keratotic scale overlying an acanthotic epidermis.

follicular ostia, a finding known as "shoulder parakeratosis." Occasional pyknotic neutrophils are present within parakeratotic foci. There is moderate acanthosis with regular elongation of the rete ridges, mild spongiosis, and focal exocytosis of lymphocytes. The dermis contains a sparse mononuclear cell infiltrate. In HIV-infected patients, the epidermis may contain dyskeratotic keratinocytes, and the dermal infiltrate may contain plasma cells. Distinction from psoriasis may be difficult. In a comparative study, features indicating seborrheic dermatitis were follicular plugging, shoulder parakeratosis and prominent lymphocytic exocytosis. Immunohistochemistry (including staining for GLUT-1 which was present in both conditions) was not helpful in differentiating psoriasis from seborrheic dermatitis (46).

Conditions to consider in the differential diagnosis:

dermatophytosis
seborrheic dermatitis
toxic shock syndrome

IIIC SUPERFICIAL DERMATITIS WITH EPIDERMAL ATROPHY (ATROPHIC DERMATITIS)

Most inflammatory dermatoses are associated with epithelial hyperplasia. Only a few chronic conditions exhibit epidermal atrophy.

1. Atrophic Dermatitis, Scant Inflammatory Infiltrates
2. Atrophic Dermatitis, Lymphocytes Predominant
3. Atrophic Dermatitis With Papillary Dermal Sclerosis

IIIC1 Atrophic Dermatitis, Scant Inflammatory Infiltrates

The epidermis is thinned, only a few cell layers thick. There is a scanty lymphocytic infiltrate about the superficial capillary–venular plexus. Aged skin is the prototype (47).

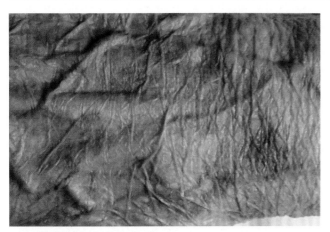

Clin. Fig. IIIC1.a

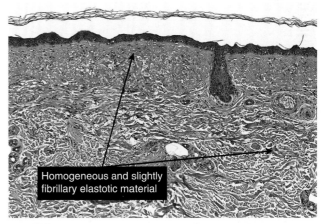

Homogeneous and slightly fibrillary elastotic material

Fig. IIIC1.a

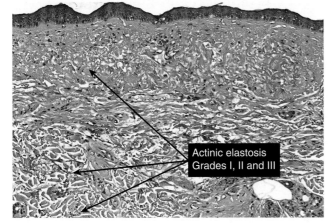

Actinic elastosis Grades I, II and III

Fig. IIIC1.b

Clin. Fig. IIIC1.a. *Aged skin.* Dorsal hand has transparent, wrinkled skin with prominent vessel and solar purpura.

Fig. IIIC1.a. *Aged skin, low power.* There is an effaced atrophic epidermis. The dermis shows marked solar elastosis with dilated thin-walled vessels. The inflammatory infiltrate is sparse.

Fig. IIIC1.b. *Aged skin, medium power.* The epidermis is evenly effaced. It overlies a dermis that has marked solar elastosis and a sparse inflammatory infiltrate. Grades of elastosis can be identified from bottom up: Grade I: Single fibers of gray elastotic material in the deep dermis where penetration of UV is less; Grade II: Bunches or "bushels" of fibers in the mid layer; Grade III: Confluent homogeneous material in the upper dermis.

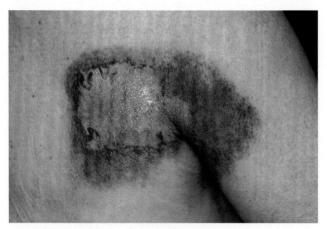

Clin. Fig. IIIC1.b

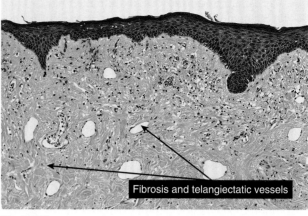

Fibrosis and telangiectatic vessels

Fig. IIIC1.c

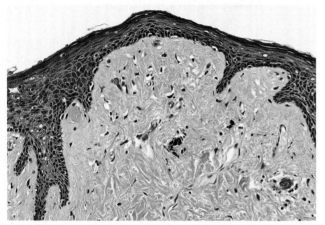

Fig. IIIC1.d

Clin. Fig. IIIC1.b. *A dark reddish patch with recent breakdown and sloughing of necrotic tissue on prior radiation site in a 59-year-old man.*

Fig. IIIC1.c. *Radiation dermatitis, low power.* The low power shows epidermal atrophy with discrete areas of acanthosis and basal layer pigmentation. The dermis is homogeneous and there is telangiectasia.

Fig. IIIC1.d. *Radiation dermatitis, medium power.* There is dermal homogenization with vascular ectasia and a sparse infiltrate about dermal vessels. The epidermis shows atrophy with basal layer pigmentation.

Conditions to consider in the differential diagnosis:

> aged skin
> chronic actinic damage
> radiation dermatitis
> porokeratosis
> acrodermatitis chronica atrophicans
> malignant atrophic papulosis
> poikiloderma atrophicans vasculare

Aged Skin

Although not an inevitable consequence of aging in the skin, actinic elastosis is a prominent feature in the sun-exposed skin of susceptible individuals. A validated grading scheme for actinic elastosis has been described (48).

Chronic Radiation Dermatitis

In late radiation dermatitis, the epidermis is irregular, with variable atrophy and hyperplasia, often with hyperkeratosis. The cells of the stratum malpighii may be disorderly, with individual cell keratinization, and some of the nuclei may be atypical. The epidermis may also have areas of irregular downward growth and may even grow around telangiectatic vessels, nearly enclosing them.

See also VF1.

IIIC2 | Atrophic Dermatitis, Lymphocytes Predominant

The epidermis is thinned, but not as marked as in aged or irradiated skin. In the dermis there are few to many lymphocytes about the superficial capillary-venular plexus.

Conditions to consider in the differential diagnosis:

> parapsoriasis/early mycosis fungoides
> lupus erythematosus
> mixed connective tissue disease
> pinta, tertiary lesions
> dermatomyositis
> poikiloderma atrophicans vasculare

Poikiloderma Atrophicans Vasculare

CLINICAL SUMMARY. Clinically, the term poikiloderma atrophicans vasculare is applied to lesions that, in the early stage, show erythema with slight, superficial scaling, a mottled pigmentation, and telangiectases. In the late stage the skin appears atrophic and the mottled pigmentation and the telangiectases are more pronounced. The condition may be seen in multiple settings, three of which are most important: (1) in association with certain genodermatoses; (2) as an early stage of mycosis fungoides (49); and (3) in association with dermatomyositis and, less commonly, lupus erythematosus. A comprehensive approach to classification and diagnosis of the various forms of poikiloderma has been proposed (50).

Genodermatoses in which the cutaneous lesions are poikilodermatous include: (1) poikiloderma congenitale of Rothmund–Thomson, with the lesions present largely on the face, hands, and feet, and occasionally also on the arms, legs, and buttocks (51); (2) Bloom syndrome, with poikiloderma-like lesions on the face, hands, and forearms (52); (3) dyskeratosis congenita, in which there may be extensive netlike pigmentation (53); and (4) Kindler syndrome which is categorized as a subtype of epidermolysis bullosa and is characterized by poikiloderma, trauma-induced skin blistering, mucosal inflammation, and photosensitivity (54).

Poikiloderma-like lesions as features of early mycosis fungoides may be seen in one of two clinical forms: either as the large plaque (>10 cm) type of parapsoriasis en plaques, also known as poikilodermatous parapsoriasis, or as parapsoriasis variegata, which shows papules arranged in a netlike pattern. Although these two types of parapsoriasis are thought to represent an early stage of mycosis fungoides, not all cases progress clinically into fully developed mycosis fungoides.

The third group of diseases in which lesions of poikiloderma atrophicans vasculare occur is represented by

dermatomyositis and SLE. Dermatomyositis is much more commonly seen as the primary disease than lupus erythematosus, and the association with dermatomyositis often is referred to as poikilodermatomyositis. In contrast to mycosis fungoides, in which poikilodermatous lesions are seen in the early stage, the lesions found in dermatomyositis and SLE generally represent a late stage.

HISTOPATHOLOGY. In early lesions of any cause, there is moderate thinning of the epidermis, with effacement of the rete ridges, and hydropic degeneration of the basal cells. In the upper dermis there is a band-like infiltrate, which in places invades the epidermis. The infiltrate consists mainly of lymphoid cells but also contains a few histiocytes. Melanophages filled with melanin as a result of pigmentary incontinence are found in varying numbers within the infiltrate. In addition, there is edema in the upper dermis and the superficial capillaries are often dilated. In the late stage the epidermis is apt to be markedly thinned and flattened, but the basal cells still show hydropic degeneration. Melanophages and edema of the upper dermis are still present, and telangiectasia may be pronounced.

The amount and type of dermal infiltrate vary with the underlying cause. In the genodermatoses and in dermatomyositis or SLE there is only slight dermal inflammation. In contrast, the inflammatory infiltrate seen in poikiloderma associated with early mycosis fungoides increases with time. Cells with large, hyperchromatic nuclei, so-called mycosis cells, are likely to be present and there is often marked epidermotropism of the infiltrate, which may result in Pautrier microabscesses (55). Even in developing lesions, the papillary dermis is expanded by fibrosis and collagen bundle thickening which increases in rough proportion to lesional age. Thus, in the earliest patches,

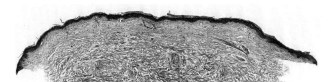

Fig. IIIC2.a

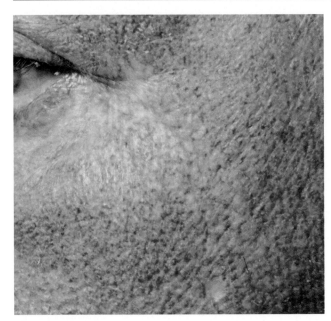

Clin. Fig. IIIC2.a

Clin. Fig. IIIC2.a. *Poikiloderma vasculare atrophicans.* Chronic skin changes in dermatomyositis reveal skin thinning, capillary dilatation, and mild pigmentary change.

Fig. IIIC2.a. *Poikiloderma atrophicans vasculare, low power.* There is a thin, keratotic scale overlying an atrophic epidermis. The papillary dermis is edematous and has a subtle diffuse infiltrate of mononuclear cells. (*continues*)

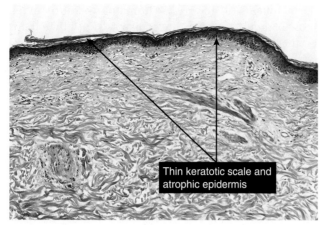

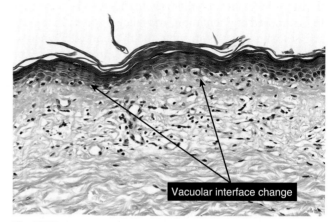

Fig. IIIC2.b   **Fig. IIIC2.c**

Fig. IIIC2.b. *Poikiloderma atrophicans vasculare, medium power.* The thinned atrophic epidermis shows basal layer vacuolar degeneration. In the papillary dermis there is an infiltrate of lymphocytes seen diffusely as well as about thin-walled dermal vessels.

Fig. IIIC2.c. *Poikiloderma atrophicans vasculare, high power.* The epidermis shows focal basal layer liquefaction degeneration and a diffuse infiltrate of lymphocytes in an edematous papillary dermis, with a few lymphocytes extending among basal keratinocytes.

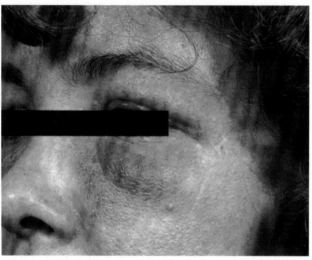

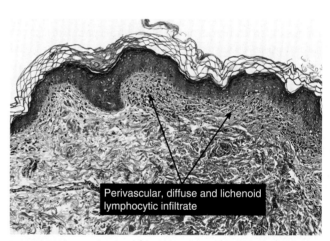

Clin. Fig. IIIC2.b   **Fig. IIIC2.d**

Clin. Fig. IIIC2.b. *Dermatomyositis.* Heliotrope lavender pruritic edematous periorbital changes in middle-aged woman indicates a search for malignancy.

Fig. IIIC2.d. *Dermatomyositis, low power.* The epidermis is little altered in this example. In the dermis there is an infiltrate of mononuclear cells. The papillary dermis is expanded and edematous.

fibrosis is noticeable but subtle, whereas the papillary dermis is coarsely fibrotic late in the patch stage or in fully developed plaques. Thickened collagen bundles often lie roughly parallel to the epidermal surface, in contrast to the vertically oriented collagen bundles that develop secondary to lichenification. The overlying epidermis is nearly normal in the earliest patch lesions, but typically shows slight, regular psoriasiform hyperplasia and hyperkeratosis, although atrophy can be seen in poikilodermatous

patches. Because the specific histologic features of MF are attenuated in poikilodermatous disease, multiple biopsies may be necessary for unequivocal diagnosis.

Dermatomyositis

Old cutaneous lesions of dermatomyositis with the clinical appearance of poikiloderma atrophicans vasculare may have a sparse to band-like infiltrate under an atrophic

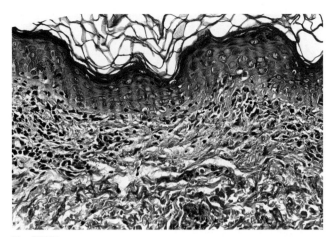

Fig. IIIC2.e

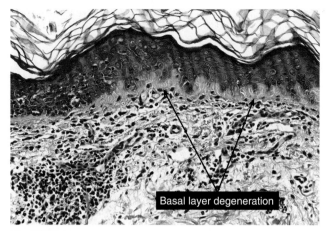

Basal layer degeneration

Fig. IIIC2.f

Fig. IIIC2.e. *Dermatomyositis, medium power.* There is a sparse lichenoid infiltrate at the dermal–epidermal junction that causes basal layer liquefaction degeneration. The papillary dermis is expanded. The infiltrate is diffuse as well as being perivascular and is lymphocytic in type.

Fig. IIIC2.f. *Dermatomyositis, high power.* The basal layer shows distinct basal layer degeneration. The papillary dermis has telangiectatic vessels, and a perivascular as well as diffuse infiltrate of lymphocytes.

epidermis with vacuolar interface change of the basal cell layer. See also IIIH2.

IIIC3 | Atrophic Dermatitis With Papillary Dermal Sclerosis

The epidermis is thinned, there can be hyperkeratosis. The dermis is homogenized and edematous, inflammation is minimal. *Lichen sclerosus et atrophicus* is prototypic (56,57).

Lichen Sclerosus Et Atrophicus

CLINICAL SUMMARY. Lichen sclerosus (LS) encompasses the disorders known as *lichen sclerosus et atrophicus*, *balanitis xerotica obliterans* (LS of the male glans and prepuce), and *kraurosis vulvae* (LS of the female labia majora, labia minora, perineum, and perianal region). Lichen sclerosus is an inflammatory disorder of unknown etiology that affects patients 6 months of age to late adulthood. In both males and females, genital involvement is the most frequent, and often the only, site of involvement. Extragenital lesions may occur with or without coexisting genital lesions. Lesions of LS are characterized by white polygonal papules that coalesce to form plaques. Comedo-like plugs on the surface of the plaque correspond to dilated appendageal ostia. The plugs may disappear as the lesion ages, leaving a smooth, porcelain-white plaque. Solitary or generalized lesions may become bullous and hemorrhagic.

HISTOPATHOLOGY. The salient histologic findings in cutaneous lesions of lichen sclerosus et atrophicus are:

(1) hyperkeratosis with follicular plugging, (2) atrophy of the stratum malpighii with hydropic degeneration of basal cells, (3) pronounced edema and homogenization of the collagen in the upper dermis, and (4) an inflammatory infiltrate in the mid-dermis. Beneath the hyperkeratotic and atrophic epidermis is a broad zone of pronounced lymphedema. Within this zone, the collagen fibers are swollen and homogeneous and contain only a few nuclei. The blood and lymph vessels are dilated, and there may be areas of hemorrhage. In areas of severe lymphedema, clinically visible subepidermal bullae may form. Except in lesions of long duration, an inflammatory infiltrate is present in the dermis. In very early lesions the infiltrate may be found in the uppermost dermis, in direct apposition to the basal layer. The histologic features in early LS may be subtle and may be more prominent in adnexa, with various combinations of acanthosis, hyperkeratosis and hypergranulosis, dystrophic hairs, and basement membrane thickening. The epithelium begins to develop irregular acanthosis, occasionally psoriasiform, and focal basement membrane thickening. Early dermal changes of homogenized collagen and wide ectatic capillaries in superficial dermal papillae are followed by the development of a lymphocytic infiltrate which can be sparse or dense, lichenoid, perivascular or interstitial, with epidermal lymphocyte exocytosis. Dermal melanophages indicate preceding destruction of pigmented keratinocytes and/or melanocytes. Biopsy specimens of early lesions rarely display all features (34). With time, a narrow zone of edema and homogenization of the collagen displaces the inflammatory infiltrate farther down, so that, in well-developed lesions, the infiltrate is found in the mid-dermis. The infiltrate can be patchy, but it is often band-like and

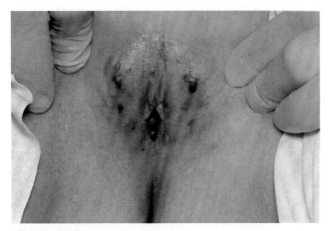

Clin. Fig. IIIC3.a

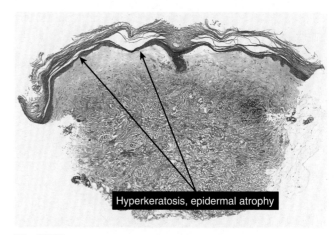

Fig. IIIC3.a

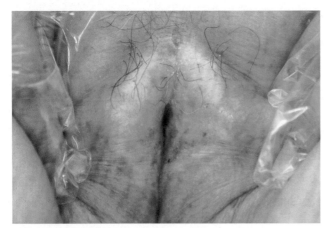

Clin. Fig. IIIC3.b

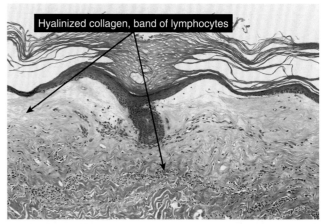

Fig. IIIC3.b

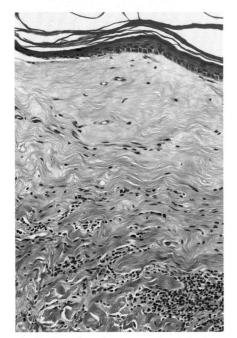

Fig. IIIC3.c

Clin. Fig. IIIC3.a. *Lichen sclerosus et atrophicus.* A "keyhole" ivory colored, sclerotic plaque with hemorrhage, which evolved in a child who had genital pruritus.

Clin. Fig. IIIC3.b. *Lichen sclerosus et atrophicus.* A more advanced lesion in an 86-year-old woman presenting as a smooth porcelain-white plaque extensively involving the vulva, which has been present for several decades.

Fig. IIIC3.a. *Lichen sclerosus et atrophicus, low power.* There is hyperkeratosis overlying an atrophic epidermis. The papillary dermis appears pale and there is an underlying perivascular infiltrate of mononuclear cells.

Fig. IIIC3.b. *Lichen sclerosus et atrophicus, medium power.* Hyperkeratosis overlies an atrophic epidermis. The papillary dermis shows homogenization and there is an underlying infiltrate of lymphocytes about dermal vessels.

Fig. IIIC3.c. *Lichen sclerosus et atrophicus, high power.* There is hyperkeratosis overlying an atrophic effaced epidermis. Underlying the area of homogenization of the papillary dermis is a perivascular as well as a diffuse (often band-like) infiltrate of lymphocytes in the reticular dermis.

composed of lymphoid cells admixed with plasma cells and histiocytes.

Conditions to consider in the differential diagnosis:

lichen sclerosus et atrophicus
thermal burns
parapsoriasis/early mycosis fungoides
poikiloderma atrophicans vasculare

IIID SUPERFICIAL DERMATITIS WITH PSORIASIFORM PROLIFERATION (PSORIASIFORM DERMATITIS)

Psoriasiform proliferation, so called because it is a characteristic feature of psoriasis, is a form of epithelial hyperplasia characterized by uniform elongation of rete ridges. Although the surface may be slightly raised to form a plaque, the epidermal proliferation tends to extend downwards into the dermis, in contrast to a papillomatous pattern in which the rete ridges are elongated upwards above the plane of the epidermal surface and a papilloma (such as a wart) is formed. The prototype is psoriasis, in which the suprapapillary plates are thinned. In most other psoriasiform conditions, the suprapapillary plates are thickened, but not as much as the elongated rete. Because of the increased epithelial turnover, there is often associated hypogranulosis and parakeratosis.

1. Psoriasiform Dermatitis, Mostly Lymphocytes
   1a. Psoriasiform Dermatitis, With Plasma Cells
   1b. Psoriasiform Dermatitis, With Eosinophils
2. Psoriasiform Dermatitis, Neutrophils Prominent (Neutrophilic/Pustular Psoriasiform Dermatitis)
3. Psoriasiform Dermatitis, With Epidermal Pallor and Necrosis ("Nutritional Pattern Dermatoses")

IIID1 Psoriasiform Dermatitis, Mostly Lymphocytes

The epidermis is evenly and regularly thickened in a psoriasiform pattern, spongiosis is variable (rare to absent in psoriasis; common in seborrheic and inflammatory dermatoses). There is an infiltrate of lymphocytes about dermal vessels. *Pityriasis rubra pilaris* is a prototypic example (58).

Pityriasis Rubra Pilaris

CLINICAL SUMMARY. Pityriasis rubra pilaris is an erythematous squamous disorder characterized by follicular plugging and perifollicular erythema that coalesces to form orange-red scaly plaques that frequently contain islands of normal-appearing skin. As the erythema extends, the follicular component is often lost, but it

persists longest on the dorsa of the proximal phalanges. The lesions spread caudally and may progress to a generalized erythroderma. Other clinical findings are palmoplantar keratoderma and scaling of the face and scalp. Most patients clear within 3 years, but some cases are more persistent, especially the circumscribed juvenile type, which is characterized by sharply demarcated lesions on the knees and elbows. Some cases, usually in adults, progress to generalized exfoliative erythroderma. Six subtypes have been identified, with Type 1 "Classical adult" the most common, and Type 6 "HIV-associated" having a poorer prognosis (59).

HISTOPATHOLOGY. The histologic picture of a fully developed erythematous lesion includes acanthosis with broad and short rete ridges, slight spongiosis, thick suprapapillary plates, focal or confluent hypergranulosis, and alternating orthokeratosis and parakeratosis oriented in both vertical and horizontal directions. In the dermis there is a mild superficial perivascular lymphocytic infiltrate and moderately dilated blood vessels.

Areas corresponding to follicular papules show dilated infundibula filled with an orthokeratotic plug and often display perifollicular shoulders of parakeratosis and a mild perifollicular lymphocytic inflammation. Erythrodermic lesions have a thinned or absent cornified layer, plasma exudates, and a diminished granular zone.

Mycosis Fungoides, Patch-Plaque Stage

CLINICAL SUMMARY. Mycosis fungoides (60,61) (MF) is a form of T-cell lymphoma that initially involves the epidermis and papillary dermis, comprising the *patch stage* of the disease. With time, the neoplastic lymphocytes often acquire the capacity to proliferate within the reticular dermis, and plaques, nodules, and tumors (*plaque* and *tumor stages*) are manifest clinically. In some patients, generally after extended periods of time, the neoplasm disseminates to extracutaneous sites such as lymph nodes and viscera. The term MF was coined by Alibert after observing mushroom-like nodules in the tumor stage of the disease. Patches of MF are usually pinkish red and slightly scaly, typically distributed on the trunk and proximal extremities. The buttocks and breasts are often involved. At least some of the patches exceed 10 cm in diameter in most patients, corresponding to the morphologic pattern of "large plaque parapsoriasis." The proportion of patients with patch stage MF that will progress to develop plaques is not precisely known but is thought to be low. Plaques of MF are sharply marginated and are usually red to reddish brown. The centers of plaques can involute, yielding annular or serpiginous morphology. Tumors of MF are morphologically similar to tumors of other cutaneous lymphomas, except that residual patch and plaques are virtually always evident.

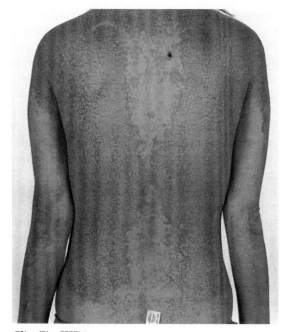

Clin. Fig. IIID1.a

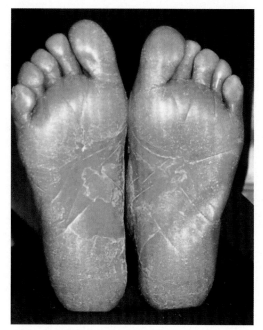

Clin. Fig. IIID1.b

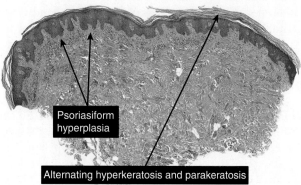

Fig. IIID1.a

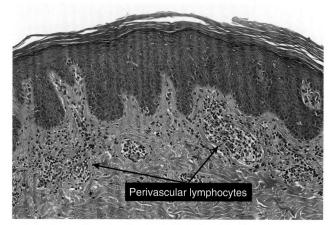

Fig. IIID1.b

Clin. Fig. IIID1.a. *Pityriasis rubra pilaris.* A 22-year-old woman developed confluent well-demarcated orange-red scaling patches with prominent keratotic follicular papules on the trunk, with "skip areas" of normal skin.

Clin. Fig. IIID1.b. *Pityriasis rubra pilaris.* "Keratodermic sandals" present with thick yellow waxy fissured sometimes painful palms and soles.

Fig. IIID1.a. *Pityriasis rubra pilaris, low power.* There is follicular hyperkeratosis with an alternating scale of ortho and parakeratin overlying an acanthotic epidermis. A perivascular infiltrate of mononuclear cells is seen in the dermis.

Fig. IIID1.b. *Pityriasis rubra pilaris, medium power.* The parakeratotic scale has alternating vertical as well as linear parakeratosis. The epidermis is acanthotic with slight spongiosis.

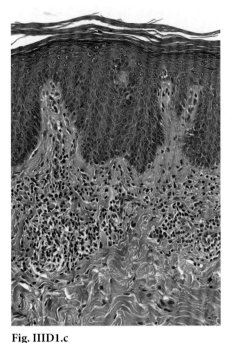

Fig. IIID1.c

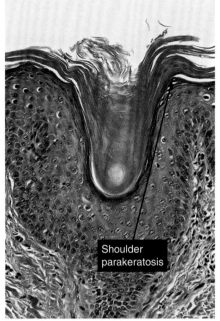

Shoulder parakeratosis

Fig. IIID1.d

Fig. IIID1.c. *Pityriasis rubra pilaris, medium power.* The papillary dermis has a sparse to moderate, perivascular infiltrate of lymphocytes.

Fig. IIID1.d. *Pityriasis rubra pilaris, high power.* There is parakeratosis dipping into the follicular orifice.

HISTOPATHOLOGY. The microscopic findings in the earliest patches of MF are subtle, consisting of a sparse intraepidermal and papillary dermal infiltrate of lymphocytes, arrayed within a fibrotic papillary dermis below an epidermis that shows slight psoriasiform hyperplasia. Because of the sparse infiltrate, multiple biopsies and close clinicopathologic correlation are often needed for diagnosis. Small numbers of lymphocytes, with relatively small but irregular nuclei, are arrayed within the epidermis with minimal associated spongiosis. The lymphocytes are often distributed in a linear array on the epidermal side of the basement membrane zone, an arrangement that has been likened to a string of pearls. Although clusters of intraepidermal lymphocytes, so-called Pautrier microabscesses, are often sought as the key to a diagnosis of MF, a pattern in which lymphocytes are dispersed among keratinocytes is more common in biopsies of macular lesions. Architectural alterations involve both the papillary dermis and the epidermis. The papillary dermis is expanded by fibrosis, whose degree increases in rough proportion to lesional age. Thickened collagen bundles often lie roughly parallel to the epidermal surface, in contrast to the vertically oriented collagen bundles that develop secondary to lichenification. The overlying epidermis typically shows slight, regular psoriasiform hyperplasia and hyperkeratosis in the more advanced lesions. Readily discernible nuclear atypia of lymphocytes is the exception rather than the rule in conventional histologic sections of patch stage disease, but at high magnification, some degree of nuclear convolution is usually

appreciable, especially among the intraepithelial lymphocytes. A working group has recently defined an algorithm for diagnosis of early MF in which clinical, histologic, immunopathologic, and molecular criteria are all considered in a point system (Table III.1) (67). This system will likely add specificity to the process, and emphasizes that none of these attributes, taken in isolation, is uniformly diagnostic.

In plaque stage MF, the papillary dermis is similarly expanded by coarse fibrosis and contains denser, bandlike infiltrates of lymphocytes, with as a rule more prominent epidermotropism. In combination with slight, regular epidermal thickening, these features account for the "lichenoid-psoriasiform" pattern that is characteristic of the late patch stage and the plaque stage. In addition to a papillary dermal infiltrate, the reticular dermis holds superficial and deep perivascular or nearly diffuse infiltrates of lymphocytes. Cytologic atypism, particularly of intraepidermal lymphocytes, is often conspicuous in biopsies from plaques, in contrast to the subtle cytologic changes evident in macular lesions.

IMMUNOPATHOLOGY. Early stages of mycosis fungoides display a predominant CD4+ T-helper 1 (Th1) cytokine profile. It is believed that a shift in cytokine profile from Th1 to Th2 accompanies disease progression. Malignant CD4+ T cells, after stimulation with immature dendritic cells, can adopt a CD4+CD25+ Treg cell phenotype, then appearing to function as immune suppressors by secreting interleukin-10 and transforming growth factor-beta (62). Rare cases of CD4–CD8+, CD4–CD8–,

TABLE III.1. Algorithm for the Diagnosis of Early MF

Criteria	Major (2 points)	Minor (1 point)
Clinical		
Persistent and/or progressive patches and plaques plus	Any 2	Any 1
(1) Non–sun-exposed location		
(2) Size/shape variation		
(3) Poikiloderma		
Histopathologic		
Superficial lymphoid infiltrate plus	Both	Either
(1) Epidermotropism without spongiosis		
(2) Lymphoid atypia[a]		
Molecular/biologic:		
Clonal TCR gene rearrangement	NA[b]	Present
Immunopathologic	NA[b]	Any 1
(1) CD2,3,5 less than 50% of T cells		
(2) CD7 less than 10% of T cells		
(3) Epidermal discordance from expression of CD2,3,5 or CD7 on dermal T cells		
NA indicates not applicable.		

[a]Lymphoid atypia is defined as cells with enlarged hyperchromatic nuclei and irregular or cerebriform nuclear contours.

[b]Not applicable since it cannot fulfill any major criteria.

Adapted from Nofal A, Salah E. Acquired poikiloderma: proposed classification and diagnostic approach. J Am Acad Dermatol 2013;69(3):e129–e140.

CD4+CD8+ immunophenotypes have been described. Hypopigmented MF is more frequent in the CD4–CD8+ group while folliculotropic MF predominates in the CD4+CD8– group (63).

CLONALITY. Identification of dominant T-cell clones in lesions or in blood can be a confirmatory diagnostic test, as determined by detection of alpha/beta or gamma/delta T-cell receptor (TCR) gene rearrangements. Clonality may be difficult to determine in early MF lesions with small neoplastic cell populations, and is found in about 50% of patch, 70% of plaque, and 80% to 100% of tumor stage lesions. The presence of a peripheral blood clone in early MF may imply a worse prognosis. Dominant T-cell clones have also been detected in substantial proportions of patients with benign inflammatory dermatoses. The detection of the same T-cell clone in different biopsy specimens is more supportive of MF (64).

CLINICOPATHOLOGIC DIAGNOSIS. In many cases, the diagnosis of MF can be made with confidence on a skin biopsy accompanied by clinical information. However, a definitive histopathologic diagnosis by light microscopy alone may be difficult to make in early MF or in erythroderma, in which inflammatory cells often predominate in the dermal infiltrate (if any is present). The International Society for Cutaneous Lymphoma has proposed a diagnostic algorithm for early mycosis fungoides (Table III.1) (65).

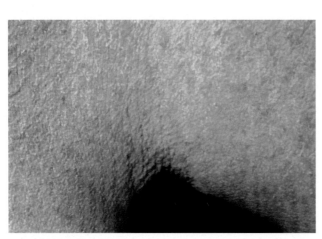

Clin. Fig. IIID1.c

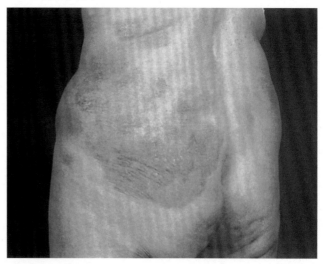

Clin. Fig. IIID1.d

Clin. Fig. IIID1.c. *Parapsoriasis/early mycosis fungoides.* Chronic pruritic maculopapular changes became increasingly indurated with erosions.

Clin. Fig. IIID1.d. *Mycosis fungoides.* A 66-year-old woman presented with a 30-year history of erythematous scaly patches and plaques with telangiectases, atrophy, and pigmentation.

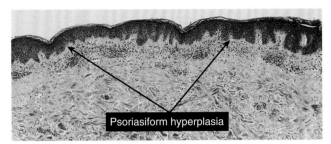

Fig. IIID1.e

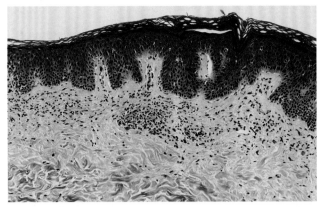

Fig. IIID1.f

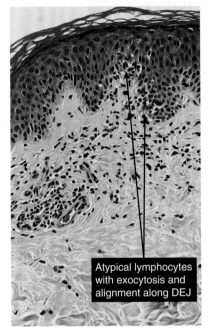

Fig. IIID1.g

Fig. IIID1.e. *Mycosis fungoides, patch stage, low power.* A thin keratin layer overlies an acanthotic epidermis. The papillary dermis is edematous. A mononuclear cell infiltrate about dermal vessels is in the upper reticular dermis.

Fig. IIID1.f. *Mycosis fungoides, patch stage, medium power.* Exocytosis of hyperchromatic lymphocytes into an acanthotic nonspongiotic epidermis is seen. The papillary dermis shows edema and a similar infiltrate that is diffuse within the papillary dermis.

Fig. IIID1.g. *Mycosis fungoides, patch stage, high power.* Exocytosis is characterized by the presence of hyperchromatic mononuclear cells within the acanthotic epidermis; in addition, the cells align along the DEJ. Clinicopathologic correlation, immunoprofiling and possibly gene rearrangement studies would be important to help establish the diagnosis in this case (see Table III.1).

Parapsoriasis

GENERAL. Parapsoriasis is a chronic dermatosis which has been divided into two categories: large-plaque parapsoriasis and small-plaque parapsoriasis. The relationship between parapsoriasis and early mycosis fungoides is not clearly defined and has been controversial. Large-plaque parapsoriasis is generally agreed to be either prelymphomatous or early established lymphoma. Small-plaque parapsoriasis, which has been known as "chronic superficial dermatitis" or "superficial persistent dermatitis," describing its salient clinical characteristics, is generally considered to be a reactive chronic dermatosis with an almost invariably benign clinical course. Ackerman stated that even small-plaque parapsoriasis should be considered to represent early mycosis fungoides (66). Although some cases of evolution have probably been described, this is rare and patients with small-plaque parapsoriasis should not be lumped together with those who have a true lymphoma with potential for life-threatening progression. Simple light microscopy even with immunohistochemical analysis for

CD4/CD8 ratio, aberrant expression of T-cell antigens, and expression of proliferation markers, is often unable to establish a more definitive diagnosis (10). Clinical and molecular criteria are then required. Criteria presented in Table III.1 may be used to help distinguish these difficult cases from early mycosis fungoides. TCR gene rearrangement studies may lack sensitivity in these paucicellular lesions (70).

Conditions to consider in the differential diagnosis:

> chronic spongiotic dermatitis
>> atopic dermatitis
>> seborrheic dermatitis
>> nummular eczema
> lichen simplex chronicus
> prurigo nodularis
> psoriasis
> psoriasiform drug eruptions
> pityriasis rosea
> exfoliative dermatitis

III   Disorders of the Superficial Cutaneous Reactive Unit

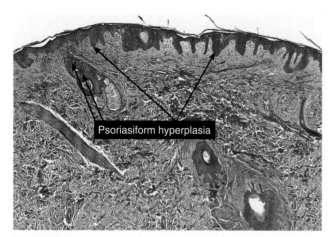

Fig. IIID1.h

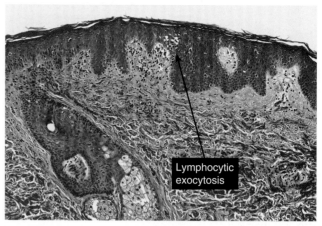

Fig. IIID1.i

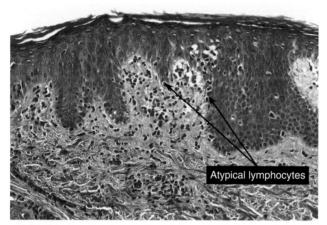

Fig. IIID1.j

Fig. IIID1.h. *Large plaque parapsoriasis/early mycosis fungoides, low power.* There is hyperkeratosis, acanthosis and spongiosis. In the papillary dermis there is a diffuse (albeit subtle) as well as perivascular infiltrate of mononuclear cells.

Fig. IIID1.i. *Parapsoriasis/early mycosis fungoides, medium power.* The lymphocytic infiltrate is patchy and perivascular in the papillary dermis, and extends into the epidermis constituting exocytosis.

Fig. IIID1.j. *Parapsoriasis/early mycosis fungoides, high power.* An orthokeratotic basket-weave layer of keratin overlies an epidermis that is acanthotic with exocytosis of hyperchromatic mononuclear cells and little or no spongiosis. The cells focally align along the junction. In the dermis there is fibrosis, a lymphocytic infiltrate, and melanophage pigmentation.

pityriasis rubra pilaris
parapsoriasis/early mycosis fungoides
verrucous hyperkeratotic mycosis fungoides
inflammatory linear verrucous epidermal nevus (ILVEN)
pellagra
necrolytic migratory erythema (chronic lesions)
acrodermatitis enteropathica
kwashiorkor
reticulated hyperpigmentations (e.g., Dowling–Degos disease)

IIID1a Psoriasiform Dermatitis, With Plasma Cells

The epidermis is evenly thickened and may be spongiotic. There may be exocytosis of lymphocytes. The stratum corneum is variable, often parakeratotic. Plasma cells are found about the superficial vessels in varying numbers, admixed with lymphocytes. Lichen simplex chronicus is a prototype.

Lichen Simplex Chronicus (See also IIIE)

CLINICAL SUMMARY. Any patient with pruritus who chronically rubs the skin may develop lichen simplex chronicus. It often develops in the setting of atopic dermatitis or allergic contact dermatitis. The lesions are pruritic, thickened plaques often with excoriation, in which the normal skin markings are accentuated, the latter finding known as lichenification. The process is commonly seen in chronic vulvar lesions (67).

HISTOPATHOLOGY. Lichen simplex chronicus is the prototype for chronic dermatitis. There is hyperkeratosis interspersed with areas of parakeratosis, acanthosis with irregular elongation of the rete ridges, hypergranulosis, and broadening of the dermal papillae. Slight spongiosis may be observed, but vesiculation is absent. There may be a sparse superficial perivascular infiltrate without exocytosis. In the papillary dermis, there is an increased number of fibroblasts and vertically oriented collagen bundles. As rubbing increases in intensity and chronicity,

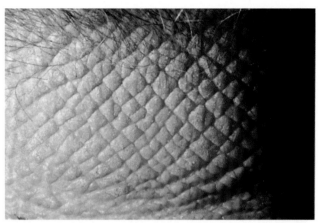

Clin. Fig. IIID1.a

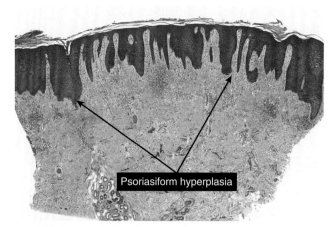

Psoriasiform hyperplasia

Fig. IIID1a.a

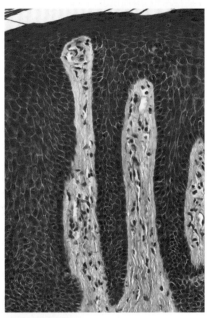

Fig. IIID1a.b

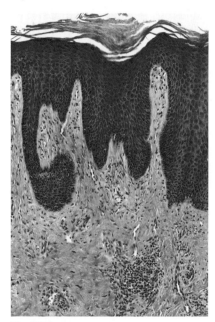

Fig. IIID1a.c

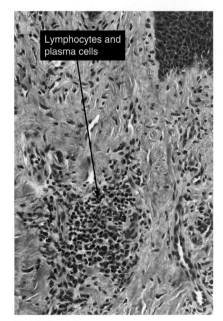

Lymphocytes and plasma cells

Fig. IIID1a.d

Clin. Fig. IIID1.a. *Lichen simplex chronicus.* Chronic "rubbing" of posterior neck led to accentuation and thickening of skin markings.

Fig. IIID1a.a. *Lichen simplex chronicus, low power.* There is a patchy parakeratotic scale overlying an irregularly acanthotic epidermis in which there is fusion of the rete ridges. The dermis is papillomatous, with a perivascular infiltrate of mononuclear cells.

Fig. IIID1a.b. *Lichen simplex chronicus, medium power.* The epidermis shows marked acanthosis without significant exocytosis. There is papillomatosis and a diffuse as well as perivascular infiltrate in the fibrocellular dermis.

Fig. IIID1a.c. *Lichen simplex chronicus, medium power.* There are vertically oriented collagen fibers in the elongated dermal papillae.

Fig. IIID1a.d. *Lichen simplex chronicus, high power.* The dermal infiltrate consists of lymphocytes and (in this case) plasma cells.

epidermal hyperplasia becomes more florid, and the fibrosis more marked.

Conditions to consider in the differential diagnosis:

arthropod bite reactions
secondary syphilis
cutaneous T-cell lymphoma (mycosis fungoides)
prurigo nodularis

IIID1b | Psoriasiform Dermatitis, With Eosinophils

The epidermis is evenly thickened and may be spongiotic, and there may be exocytosis of inflammatory cells, including eosinophils. Eosinophils are easily identified in the dermis and may be numerous in some conditions (e.g., incontinentia pigmenti). *Chronic spongiotic dermatitis* is prototypic (see also IIIB.1a and IIIE).

Chronic Spongiotic Dermatitis

In *chronic spongiotic dermatitis* (e.g., chronic contact dermatitis), there is hyperkeratosis with areas of parakeratosis, often hypergranulosis, and moderate to marked psoriasiform acanthosis. Although spongiosis may be present focally, it is minimal. The inflammatory infiltrate is sparse, often with scattered eosinophils, and papillary dermal fibrosis may be a prominent feature. With chronic rubbing and scratching, the pathology becomes that of lichen simplex chronicus (see also IIIE).

Conditions to consider in the differential diagnosis:

chronic spongiotic dermatitis
chronic allergic dermatitis
chronic atopic dermatitis
exfoliative dermatitis
cutaneous T-cell lymphoma
incontinentia pigmenti, verrucous stage

IIID2 | Psoriasiform Dermatitis, Neutrophils Prominent (Neutrophilic/Pustular Psoriasiform Dermatitis)

The epidermis is evenly thickened, and there is exocytosis (migration of inflammatory cells through the epidermis) of neutrophils. These may collect into abscesses in the epidermis at the level of the stratum corneum (Munro microabscess). The stratum corneum is thickened, parakeratotic and contains neutrophils. *Psoriasis vulgaris* is the prototype (68–70).

Psoriasis Vulgaris

CLINICAL SUMMARY. Psoriasis is a common chronic skin disease which affects approximately 2% of the population. The disease is best placed within the spectrum of immune-related diseases, characterized by chronic inflammation and the absence of infectious agents or antigens (71). Psoriasis vulgaris accounts for the majority of patients with the disease, and is

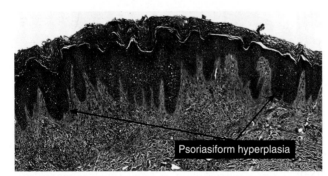

Fig. IIID1b.a

Fig. IIID1b.a. *Chronic spongiotic dermatitis, medium power.* There is hyperkeratosis with even acanthosis. The epidermis, covered by an orthokeratotic scale is acanthotic and shows fusion of the rete ridges. The dermis shows vascular ectasia and a perivascular mononuclear cell infiltrate. The reaction pattern is that of lichen simplex chronicus.

Fig. IIID1b.b. *Chronic spongiotic dermatitis, high power.* The papillary dermis shows fibrosis. The infiltrate in the dermis consists of lymphocytes, often with plasma cells and with eosinophils. The latter finding is consistent with an allergic etiology.

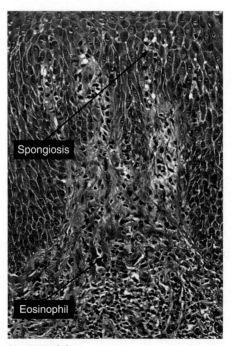

Fig. IIID1b.b

characterized by pink to red papules and plaques which are of variable size, sharply demarcated, dry, and usually covered with layers of fine, silvery scales. As the scales are removed by gentle scraping, fine bleeding points usually are seen, the so-called Auspitz sign. The scalp, sacral region, and extensor surfaces of the extremities are commonly involved, although in some patients the flexural and intertriginous areas (inverse psoriasis) are mainly affected. An acute variant, guttate or eruptive psoriasis, is often seen in younger patients and is characterized by an abrupt eruption of small lesions associated with acute group A beta-hemolytic streptococcal infections. Involvement of the nails is common, and can present with splinter hemorrhages, oil spots, pitting, onycholysis and subungual hyperkeratosis. In severe cases the disease may affect the entire skin and present as generalized erythrodermic psoriasis. Pustules generally are absent in psoriasis vulgaris, although pustules on palms and soles occasionally occur, and rarely, severe psoriasis vulgaris develops into generalized pustular psoriasis. Oral lesions such as stomatitis areata migrans (geographic stomatitis) and benign migratory glossitis may be seen in psoriasis. Psoriatic arthritis characteristically involves the terminal interphalangeal joints, but frequently the large joints are also affected so that a clinical differentiation from rheumatoid arthritis often is impossible, although rheumatoid factor generally is absent.

HISTOPATHOLOGY. The histology varies considerably with the stage of the lesion and usually is diagnostic only in early, scaling papules and near the margin of advancing plaques. At first, there is capillary dilatation and edema in the papillary dermis, with a lymphocytic infiltrate surrounding the capillaries. Keratinocytes in psoriasis appear to be sensitive to the effects of T-cell activation and cytokine production, interferon (IFN)-gamma and TNF-alpha, by responding with psoriasiform hyperplasia (72). The lymphocytes extend into the lower epidermis, where slight spongiosis develops. Then focal changes occur in the upper epidermis, where granular cells become vacuolated and disappear, and mounds of parakeratosis are formed. Neutrophils usually are seen at the summits of some of the mounds of parakeratosis and scattered through an otherwise orthokeratotic cornified layer, representing the earliest manifestation of Munro microabscesses. When there is marked exocytosis of neutrophils, they may aggregate in the uppermost portion of the spinous layer to form small spongiform pustules of Kogoj. A spongiform pustule has aggregates of neutrophils within the interstices of a sponge-like network formed by degenerated and thinned epidermal cells. Munro microabscesses are located within parakeratotic areas of the cornified layer, and

consist of accumulations of neutrophils and pyknotic nuclei of neutrophils that have migrated there from capillaries in the papillae through the suprapapillary epidermis. Lymphocytes remain confined to the lower epidermis, which, as more and more mitoses occur, becomes increasingly hyperplastic. The epidermal changes at first are focal but later on become confluent, leading clinically to plaques.

In the fully developed lesions of psoriasis, as best seen at the margin of enlarging plaques, the histologic picture is characterized by (1) acanthosis with regular elongation of the rete ridges with thickening in their lower portion, (2) thinning of the suprapapillary epidermis with the occasional presence of small spongiform pustules, (3) pallor of the upper layers of the epidermis, (4) diminished to absent granular layer, (5) confluent parakeratosis, (6) the presence of Munro microabscesses, (7) elongation and edema of the dermal papillae, and (8) dilated and tortuous capillaries. Of all these, the spongiform pustules of Kogoj and Munro microabscesses are most consistent with psoriasis, and, in their absence, the diagnosis rarely can be made with certainty on a histologic basis. Spongiform pustules are not pathognomonic of psoriasis, being seen also on occasion in candidiasis, reactive arthritis or Reiter syndrome, geographic tongue, and rarely in secondary syphilis.

Distinction from seborrheic dermatitis can be difficult. In a comparative study, features favoring psoriasis include mounds of parakeratosis with neutrophils, spongiform micropustules of Kogoj, clubbed and evenly elongated rete ridges, and increased mitotic figures (≥6/high-powered field) (50).

Guttate Psoriasis

An acute variant of psoriasis, guttate or eruptive psoriasis, is often seen in younger patients and is characterized by an abrupt eruption of small lesions associated with acute group infections with group A beta-hemolytic streptococci. It is generally accepted that guttate psoriasis has a better prognosis than other types of psoriasis because it involutes rapidly and usually has a longer remission period; however, some cases persist and progress to plaque-type psoriasis (73).

Conditions to consider in the differential diagnosis:

> psoriasis vulgaris
> pustular psoriasis
> keratoderma blenorrhagicum
> reactive arthritis—Reiter syndrome
> pustular drug eruption
> geographic tongue (lingua geographica)
> candidiasis
> pustular secondary syphilis (rare)
> dermatophytosis

III Disorders of the Superficial Cutaneous Reactive Unit

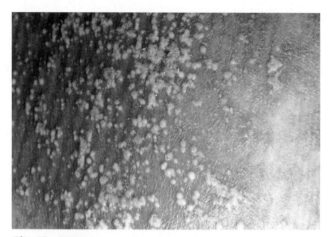

Clin. Fig. IIID2.a

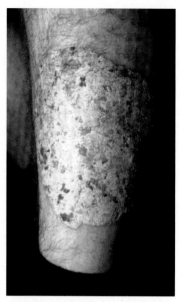

Clin. Fig. IIID2.b

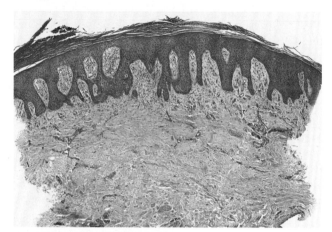

Fig. IIID2.a

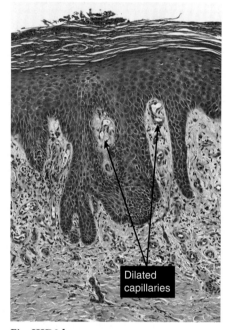

Dilated capillaries

Fig. IIID2.b

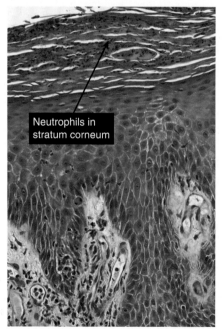

Neutrophils in stratum corneum

Fig. IIID2.c

Clin. Fig. IIID2.a. *Pustular psoriasis.* Rapid development of sterile pustules complicated a case of erythroderma.

Clin. Fig. IIID2.b. *Psoriasis, plaque lesion.* Well-demarcated erythematous plaque with a thick, white silvery scale on extensor surfaces.

Fig. IIID2.a. *Psoriasis vulgaris, low power.* The hyperkeratotic scale is composed of ortho and parakeratin. The epidermis is evenly acanthotic. There is papillomatosis which can give an "inverted clubs" appearance of the epidermis and dermal papillae, and an infiltrate about dermal vessels and in the dermal papillae.

Fig. IIID2.b. *Psoriasis vulgaris, medium power.* The parakeratotic scale contains fragments of neutrophils. The epidermis shows even acanthosis with some rete ridge fusion. The papillary dermis is edematous and well vascularized.

Fig. IIID2.c. *Psoriasis vulgaris, high power.* The scale contains a collection of polymorphonuclear leukocytes and parakeratin. The epidermis is acanthotic. The papillary dermis is well vascularized with discrete areas of hemorrhage.

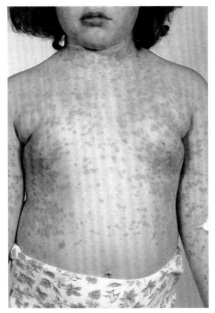

Clin. Fig. IIID2.c

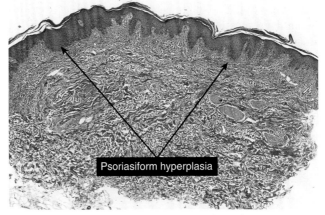

Fig. IIID2.d

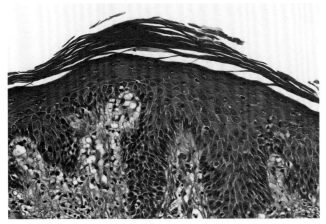

Fig. IIID2.e

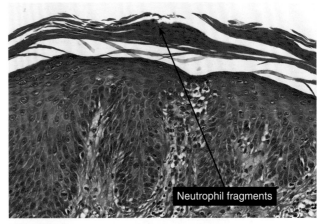

Fig. IIID2.f

Clin. Fig. IIID2.c. *Guttate psoriasis.* Eruptive "drop-like" and small plaques which cleared following therapy for beta-hemolytic streptococcal infection.

Fig. IIID2.d. *Guttate psoriasis, low power.* Psoriasiform hyperplasia and a parakeratotic scale.

Fig. IIID2.e. *Guttate psoriasis, medium power.* Parakeratotic scale and slight epidermal spongiosis.

Fig. IIID2.f. *Guttate psoriasis, high power.* There is a focal collection of neutrophils in the parakeratotic stratum corneum.

IIID3 Psoriasiform Dermatitis, With Epidermal Pallor and Necrosis ("Nutritional Pattern" Dermatoses)

In this group of conditions, often associated with nutritional deficiency, the epidermis is thickened with elongated rete ridges, especially in chronic lesions, and in many cases there is characteristic pallor and individual or confluent necrosis of superficial keratinocytes, attributable to deficiency of essential nutrients, or idiopathic in some cases. The histologic findings may be indistinguishable between necrolytic acral erythema, necrolytic migratory erythema, fatty acid deficiency, zinc deficiency (acrodermatitis enteropathica), pellagra, and biotin deficiency. These diagnoses must be excluded clinically. Necrolytic migratory erythema is prototypic (74).

Necrolytic Migratory Erythema (Glucagonoma Syndrome)

CLINICAL SUMMARY. Necrolytic migratory erythema is the name given to the cutaneous manifestations of a glucagon-secreting pancreatic carcinoma originating from alpha islet cells (74,75). Due to elevated serum glucagon, patients have sustained gluconeogenesis, which results in negative nitrogen balance with amino acid degradation. This gives a clinical picture similar to nutritional deficiencies such as acrodermatitis enteropathica and pellagra. The skin lesions are characteristically distributed periorofically on the face, the perineum and genitals, and shins, feet, and ankles. There are erythematous patches and plaques that may appear circinate due to peripheral spreading. Flaccid blisters may develop that rupture easily, leaving erosions. Lesions heal rapidly while new ones continually develop, resulting in daily fluctuations in the appearance of the eruption. Mucosal lesions may be manifested by cheilitis and glossitis. Nails may be involved and become brittle. The eruption can precede other findings of a pancreatic tumor by years, and in approximately 50% of patients, metastases are present at the time of diagnosis.

Nonskin manifestations of the glucagonoma syndrome include weight loss, anemia, glucose intolerance, and adult-onset diabetes. Surgical resection of the tumor or infusion of amino acids can produce resolution of skin lesions. Conditions other than glucagonoma including various carcinomas, cirrhosis, and glucagon cell adenomatosis, a benign condition that may nevertheless have devastating endocrine effects, have been reported to give a similar rash (76).

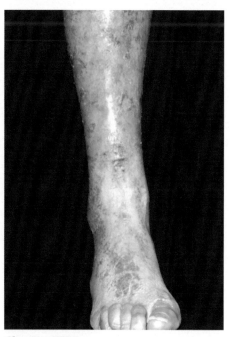

Clin. Fig. IIID3.a

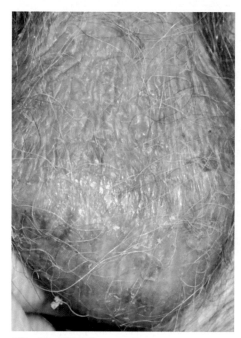

Clin. Fig. IIID3.b

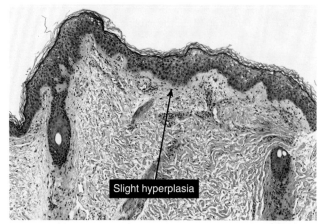

Slight hyperplasia

Fig. IIID3.a

Clin. Fig. IIID3.a. *Necrolytic migratory erythema.* Note the erosions on the lower extremities.

Clin. Fig. IIID3.b. *Necrolytic migratory erythema.* Note erosions on the scrotum. Biopsy confirmed the diagnosis. Resection of the glucagonoma resulted in resolution of this patient's burning skin lesions.

Fig. IIID3.a. *Necrolytic migratory erythema, low power.* More acute lesions may show mild acanthosis, and there is hypogranulosis with pallor of the upper epidermis.

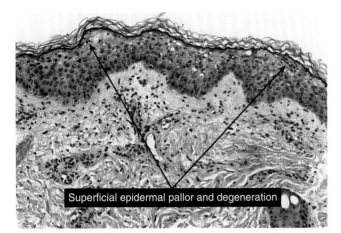

Fig. IIID3.b

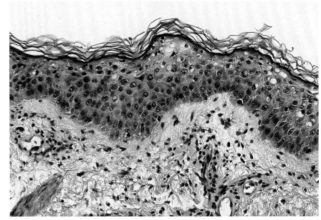

Fig. IIID3.c

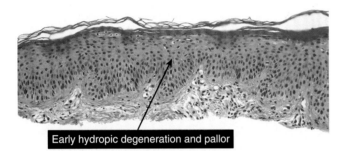

Fig. IIID3.d

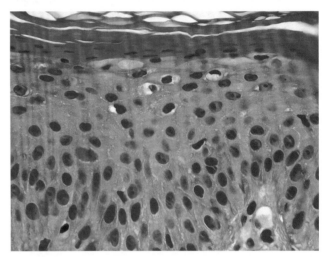

Fig. IIID3.e

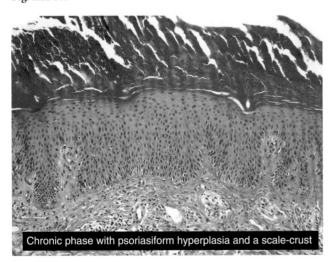

Fig. IIID3.f

Fig. IIID3.b,c. *Necrolytic migratory erythema, medium and high power.* Keratinocytes in the upper stratum spinosum show early hydropic degeneration. Maturation of keratinocytes is somewhat disordered.

Fig. IIID3.d,e. *Necrolytic migratory erythema, medium and high power.* In a later phase there is a thin layer of parakeratosis, with hydropic degeneration and pallor of superficial keratinocytes.

Fig. IIID3.f. *Necrolytic migratory erythema, medium power.* A chronic lesion with a necrotic scale-crust, parakeratosis and epidermal hyperplasia.

HISTOPATHOLOGY. A fresh, acute lesion yields the most diagnostic information, as it characteristically shows necrosis of the upper layers of the epidermis, which can then detach from the viable layers beneath. Keratinocytes undergoing necrosis may show hydropic swelling, pallor, or eosinophilia with nuclear pyknosis. Neutrophils enter the epidermis and may produce a subcorneal pustule, while in the superficial dermis there is a perivascular lymphocytic infiltrate and often papillary dermal edema. In chronic lesions there is psoriasiform epidermal hyperplasia. All phases can show architectural disarray with vacuolar change and a diminished granular cell layer. The stratum corneum often shows broad areas of parakeratosis.

Necrolytic Acral Erythema

CLINICAL SUMMARY. Necrolytic acral erythema (NAE) is a papulosquamous eruption that occurs in

III Disorders of the Superficial Cutaneous Reactive Unit

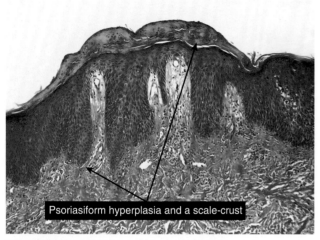

Psoriasiform hyperplasia and a scale-crust

Fig. IIID3.g

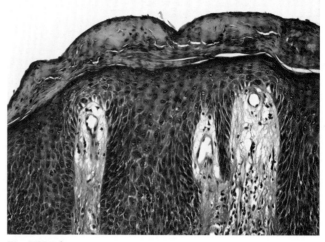

Fig. IIID3.h

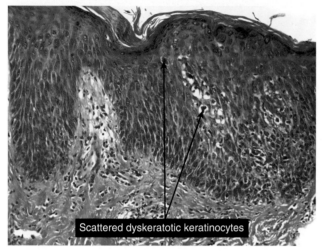

Scattered dyskeratotic keratinocytes

Fig. IIID3.i

Fig. IIID3.g. *Necrolytic acral erythema, medium power.* There is psoriasiform epidermal hyperplasia with a thickened ortho and parakeratotic stratum corneum. There is a mild perivascular mixed inflammatory infiltrate in the superficial dermis.

Fig. IIID3.h. *Necrolytic acral erythema, high power.* There are areas of hypogranulosis and/or pallor of the upper epidermal layers. There may be edema of the papillary dermis, as here.

Fig. IIID3.i. *Necrolytic acral erythema, medium power.* The epidermis may also show scattered dyskeratotic keratinocytes.

association with hepatitis C virus infection (77,78). Many of the described cases have occurred in Egypt, however it has also been reported in the United States. The condition may appear before the discovery of the hepatitis C infection (79). Early lesions may present with erosions and flaccid blisters. Fully evolved lesions are erythematous, dusky, hyperpigmented plaques with a darker peripheral rim. Hyperkeratosis may be prominent. The characteristic distribution is involvement of the distal extremities, however proximal extremities and truncal lesions have also been described.

HISTOPATHOLOGY. Histopathologic findings of NAE include psoriasiform epidermal hyperplasia, hyperkeratosis with parakeratosis, and a diminished granular cell layer. Characteristic findings also include individual keratinocyte necrosis and pallor of the superficial epidermal

layer. Vacuolar alteration may be present. The dermis reveals a superficial perivascular mononuclear cell infiltrate. There are overlapping histologic features with psoriasis, however the presence of spongiform pustules would favor a diagnosis of psoriasis; individual keratinocyte necrosis favors NAE.

Pellagra

CLINICAL SUMMARY. Pellagra was first discovered as a potential complication of diet dominated by corn-meal, a cheap energy-rich food source that fails to provide adequate levels of niacin (nicotinic acid, vitamin B_3) (80). Other causes include general malnutrition, often associated with alcoholism, metabolic enzyme deficiency (Hartnup disease), metabolic "steal" of nutrients by tumors, malabsorption, and certain drugs. The features of pellagra include the "four Ds": dermatitis, diarrhea, dementia and,

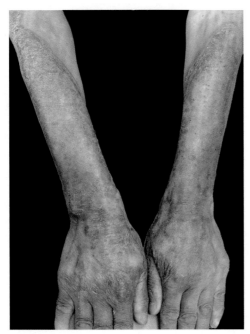

Clin. Fig. IIID3.c

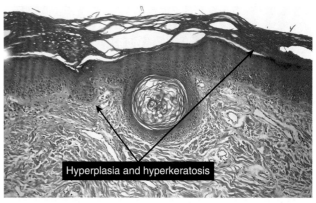

Fig. IIID3.j

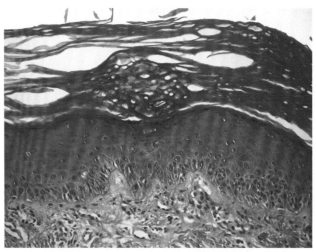

Fig. IIID3.k

Clin. Fig. IIID3.c. *Pellagra.* Hyperpigmentation with scaling, thickening, and roughness of the skin with a photo distribution in a 51-year-old man with chronic alcoholism.

Fig. IIID3.j. *Pellagra, low power.* Skin biopsy from a patient with carcinoid syndrome. There is hyperkeratosis and there may be mild keratotic follicular plugging.

Fig. IIID3.k. *Pellagra, high power.* The hyperkeratosis is composed of orthokeratin, but parakeratosis can be seen. There may be architectural disarray of the epidermis.

---

if left untreated, death. The dermatitis is related to extreme photosensitivity.

The rash is typically bilateral, symmetrical and limited to exposed sites of solar exposure. It is well-defined and usually most prominent on the dorsum of hands, "V" of the neck, face, radial aspects of the forearms, and exposed skin on legs and feet. The early clinical features at this stage closely resemble sunburn with erythema and skin edema as dominant signs. Vesicles may occur in acute and severe attacks. In contrast to sunburn, where erythema and swelling typically fade within days, in pellagra the skin becomes darker with scaling and prominent hyperpigmentation. In long-established disease, hyperpigmentation increases and becomes the dominant cutaneous sign, in association with skin thickening, dryness and roughness. Painful fissures involve palms and soles.

HISTOPATHOLOGY. The histologic features are nondiagnostic, but can include psoriasiform epidermal hyperplasia with hyperkeratosis. In one study, histologic features ranged from mild lymphocytic inflammation and moderate vacuolization to severe cases with extensive necrosis of keratinocytes. Langerhans cells have been found to be reduced in the affected skin (81).

Conditions to consider in the differential diagnosis:

necrolytic migratory erythema
fatty acid deficiency
acrodermatitis enteropathica
pellagra
biotin deficiency
psoriasis
graft-versus-host disease
subacute cutaneous lupus erythematosus
dermatomyositis
pityriasis rubra pilaris
toxic drug eruptions
cystic fibrosis associated dermatitis

III　Disorders of the Superficial Cutaneous Reactive Unit

IIIE SUPERFICIAL DERMATITIS WITH IRREGULAR EPIDERMAL PROLIFERATION ("HYPERTROPHIC DERMATITIS")

Irregular thickening and thinning of the epidermis is seen in some reactive conditions, but the possibility of squamous cell carcinoma should also be considered. As in other conditions associated with increased epithelial turnover, there may be hypogranulosis and parakeratosis.

1. Hypertrophic Dermatitis, Lymphocytes Predominant
   1a. Irregular Epidermal Proliferation, Plasma Cells Present
2. Irregular Epidermal Proliferation, Neutrophils Prominent
3. Irregular Epidermal Proliferation, Above A Neoplasm

IIIE1 Hypertrophic Dermatitis, Lymphocytes Predominant

The epidermis is irregularly thickened, with areas of normal thickness, of acanthosis and of thinning. Lymphocytes are the predominant inflammatory cell about the dermal vessels. *Prurigo nodularis* is a prototype.

Prurigo Nodularis

CLINICAL SUMMARY. Prurigo nodularis (82) is a chronic skin dermatitis characterized by discrete, raised, firm hyperkeratotic papulonodules, usually from 5 to 12 mm in diameter but occasionally larger. They occur chiefly on the extensor surfaces of the extremities and are intensely pruritic. The disease usually begins in middle age and women are more frequently affected than men. Prurigo nodularis may coexist with lesions of lichen simplex chronicus and there may be transitional lesions. The cause remains unknown but

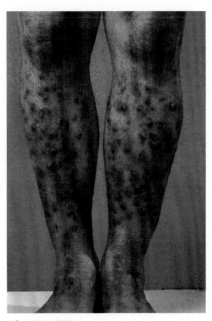

Clin. Fig. IIIE.1

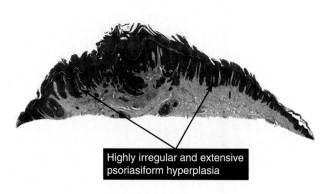

Highly irregular and extensive psoriasiform hyperplasia

Fig. IIIE1.a

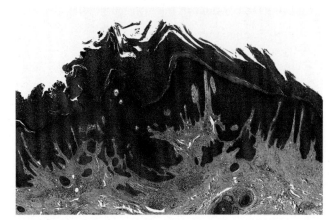

Fig. IIIE1.b

Clin. Fig. IIIE.1. *Prurigo nodularis.* Hyperpigmented ill-defined papules and nodules in accessible body sites result from repeated picking and scratching.

Fig. IIIE1.a. *Prurigo nodularis/lichen simplex chronicus, low power.* There is marked irregular hyperplasia of the epidermis as well as hyperkeratosis. At the periphery of prurigo nodularis, the changes are those of lichen simplex chronicus.

Fig. IIIE1.b. *Prurigo nodularis/lichen simplex chronicus, medium power.* At higher magnification there may be hypergranulosis and the hyperplastic epithelium is composed of bland-appearing keratinocytes without cytologic atypia. In a fully-evolved case, there is irregular downward proliferation of the epidermis and adnexal epithelium approaching pseudocarcinomatous hyperplasia.

local trauma, insect bites, atopic background, metabolic or systemic diseases, have been implicated as predisposing factors in some cases. An association with *H. pylori* infection of the stomach has been described (83).

HISTOPATHOLOGY. There are pronounced hyperkeratosis and irregular acanthosis. There may be papillomatosis and irregular downward proliferation of the epidermis and adnexal epithelium approaching pseudoepitheliomatous (pseudocarcinomatous) hyperplasia. In the papillary dermis, there is a predominantly lymphocytic inflammatory infiltrate and vertically oriented collagen bundles. Occasionally, prominent neural hyperplasia may be observed; however, this is an uncommon finding and is not considered to be an essential feature for the diagnosis of prurigo nodularis. Eosinophils and marked eosinophil degranulation may be seen more frequently in patients with an atopic background. Plasma cells may be present in many examples. In a systematic analysis of 136 cases, findings highly characteristic for PN included the presence of thick compact orthohyperkeratosis; the "hairy palm sign" (folliculosebaceous units in nonvolar skin in conjunction with a thick and compact cornified layer, like that of volar skin); irregular epidermal hyperplasia or pseudoepitheliomatous hyperplasia; focal parakeratosis; hypergranulosis; fibrosis of the papillary dermis with vertically arranged collagen fibers; increased number of fibroblasts and capillaries; a superficial, perivascular and/or interstitial inflammatory infiltrate of lymphocytes, macrophages and, to a lesser extent, eosinophils and neutrophils (84).

Conditions to consider in the differential diagnosis:

> lichen simplex chronicus
> inflammatory linear verrucous nevus (ILVEN, psoriasiform category)
> prurigo nodularis
> lichen simplex chronicus
> incontinentia pigmenti, verrucous stage
> pellagra (niacin deficiency)
> Hartnup disease

IIIE1a | Irregular Epidermal Proliferation, Plasma Cells Present

The epidermis is irregularly acanthotic. Plasma cells are found about the dermal vessels admixed with lymphocytes.

Actinic Keratosis (See also IIA1)

See Figs. IIIE1a.a,b.

Conditions to consider in the differential diagnosis:

> actinic keratosis
> squamous cell carcinoma *in situ* and invasive
> basal cell carcinoma
> pseudoepitheliomatous hyperplasia
> lichen simplex chronicus
> prurigo nodularis
> erythroplasia of Queyrat

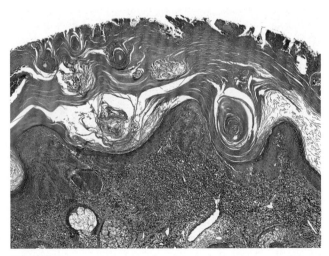

Fig. IIIE1a.a

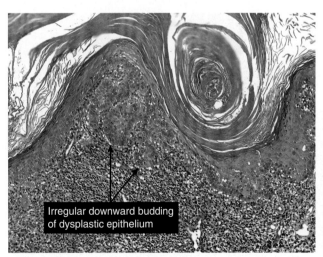

Irregular downward budding of dysplastic epithelium

Fig. IIIE1a.b

Fig. IIIE1a.a. *Hypertrophic actinic keratosis, medium power.* There is an ortho and parakeratotic scale overlying an acanthotic epidermis that shows loss of natural maturation. The dermis has a dense infiltrate of mononuclear cells and discrete hemorrhage.

Fig. IIIE1a.b. *Hypertrophic actinic keratosis, high power.* There is atypical epidermal proliferation in which there is no distinction between basal cells and epidermal keratinocytes. The dermis contains an infiltrate of plasma cells, lymphocytes and there is vascular ectasia.

rupial secondary syphilis, condyloma lata
yaws, primary or secondary
pinta, primary or secondary lesions
pemphigus vegetans

IIIE2 | Irregular Epidermal Proliferation, Neutrophils Prominent

The epidermis has focal areas of acanthosis, neutrophils
can be seen as exocytotic cells, and are found in the dermis
in abscesses and about dermal vessels without there being
a primary vasculitis. Most examples of these epithelial
reactions are associated with inflammation that involves
the reticular dermis as well as the papillary dermis, such as
deep fungus infections, and also halogenodermas. Keratoacanthoma is a neoplastic example.

Keratoacanthoma (See also VIB1)

Collections of neutrophils are commonly seen in keratoacanthomas, and could simulate an inflammatory condition in a superficial biopsy.

Deep Fungus Infection (See also VD1)

See Fig. IIIE2.b.

Conditions to consider in the differential diagnosis:

deep fungal infections (superficial biopsy, see also VD1)
halogenodermas
botryomycosis

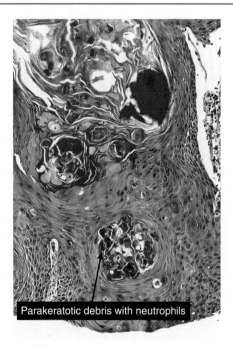

Fig. IIIE2.a

Fig. IIIE2.a. *Keratoacanthoma, high power.* Intratumoral
abscesses of polymorphonuclear leukocytes are a common feature in keratoacanthomas.

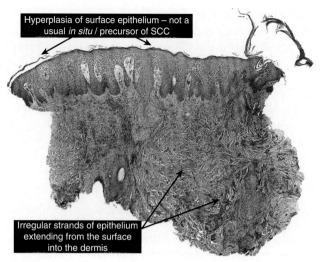

Hyperplasia of surface epithelium – not a
usual *in situ* / precursor of SCC

Irregular strands of epithelium
extending from the surface
into the dermis

Fig. IIIE2.b

Fig. IIIE2.b. *Pseudoepitheliomatous hyperplasia.* A biopsy of a
violaceous nodule revealed an irregular proliferation of mature
squamous epithelium extending into the dermis, simulating an
invasive squamous cell carcinoma. Culture was positive for Rhi-
zopus fungus, and a subsequent excision revealed colonies of
organisms with abscess formation.

keratoacanthoma
impetigo contagiosa
granuloma inguinale

IIIE3 | Irregular Epidermal Proliferation, Above A Neoplasm

The epidermis is irregularly acanthotic. There is an associated neoplastic infiltrate, in the epidermis or dermis, or in
both. Most of these neoplasms involve the reticular dermis as well as the papillary dermis (see also section VI).

Verrucous Melanoma (See also VIB3)

In a series of lesions classified as verrucous nevoid and
keratotic malignant melanomas, a clinical diagnosis of
benign lesions (warty nevi, papillomas, seborrheic keratoses and cysts) had been made in over 50% of the cases.
Microscopically, these lesions exhibited a spectrum of
nevoid and/or keratotic features such as symmetry, exophytic and papilliferous growth pattern, hyperkeratosis
and pseudoepitheliomatous hyperplasia. Most also had
lateral intraepidermal spread and were composed of large
epithelioid cells exhibiting various degrees of cellular
pleomorphism. Initially, 10% of the cases were histologically diagnosed as benign, however 7 of 20 patients with
these lesions ultimately died of their disease (85).

Conditions to consider in the differential diagnosis:

malignant melanoma ("verrucous" pattern)
granular cell tumor

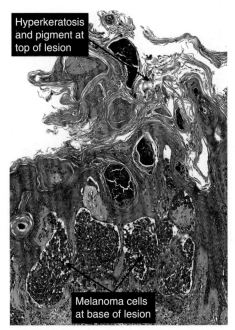

Hyperkeratosis and pigment at top of lesion

Melanoma cells at base of lesion

Fig. IIIE3.a

Fig. IIIE3.a. *Verrucous melanoma.* There is verrucous epidermal hyperplasia, associated with a proliferation of neoplastic melanocytes.

IIIF SUPERFICIAL DERMATITIS WITH LICHENOID INFILTRATES (LICHENOID DERMATITIS)

Lichenoid inflammation is a dense "band-like" infiltrate of small lymphocytes clustered about the dermal–epidermal junction and obscuring the interface. The epidermis is variable in its thickness, amount of exocytotic lymphocytes, and the integrity of the basal cell zone (liquefaction degeneration). Hypergranulosis due to delayed epidermal maturation is a commonly associated feature. For the same reason, there may be orthokeratotic hyperkeratosis. Apoptotic or necrotic keratinocytes are often present. In lichen planus, these are called Civatte bodies. Pigmentary incontinence (melanin-laden macrophages in the papillary dermis) is common, as in any condition in which there is destruction of basal keratinocytes.

1. Lichenoid Dermatitis, Lymphocytes Exclusively
2. Lichenoid Dermatitis, Lymphocytes Predominant
   2a. Lichenoid Dermatitis, Eosinophils Present
   2b. Lichenoid Dermatitis, Plasma Cells Present
   2c. Lichenoid Dermatitis, With Melanophages
3. Lichenoid Dermatitis, Histiocytes Predominant
4. Lichenoid Dermatitis, Mast Cells Predominant
5. Lichenoid Dermatitis With Dermal Fibroplasia

IIIF1 Lichenoid Dermatitis, Lymphocytes Exclusively

The band-like infiltrate is composed almost exclusively of lymphocytes. Eosinophils and plasma cells are essentially absent. *Lichen planus* is the prototype (86).

Lichen Planus

CLINICAL FEATURES. Lichen planus is a subacute or a chronic dermatosis that may involve skin, mucous membranes, hair follicles, and nails. In glabrous skin, the eruption is characterized by small, flat-topped, shiny, polygonal, violaceous papules that may coalesce into plaques. The papules often show a network of white lines known as Wickham striae. Itching is usually pronounced. The disease has a predilection for the flexor surfaces of the forearms, legs, and the glans penis. The eruption may be localized or extensive and Koebner phenomenon (exacerbation or elicitation of lesions by trauma) is commonly seen. A common variant is *hypertrophic lichen planus*, which is usually found on the shins and consists of thickened, often verrucous plaques. Associations of LP include stress/anxiety, hepatitis C virus (HCV), autoimmune diseases, internal malignancies, dyslipidemia, and viral infections (87,95). A longitudinal follow-up study of patients with oral lichen planus demonstrated a significant increase in the risk for oral squamous cell carcinoma (88), suggesting that this may be a premalignant lesion; however distinction of oral lichen planus from lichenoid inflammation in an already established squamous dysplasia of the oral mucosa can be difficult. Cutaneous lichen planus is not considered a premalignant condition.

HISTOPATHOLOGY. Typical papules of lichen planus show (1) compact orthokeratosis with very few, if any, parakeratotic cells, a fact that is important for the diagnosis, (2) wedge-shaped hypergranulosis with coarse and abundant keratohyalin granules, (3) irregular acanthosis giving rise to dome-shaped dermal papillae and to pointed or "saw-toothed" rete ridges, (4) damage to the basal cell layer with vacuolar degeneration and apoptosis of the basal cells giving rise to the characteristic round eosinophilic apoptotic bodies (as colloid, hyaline, cytoid, or Civatte bodies), and (5) a band-like dermal lymphocytic infiltrate which is composed almost entirely of lymphocytes intermingled with macrophages. A few eosinophils and/or plasma cells may be seen in close approximation to the epidermis, but these are rare except in some examples of hypertrophic lichen planus. Wickham striae are believed to be caused by a focal increase in the thickness of the granular layer and of the total epidermis. Occasionally, small areas of artifactual separation between the epidermis and the dermis, known as Max–Josef spaces, are seen. In some instances, the separation occurs *in vivo* and subepidermal blisters form (*bullous lichen planus*). These vesicles form as a result of extensive damage to the basal

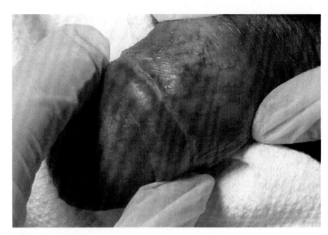

Clin. Fig. IIIF1.a

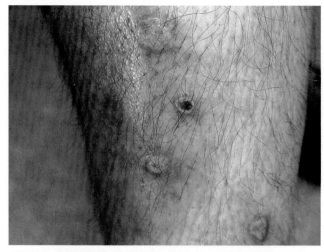

Clin. Fig. IIIF1.b

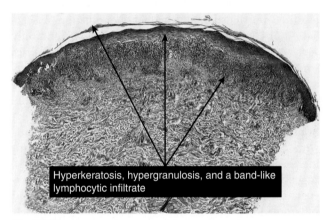

Hyperkeratosis, hypergranulosis, and a band-like lymphocytic infiltrate

Fig. IIIF1.a

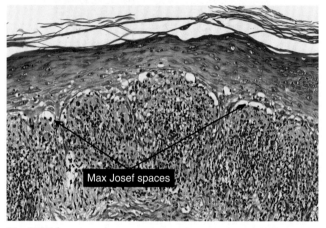

Max Josef spaces

Fig. IIIF1.b

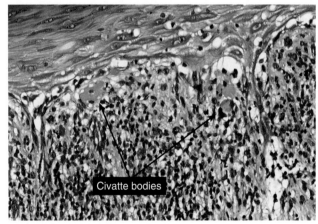

Civatte bodies

Fig. IIIF1.c

Clin. Fig. IIIF1.a. *Lichen planus.* 1 to 5 mm violaceous polygonal papules on coronal sulcus with Wickham striae followed longstanding lacy changes on buccal mucosa.

Clin. Fig. IIIF1.b. *Lichen planus.* Multiple flat-topped violaceous polygonal papules on the lower leg in a 41-year-old man.

Fig. IIIF1.a. *Lichen planus, low power.* There is a band-like infiltrate that occupies the papillary dermis and obscures the dermal–epidermal interface. A thin keratin scale covers the epidermis.

Fig. IIIF1.b. *Lichen planus, medium power.* The infiltrate of lymphocytes at the dermal–epidermal interface obscures and obliterates basal cells. There are also areas of separation. The epidermis is thickened and there is hypergranulosis.

Fig. IIIF1.c. *Lichen planus, high power.* There is focal hypergranulosis with overlying hyperkeratosis. The infiltrate consists of lymphocytes with the presence of eosinophilic bodies (Civatte bodies) within the inflammatory infiltrate.

cells. In old lesions the cellular infiltrate decreases in density, but the number of macrophages increases. In areas in which a basal cell layer has reformed, the dermal infiltrate no longer lies in close approximation to the epidermis. Chronic lesions may show considerable acanthosis, papillomatosis, and hyperkeratosis (*hypertrophic lichen planus*). LP is a T-cell–mediated autoimmune disease, involving T-helper and T-cytotoxic lymphocytes, natural killer (NK) cells, and dendritic cells. T-cell activation is central to the pathogenesis of LP (95).

Graft-Versus-Host Disease

Graft-versus-host disease (89) presents with both lichenoid and vacuolar dermatitis, see also IIIH1:

CLINICAL FEATURES: Graft-versus-host disease (GVHD) occurs in situations in which donor immunocompetent T cells are transferred into allogeneic hosts incapable of rejecting them. The sources of the T cells include primarily peripheral blood stem cell and bone marrow transplants and, infrequently, unirradiated blood products, solid organ transplants, and maternofetal lymphocyte engraftment. A graft versus tumor response also occurs and is an important component of the therapeutic regimen.

The condition can be divided into an acute and a chronic phase. Acute GVHD typically occurs between 7 and 21 days after transplantation but may be seen as late as 3 months; chronic GVHD arises after a mean of 4 months, but may occur as soon as 40 days' post transplantation. Many patients have both phases, either merging with one another or separated by an asymptomatic period. In the *acute phase*, the classic triad includes skin lesions, hepatic dysfunction, and diarrhea. The eruption is characterized by extensive macular erythema, a morbilliform eruption, purpuric lesions, violaceous scaly papules and plaques, bullae, or in rare cases a toxic epidermal necrolysis–like epidermal detachment. There is a predilection for the cheeks, ears, neck, upper chest, and palms and soles. Occasionally, follicular papules are seen simulating a folliculitis. In the *chronic phase,* an early lichenoid stage and a late sclerodermoid stage can be distinguished. Each stage can occur without the other. Although usually generalized, the involvement is in rare instances localized to a few areas. In the lichenoid stage, both the cutaneous and oral lesions may be clinically similar to those in lichen planus. In addition, the skin may show extensive erythema and irregular hyperpigmentation. A poikiloderma phase may precede the eventual sclerodermoid stage. Other late manifestations include a lupus erythematosus-like eruption, cicatricial alopecia, chronic ulcerations, pyogenic granuloma and angiomatous lesions.

HISTOPATHOLOGY. In 2006, the National Institutes of Health Consensus Development Project Pathology Working Group proposed histologic criteria for GVHD. Their minimal histologic criteria for active cutaneous GVHD required apoptosis within the basilar or lower spinosum layers of the epidermis, outer root sheath of the hair follicle or acrosyringium. Marked apoptotic activity was defined as more than 5 epidermal apoptotic bodies per section from a 4-mm punch biopsy. It was noted that no single histologic feature is pathognomonic of cutaneous GVHD. Both acute and chronic GVHD feature an interface dermatitis that can be characterized by either a lichenoid pattern of lymphocytic inflammation (with or without lymphocyte satellitosis) or primarily vacuolar changes of the basilar layer. In traditional grading of acute GVHD, grade I is characterized by vacuolar change, grade II by keratinocyte necrosis, grade III by focal separation at the DEJ, and grade IV by bullae. Epidermal compact orthokeratosis, hypergranulosis, and acanthosis are consistent with a diagnosis of lichenoid GVHD. In the late sclerodermoid phase, the epidermis is atrophic, with the keratinocytes being small, flattened, and hyperpigmented. Basal layer vacuolization, inflammation, and colloid body formation are rare or absent. The dermis is thickened, with sclerosis extending into the subcutaneous tissue resulting in septal hyalinization. The adnexal structures are destroyed. Lichen sclerosus and eosinophilic fasciitis-like lesions complete the spectrum of chronic cutaneous GVH (76). Accurate diagnosis requires correlation with clinical information (90).

PATHOGENESIS. Acute and chronic forms of the disease have a different pathogenesis. In acute GVHD, it is believed that preparative regimen before the infusion of the graft cause extensive tissue damage, which releases inflammatory cytokines and exposes recipient major histocompatibility complex (MHC) antigens. Recognition of the host antigen by donor T cells, and activation and proliferation of them are crucial in the initial phase. In the skin, young rete ridge keratinocytes, follicular stem cells, and Langerhans cells are preferred targets. Less is understood about the pathophysiology of chronic GVHD. The role of donor T cells against the recipient's tissue has been demonstrated.

DIFFERENTIAL DIAGNOSIS. The acute phase of GVHD is similar to erythema multiforme, with scattered necrotic keratinocytes and the formation of subepidermal clefts through hydropic degeneration of basal cells. In severe cases, the fulminant lesions resemble TEN. These patients are also at increased risk for drug eruptions, chemotherapy-induced eruptions and radiation dermatitis, all of which may be indistinguishable from acute GVHD. If there is follicular dyskeratosis, the diagnosis is much more likely to be acute GVHD. The presence of eosinophils is not necessarily in favor of drug reaction, as eosinophils are occasionally observed in GVHD (91).

The *eruption of lymphocyte recovery* occurs predominantly in patients after receiving cytoreductive therapy (without bone marrow transplant) for acute myelogenous leukemia. The eruption is typically morbilliform and develops between 6 and 21 days of chemotherapy, correlating with the earliest recovery of lymphocytes to the circulation. In contrast to patients with GVHD, these patients do not develop diarrhea or liver abnormalities. Resolution occurs over several days. Histopathologically, a superficial perivascular mononuclear cell infiltrate, basal vacuolization, spongiosis, and rare dyskeratotic keratinocytes are present. The changes may be indistinguishable from those of early allogeneic or autologous GVHD, and clinical information is essential. The systemic administration of recombinant cytokines prior to marrow recovery leads to a relatively heavy lymphocytic infiltrate with nuclear pleomorphism and hyperchromasia. Distinguishing between the lichenoid lesions of GVHD and lichen planus is often impossible. However, late sclerotic lesions can be differentiated from scleroderma by the marked atrophy of the epidermis. Active synthesis of collagen takes place largely in the upper third of the dermis; in scleroderma, collagen is synthesized mainly in the lower dermis and in the subcutaneous tissue.

Mycosis Fungoides, Patch/Plaque Stage

Clinical features and histopathology of patch and plaque stage mycosis fungoides, which may present as a lichenoid infiltrate, are discussed elsewhere (IIID1). A lichenoid infiltrate which may be dense or sparse, as here, is a common presentation and typically involves lymphocytes "tagging" along the interface.

Conditions to consider in the differential diagnosis:

lichen planus–like keratosis (benign lichenoid keratosis)
lichen planus
lupus erythematous, lichenoid forms
mixed connective tissue disease

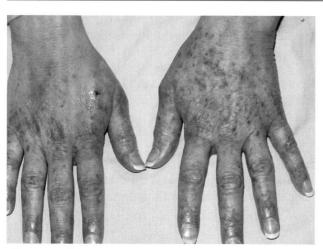

Clin. Fig. IIIF1.c

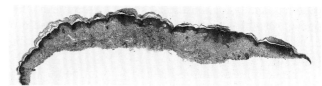

Fig. IIIF1.d

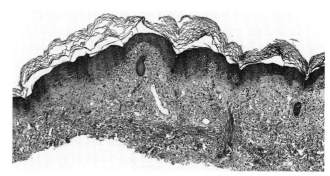

Fig. IIIF1.e

Clin. Fig. IIIF1.c. *Graft-versus-host disease.* Note lichenoid papules that are symmetrically distributed.

Fig. IIIF1.d. *Graft-versus-host disease, lichenoid, low power.* There is an inflammatory infiltrate in the superficial dermis.

Fig. IIIF1.e. *Graft-versus-host disease, lichenoid, medium power.* The stratum corneum is normal, indicative of a recent onset. Lymphocytes are seen "tagging" at the dermal-epidermal junction in a lichenoid pattern. Lymphocytes and a few melanophages are present in the papillary dermis.

Fig. IIIF1.f. *Graft-versus-host disease, lichenoid, high power.* There is vacuolar alteration at the dermal-epidermal junction, and there are many necrotic (apoptotic) keratinocytes near the interface. Lymphocytes are adherent to some of the eosinophilic apoptotic keratinocytes, constituting so-called "satellite-cell necrosis."

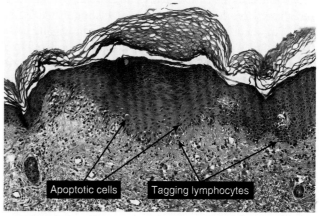

Fig. IIIF1.f

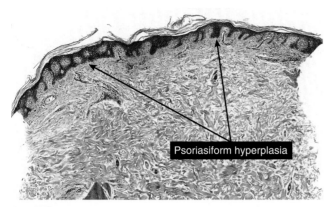

Fig. IIIF1.g

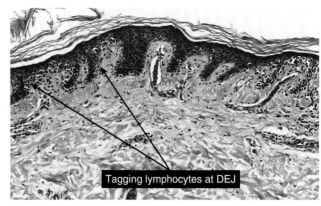

Fig. IIIF1.h

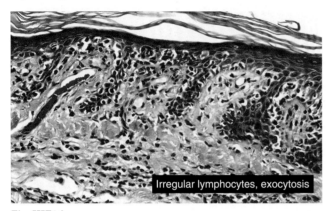

Fig. IIIF1.i

Fig. IIIF1.g. *Mycosis fungoides, patch/plaque stage, low power.* In this example, the infiltrate is sparser than most lichenoid inflammatory infiltrates.

Fig. IIIF1.h. *Mycosis fungoides, patch/plaque stage, medium power.* Lymphocytes at the dermal–epidermal junction enter the epidermis with minimal spongiosis.

Fig. IIIF1.i. *Mycosis fungoides, patch/plaque stage, high power.* Although lymphoid atypia is not striking in this early lesion, there is some irregularity of nuclear contour. There is prominent "tagging" of lymphocytes along the interface.

acrodermatitis chronica atrophicans
poikiloderma atrophicans vasculare
pigmented purpuric dermatitis, lichenoid type (Gougerot–Blum)
graft-versus-host disease (GVH), lichenoid stage
erythema multiforme
pityriasis lichenoides et varioliformis acuta (PLEVA), early lesions
parapsoriasis/mycosis fungoides, patch/plaque stage
Sezary syndrome

IIIF2 | Lichenoid Dermatitis, Lymphocytes Predominant

The band-like lichenoid infiltrate is composed almost exclusively of lymphocytes. A few plasma cells and eosinophils may also be present. *Lichen planus–like keratosis* is a prototype (92,93).

Lichen Planus–Like Keratosis (Benign Lichenoid Keratosis)

CLINICAL SUMMARY. Lichen planus–like keratosis (LPLK), also known as "benign lichenoid keratosis (BLK)," or lichenoid keratosis (LK), is a common lesion that occurs predominantly on the trunk and upper extremities of adults between the fifth and seventh decades, and consists of a nearly always solitary nonpruritic papule or slightly indurated plaque. It usually measures 5 to 20 mm in diameter and its color varies from bright red to violaceous to brown. Its surface may be smooth or slightly verrucous. LPLK probably represents the inflammatory stage of involuting solar lentigines. Clinically it can mimic a basal cell carcinoma and is often biopsied to evaluate for this possibility.

HISTOPATHOLOGY. Histologic examination shows, at least in a part of the lesion, a lichenoid pattern that may be indistinguishable from lichen planus (94). As in lichen planus, there is vacuolar alteration of the basal cell layer and a band-like lymphocytic infiltrate that obscures the dermal–epidermal junction. Necrotic keratinocytes are commonly seen and may be numerous. As in lichen planus, the epidermis often shows increased eosinophilia, hypergranulosis, and hyperkeratosis. In contrast to lichen planus, however, parakeratosis is fairly common, and eosinophils and plasma cells may be present in the infiltrate. In a study of 1,040 cases five different pathologic subtypes were identified: a classic type; a bullous type; an atypical type with cytologically atypical lymphocytes; an early or interface type; and a late regressed or atrophic type (95). A residual solar lentigo at the edge of the lesion

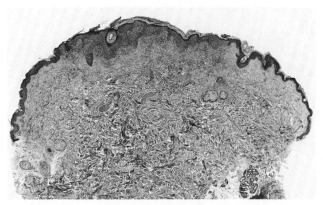

Fig. IIIF2.a

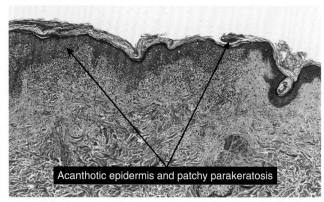

Acanthotic epidermis and patchy parakeratosis

Fig. IIIF2.b

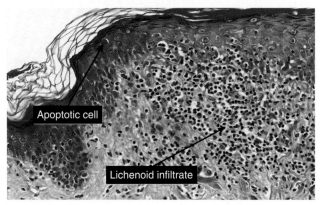

Apoptotic cell

Lichenoid infiltrate

Fig. IIIF2.c

Fig. IIIF2.a. *Lichen planus–like keratosis, low power.* The features seen are those of a dense, band-like infiltrate in an expanded papillary dermis that obscures the dermal–epidermal interface. The infiltrate is lymphocytic and fills the papillary dermis.

Fig. IIIF2.b. *Lichen planus–like keratosis, medium power.* The dermis has a dense infiltrate of lymphocytes that are exocytotic to the proliferative epidermis, destroying the basal keratinocytes.

Fig. IIIF2.c. *Lichen planus–like keratosis, high power.* There is a dense infiltrate of lymphocytes that is exocytotic to the epidermis, and obscures the dermal–epidermal junction.

supports the diagnosis of LPLK. If marked keratinocytic atypia is found in association with a lichenoid inflammatory pattern, a lichenoid actinic keratosis should be considered in the differential diagnosis. A regressed melanoma should also be considered; a complete or near-complete loss of melanocytes within the epidermis demonstrated by immunohistochemistry, and the presence of a dense band-like distribution of dermal melanophages favor a regressed melanoma, while necrotic epidermal keratinocytes favor an LPLK (96).

Conditions to consider in the differential diagnosis:

lichen planus–like keratosis (benign lichenoid keratosis)
parapsoriasis/mycosis fungoides, patch/plaque stage
Sezary syndrome
paraneoplastic pemphigus
secondary syphilis
halo nevus
lichenoid tattoo reaction
lichen striatus

IIIF2a Lichenoid Dermatitis, Eosinophils Present

Eosinophils are found in the lichenoid dermal infiltrate, about the dermal vessels and in some instances around the adnexal structures. *Lichenoid drug eruptions* are prototypic (97). Langerhans cell histiocytosis is an important differential diagnosis.

Lichenoid Drug Eruptions

CLINICAL SUMMARY. Lichenoid drug eruption is clinically similar to lichen planus. Erythematous to violaceous papules and plaques develop on the trunk and extremities in association with drug ingestion. Implicated agents include gold, antihypertensive medications (especially captopril), penicillamine, and chloroquine, and many others.

HISTOPATHOLOGY. Lichenoid drug eruption is similar to lichen planus histologically (98). In comparison with erythema multiforme and TEN, lichenoid drug eruptions are more heavily inflamed with a more prominent interstitial pattern. Differentiation from lichen planus may not be possible. Numerous eosinophils, parakeratosis, and perivascular inflammation around the mid and deep dermal plexuses are generally absent in lichen planus and should prompt consideration of a lichenoid drug eruption.

Conditions to consider in the differential diagnosis:

lichenoid drug eruptions
lichenoid actinic keratoses

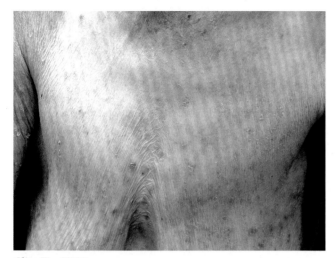

Clin. Fig. IIIF2.a

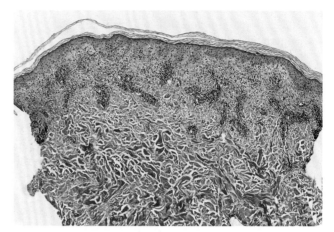

Fig. IIIF2a.a

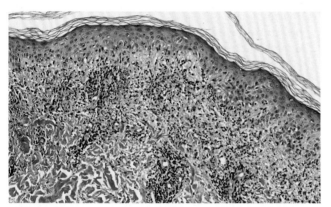

Fig. IIIF2a.b

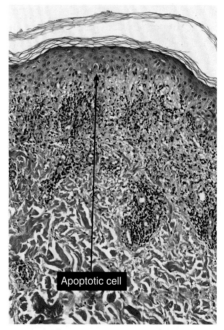

Apoptotic cell

Fig. IIIF2a.c

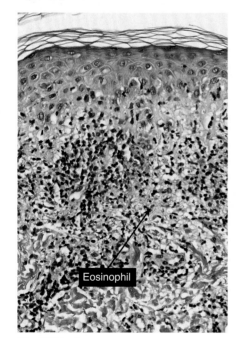

Eosinophil

Fig. IIIF2a.d

Clin. Fig. IIIF2.a. *Lichenoid drug eruption.* Erythematous papulosquamous lesions which were widespread over the body after taking antituberculosis medication for 3 months in a 76-year-old woman.

Fig. IIIF2a.a. *Lichenoid drug eruption, low power.* There is orthokeratosis and a relatively undisturbed epidermis, indicative of a lesion of very recent onset. The papillary dermis is filled with an infiltrate of mononuclear cells that obscures the dermal–epidermal interface. The inflammatory infiltrate extends to the mid-reticular dermis about dermal vessels.

Fig. IIIF2a.b. *Lichenoid drug eruption, medium power.* The papillary dermis is edematous and filled with an infiltrate of mononuclear cells.

Fig. IIIF2a.c. *Lichenoid drug eruption, medium power.* The inflammatory infiltrate in the dermis consists of lymphocytes, histiocytes, and eosinophils. These cells are seen as exocytotic cells into the irregularly acanthotic epidermis.

Fig. IIIF2a.d. *Lichenoid drug eruption, high power.* Eosinophils are seen in the infiltrate. The epidermis shows some disorganization and exocytosis, with apoptotic "Civatte" bodies. The presence of a few apoptotic cells in a superficial inflammatory infiltrate is a clue to a drug eruption.

lichen planus, hypertrophic
arthropod bite reactions
CTCL, mycosis fungoides, patch/plaque stage
Langerhans cell histiocytosis (Letterer–Siwe)
mastocytosis/telangiectasia eruptiva macularis perstans

IIIF2b Lichenoid Dermatitis, Plasma Cells Present

Plasma cells are found in the lichenoid infiltrate; their number is variable, but they do not as a rule comprise the major portion of the dermal infiltrate. *Lichenoid actinic keratosis* is a prototype (71).

Lichenoid Actinic Keratosis

(See also IIA.1.) A variant of the hypertrophic type of actinic keratosis, which demonstrates nuclear atypia, irregular acanthosis and hyperkeratosis, the presence of basal cell liquefaction, degeneration of the basal cell layer, and a band-like "lichenoid" infiltrate in close apposition to the epidermis. Fairly numerous eosinophilic, homogeneous apoptotic Civatte-like bodies may be seen in the upper dermis. The presence of nuclear atypia distinguishes these lesions from lichen planus and BLK. Care

should also be taken to distinguish these lesions from melanoma *in situ* in sun-damaged skin. Melan A staining can be positive in nonmelanocytic cells including "pseudomelanocytic nests" of antigen-positive cells that may be keratinocytes or histiocytes located at the dermal–epidermal junction (99). This reaction pattern should not be over interpreted. Concurrent use of a Sox10 stain will demonstrate no increase of melanocytes in these nests.

Secondary Syphilis

The presence of plasma cells in an infiltrate is unusual, and should raise suspicion of syphilis, as well as collagen vascular disease and neoplasia (100). See also IIIA1c.

Conditions to consider in the differential diagnosis:

lichenoid actinic keratosis
Bowen disease
erythroplasia of Queyrat
keratosis lichenoides chronica
secondary syphilis
pinta, primary or secondary lesions
arthropod bite reaction
CTCL, mycosis fungoides, patch/plaque stage
Zoon's plasma cell balanitis

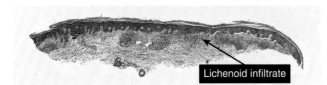

Fig. IIIF2b.a

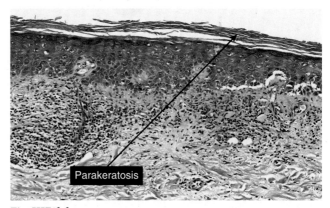

Fig. IIIF2b.b

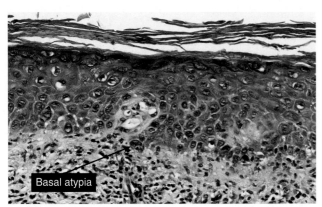

Fig. IIIF2b.c

Fig. IIIF2b.a. *Lichenoid actinic keratosis, low power.* There is an ortho and parakeratotic scale overlying an evenly acanthotic epidermis. In the papillary dermis there is a nodular as well as diffuse lichenoid inflammatory infiltrate that obscures the dermal–epidermal interface.

Fig. IIIF2b.b. *Lichenoid actinic keratosis, medium power.* The basal cell zone is obliterated by the inflammatory infiltrate. The cells are lymphocytes and are exocytotic to the irregularly thickened epidermis. Necrotic keratinocytes are seen within this epidermis.

Fig. IIIF2b.c. *Lichenoid actinic keratosis, medium power.* The epidermis shows subtle keratinocyte atypia (best seen away from the more intense part of the lichenoid inflammation) with an overlying ortho and parakeratotic scale. Within the dermal infiltrate, there are lymphocytes and often plasma cells.

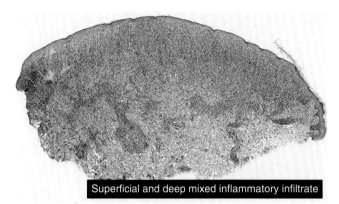

Superficial and deep mixed inflammatory infiltrate

Fig. IIIF2b.d

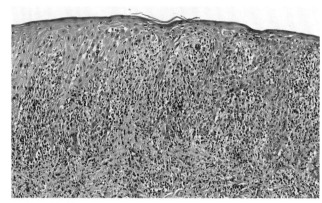

Fig. IIIF2b.e

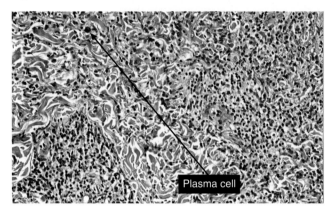

Plasma cell

Fig. IIIF2b.f

Fig. IIIF2b.d. *Secondary syphilis, low power.* There is a prominent band-like lichenoid and a dense superficial and deep perivascular and interstitial infiltrate of mononuclear cells.

Fig. IIIF2b.e. *Secondary syphilis, medium power.* There is a mixed infiltrate of lymphocytes and plasma cells, with lichenoid inflammation and Civatte-like bodies.

Fig. IIIF2b.f. *Secondary syphilis, high power.* The infiltrate includes plasma cells, and nodular clusters of lymphocytes. Germinal centers may be present.

IIIF2c **Lichenoid Dermatitis, With Melanophages**

Most of the conditions listed as lichenoid dermatoses may be associated with release of pigment from damaged basal keratinocytes into the papillary dermis "pigmentary incontinence." Very prominent melanophages, especially if in a fair-skinned individual, should prompt consideration of a regressed melanoma (107). If a specific dermatosis cannot be identified, the appearances may be classified as postinflammatory hyperpigmentation (see IIA.1e).

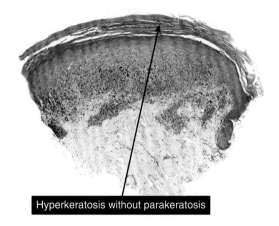

Hyperkeratosis without parakeratosis

Fig. IIIF2c.a

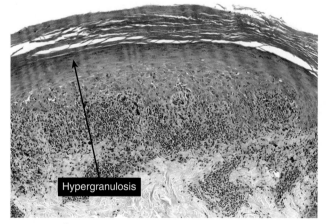

Hypergranulosis

Fig. IIIF2c.b

Fig. IIIF2c.a. *Lichen planus, low power.* There is a thick orthokeratotic scale overlying an epidermis that is thinned and effaced. The papillary dermis is expanded and occupied by an infiltrate of mononuclear cells.

Fig. IIIF2c.b. *Lichen planus, medium power.* Hyperkeratosis overlies an effaced epidermis, with hypergranulosis. In the dermis there is an inflammatory infiltrate of lymphocytes as well as brown pigmented melanophages. (*continues*)

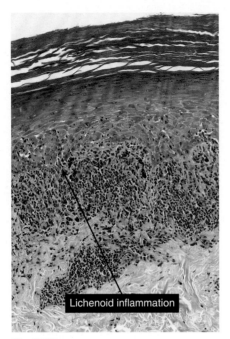

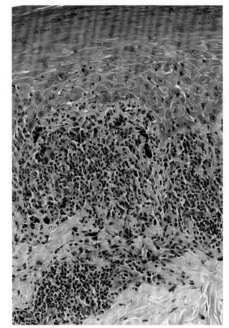

Fig. IIIF2c.c   **Fig. IIIF2c.d**

Fig. IIIF2c.c,d. *Lichen planus, high power.* The dermal–epidermal interface is obliterated by the inflammatory infiltrate that consists of lymphocytes and many melanophages.

Conditions to consider in this category:

> postinflammatory hyperpigmentation
> regressed melanoma or other pigmented lesion

IIIF3 | Lichenoid Dermatitis, Histiocytes Predominant

Histiocytes are the predominant cell type in the dermal infiltrate. *Lichen nitidus* is the prototype (101).

Lichen Nitidus

CLINICAL SUMMARY. This chronic, usually asymptomatic, dermatitis begins commonly in childhood or early adulthood and is characterized by round, flat-topped, flesh-colored papules 2 to 3 mm in diameter that may occur in groups but do not coalesce. The lesions appear frequently as a localized eruption affecting predominantly the arms, trunk, or penis with a few cases reported to occur on palms, soles, nails, and mucous membranes. The clinical course is unpredictable; in some patients the eruption may become generalized and in others spontaneous resolution may be seen.

HISTOPATHOLOGY. Histologically, the papules have a parakeratotic "cap," epidermal atrophy, liquefaction degeneration of the basal layer, and a dermal infiltrate of lymphocytes, epithelioid cells, and sometimes giant cells (78). Each papule consists of a well-circumscribed mixed-cell granulomatous infiltrate that is closely attached to the lower surface of the epidermis and confined to a widened dermal papilla. The dermal infiltrate is composed of lymphocytes, numerous foamy or epithelioid histiocytes, and a few multinucleated giant cells. The infiltrate often extends slightly into the overlying epidermis, which is flattened and shows vacuolar alteration of the basal cell layer, focal subepidermal clefting, a diminished granular layer, and focal parakeratosis. Transepidermal perforation of the infiltrate through the thinned epidermis may occur. At each lateral margin of the infiltrate, rete ridges tend to extend downward and seem to clutch the infiltrate in the manner of a "claw clutching a ball." Follicular involvement has been described. The differential diagnosis includes *giant cell lichenoid dermatitis* which is thought to be an unusual lichenoid drug eruption, characterized by areas of epidermal hyperplasia and atrophy with focal vacuolar alteration of the basal layer, exocytosis and cytoid body formation. The dermis contains a band-like, mononuclear cell infiltrate at the dermoepidermal junction with admixed eosinophils, plasma cells and large multinucleate cells (102).

Conditions to consider in the differential diagnosis:

> lichen nitidus
> giant cell lichenoid dermatitis
> sarcoidosis
> actinic reticuloid/chronic actinic dermatitis
> Langerhans cell histiocytosis (Letterer–Siwe, Hand—
>   Schuller–Christian)
> granulomatous slack skin

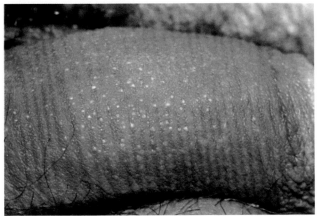

Clin. Fig. IIIF.3

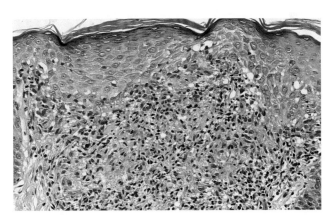

Fig. IIIF3.a

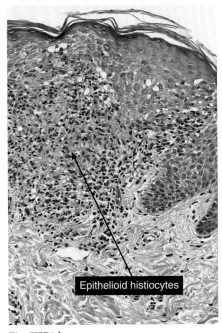

Epithelioid histiocytes

Fig. IIIF3.b

Fig. IIIF3.c

Clin. Fig. IIIF.3. *Lichen nitidus.* Myriads of minute flesh-colored papules on the shaft of the penis.

Fig. IIIF3.a. *Lichen nitidus, low power.* There is a localized nodular infiltrate in a focally expanded papillary dermis. The epidermis surrounding the infiltrate is focally acanthotic.

Fig. IIIF3.b. *Lichen nitidus, medium power.* In an expanded dermal papilla there is a mixed inflammatory infiltrate of lymphocytes and histiocytes.

Fig. IIIF3.c. *Lichen nitidus, high power.* The nodular infiltrate within the expanded papillary dermis consists of histiocytes surrounded by a mantle of lymphocytes.

IIIF4 | Lichenoid Dermatitis, Mast Cells Predominant

Mast cells are the predominant cell type in the dermis. They are frequently accompanied by eosinophils. Urticaria pigmentosa is a prototypic form of mastocytosis (20,103) (see also IIIA2).

Urticaria Pigmentosa, Lichenoid Examples

In the diffuse, erythrodermic type of urticaria pigmentosa, and in some papulonodular lesions, there is a dense, band-like infiltrate of mast cells in the upper dermis that may obscure the dermal–epidermal junction in a lichenoid pattern. Eosinophils may be present in small numbers.

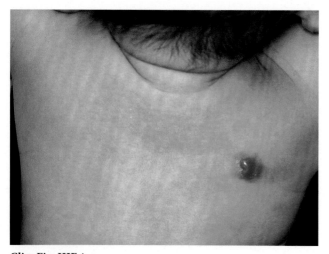

Clin. Fig. IIIF.4

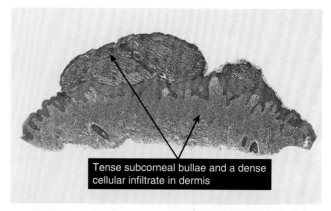

Tense subcorneal bullae and a dense cellular infiltrate in dermis

Fig. IIIF4.a

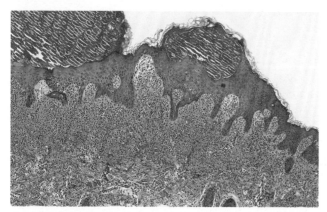

Fig. IIIF4.b

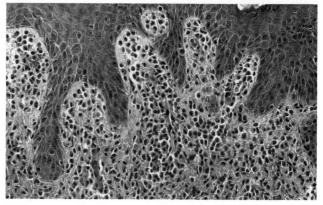

Fig. IIIF4.c

Clin. Fig. IIIF.4. *Bullous mastocytosis.* A brown nodule since birth with an overlying bulla of recent onset in a 4-month-old boy.

Fig. IIIF4.a. *Mastocytosis, low power.* There is a band-like infiltrate of mast cells and lymphocytes in the papillary dermis. The overlying epidermis is acanthotic. There is a subcorneal bulla which may be the result of re-epithelialization at its base.

Fig. IIIF4.b. *Mastocytosis, medium power.* A diffuse infiltrate of mast cells and lymphocytes is seen in an edematous papillary dermis. The overlying epidermis is acanthotic. Interface damage is not prominent.

Fig. IIIF4.c. *Mastocytosis, high power.* The infiltrate in the dermis consists of many mast cells as well as scattered eosinophils.

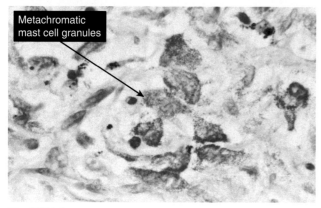

Metachromatic mast cell granules

Fig. IIIF4.d

Fig. IIIF4.d. *Mastocytosis, high power, Giemsa stain.* Metachromatic granules are seen within dermal mast cells.

IIIF5 | Lichenoid Dermatitis With Dermal Fibroplasia

Lymphocytes are the predominant cell type often with an admixture of eosinophils, plasma cells, and histiocytes. In pigmented skin types and in regressed pigmented lesions, melanophages may be prominent. Mycosis fungoides is prototypic (see also IIID).

Mycosis Fungoides, Patch Stage

See Figs. IIIF5.a–d.

Conditions to consider in the differential diagnosis:

mycosis fungoides, patch-plaque stage
lichenoid keratosis

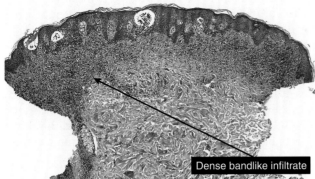

Fig. IIIF5.a

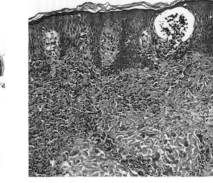

Fig. IIIF5.b

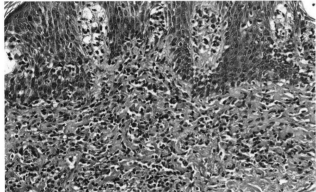

Fig. IIIF5.c

Fig. IIIF5.d

Fig. IIIF5.a. *Mycosis fungoides, atrophic patch stage, low power.* There is psoriasiform epidermal hyperplasia, and there is a dense infiltrate in the dermis.

Fig. IIIF5.b. *Mycosis fungoides, atrophic patch stage, high power.* A linear array of lymphocytes is disposed on the epidermal side of the basement membrane zone. There is delicate fibroplasia in the papillary dermis (the "Fettucine sign" of Ackerman).

Fig. IIIF5.c. *Mycosis fungoides, late plaque stage, high power.* There is exocytosis of irregular lymphocytes into the epidermis.

Fig. IIIF5.d. *Mycosis fungoides, late plaque stage, high power.* Pautrier microabscesses are seen as collections of irregular lymphocytes in the epidermis, typically without spongiosis.

actin keratosis
regressed pigmented lesions including regressed melanomas

IIIG SUPERFICIAL VASCULITIS AND VASCULOPATHIES

Endothelial swelling, eosinophilic degeneration of the vessel wall ("fibrinoid necrosis"), and infiltration of the vessel wall by neutrophils, with nuclear fragmentation or leukocytoclasia resulting in "nuclear dust," define true vasculitis. There are extravasated red cells in the vessel walls and adjacent dermis. If the vasculitis is severe, ulceration or subepidermal separation ("bullous vasculitis") can occur. "Lymphocytic vasculitis" in which there is no vessel wall

damage is a controversial term and is discussed under lymphocytic infiltrates. A "vasculopathy" includes any abnormality of the vessel wall that does not meet the criteria above for vasculitis, such as fibrosis or hyalinization of the vessel wall without inflammation or necrosis.

1. Neutrophilic Vasculitis
2. Mixed Cell and Granulomatous Vasculitis
3. Vasculopathies With Lymphocytic Inflammation
4. Vasculopathies With Scant Inflammation
5. Thrombotic, Embolic and Other Microangiopathies

IIIG1 Neutrophilic Vasculitis

In the dermis, vessels are necrotic, fibrinoid is present and there are perivascular and intravascular neutrophils with leukocytoclasia and nuclear dust. Vasculitis can be classified as affecting small, medium or large vessels, and can be superficial or deep, or single organ versus multi-organ, and also as being associated with antinuclear cytoplasmic antibodies (ANCA) or not. The classification of cutaneous vasculitis has been recently reviewed in a consensus document (104). *Cutaneous necrotizing (leukocytoclastic) vasculitis* is the prototype (105–107).

Cutaneous Necrotizing (Leukocytoclastic) Vasculitis

CLINICAL SUMMARY. A large number of different disease processes can be accompanied by small-vessel vasculitis with predominantly neutrophilic infiltrates. The clinical hallmark is palpable purpura which may be the clinical appearance of dermal leukocytoclastic small-vessel vasculitis secondary to infection (e.g., gonococcal meningococcal or rickettsial sepsis), immune-complex–mediated vasculitis (e.g., serum sickness, cryoglobulinemia or Henoch–Schönlein purpura), ANCA-associated vasculitis (e.g., Wegener granulomatosis), allergic vasculitis (e.g., reaction to a drug), vasculitis associated with connective tissue diseases, or a paraneoplastic phenomenon. It is important therefore, to interpret the histologic findings in the context of clinical information to reach an appropriate diagnosis. Often, additional laboratory data, such as from microbiologic cultures, special stains for organisms, or immunofluorescence or serologic studies, are needed. Because the treatment for infectious vasculitides is so radically different from the treatment for immune-mediated diseases, the most important diagnostic step in the evaluation of a vasculitis is to rule out an infectious process. If noninfectious vasculitis is suspected, evidence for systemic vasculitis should be sought. Clinical

findings—such as hematuria, arthritis, myalgia, enzymatic assays for muscle or liver enzymes, and serologic analysis for ANCAs, antinuclear antibodies, cryoglobulins, hepatitis B and C antibodies, IgA-fibronectin aggregates, and complement levels—are important to further delineate the disease process. Exposure to a potential allergen, such as a drug, that might have elicited a hypersensitivity reaction should be sought. It is also important to address the possibility that the histologic findings of vasculitis may be a secondary phenomenon, as, for example, in ulceration from localized trauma.

HISTOPATHOLOGY OF NEUTROPHILIC SMALL-VESSEL VASCULITIS. Neutrophilic small-vessel vasculitis is a reaction pattern of small dermal vessels, almost exclusively postcapillary venules, characterized by a combination of vascular damage and an infiltrate composed largely of neutrophils. Because there is often fragmentation of nuclei (karyorrhexis or leukocytoclasia), the term *leukocytoclastic vasculitis* (LCV) is frequently used. Depending on its severity, this process may be subtle and limited to the superficial dermis or be pandermal and florid and associated with necrosis and ulceration. If edema is prominent, a subepidermal blister may form. If the neutrophilic infiltrate is dense and there is pustule formation, the term *pustular vasculitis* may be applied. In a typical case of LCV, the dermal vessels have swelling of the endothelial cells and deposits of strongly eosinophilic strands of fibrin within and around their walls, giving the vessel walls a "smudgy" appearance referred to as *fibrinoid degeneration*. Actual necrosis of the perivascular collagen, however, is seen only rarely in conjunction with ulcerative lesions. If the vascular changes are severe, the vessel lumen

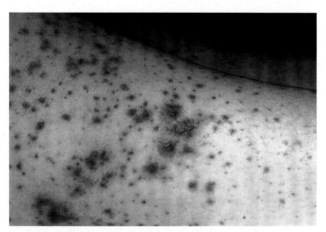

Clin. Fig. IIIG1.a

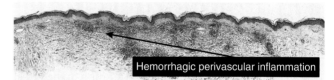

Fig. IIIG1.a

Clin. Fig. IIIG1.a. *Leukocytoclastic vasculitis.* Palpable purpuric tender papules on the legs of a 25-year-old woman resolved after therapy for streptococcal pharyngitis.

Fig. IIIG1.a. *Leukocytoclastic vasculitis, low power.* In the papillary dermis there is hemorrhage and an infiltrate about dermal vessels.

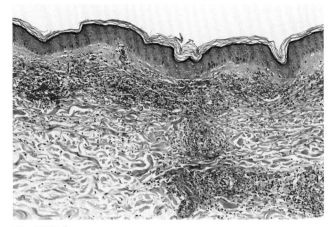

Fig. IIIG1.b

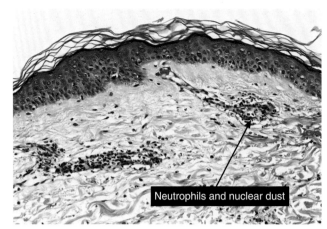

Neutrophils and nuclear dust

Fig. IIIG1.c

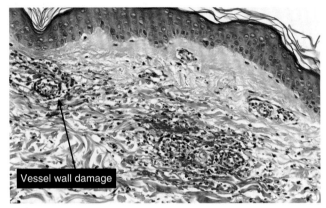

Vessel wall damage

Fig. IIIG1.d

Fig. IIIG1.b. *Leukocytoclastic vasculitis, medium power.* The dermis is edematous and shows a distinct perivascular inflammatory infiltrate of lymphocytes, polymorphonuclear leukocytes and hemorrhage.

Fig. IIIG1.c. *Leukocytoclastic vasculitis, medium power.* There is vascular destruction with an infiltrate of fragmented neutrophils and eosinophils, scattered hemorrhage, and lymphocytes.

Fig. IIIG1.d. *Leukocytoclastic vasculitis, high power.* Eosinophilic homogenous fibrinoid material is seen within the walls of vascular structures. The inflammatory infiltrate consists of lymphocytes, polymorphonuclear leukocytes and fragmented polymorphonuclear leukocytes (leukocytoclasia).

may be occluded. The cellular infiltrate consists mainly of neutrophils and of varying numbers of eosinophils and mononuclear cells. The infiltrate also is scattered throughout the upper dermis in association with fibrin deposits between and within collagen bundles. Extravasation of erythrocytes (purpura) is commonly present.

Septic Vasculitis (Gonococcemia)

Vasculitis is not uncommonly associated with sepsis. In a large study, an underlying severe bacterial infection was diagnosed in 27 of 766 cases presenting with cutaneous vasculitis (3.5%). These patients with infections were older, with male predominance, and more often had fever, constitutional symptoms, focal infectious features, and leukocytosis with left shift, and anemia (108).

Conditions to consider in the differential diagnosis:

cutaneous necrotizing (leukocytoclastic) vasculitis
Henoch–Schoenlein purpura
cryoglobulinemia
connective tissue associated (RA, LE)
septicemia esp. meningococcemia/gonococcemia
urticarial vasculitis
erythema elevatum diutinum
miscellaneous
microscopic polyarteritis nodosa
vasculitis in exanthemic pustulosis (drug-induced)

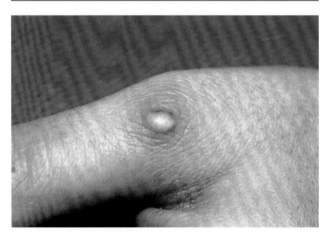

Clin. Fig. IIIG1.b

Clin. Fig. IIIG1.b. *Gonococcemia.* A 25-year-old woman developed hemorrhagic pustules of palms, knees and elbows, associated with joint tenderness and swelling. Blood and vaginal cultures were positive. (*continues*)

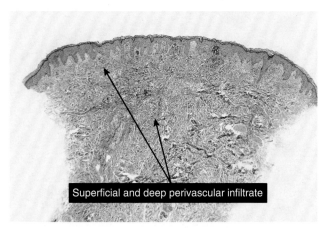

Fig. IIIG1.e

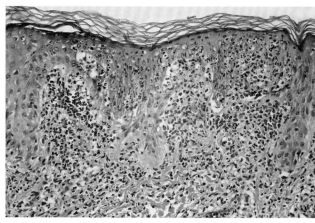

Fig. IIIG1.f

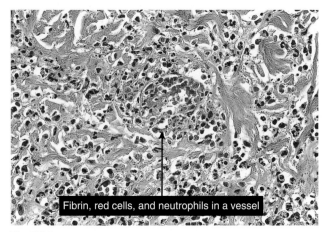

Fig. IIIG1.g

Fig. IIIG1.e. *Gonococcemia, low power.* A perivascular and diffuse infiltrate of mixed cells with prominent hemorrhage in the upper and mid dermis.

Fig. IIIG1.f. *Gonococcemia, medium power.* Mixed inflammatory cells with prominent hemorrhage in the dermis and extending into the epidermis, with vacuolar change and eosinophilic degeneration of the epidermis, probably due to ischemia. In a slightly more advanced lesion, a necrotic hemorrhagic bulla is often produced.

Fig. IIIG1.g. *Gonococcemia, high power.* An inflammatory and thrombotic microangiopathy, with fibrin in the lumen of a small vessel, and neutrophils in its wall.

IIIG2 | Mixed Cell and Granulomatous Vasculitis

There is vessel wall damage, and a mixed infiltrate in the dermis that includes eosinophils, plasma cells, histiocytes and giant cells. *Granuloma faciale* is prototypic (109).

Granuloma Faciale

CLINICAL SUMMARY. Granuloma faciale presents clinically as one or several asymptomatic, soft, brown-red, slowly enlarging papules or plaques, almost always on the face.

HISTOPATHOLOGY. There is a dense polymorphous infiltrate, mainly in the upper half of the dermis, but occasionally extending even into the subcutaneous tissue. The infiltrate is typically separated from the epidermis or the pilosebaceous appendages by a narrow "grenz" zone of normal collagen, and the pilosebaceous structures tend to remain intact. The infiltrate consists in large part of neutrophils and eosinophils, but mononuclear cells, plasma cells, and mast cells are also present. Frequently, there is leukocytoclasia with formation of nuclear dust, especially

in the vicinity of the capillaries, and often there is some evidence of vasculitis with deposition of fibrinoid material within and around vessel walls. Occasionally, some hemorrhage is noted. Foam cells are sometimes observed as well as areas of fibrosis in older lesions. Direct immunofluorescence data suggest an immune-complex–mediated event with deposition of mainly IgG in and around vessels. The distinction between granuloma faciale and erythema elevatum diutinum may be difficult; in a recent study only 4 of 26 criteria distinguished between the two conditions—the density of the infiltrate, and the number of plasma cells and eosinophils were higher in granuloma faciale, while granulomas were never found in granuloma faciale but were present in some cases of erythema elevatum diutinum. A grenz zone was observed in about three quarters of the cases in both groups (110).

Conditions to consider in the differential diagnosis:

Churg–Strauss vasculitis
Wegener granulomatosis
giant-cell arteritis
granuloma faciale
Buerger disease

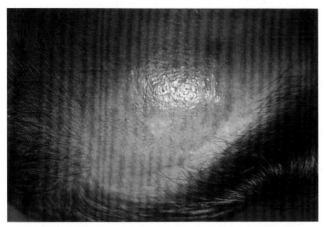

Clin. Fig. IIIG.2

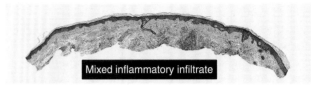

Mixed inflammatory infiltrate

Fig. IIIG2.a

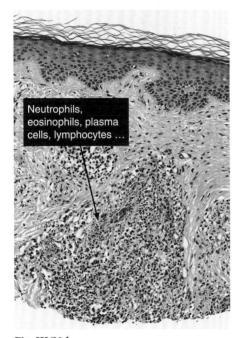

Neutrophils, eosinophils, plasma cells, lymphocytes …

Plasma cell; eosinophil

Fig. IIIG2.b

Fig. IIIG2.c

Clin. Fig. IIIG.2. *Granuloma faciale.* A boggy erythematous plaque on the scalp in a middle-aged man.

Fig. IIIG2.a. *Granuloma faciale, low power.* There is a dense diffuse dermal infiltrate spanning the reticular dermis.

Fig. IIIG2.b. *Granuloma faciale, medium power.* There is a small grenz or clear zone between the epidermis and the dermal infiltrate.

Fig. IIIG2.c. *Granuloma faciale, low power.* The infiltrate is composed of mixed inflammatory cells including neutrophils, eosinophils, lymphocytes, and histiocytes.

IIIG3   Vasculopathies With Lymphocytic Inflammation

A histologic diagnosis of a "lymphocytic vasculitis" may be made if there is sufficient evidence of vascular damage and the inflammatory infiltrate is predominantly lympho- cytic. Often, the vascular damage is subtle and in many cases there may be disagreement as to whether or not the term "vasculitis" is warranted. Clear-cut evidence of vasculitis requires the presence of an inflammatory infil- trate together with fibrinoid necrosis of the vascular wall. These changes are not often seen in combination with a strictly lymphocytic infiltrate. The purpuric dermatoses are exemplary of a pattern of vasculopathy that usually falls short of frank vasculitis, in association with a lym- phocytic infiltrate that may involve the vessel walls (111).

Pigmented Purpuric Dermatoses

CLINICAL SUMMARY. Historically, four variants of purpura pigmentosa chronica have been described: purpura annularis telangiectoides of Majocchi, progressive pigmentary dermatosis of Schamberg, pigmented purpuric dermatitis of Gougerot and Blum, and eczematoid-like purpura of Doucas and Kapetanakis. They are all closely related and often cannot be reliably distinguished on clinical and histologic grounds. Therefore, their classification as distinct entities is not necessary. It is likely that lichen aureus is a closely related variant as well, because the clinical lesion suggests a purpuric component and the histologic findings are similar to those of the other four variants of pigmented purpuric dermatitis (PPD). The general terms "pigmented purpuric dermatitis," "chronic purpuric dermatitis," and "purpura pigmentosa chronica" appear suitable for this disease spectrum. These lesions have been found in some cases to be associated with hepatitis B and C infection (112).

Clinically, the primary lesion consists of discrete telangiectatic puncta as a result of capillary dilatation, and pigmentation as a result of hemosiderin deposits. In some cases, telangiectasia (Majocchi disease) predominates; in others, pigmentation (Schamberg disease) predominates. In Majocchi disease, the lesions are usually irregular in shape and occur predominantly on the lower legs. In some cases, the findings may mimic those of stasis. Not infrequently, clinical signs of inflammation are present, such as erythema, papules, and scaling (Gougerot–Blum disease) or papules, scaling, and lichenification (eczematoid-like purpura). The disorder is often limited to the lower extremities, but it may be extensive. Mild pruritus may be present. A localized variant of PPD is lichen aureus, in which one or a few closely set, flat papules or macules of a rust, copper, or orange color are present, most commonly on the legs.

HISTOPATHOLOGY. The basic process is a lymphocytic perivascular infiltrate limited to the papillary dermis. Epidermal alterations may include slight acanthosis and basal layer vacuolopathy. There is variability in the pattern of the dermal infiltrate. In some instances, the infiltrate may assume a bandlike or lichenoid pattern, particularly in the lichenoid variant of Gougerot–Blum disease, and may involve the reticular dermis in a perivascular distribution. Evidence of vascular damage may be present. However, the extent of vascular injury is usually mild and often insufficient to justify the term "vasculitis." Vascular damage commonly consists only of endothelial cell swelling and dermal hemorrhage. Extravasated red blood cells are usually found

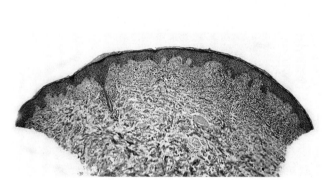

Fig. IIIG3.a

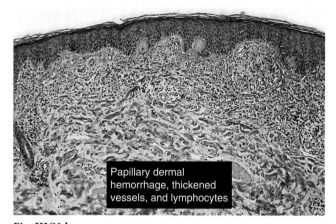

Fig. IIIG3.b

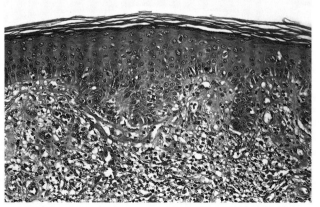

Fig. IIIG3.c

Fig. IIIG3.a. *Pigmented purpuric dermatosis, low power.* There is hyperkeratosis overlying an acanthotic epidermis. The papillary dermis is expanded with an infiltrate about dermal vessels.

Fig. IIIG3.b. *Pigmented purpuric dermatosis, medium power.* Tufted collections of thick-walled vessels are in an edematous expanded papillary dermis. Hemorrhage is present.

Fig. IIIG3.c. *Pigmented purpuric dermatosis, high power.* The papillary dermal hemorrhage is associated with prominent vessels.

in the vicinity of the capillaries. Less commonly one may observe deposition of fibrinoid material in vessel walls. In some instances, the infiltrate involves the epidermis and may be associated with mild spongiosis and patchy parakeratosis. This is observed particularly in some cases of pigmented purpuric lichenoid dermatitis and eczematoid-like purpura. The pattern of the infiltrate often is not strictly confined to the perivascular area and may infiltrate the adjacent papillary dermis (between vessels).

In old lesions, the capillaries often show dilatation of their lumen and proliferation of their endothelium. Extravasated red blood cells may no longer be present, but one frequently finds varying amounts of hemosiderin. The inflammatory infiltrate is less pronounced than in the early stage.

In lichen aureus, a dense lymphohistiocytic infiltrate is present in the superficial dermis, typically distributed in a band-like fashion and often associated with an increase in dermal capillaries. Exocytosis of mononuclear cells into the epidermis may be seen. Scattered within the infiltrate are hemosiderin-laden macrophages. An iron stain can be helpful in demonstrating these.

Conditions to consider in the differential diagnosis:

arthropod bites
hypersensitivity reactions to drugs
urticarial vasculitis
pigmented purpuric dermatoses
autoimmune and connective tissue diseases
pernio (chilblains)
polymorphous light eruption
atrophie blanche
viral processes

cutaneous T-cell infiltrates
pityriasis lichenoides et varioliformis acuta (PLEVA)
pityriasis lichenoides chronica (PLC)
lymphomatoid papulosis (LyP)

IIIG4 | Vasculopathies With Scant Inflammation

There is fibrosis or hyalinization of the vessel walls, with few inflammatory cells. *Stasis dermatitis* is a prototype.

Stasis Dermatitis

CLINICAL SUMMARY. Patients with long-standing venous insufficiency and lower-extremity edema may develop pruritic, erythematous, scaly papules and plaques on the lower legs, often in association with brown pigmentation and hair loss (113).

HISTOPATHOLOGY. The epidermis is hyperkeratotic with areas of parakeratosis, acanthosis, and focal spongiosis. The superficial dermal vessels may be arranged in lobular aggregates. The proliferation may be florid, mimicking Kaposi sarcoma (acroangiodermatitis). Inflammation may be minimal or there may be a superficial, perivascular lymphohistiocytic infiltrate that around plump, thickened capillaries and venules. The reticular dermis is often fibrotic. Hemosiderin is usually present superficially but may be identified about the deep vascular plexus as well.

Stasis Dermatitis

See Clin. Fig. IIIG4.a and Figs. IIIG4.a–c.

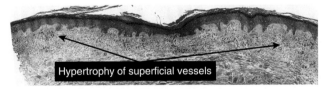

Fig. IIIG4.a

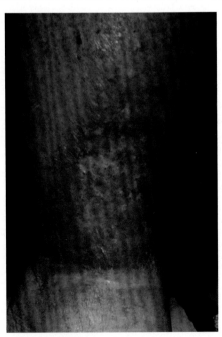

Clin. Fig. IIIG4.a

Clin. Fig. IIIG4.a. *Stasis dermatitis.* Lower leg brawny, violaceous pigmentation, edema, and "bottle neck" deformity resulted from chronic venous insufficiency in an elderly woman.

Fig. IIIG4.a. *Stasis dermatitis, low power.* There is hyperkeratosis overlying an acanthotic epidermis. The papillary dermis is expanded with a scant infiltrate about the prominent dermal vessels. (*continues*)

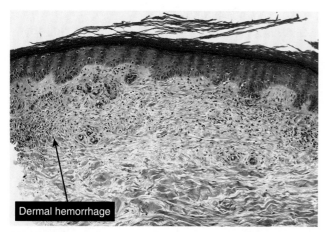

Fig. IIIG4.b

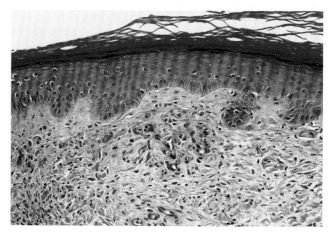

Fig. IIIG4.c

Fig. IIIG4.b. *Stasis dermatitis, medium power.* Tufted collections of thick-walled vessels are in an edematous expanded papillary dermis. Hemorrhage is present.

Fig. IIIG4.c. *Stasis dermatitis, high power.* The papillary dermal hemorrhage is well defined and is associated with vascular proliferation and hypertrophy.

Conditions to consider in the differential diagnosis:

> stasis dermatitis
> atrophie blanche (segmental hyalinizing vasculitis)
> malignant atrophic papulosis (Degos)
> cryoglobulinemia (type I)
> Mondor disease
> pigmented purpuric dermatoses (Majocchi–Schamberg/
> 	Gougerot–Blum)

IIIG5 | Thrombotic, Embolic and Other Microangiopathies

There are thrombi or emboli within the lumens of small vessels, *constituting thrombotic microangiopathy* (114). In other microangiopathies, the vessel walls may be thickened with compromise of the lumen (amyloidosis, calciphylaxis). The *antiphospholipid syndromes* are prototypic (115).

Lupus Anticoagulant and Antiocardiolipin Syndromes

CLINICAL SUMMARY. The *antiphospholipid syndrome* (APS), formerly known as anticardiolipin syndrome (116), occurs in patients with SLE and other autoimmune diseases who develop autoantibodies that can prolong phospholipid-dependent coagulation tests. Many of the immunoglobulins associated with APS are directed against certain plasma proteins and proteins expressed on, or bound to, the surface of vascular endothelial cells or platelets, and involved in coagulant processes (117). These antiphospholipid antibodies (APA) are directed against phospholipid-protein complexes and include lupus anticoagulant, anticardiolipin antibodies, and anti-beta-2 glycoprotein I antibodies.

APS is a common cause of acquired thrombophilia and is characterized by venous or arterial thromboembolism (118). These immunoglobulins occur in association with SLE and other autoimmune diseases, but are found unassociated with them as well. The lupus anticoagulant occurs in about 10% of SLE patients. Affected patients are at greater risk for thromboembolic disease including deep venous thrombosis, pulmonary emboli, and other large vessel thrombosis. Other associated findings are recurrent fetal wastage, renal vascular thrombosis, thrombosis of dermal vessels, and thrombocytopenia. Anticardiolipin antibody occurs five times more often than lupus anticoagulant antibody. It is associated with recurrent arterial and venous thrombosis, valvular abnormalities, cerebrovascular thromboses, and essential hypertension (Sneddon syndrome) (119). Other cutaneous findings include livedo reticularis, necrotizing purpura, disseminated intravascular coagulation, and stasis ulcers of the ankles. In severe forms of coagulopathies, large areas of ecchymosis may be present, typically located on the extremities. Large hemorrhagic bullae may overlie the ecchymoses, and some of the ecchymotic areas may undergo necrosis.

HISTOPATHOLOGY. The histologic features are nonspecific. In mild forms, the only histologic manifestation may be dermal hemorrhage—that is, extravasation of red blood cells into perivascular connective tissue. With increasing severity of the disease process, intravascular fibrin thrombi may be found. In severe cases, thrombotic vascular occlusion may lead to hemorrhagic infarcts, epidermal and dermal necrosis, or subepidermal bulla formation.

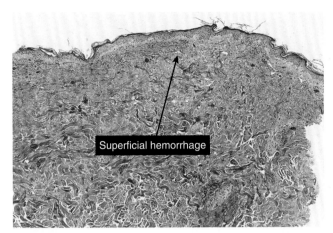

Fig. IIIG5.a

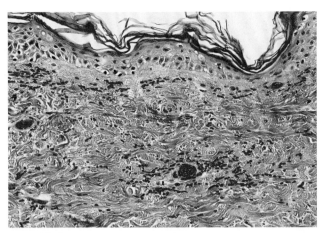

Fig. IIIG5.b

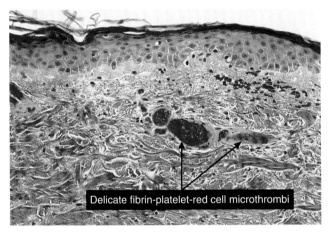

Fig. IIIG5.c

Fig. IIIG5.a. *Noninflammatory thrombi, low power.* There is an effaced epidermis with an overlying keratotic scale. The dermis shows hemorrhage with its greatest concentration in the papillary dermis but also within the reticular dermis.

Fig. IIIG5.b. *Noninflammatory thrombi, medium power.* The papillary dermis is edematous with hemorrhage. Vessels are engorged with red cell—fibrin thrombi.

Fig. IIIG5.c. *Noninflammatory thrombi, high power.* Dermal vessels show red cell—fibrin thrombi without an inflammatory response.

Cryoglobulinemia

CLINICAL SUMMARY. There are three major types of cryoglobulinemia (120): in type I cryoglobulinemia, monoclonal IgG or IgM cryoglobulins are found, often associated with lymphoma, leukemia, Waldenstrom macroglobulinemia, or multiple myeloma, or without known underlying disease. In type II cryoglobulinemia, the cryoprecipitate consists of both monoclonal and polyclonal immunoglobulins, with one member of the complex acting as an antibody against the other. These cryoglobulins are circulating immune complexes. The most common combination is IgG–IgM. In type III cryoglobulinemia, the immunoglobulins are polyclonal. Type II and III or mixed cryoglobulinemias are frequently associated with connective tissue disorders, such as lupus erythematosus, rheumatoid arthritis, and Sjögren syndrome, or may be related to infection—in particular, hepatitis C infection. Idiopathic forms of type II and III cryoglobulinemias are also termed essential mixed cryoglobulinemia.

Clinically, cutaneous lesions in patients with cryoglobulinemia may manifest as chronic palpable purpura, urticaria-like lesions, livedo reticularis, acrocyanosis, digital gangrene, and leg ulcers. Raynaud phenomenon is common. Systemic manifestations may include arthralgia, hepatosplenomegaly, lymphadenopathy, and glomerulonephritis.

HISTOPATHOLOGY. In type I cryoglobulinemia, amorphous material (precipitated cryoglobulins) is deposited subjacent to endothelium and throughout the vessel wall as well as within the vessel lumen, resulting in a thrombus-like appearance. These precipitates stain pink with hematoxylin and eosin and bright red with PAS stain, as opposed to less intense staining of fibrinoid material. Some capillaries are filled with red blood cells, and extensive extravasation of erythrocytes may be present. An inflammatory infiltrate is usually lacking in contrast to mixed cryoglobulinemia, which typically shows an LCV (cryoglobulinemic vasculitis) (121). PAS-positive intramural and intravascular cryoprecipitates may be found also in mixed cryoglobulinemia, although less frequently than in type I cryoglobulinemia.

Other small-vessel vasculitides with the histologic pattern of an LCV may be found in association with Waldenström hyperglobulinemia (hyperglobulinemic purpura)

III Disorders of the Superficial Cutaneous Reactive Unit

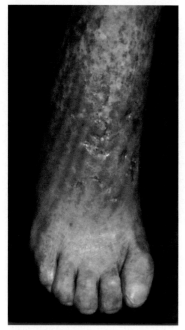

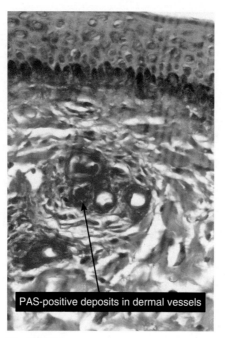

PAS-positive deposits in dermal vessels

Clin. Fig. IIIG5.a. *Cryoglobulinemia.* A 73-year-old woman developed edema and reticulated erythema with extremely painful ulcerations of the lower legs and feet.

Fig. IIIG5.d. *Cryoglobulinemia, medium power (PAS stain).* PAS-positive bright red cryoprecipitates are present in small dermal vessels. An inflammatory infiltrate is generally lacking in type I cryoglobulinemia, caused by deposition of monoclonal immunoglobulins, usually in association with an underlying lymphoproliferative disorder (R. Barnhill and K. Busam).

Clin. Fig. IIIG5.a   Fig. IIIG5.d

and in Schnitzler syndrome, which manifests as chronic urticaria with macroglobulinemia (usually monoclonal IgM) and other paraproteinemias.

Conditions to consider in the differential diagnosis:

disseminated intravascular coagulation
thrombotic thrombocytopenic purpura
cryoglobulinemia/macroglobulinemia
antiphospholipid syndrome
lupus anticoagulant and antiocardiolipin syndromes
connective tissue disease (rheumatoid, mixed)
calciphylaxis
amyloidosis
porphyria cutanea tarda and other porphyrias
cholesterol emboli

 SUPERFICIAL DERMATITIS WITH INTERFACE VACUOLES (INTERFACE DERMATITIS)

Lymphocytes approximate the dermal–epidermal junction. Cellular degeneration and edema in the basal cell zone produces interface vacuoles. The dermis usually has perivascular lymphocytes and there may be pigment incontinence.

1. Vacuolar Dermatitis, Apoptotic/Necrotic Cells Prominent
2. Vacuolar Dermatitis, Apoptotic Cells Usually Absent
3. Vacuolar Dermatitis, Variable Apoptosis
4. Vacuolar Dermatitis, Basement Membranes Thickened

IIIH1 **Vacuolar Dermatitis, Apoptotic/ Necrotic Cells Prominent**

Lymphocytes approximate the dermal–epidermal junction. Vacuolar degeneration is present in the basal cell zone. Apoptotic keratinocytes are found in the epidermis in variable numbers, visualized as round eosinophilic anuclear structures. The dermis usually has perivascular lymphocytes and may show pigment incontinence. *Erythema multiforme* is the prototype (122).

Erythema Multiforme

CLINICAL SUMMARY. Erythema multiforme (EM) is an acute, self-limited dermatosis characterized by multiform lesions, including macules, papules, vesicles, and bullae, typically with target or iris lesions that have the form of a bull's-eye surrounded by a ring of erythema. The disease may be divided into a minor and major form, the latter also known as Stevens–Johnson syndrome (SJS). The most frequent etiology in erythema multiforme is infection, *Herpes simplex virus* and drugs being the most common agents. In viral and idiopathic but not in drug-induced cases, HSV DNA has been detected in lesions of erythema multiforme by PCR (123). In SJS, medications, in particular sulfonamides, are the offending agents in most patients. Patients with herpes simplex virus–associated erythema multiforme have recurrent lesions, affecting primarily the oral mucosa or the extremities, with typical target or iris lesions. Those with drug-induced SJS have truncal involvement, a more purpuric macular eruption, and atypical target lesions. Patients often present

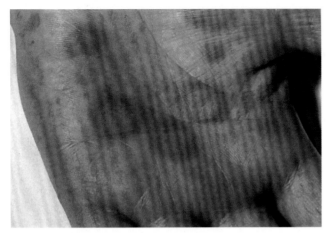

Clin. Fig. IIIH1.a

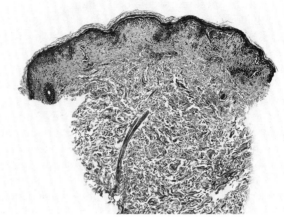

Fig. IIIH1.a

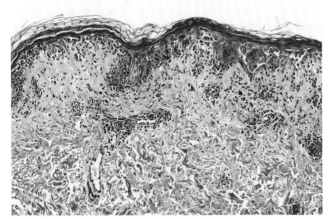

Fig. IIIH1.b

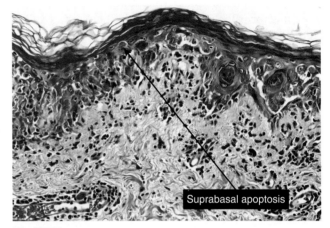

Suprabasal apoptosis

Fig. IIIH1.c

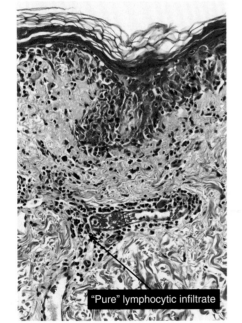

"Pure" lymphocytic infiltrate

Fig. IIIH1.d

Clin. Fig. IIIH1.a. *Erythema multiforme.* Steroid responsive "target" papules characterized by central bullae with surrounding erythema appeared after antibiotic therapy.

Fig. IIIH1.a. *Erythema multiforme, low power.* The epidermis is effaced and there is a dense perivascular infiltrate of mononuclear cells.

Fig. IIIH1.b. *Erythema multiforme, medium power.* The epidermis shows spongiosis and exocytosis. The reticular and papillary dermis has a dense infiltrate of lymphocytes with scattered areas of hemorrhage.

Fig. IIIH1.c. *Erythema multiforme, medium power.* The epidermis shows necrotic/apoptotic keratinocytes, vacuolar degeneration at the basal cell zone and a lichenoid inflammatory infiltrate of lymphocytic cells.

Fig. IIIH1.d. *Erythema multiforme, high power.* There is basket-weave orthokeratin overlying an epidermis that shows exocytosis, basal layer liquefaction degeneration and necrotic keratinocytes. The dermal vessels are thickened and there is an infiltrate of lymphocytes without eosinophils or plasma cells.

with fever. Involvement of the oral, conjunctival, nasal, and genital mucosa is common. In *toxic epidermal necrolysis* (TEN, Lyell syndrome), which frequently overlaps with SJS and is usually regarded as a severe form of erythema multiforme, a widespread blotchy erythema develops. This is soon followed by the development of large, flaccid bullae and detachment of the epidermis in large sheets, leaving the dermis exposed and giving a moist, eroded appearance. The disease has a high mortality rate because of fluid loss and sepsis. In nearly 90% of cases it is caused by medications, most commonly sulfonamides. The *"cytotoxic" or "erythema multiforme-like" drug eruptions* overlap histologically with authentic erythema multiforme and with TEN, both of which may be drug-induced. Medications associated with increased risk for these entities include sulfonamides, trimethoprim-sulfamethoxazole, phenobarbital, carbamazepine, phenytoin, oxicam nonsteroidal anti-inflammatory agents, allopurinol, chlormezanone, and corticosteroids.

HISTOPATHOLOGY. EM is considered the prototype of the vacuolar and cytotoxic/apoptotic form of interface dermatitis. Because of its acute nature, there is an orthokeratotic stratum corneum. The earliest changes include vacuolization of the basal cell layer, tagging of lymphocytes along the dermoepidermal junction, and a sparse, superficial, perivascular lymphoid infiltrate. Mild spongiosis and exocytosis are seen. Necrosis of individual keratinocytes ("apoptosis") occurs in the stratum malpighii, and is the hallmark of EM. Satellite cell necrosis, characterized by intraepidermal lymphocytes in close association with apoptotic keratinocytes, is frequently present. In more papular, edematous lesions, there is papillary dermal edema and more significant spongiosis and inflammation. Intraepidermal vesicles associated with exocytosis may be noted on occasion. Although some authors have noted a significant number of eosinophils in drug-induced EM, this has not been noted by others. In addition to the clinical differences, some histologic differences have been noted between drug-induced and herpes simplex–associated EM. In the former, there is more widespread keratinocyte necrosis, microscopic blister formation, and more pigmentary incontinence. In cases associated with herpes simplex virus infection, there is

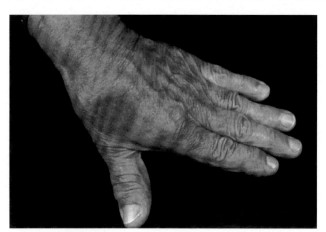

Clin. Fig. IIIH1.b

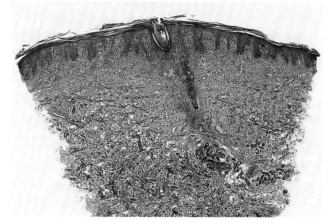

Fig. IIIH1.e

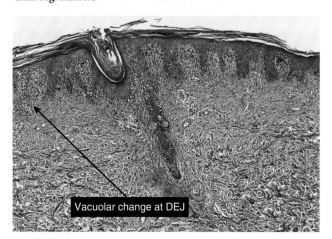

Vacuolar change at DEJ

Fig. IIIH1.f

Clin. Fig. IIIH1.b. *Fixed drug eruption.* Challenge with sulfa drug resulted in recurrence of "burning" dusky vesiculated plaque on the dorsal hand. Histology (not illustrated) typically shows apoptotic dermatitis with pigmentary incontinence.

Fig. IIIH1.e,f. *Fixed drug eruption.* There is hyperkeratosis and there is a lichenoid inflammatory infiltrate in the dermis.

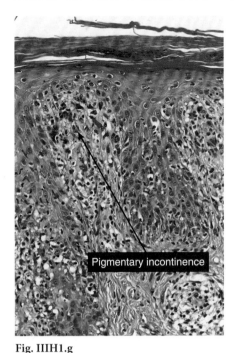

Fig. IIIH1.g

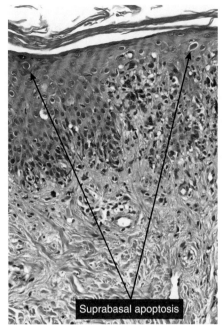

Fig. IIIH1.h

Fig. IIIH1.g,h. *Fixed drug eruption.* Vacuolar alteration is present at the dermal–epidermal junction. Mostly in the suprabasal epidermis, there are scattered apoptotic keratinocytes.

more spongiosis, exocytosis, liquefaction degeneration of the basal layer, and papillary dermal edema. Nuclear dust may be identified in the papillary dermis in the latter.

In TEN, in bullous lesions, and in the central portion of target lesions, there are numerous necrotic keratinocytes, even with full-thickness epidermal necrosis, and a subepidermal bulla. The dermal inflammatory infiltrate is more sparse in TEN than in EM, however there is considerable overlap. Extravasated erythrocytes are commonly found within the blister cavity. Melanophages within the papillary dermis occur in late lesions.

It is not reliably possible for any given biopsy to be pathognomonic of either EM, TEN or SJS, or another EM-like condition, and an appropriate interpretation is as "consistent with erythema multiforme and related disorders," with a note that the differential diagnosis includes these three groups.

Fixed Drug Eruption

Fixed drug eruption is a well-defined, circular or ovoid, hyperpigmented plaque that recurs as one or a few lesions always in fixed locations upon ingestion of a drug (124). It commonly occurs on the genitals, lips, trunk, and hands. The reasons for the site preferences are unknown.

The histopathology is comparable to that of erythema multiforme.

Graft-Versus-Host Disease, Acute

The two major patterns of GVHD are a lichenoid pattern, discussed in IIIG1, and a vacuolar-interface pattern, illustrated here.

Conditions to consider in the differential diagnosis:

erythema multiforme
toxic epidermal necrolysis (Lyell syndrome)
Stevens–Johnson Syndrome
fixed drug eruption
phototoxic drug eruption
radiation dermatitis
sunburn reaction
thermal burn
pityriasis lichenoides et varioliformis acuta (PLEVA)
GVHD, acute
eruption of lymphocyte recovery
bullous vasculitis

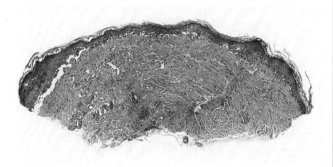

Fig. IIIH1.i

Fig. IIIH1.i. *Graft-versus-host disease, acute.* In this Grade 3 graft-versus-host reaction, subepithelial separation has resulted from confluent vacuolar change. (*continues*)

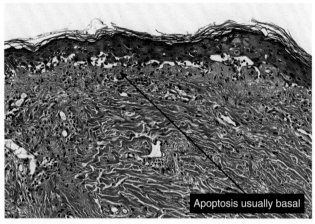

Fig. IIIH1.j

Fig. IIIH1.k

Fig. IIIH1.j,k. *Graft-versus-host disease, acute.* Lymphocytes tagging at the dermal–epidermal junction and eliciting "satellite-cell necrosis" of keratinocytes.

IIIH2 | Vacuolar Dermatitis, Apoptotic Cells Usually Absent

There is basilar keratinocyte vacuolar destruction, apoptotic cells are rare or absent. The dermis has perivascular lymphocytes and may show pigment incontinence. *Dermatomyositis* is a prototype (125,126).

Dermatomyositis

CLINICAL SUMMARY. Dermatomyositis manifests as an inflammatory myopathy with characteristic cutaneous findings, which has peaks of incidence in children and adults aged 45 to 65. In the absence of cutaneous findings, the diagnosis of polymyositis is applied. The cutaneous disease alone, without muscular involvement, has been termed *amyopathic dermatomyositis* or *dermatomyositis sine myositis*. In some instances, the cutaneous eruption precedes the development of muscular weakness by many months or even by several years. Diagnostic criteria for dermatomyositis include proximal symmetric muscle weakness, elevated muscle enzymes, lack of neuropathy on electromyography, consistent muscle biopsy changes, and cutaneous findings.

Two distinctive cutaneous lesions are found in dermatomyositis. One is violaceous, slightly edematous periorbital patches that primarily involve the eyelids, known as the *heliotrope rash*. The other is discrete redpurple papules over the bony prominences, particularly the knuckles, knees, and elbows, known as *Gottron papules*. These may evolve into atrophic plaques with pigmentary alterations and telangiectasia and are then known as *Gottron sign*. Other cutaneous findings include periungual telangiectasia, hypertrophy of cuticular tissues of the nail unit associated with splinter hemorrhages, as well as photosensitivity, and poikiloderma. There may be subcutaneous and periarticular

calcification, usually centered in the proximal muscles of the shoulders and pelvic girdle.

Controversy exists over the association of dermatomyositis with malignancy. The pathogenesis of the disease is uncertain. Associated antibodies include PM1, Jo1 (correlates with pulmonary fibrosis), Ku (associated with sclerodermatomyositis), and M2.

HISTOPATHOLOGY. The erythematous-edematous lesions of the skin in dermatomyositis may have only nonspecific inflammation. However, quite frequently the histologic changes are indistinguishable from those seen in SLE. There may be epidermal atrophy, basement membrane degeneration, vacuolar alteration of basilar keratinocytes, a sparse lymphocytic inflammatory infiltrate around blood vessels, and interstitial mucin deposition. With severe inflammation, there may be subepidermal fibrin deposition. Immune complexes are not detected at the dermal–epidermal junction as in lupus erythematosus. Old cutaneous lesions with the clinical appearance of poikiloderma atrophicans vasculare usually show a band-like infiltrate under an atrophic epidermis with vacuolar interface change of the basal cell layer. The Gottron papules overlying the knuckles also have vacuolization of the basal cell layer, but acanthosis rather than epidermal atrophy. Subcutaneous tissue may contain focal areas of panniculitis associated with mucoid degeneration of fat cells in early lesions. Extensive areas of calcification may be present in the subcutis at a later stage.

Three types of muscle biopsy changes may be observed in active disease: (1) interstitial lymphohistiocytic inflammatory infiltrates; (2) segmental muscle fiber necrosis; or (3) vasculopathy, characterized by immune complex deposition in vessel walls. Old lesions usually show nonspecific atrophy of the muscle fibers and diffuse interstitial fibrosis with relatively little inflammation. Changes in

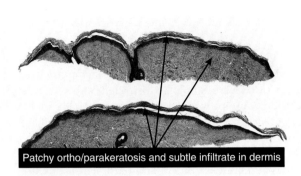

Fig. IIIH2.a

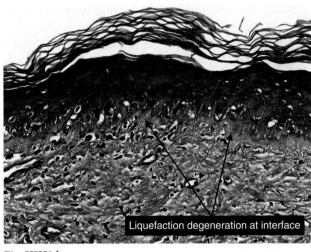

Fig. IIIH2.b

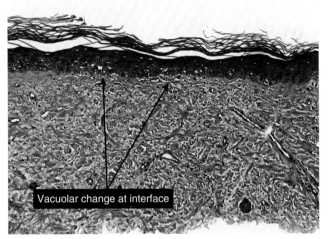

Fig. IIIH2.c

Fig. IIIH2.a. *Dermatomyositis, low power.* There is slight patchy orthokeratosis and parakeratosis overlying an effaced epidermis. In the dermis there is a subtle and patchy lichenoid inflammatory infiltrate.

Fig. IIIH2.b. *Dermatomyositis, high power.* Vacuolar change is seen at the basal cell zone and there is exocytosis of lymphocytes.

Fig. IIIH2.c. *Dermatomyositis, high power.* There is a sparse lymphocytic infiltrate with slight exocytosis and basal layer liquefaction degeneration.

organs other than the skin and the striated muscles occur only rarely in dermatomyositis, in contrast to SLE and systemic scleroderma.

Conditions to consider in the differential diagnosis:

dermatomyositis
morbilliform viral exanthem
poikiloderma vasculare atrophicans
paraneoplastic pemphigus
erythema dyschromicum perstans
pinta, tertiary stage

IIIH3 | Vacuolar Dermatitis, Variable Apoptosis

Vacuolar degeneration is associated with variable numbers of apoptotic cells in the epidermis. The dermis may have increased ground substance and there may be pigmentary incontinence. See also IIIH.1.

Subacute Cutaneous Lupus Erythematosus

CLINICAL SUMMARY. Lupus erythematosus may affect multiple organ systems and has a broad range of clinical manifestations (127). It may take the form of an isolated cutaneous eruption or a fatal systemic illness. A combination of clinical and laboratory data has been set forth as "Criteria for the Classification of Systemic Lupus Erythematosus" by the American Rheumatism Association (ARA). These criteria, developed for classification of patients with SLE as opposed to other rheumatic diseases, are also widely used to diagnose patients with lupus erythematosus. A person is judged to have SLE if any four or more of the 11 following criteria are present serially or simultaneously: Malar rash; Discoid rash; Photosensitivity; Oral ulcers; Arthritis involving two or more peripheral joints; Serositis (pleurisy or pericarditis); Renal disorder (nephritic or nephrotic); Neurologic disorders (seizures or psychosis); Hematologic disorders (hemolytic anemia, leukopenia, lymphopenia, thrombocytopenia); Immunologic disorders (positive LE-cell test, anti-DNA abnormal titer, antibody to Sm nuclear antigen, or false-positive serologic test for syphilis); Antinuclear antibody. Furthermore, a diagnosis of SLE is indicated in any patient who has at least three of the following four symptoms: (1) a cutaneous eruption consistent with lupus erythematosus, (2) renal involvement, (3) serositis, or (4) joint involvement. A diagnosis of SLE requires confirmation by laboratory tests. Molecular and genetic markers including polymorphisms of HLA, TNF-alpha and complement molecules have been summarized (128).

Cutaneous changes of lupus erythematosus may be subdivided according to the morphology of the clinical lesion and/or its duration (acute, subacute, or chronic). Differentiation between LE subtypes is based upon the constellation of clinical, histologic, and immunofluorescence findings.

Subacute cutaneous lupus erythematosus (SCLE) represents about 9% of all cases of lupus erythematosus. Some cases are drug-induced and are indistinguishable from the idiopathic cases (129). It is characterized by extensive erythematous, symmetric nonscarring and nonatrophic lesions that arise abruptly on the upper trunk, extensor surfaces of the arms, and dorsa of the hands and fingers. This eruption has two clinical variants: (1) papulosquamous lesions and (2) annular to polycyclic lesions. Frequently both types of lesions are seen. In some instances, vesicular and discoid lesions with scarring may coexist. Patients with SCLE may have mild systemic involvement, particularly arthralgias.

HISTOPATHOLOGY. Histologic changes in SCLE consist of hydropic degeneration of the basilar epithelial layer, sometimes severe enough to form clefts and subepidermal vesicles, commonly with colloid (apoptotic) bodies in the lower epidermis and papillary dermis. There is often fairly prominent edema of the dermis, and there may be focal extravasation of erythrocytes and dermal fibrinoid deposits. Hyperkeratosis and inflammatory infiltrate are less prominent than in discoid lesions.

Conditions to consider in the differential diagnosis:

cytotoxic drug eruptions
systemic lupus erythematosus
drug-induced lupus

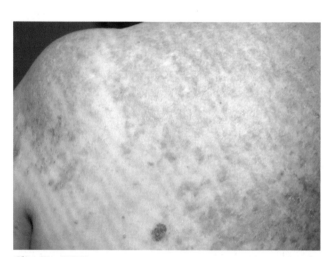

Clin. Fig. IIIH3.a

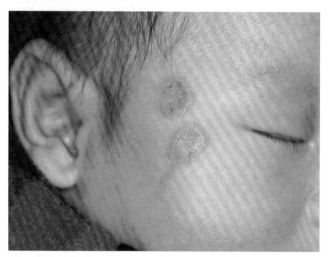

Clin. Fig. IIIH3.b

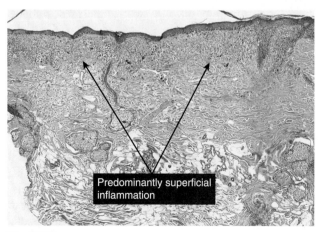

Fig. IIIH3.a

Clin. Fig. IIIH3.a. *Subacute cutaneous lupus erythematosus.* Scaling papules and plaques on the back, shoulders, and forearms are characteristic of the papulosquamous variant.

Clin. Fig. IIIH3.b. *Subacute cutaneous lupus erythematosus.* Annular lesions on the face of a one-month-old boy whose mother has systemic lupus erythematosus.

Fig. IIIH3.a. *Subacute lupus erythematosus, low power.* There is a patchy orthokeratotic scale overlying a relatively unaltered epidermis. The papillary dermis is expanded, edematous and contains a moderate perivascular and diffuse lymphocytic infiltrate.

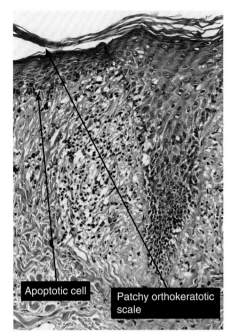

Fig. IIIH3.b

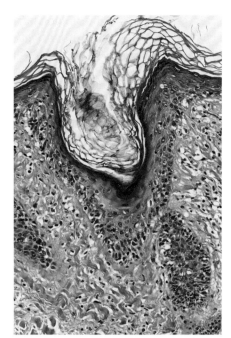

Fig. IIIH3.c

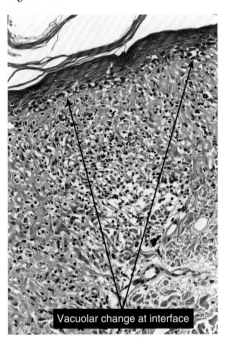

Fig. IIIH3.d

Fig. IIIH3.b. *Subacute lupus erythematosus, medium power.* The lymphocytic infiltrate in the papillary dermis obscures the dermal–epidermal interface and is exocytotic to the acanthotic epidermis. Melanophage pigment is seen within the upper reticular dermis. A rare apoptotic cell is present in the epidermis.

Fig. IIIH3.c. *Subacute lupus erythematosus, high power.* There is prominent vacuolar change at the interface, without basement membrane thickening. There is a dense infiltrate in the papillary dermis that is diffuse as well as perivascular and consists of lymphocytes and pigmented melanophages.

Fig. IIIH3.d. *Subacute lupus erythematosus, medium power.* Inflammation may extend in the subcutis and includes lymphocytes and plasma cells.

IIIH4 | **Vacuolar Dermatitis, Basement Membranes Thickened**

Vacuolar degeneration is associated with variable numbers of apoptotic cells in the epidermis. The basement membrane zone is thickened by deposition of eosinophilic hyaline material. *Discoid lupus erythematosus* is the prototype (130).

Discoid Lupus Erythematosus

CLINICAL SUMMARY. Characteristically, lesions of discoid lupus erythematosus (DLE) consist of well-demarcated, erythematous, slightly infiltrated, "discoid" plaques that often show adherent thick scales and follicular plugging. The lesions are often limited to the face, where the malar areas and the nose are predominantly affected. In addition, the scalp, ears, oral mucosa, and vermilion border of the lips may be involved. In patients with *disseminated discoid lupus erythematosus,* lesions are seen predominantly on the upper trunk and upper limbs, usually with lesions also on the head. Early and active lesions usually display surrounding erythema. Old lesions often appear atrophic and have hypo- or hyperpigmentation. Occasionally lesions may show verrucous hyperkeratosis, especially at their periphery. Hypopigmentation within previously affected areas is frequent.

HISTOPATHOLOGY. In most instances of *discoid lesions,* a diagnosis of lupus erythematosus is possible on the basis of a combination of histologic findings (131). Changes may be apparent at all levels of the skin, but all need not be present in every case. The findings may be summarized as follows: (1) *Stratum corneum*: hyperkeratosis with follicular and sometimes eccrine duct plugging. Parakeratosis is not conspicuous, and may be absent; (2) *Epithelium*: thinning and flattening of the stratum malpighii, interface change with vacuolar degeneration of basal cells, dyskeratosis and squamotization of basilar keratinocytes. In the absence of vacuolar change (hydropic degeneration), a histologic diagnosis of lupus erythematosus should be made with caution and only when other histologic findings greatly favor a diagnosis of LE. In

addition to liquefaction degeneration, basal keratinocytes may show individual cell necrosis (apoptosis) and acquire elongate contours like their superficial counterparts, rather than retaining their normal columnar appearance (squamotization). Frequently, the undulating rete ridge pattern is lost and is replaced by a linear array of squamotized keratinocytes; (3) *Basement membrane*: thickening and tortuosity. This change, which correlates with locations of immunoreactant deposits, is more apparent with PAS stains, and may be found along follicular–dermal junctions and capillary walls as well. In areas of pronounced hydropic degeneration of the basal cells, the PAS-positive subepidermal basement zone may be fragmented and even absent; (4) *Stroma*: a predominantly lymphocytic infiltrate (often with plasma cells), arranged along the dermal–epidermal junction, around blood vessels, hair follicles and eccrine coils, and in an interstitial pattern often into the deep reticular dermis; interstitial mucin deposition; edema, vasodilatation, slight extravasation of erythrocytes; (5) *Subcutaneous*: slight extension of the inflammatory infiltrate may be present.

Conditions to consider in the differential diagnosis:

discoid lupus erythematosus
dermatomyositis

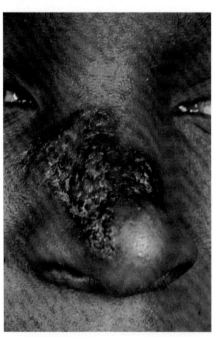

Clin. Fig. IIIH.4

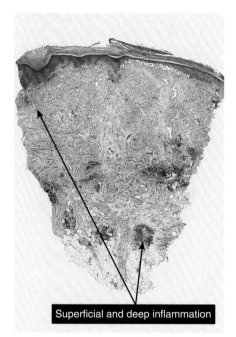

Superficial and deep inflammation

Fig. IIIH4.a

Clin. Fig. IIIH.4. *Discoid lupus.* A 29-year-old man developed pigmented plaques with central depression, atrophy and carpet tack plugging on the nose, auditory canals and scalp.

Fig. IIIH4.a. *Discoid lupus erythematosus, low power.* The epidermis is focally atrophic and effaced, and focally hyperplastic, with overlying hyperkeratosis. The reticular dermis is edematous and there is an infiltrate about dermal vessels that extends into the lower reticular dermis and the subcutaneous fat.

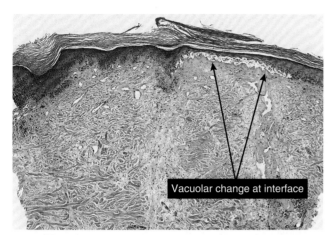

Fig. IIIH4.b

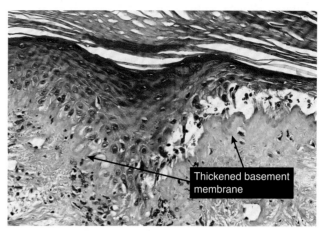

Fig. IIIH4.c

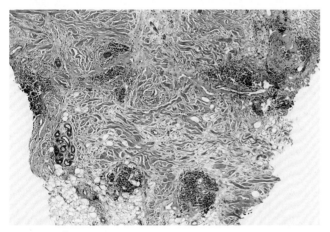

Fig. IIIH4.d

Fig. IIIH4.b. *Discoid lupus erythematosus, medium power.* The epidermis has basal layer vacuolar degeneration. An eosinophilic homogenized thickened basement membrane is at the dermal–epidermal interface. In the dermis is vascular ectasia, a lymphocytic infiltration and melanophage pigmentation.

Fig. IIIH4.c. *Discoid lupus erythematosus, high power.* The eosinophilic well-defined thickened basement membrane is seen at the dermal–epidermal interface, along with the prominent vacuolar change.

Fig. IIIH4.d. *Discoid lupus erythematosus, medium power.* Deep perivascular and periadnexal inflammation are commonly seen.

References

1. Drago F, Rampini E, Rebora A. Atypical exanthems: morphology and laboratory investigations may lead to an aetiological diagnosis in about 70% of cases. *Br J Dermatol* 2002;147(2): 255–260.
2. Rigopoulos D, Paparizos V, Katsambas A. Cutaneous markers of HIV infection. *Clin Dermatol* 2004;22(6):487–498.
3. Cedeno-Laurent F, Gómez-Flores M, Mendez N, et al. New insights into HIV-1-primary skin disorders. *J Int AIDS Soc* 2011;14:5.
4. Hulsebosch HJ, Claessen FAP, Van Ginkel CJW, et al. Human immunodeficiency virus exanthem. *J Am Acad Dermatol* 1990; 23(3 Pt 1):483–486.
5. Soeprono FF, Schinella RA, Cockerell CJ, et al. Seborrheic-like dermatitis of acquired immunodeficiency syndrome. *J Am Acad Dermatol* 1986;14(2 Pt 1):242–248.
6. James WD, Redfield RR, Lupton GP, et al. A papular eruption associated with human T-cell lymphotropic virus type III disease. *J Am Acad Dermatol* 1985;13(4):563–566.
7. Liersch J, Omaj R, Schaller J. Histopathological and immunohistochemical characteristics of measles exanthema: a study of a series of 13 adult cases and review of the literature. *Am J Dermatopathol* 2019. [Epub ahead of print]
8. Prohic A, Jovovic Sadikovic T, Krupalija-Fazlic M, et al. Malassezia species in healthy skin and in dermatological conditions. *Int J Dermatol* 2016;55(5):494–504.
9. Winfield H, Jaworsky C. Connective tissue diseases. In: Elder DE, Elenitsas R, Rosenbach M, Murphy GF, Rubin AI, Xu X, eds. *Lever's Histopathology of the Skin*. 11th ed. Philadelphia, PA: Wolters Kluwer; 2015:329–364.
10. Bordignon M, Belloni-Fortina A, Pigozzi B, et al. The role of immunohistochemical analysis in the diagnosis of parapsoriasis. *Acta Histochem* 2011;113(2):92–95.
11. Kossard S, Hamann I, Wilkinson B. Defining urticarial dermatitis: a subset of dermal hypersensitivity reaction pattern. *Arch Dermatol* 2006;142(1):29–34.
12. Hoetzenecker W, Nägeli M, Mehra ET, et al. Adverse cutaneous drug eruptions: current understanding. *Semin Immunopathol* 2016;38(1):75–86.
13. Gerson D, Sriganeshan V, Alexis JB. Cutaneous drug eruptions: a 5-year experience. *J Am Acad Dermatol* 2008;59(6):995–999.
14. Radonjic-Hoesli S, Hofmeier KS, Micaletto S, et al. Urticaria and angioedema: an update on classification and pathogenesis. *Clin Rev Allergy Immunol* 2018;54(1):88–101.
15. Bisno AL, Stevens DL. Streptococcal infections of skin and soft tissues. *New Engl J Med* 1996;334(4):240–245.

16. Rosen T, Brown TJ. Cutaneous manifestations of sexually transmitted diseases. *Med Clin North Am* 1998;82(5):1081–1104, vi.

17. Abell E, Marks R, Wilson Jones E. Secondary syphilis. A clinicopathological review. *Br J Dermatol* 1975;93(1):53–61.

18. Flamm A, Parikh K, Xie Q, et al. Histologic features of secondary syphilis: a multicenter retrospective review. *J Am Acad Dermatol* 2015;73(6):1025–1030.

19. Müller H, Eisendle K, Bräuninger W, et al. Comparative analysis of immunohistochemistry, polymerase chain reaction and focus-floating microscopy for the detection of Treponema pallidum in mucocutaneous lesions of primary, secondary and tertiary syphilis. *Br J Dermatol* 2011;165(1):50–60.

20. Duprez R, Lacoste V, Brière J, et al. Evidence for a multiclonal origin of multicentric advanced lesions of Kaposi sarcoma. *J Natl Cancer Inst* 2007;99(14):1086–1094.

21. Lebbe C, Garbe C, Stratigos AJ, et al; European Dermatology Forum (EDF), the European Association of Dermato-Oncology (EADO) and the European Organisation for Research and Treatment of Cancer (EORTC). Diagnosis and treatment of Kaposi's sarcoma: European consensus-based interdisciplinary guideline (EDF/EADO/EORTC). *Eur J Cancer* 2019;114:117–127.

22. Gonzalez LM, Allen R, Janniger CK, et al. Pityriasis rosea: an important papulosquamous disorder. *Int J Dermatol* 2005; 44(9):757–764.

23. Panizzon R, Bloch PH. Histopathology of pityriasis rosea Gibert: qualitative and quantitative light-microscopic study of 62 biopsies of 40 patients. *Dermatologica* 1982;165(6): 551–558.

24. Drago F, Ciccarese G, Rebora A, et al. Pityriasis rosea: a comprehensive classification. *Dermatology* 2016;232(4):431–437.

25. Mobini N, Toussaint S, Kamino H. Noninfectious erythematous, papular and squamous diseases. In: Elder DE, Elenitsas R, Johnson BL, Murphy GF, eds. *Lever's Histopathology of the Skin*. 9th ed. Philadelphia, PA: Lippincott Williams & Wilkins; 2005:192–193.

26. Aytekin S, Balci G, Duzgun OY. Febrile ulceronecrotic Mucha-Habermann disease: a case report and a review of the literature. *Dermatol Online J* 2005;11(3):31.

27. Zaaroura H, Sahar D, Bick T, et al. Relationship between pityriasis lichenoides and mycosis fungoides: a clinicopathological, immunohistochemical, and molecular study. *Am J Dermatopathol* 2018;40(6):409–415.

28. Dereure O, Levi E, Kadin ME. T cell clonality in pityriasis lichenoides et varioliformis acuta: a heteroduplex analysis of 20 cases. *Arch Dermatol* 2000;136(12):1483–1486.

29. Simon M Jr. Pigmented purpuric dermatosis. *Acta Derm Venereol* 1992;72(3):235.

30. Magro CM, Schaefer JT, Crowson AN, et al. Pigmented purpuric dermatosis: classification by phenotypic and molecular profiles. *Am J Clin Pathol* 2007;128(2):218–229.

31. Huang YK, Lin CK, Wu YH. The pathological spectrum and clinical correlation of pigmented purpuric dermatosis—A retrospective review of 107 cases. *J Cutan Pathol* 2018;45(5):325–332.

32. Stratigos AJ, Katsambas AD. Optimal management of recalcitrant disorders of hyperpigmentation in dark-skinned patients. *Am J Clin Dermatol* 2004;5(3):161–168.

33. Silpa-Archa N, Kohli I, Chaowattanapanit S, et al. Postinflammatory hyperpigmentation: a comprehensive overview: epidemiology, pathogenesis, clinical presentation, and noninvasive assessment technique. *J Am Acad Dermatol* 2017;77(4):591–605.

34. Longley J, Duffy TP, Kohn S. The mast cell and mast cell disease. *J Am Acad Dermatol* 1995;32(4):545–561; quiz 562–564.

35. Falchi L, Verstovsek S. Kit mutations: new insights and diagnostic value. *Immunol Allergy Clin North Am* 2018;38(3):411–428.

36. Hollmann TJ, Brenn T, Hornick JL. CD25 expression on cutaneous mast cells from adult patients presenting with urticaria pigmentosa is predictive of systemic mastocytosis. *Am J Surg Pathol* 2008;32(1):139–145.

37. Wildemore JK, Junkins-Hopkins JM, James WD. Evaluation of the histologic characteristics of patch test confirmed allergic contact dermatitis. *J Am Acad Dermatol* 2003;49(2):243–248.

38. Lachapelle JM. Comparative histopathology of allergic and irritant patch test reactions in man. Current concepts and new prospects. *Arch Belg Dermatol Syphiligr* 1973;29(1):83–92.

39. Bonamonte D, Foti C, Vestita M, et al. Nummular eczema and contact allergy: a retrospective study. *Dermatitis* 2012;23(4): 153–157.

40. Pižem J, Stojanovič L, Luzar B. Melanocytic lesions with eczematous reaction (Meyerson's phenomenon)—a histopathologic analysis of 64 cases. *J Cutan Pathol* 2012;39(10):901–910.

41. Girard C, Beesses D, Blatire V, et al. Meyerson's phenomenon induced by interferon-alpha plus ribavirin in hepatitis C infection. *Brit J Dermatol* 2005;152(1):182–183.

42. Vega J, Rodríguez MA, Martínez M. Eczematous halo reaction in congenital pigmented nevus. *Int J Dermatol* 2003;42(11):895.

43. Elenitsas R, Halpern AC. Eczematous halo reaction in atypical nevi. *J Am Acad Dermatol* 1996;34(2 Pt 2):357–361.

44. Schnuch A, Westphal G, Mössner R, et al. Genetic factors in contact allergy—review and future goals. *Contact Dermatitis* 2011;64(1):2–23.

45. Pinkus H, Mehregan AH. The primary histologic lesion of seborrheic dermatitis and psoriasis. *J Invest Dermatol* 1966;46(1): 109–116.

46. Park JH, Park YJ, Kim SK, et al. Histopathological differential diagnosis of psoriasis and seborrheic dermatitis of the scalp. *Ann Dermatol* 2016;28(4):427–432.

47. Bhawan J, Andersen W, Lee J, et al. Photoaging versus intrinsic aging: a morphologic assessment of facial skin. *J Cutan Pathol* 1995;22(2):154–159.

48. Landi MT, Bauer J, Pfeiffer RM, et al. MC1R germline variants confer risk for BRAF-mutant melanoma. *Science* 2006;313 (5786):521–522.

49. Haeffner AC, Smoller BR, Zepter K, et al. Differentiation and clonality of lesional lymphocytes in small plaque parapsoriasis. *Arch Dermatol* 1995;131(3):321–324.

50. Nofal A, Salah E. Acquired poikiloderma: proposed classification and diagnostic approach. *J Am Acad Dermatol* 2013;69(3): e129–e140.

51. Venos EM, Collins M, Jane WD. Rothmund-Thomson syndrome: review of the world literature. *J Am Acad Dermatol* 1992;27(5 Pt 1):750–762.

52. Gretzula JL, Hevia O, Weber PJ. Bloom's syndrome. *J Am Acad Dermatol* 1987;17(3):479–488.

53. Dokal I, Luzzatto L. Dyskeratosis congenita is a chromosomal instability disorder. *Leuk Lymphoma* 1995;15(1–2):1–7.

54. Lai-Cheong JE, McGrath JA. Kindler syndrome. *Dermatol Clin* 2010;28(1):119–124.

55. Howard MS, Smoller BR. Mycosis fungoides: classic disease and variant presentations. *Semin Cutan Med Surg* 2000;19(2): 91–99.

56. Regauer S, Liegl B, Reich O. Early vulvar lichen sclerosus: a histopathological challenge. *Histopathology* 2005;47(4): 340–347.

57. Fistarol SK, Itin PH. Diagnosis and treatment of lichen sclerosus: an update. *Am J Clin Dermatol* 2013;14(1):27–47.

58. Sorensen KB, Thestrup-Pedersen K. Pityriasis rubra pilaris: a retrospective analysis of 43 patients. *Acta Derm Venereol* 1999; 79(5):405–406.

59. Roenneberg S, Biedermann T. Pityriasis rubra pilaris: algorithms for diagnosis and treatment. *J Eur Acad Dermatol Venereol* 2018;32(6):889–898.

60. Burg B, Dummer R, Nestle FO, et al. Cutaneous lymphomas consist of a spectrum of nosologically different entities including mycosis fungoides and small plaque parapsoriasis. *Arch Dermatol* 1996;132(5):567–572.

61. Pimpinelli N, Olsen EA, Santucci M, et al. Defining early mycosis fungoides. *J Am Acad Dermatol* 2005;53(6): 1053–1063.

62. Querfeld C, Rosen ST, Guitart J, et al. The spectrum of cutaneous T-cell lymphomas: new insights into biology and therapy. *Curr Opin Hematol* 2005;12(4):273–278.

63. Jaque A, Mereniuk A, Walsh S, et al. Influence of the phenotype on mycosis fungoides prognosis, a retrospective cohort study of 160 patients. *Int J Dermatol* 2019;58(8):933–939.

64. Jawed SI, Myskowski PL, Horwitz S, et al. Primary cutaneous T-cell lymphoma (mycosis fungoides and Sézary syndrome): part I. Diagnosis: clinical and histopathologic features and new molecular and biologic markers. *J Am Acad Dermatol* 2014;70(2):205.e1–e16; quiz 221–222.

65. Olsen E, Vonderheid E, Pimpinelli N, et al; ISCL/EORTC. Revisions to the staging and classification of mycosis fungoides and Sezary syndrome: a proposal of the International Society for Cutaneous Lymphomas (ISCL) and the cutaneous lymphoma task force of the European Organization of Research and Treatment of Cancer (EORTC). *Blood* 2007;110(6):1713–1722.

66. Ackerman AB. If small plaque (digitate) parapsoriasis is a cutaneous T-cell lymphoma, even an 'abortive' one, it must be mycosis fungoides! *Arch Dermatol* 1996;132(5):562–566.

67. O'Keefe RJ, Scurry JP, Dennerstein G, et al. Audit of 114 nonneoplastic vulvar biopsies. *Br J Obstet Gynaecol* 1995;102(10): 780–786.

68. Trozak DJ. Histologic grading system for psoriasis vulgaris. *Int J Dermatol* 1994;33(5):380–381.

69. Altman EM, Kamino H. Diagnosis: psoriasis or not? What are the clues? *Semin Cutan Med Surg* 1999;18(1):25–35.

70. Boehncke WH, Schön MP. Psoriasis. *Lancet* 2015;386(9997): 983–994.

71. Nestle FO, Kaplan DH, Barker J. Psoriasis. *N Engl J Med* 2009; 361(5):496–509.

72. Bos JD, de Rie MA, Teunissen MB, et al. Psoriasis: dysregulation of innate immunity. *Br J Dermatol* 2005;152(6): 1098–1107.

73. Ko HC, Jwa SW, Song M, et al. Clinical course of guttate psoriasis: long-term follow-up study. *J Dermatol* 2010;37(10): 894–899.

74. Chastain MA. The glucagonoma syndrome: a review of its features and discussion of new perspectives. *Am J Med Sci* 2001; 321(5):306–320.

75. Domen RE, Shaffer MB Jr, Finke J, et al. The glucagonoma syndrome. *Arch Intern Med* 1980;140(2):262–263.

76. Otto AI, Marschalko M, Zalatnai A, et al. Glucagon cell adenomatosis: a new entity associated with necrolytic migratory erythema and glucagonoma syndrome. *J Am Acad Dermatol* 2011;65(2):458–459.

77. El Darouti M, Abu El Ela A. Necrolytic acral erythema: a cutaneous marker of viral hepatitis C. *Int J Dermatol* 1996;35(4): 252–256.

78. Abdallah MA, Ghozzi MY, Monib HA, et al. Necrolytic acral erythema: a cutaneous sign of hepatitis C virus infection. *J Am Acad Dermatol* 2005;53(2):247–251.

79. Halpern AV, Peikin SR, Ferzli P, et al. Necrolytic acral erythema: an expanding spectrum. *Cutis* 2009;84(6):301–304.

80. Wan P, Moat S, Anstey A. Pellagra: a review with emphasis on photosensitivity. *Br J Dermatol* 2011;164(6):1188–1200.

81. Yamaguchi S, Miyagi T, Sogabe Y, et al. Depletion of epidermal Langerhans cells in the skin lesions of pellagra patients. *Am J Dermatopathol* 2017;39(6):428–432.

82. Rowland Payne CME, Wilkinson JD, McKee PH, et al. Nodular prurigo: a clinicopathological study of 46 patients. *Br J Dermatol* 1985;113(4):431–439.

83. Neri S, Ierna D, D'Amico RA, et al. Helicobacter pylori and prurigo nodularis. *Hepatogastroenterology* 1999;46(28): 2269–2272.

84. Weigelt N, Metze D, Ständer S. Prurigo nodularis: systematic analysis of 58 histological criteria in 136 patients. *J Cutan Pathol* 2010;37(5):578–586.

85. Blessing K, Evans AT, al-Nafussi A. Verrucous naevoid and keratotic malignant melanoma: a clinico-pathological study of 20 cases. *Histopathology* 1993;23(5):453–458.

86. Gorouhi F, Davari P, Fazel N. Cutaneous and mucosal lichen planus: a comprehensive review of clinical subtypes, risk factors, diagnosis, and prognosis. *Scientific World Journal* 2014; 2014:742826.

87. Lodi G, Giuliani M, Majorana A, et al. Lichen planus and hepatitis C virus: a multicentre study of patients with oral lesions and a systematic review. *Br J Dermatol* 2004;151(6):1172–1181.

88. Bombeccari GP, Guzzi G, Tettamanti M, et al. Oral lichen planus and malignant transformation: a longitudinal cohort study. *Oral Surg Oral Med Oral Pathol Oral Radiol Endod* 2011;112(3):328–334.

89. Schaffer JV. The changing face of graft-versus-host disease. *Semin Cutan Med Surg* 2006;25(4):190–200.

90. Ziemer M, Haeusermann P, Janin A, et al. Histopathological diagnosis of graft-versus-host disease of the skin: an interobserver comparison. *J Eur Acad Dermatol Venereol* 2014;28(7): 915–924.

91. Weaver J, Bergfeld WF. Quantitative analysis of eosinophils in acute graft-versus-host disease compared with drug hypersensitivity reactions. *Am J Dermatopathol* 2010;32(1):31–34.

92. Jang KA, Kim SH, Choi JH, et al. Lichenoid keratosis: a clinicopathologic study of 17 patients. *J Am Acad Dermatol* 2000; 43(3):511–516.

93. Prieto VG, Casal M, McNutt NS. Immunohistochemistry detects differences between lichen planus-like keratosis, lichen planus, and lichenoid actinic keratosis. *J Cutan Pathol* 1993;20(2): 143–147.

94. Prieto VG, Casal M, McNutt NS. Lichen planus-like keratosis. A clinical and histological reexamination. *Am J Surg Pathol* 1993;17(3):259–263.

95. Morgan MB, Stevens GL, Switlyk S. Benign lichenoid keratosis: a clinical and pathologic reappraisal of 1040 cases. *Am J Dermatopathol* 2005;27(5):387–392.

96. Chan AH, Shulman KJ, Lee BA. Differentiating regressed melanoma from regressed lichenoid keratosis. *J Cutan Pathol* 2017;44(4):338–341.

97. Van den Haute V, Antoine JL, Lachapelle JM. Histopathological discriminant criteria between lichenoid drug eruption and idiopathic lichen planus: retrospective study on selected samples. *Dermatologica* 1989;179(1):10–13.

98. Halevy S, Shai A. Lichenoid drug eruptions. *J Am Acad Dermatol* 1993;29(2 Pt 1):249–255.

99. Beltraminelli H, Shabrawi-Caelen LE, Kerl H, et al. Melan-a-positive "pseudomelanocytic nests": a pitfall in the histopathologic and immunohistochemical diagnosis of pigmented lesions on sun-damaged skin. *Am J Dermatopathol* 2009;31(3):305–308.

100. Yamashita M, Fujii Y, Ozaki K, et al. Human immunodeficiency virus-positive secondary syphilis mimicking cutaneous T-cell lymphoma. *Diagn Pathol* 2015;10:185.

101. Lapins JA, Willoughby C, Helwig EB. Lichen nitidus: a study of forty-three cases. *Cutis* 1978;21(5):634–637.

102. Goldberg LJ, Goldberg N, Abrahams I, et al. Giant cell lichenoid dermatitis: a possible manifestation of sarcoidosis. *J Cutan Pathol* 1994;21(1):47–51.

103. Valent P, Horny HP, Escribano L, et al. Diagnostic criteria and classification of mastocytosis: a consensus proposal. *Leuk Res* 2001;25(7):603–625.

104. Sunderkötter CH, Zelger B, Chen KR, et al. Nomenclature of cutaneous vasculitis: dermatologic addendum to the 2012 revised International Chapel Hill Consensus Conference Nomenclature of Vasculitides. *Arthritis Rheumatol* 2018;70(2):171–184.

105. Gonzalez-Gay MA, Garcia-Porrua C, Pujol RM. Clinical approach to cutaneous vasculitis. *Curr Opin Rheumatol* 2005;17(1):56–61.

106. Carlson JA, Chen KR. Cutaneous vasculitis update: small vessel neutrophilic vasculitis syndromes. *Am J Dermatopathol* 2006;28(6):486–506.

107. Demirkesen C. Approach to cutaneous vasculitides with special emphasis on small vessel vasculitis: histopathology and direct immunofluorescence. *Curr Opin Rheumatol* 2017;29(1):39–44.

108. Loricera J, Blanco R, Hernández JL, et al. Cutaneous vasculitis associated with severe bacterial infections. A study of 27 patients from a series of 766 cutaneous vasculitis. *Clin Exp Rheumatol* 2015;33(2 Suppl 89):S-36–43.

109. Ortonne N, Wechsler J, Bagot M, et al. Granuloma faciale: a clinicopathologic study of 66 patients. *J Am Acad Dermatol* 2005;53(6):1002–1009.

110. Ziemer M, Koehler MJ, Weyers W. Erythema elevatum diutinum—a chronic leukocytoclastic vasculitis microscopically indistinguishable from granuloma faciale? *J Cutan Pathol* 2011;38(11):876–883.

111. Sardana K, Sarkar R, Sehgal VN. Pigmented purpuric dermatoses: an overview. *Int J Dermatol* 2004;43(7):482–488.

112. Dessoukey MW, Abdel-Dayem H, Omar MF, et al. Pigmented purpuric dermatosis and hepatitis profile: a report on 10 patients. *Int J Dermatol* 2005;44(6):486–488.

113. Sundaresan S, Migden MR, Silapunt S. Stasis dermatitis: pathophysiology, evaluation, and management. *Am J Clin Dermatol* 2017;18(3):383–390.

114. Robboy SJ, Mihm MC, Colman RC, et al. The skin in disseminated intravascular coagulation. Prospective analysis of thirty-six cases. *Br J Dermatol* 1973;88(3):221–229.

115. Sipek-Dolnicar A, Hojnik M, Bozic B, et al. Clinical presentations and vascular histopathology in autopsied patients with systemic lupus erythematosus and anticardiolipin antibodies. *Clin Exp Rheumatol* 2002;20(3):335–342.

116. Noureldine MHA, Nour-Eldine W, Khamashta MA, et al. Insights into the diagnosis and pathogenesis of the antiphospholipid syndrome. *Semin Arthritis Rheum* 2019;48(5):860–866.

117. Cervera R. Antiphospholipid syndrome. *Thromb Res* 2017;151 Suppl 1:S43–S47.

118. Sangle NA, Smock KJ. Antiphospholipid antibody syndrome. *Arch Pathol Lab Med* 2011;135(9):1092–1096.

119. Samanta D, Cobb S, Arya K. Sneddon syndrome: a comprehensive overview. *J Stroke Cerebrovasc Dis* 2019;28(8):2098–2108.

120. Cohen SJ, Pittelkow MR, Su WP. Cutaneous manifestations of cryoglobulinemia: clinical and histopathologic study of seventy-two patients. *J Am Acad Dermatol* 1991;25(1 Pt 1):21–27.

121. Cacoub P, Comarmond C, Domont F, et al. Cryoglobulinemia vasculitis. *Am J Med* 2015;128(9):950–955.

122. Rzany B, Hering O, Mockenhaupt M, et al. Histopathological and epidemiological characteristics of patients with erythema exudativum multiforme major, Stevens-Johnson syndrome and toxic epidermal necrolysis. *Br J Dermatol* 1996;135(1):6–11.

123. Ng PP, Sun YJ, Tan HH, et al. Detection of herpes simplex virus genomic DNA in various subsets of Erythema multiforme by polymerase chain reaction. *Dermatology* 2003;207(4):349–353.

124. Flowers H, Brodell R, Brents M, et al. Fixed drug eruptions: presentation, diagnosis, and management. *South Med J* 2014;107(11):724–727.

125. Krathen MS, Fiorentino D, Werth VP. Dermatomyositis. *Curr Dir Autoimmun* 2008;10:313–332.

126. Mainetti C, Terziroli Beretta-Piccoli B, Selmi C. Cutaneous manifestations of dermatomyositis: a comprehensive review. *Clin Rev Allergy Immunol* 2017;53(3):337–356.

127. Kuhn A, Sontheimer RD. Cutaneous lupus erythematosus: molecular and cellular basis of clinical findings. *Curr Dir Autoimmun* 2008;10:119–140.

128. Millard TP, McGregor JM. Molecular genetics of cutaneous lupus erythematosus. *Clin Exp Dermatol* 2001;26(2):184–191.

129. Lowe G, Henderson CL, Grau RH, et al. A systematic review of drug-induced subacute cutaneous lupus erythematosus. *Br J Dermatol* 2011;164(3):465–472.

130. David-Bajar KM, Bennion SD, DeSpain JD, et al. Clinical, histologic, and immunofluorescent distinctions between subacute cutaneous lupus erythematosus and discoid lupus erythematosus. *J Invest Dermatol* 1992;99(3):251–257.

131. Elman SA, Joyce C, Nyberg F, et al. Development of classification criteria for discoid lupus erythematosus: results of a Delphi exercise. *J Am Acad Dermatol* 2017;77(2):261–267.

Acantholytic, Vesicular, and Pustular Disorders

IV

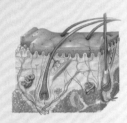

Keratinocytes may separate from each other on the basis of immunologic antigen–antibody–mediated damage resulting in separation and rounding-up of keratinocyte cell bodies (acantholysis), on the basis of edema and inflammation (spongiosis), or perhaps on the basis of structural deficiencies of cell adhesion (Darier disease). These processes produce intraepidermal spaces (vesicles, bullae, pustules).

IVA SUBCORNEAL AND/OR INTRACORNEAL SEPARATION

There is separation within or just below the stratum corneum. Inflammatory cells may be sparse, or may consist predominantly of neutrophils.

1. Sub/Intracorneal Separation, Scant Inflammatory Cells
2. Sub/Intracorneal Separation, Neutrophils Prominent
3. Sub/Intracorneal Separation, Eosinophils Predominant

IVA1 Sub/Intracorneal Separation, Scant Inflammatory Cells

There is separation within or just below the stratum corneum, associated with scant inflammation, usually lymphocytic. Pemphigus foliaceus is prototypic (1,2).

Pemphigus Foliaceus

Usually developing in middle-aged individuals, pemphigus foliaceus may have a chronic generalized course or may rarely present as an exfoliative dermatitis. The disorder is caused by autoantibodies to a desmosomal protein, desmoglein 1, causing dyshesion in the outer spinous and granular epidermal layers. Some cases may be related to exposure to drugs such as penicillamine (3). Patients present with flaccid bullae that usually arise on an erythematous base. Erythema, oozing, and crusting

are present. Because of their superficial location, the blisters break easily, leaving shallow erosions rather than the denuded areas seen in pemphigus vulgaris. Oral lesions do not occur. The Nikolsky sign is positive, and Tzanck preparation reveals acantholytic granular keratinocytes. Fogo selvagem (endemic pemphigus foliaceus which occurs in Brazil) is clinically, histologically, and immunologically indistinguishable from pemphigus foliaceus (4).

HISTOPATHOLOGY. The earliest change consists of acantholysis in the upper epidermis, within or adjacent to the granular layer, leading to a subcorneal bulla in some instances. More commonly, enlargement of the cleft leads to detachment of the stratum corneum without bulla formation. The number of acantholytic keratinocytes is usually small, often requiring a careful search to identify them. Secondary clefts may develop, leading to detachment of the epidermis in its midlevel. These clefts may extend to above the basal layer, rarely giving rise to limited areas of suprabasal separation. In the setting of a subcorneal blister, dyskeratotic granular keratinocytes are diagnostic for this disorder. Eosinophilic spongiosis may be prominent with intraepidermal eosinophilic pustules. Thus the histologic features of pemphigus foliaceus may have three patterns: (1) eosinophilic spongiosis, (2) a subcorneal blister, often with few acantholytic keratinocytes, and (3) a subcorneal blister with dyskeratotic granular keratinocytes, diagnostic for this disorder. The character of the inflammatory infiltrate observed is variable. Most commonly the histologic differential diagnoses considered for pemphigus foliaceus are staphylococcal scalded skin and bullous impetigo.

Direct immunofluorescence (DIF) in pemphigus foliaceus demonstrates cell surface membrane staining with antibodies to IgG. The staining may be confined to the upper epidermal layers or it may involve all epidermal layers, indistinguishable from pemphigus vulgaris. Indirect immunofluorescence (IIF) can also be utilized to detect circulating antibodies in the patient's blood. In pemphigus foliaceus, normal human skin has a higher sensitivity as a substrate than monkey esophagus (5). Enzyme-linked immunosorbent assay (ELISA) testing provides a quantitative and very sensitive method for detecting serum anti-dsg-1 antibodies. Sensitivities and specificities have been reported in the range of 92% to 100% (6).

Conditions to consider in the differential diagnosis:

staphylococcal scalded skin
bullous impetigo
miliaria crystallina
exfoliative dermatitis
pemphigus foliaceus
pemphigus erythematosus
necrolytic migratory erythema
pellagra
acrodermatitis enteropathica

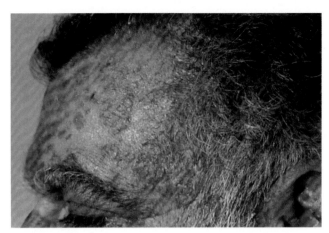

Clin. Fig. IVA1.a

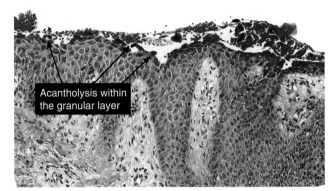

Fig. IVA1.b

Fig. IVA1.a

Clin. Fig. IVA1.a. *Pemphigus foliaceus.* A middle-aged male with crusted plaques required systemic cortico-steroids and immunosuppressive therapy to control his blistering disease. (W. Witmer.)

Fig. IVA1.a. *Pemphigus foliaceus, low power.* A blister forms in the superficial epidermis and there is a sparse dermal infiltrate.

Fig. IVA1.b. *Pemphigus foliaceus, high power.* The absence of a stratum corneum, and the presence of a few acantholytic cells, may be subtle clues to the diagnosis of pemphigus foliaceus. If there is an intact blister, it is seen as an intraepidermal blister within the granular cell layer and is devoid of an associated neutrophilic infiltrate. This feature is important in differentiating pemphigus foliaceus from impetigo/impetiginization.

IVA2 Sub/Intracorneal Separation, Neutrophils Prominent

There is separation in or just below the stratum corneum. Neutrophils are prominent in the stratum corneum and in the superficial epidermis, and can often be found in the dermis. *Impetigo contagiosa* is a prototypic example (7,8).

Impetigo Contagiosa

CLINICAL SUMMARY. Impetigo contagiosa is primarily an endemic disease of preschool-age children that may occur in epidemics. It is an acute, highly contagious infection of the superficial layers of the epidermis that is usually caused by either *Streptococcus pyogenes* or *Staphylococcus aureus*. Very early lesions consist of vesicopustules that

rupture quickly and are followed by heavy, yellow crusts. Most of the lesions are located in exposed areas. An occasional sequel is acute glomerulonephritis, which usually has a favorable long-term prognosis.

HISTOPATHOLOGY. The vesicopustule of impetigo contagiosa arises in the upper layers of the epidermis above, within, or below the granular layer. It contains numerous neutrophils. Not infrequently, a few acantholytic cells can be observed at the floor of the vesicopustule. Often, gram-positive cocci are present, both within neutrophils and extracellularly. The stratum malpighii underlying the bulla is spongiotic, and neutrophils often can be seen migrating through it. The upper dermis contains a moderately severe inflammatory

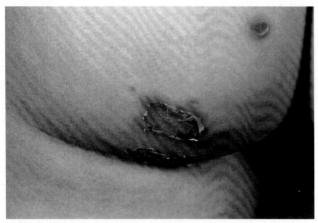

Clin. Fig. IVA2.a

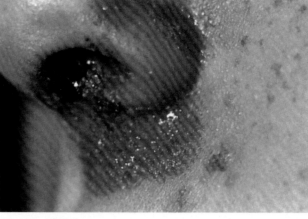

Clin. Fig. IVA2.b

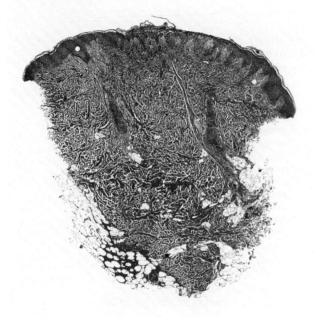

Fig. IVA2.a

Clin. Fig. IVA2.a. *Bullous impetigo.* This 4-year-old female developed culture-positive staphylococcal aureus erosions with a collaret of superficial desquamated skin on her buttock. Response to antibiotic therapy was dramatic.

Clin. Fig. IVA2.b. *Impetigo contagiosa.* Classic honey-colored crusts secondary to rupture of vesicopustules are seen in the nasal area of a child, an area commonly colonized with *Staphylococcal aureus.*

Fig. IVA2.a. *Impetigo contagiosa, medium power.* Neutrophils are seen in the upper epidermis, forming a subcorneal pustule. There is a superficial mixed infiltrate within the dermis.

infiltrate of neutrophils and lymphoid cells. At a later stage, when the bulla has ruptured, the horny layer is absent, and a crust composed of serous exudate and the nuclear debris of neutrophils may be seen covering the stratum malpighii.

Staphylococcal Scalded Skin Syndrome

CLINICAL SUMMARY. Staphylococcal scalded skin syndrome (Ritter disease) is clinically and histologically distinct from impetigo contagiosa (9). It occurs largely in the newborn and in children younger than 5 years, and rarely in older individuals often in association with immunodeficiency or renal insufficiency, and from bullous impetigo (10). The disease begins abruptly with diffuse erythema and fever. Large, flaccid bullae filled with

clear fluid form and rupture almost immediately. Large sheets of superficial epidermis separate and exfoliate. The disease is rarely fatal in children. In neonates with generalized lesions, and in adults with severe underlying diseases, the prognosis is worse. Both bullous impetigo and staphylococcal scalded skin syndrome are transmissible and can cause epidemics in nurseries, where they may occur together. The blisters in bullous impetigo and the scalded skin syndrome are caused by exfoliative toxin (exfoliatin, types A or B) released by staphylococcus, and targeting desmoglein 1 which is important for adhesion of the stratum corneum (11). In patients with bullous impetigo, the toxin produces blisters locally at the site of infection, whereas in cases of the scalded skin syndrome, it circulates throughout the body, causing blisters at sites distant from the infection (3). In these

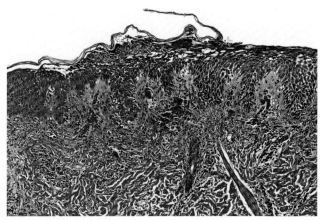

Fig. IVA2.b

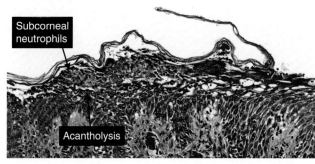

Fig. IVA2.c

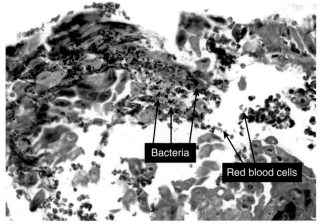

Fig. IVA2.d

Fig. IVA2.b,c. *Impetigo contagiosa, low and high power.* The subcorneal blister is filled with neutrophils. The stratum corneum is thickened and crusted.

Fig. IVA2.d. *Impetigo contagiosa, high power.* Gram stain demonstrates bacterial colonies within the stratum corneum.

two conditions, the bullae contain only few inflammatory cells, whereas in impetigo contagiosa the blisters are filled with neutrophils.

An important difference between the two diseases is that no staphylococci can be grown from the bullae of the staphylococcal scalded skin syndrome, in contrast to those of bullous impetigo. In staphylococcal scalded skin syndrome, the staphylococci are present at a distant focus, often a purulent conjunctivitis, rhinitis, or pharyngitis or rarely a cutaneous infection or a septicemia.

HISTOPATHOLOGY. In both bullous impetigo and staphylococcal scalded skin syndrome, the cleavage plane of the bulla, like that in impetigo contagiosa, lies in the uppermost epidermis either below or, less commonly, within the granular layer. A few acantholytic cells are often seen adjoining the cleavage plane. In contrast to impetigo contagiosa, however, there are few or no inflammatory cells within the bulla cavity. In bullous impetigo, the upper dermis may show a polymorphous infiltrate, whereas in the staphylococcal scalded skin syndrome the dermis is usually free of inflammation.

Folliculitis With Subcorneal Pustule Formation

A superficial biopsy of folliculitis could mimic a subcorneal pustule.

Acute Generalized Exanthematous Pustulosis

CLINICAL FEATURES. The majority of these cases have been associated with medications and may have previously been called pustular drug eruption. (See also Section IVB3.) Various drugs are implicated in acute generalized exanthematous pustulosis (AGEP) (12), and also food such as Rhus soup, a Korean delicacy. Widespread nonfollicular, sterile, pustules develop within a period of hours after administration of the offending agent. Although enteroviral infection and mercury exposure are cited as causes, antibacterial antibiotics are most often implicated with a broad range of other medications as well, including acetaminophen and terbinafine. The involvement of drug-specific T cells in the pathogenesis can be confirmed by positive skin patch tests and lymphocyte transformation tests. Fever, leukocytosis, purpura,

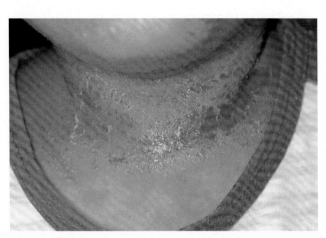

Clin. Fig. IVA2.c

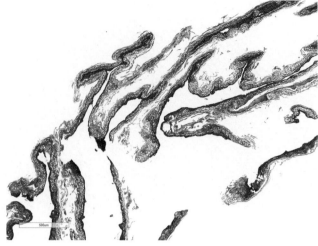

Fig. IVA2.e

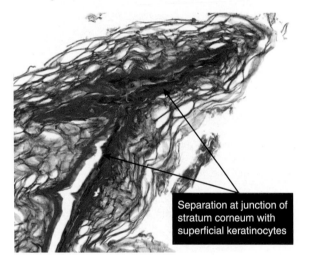

Separation at junction of stratum corneum with superficial keratinocytes

Fig. IVA2.f

Clin. Fig. IVA2.c. *Staphylococcal scalded skin syndrome.* A 2-year-old boy suddenly developed flaccid bulla on the erythematous patch with erosion and oozing after URI symptoms for 1 week.

Fig. IVA2.e. *Staphylococcal scalded skin syndrome.* Strips of desquamated material were sent for histology. There is separation beneath the stratum corneum.

Fig. IVA2.f. *Staphylococcal scalded skin syndrome.* At higher magnification, the locus action of the exfoliative toxin is visualized as a red band beneath the basket-weave keratin.

and occasionally clinical features suggesting erythema multiforme accompany the pustules. The pathophysiology of AGEP is unclear, but involvement of innate and acquired immune cells together with resident keratinocytes, recruiting and activating neutrophils through cytokine/chemokine mediators such as IL-17, IL-36, GM-CSF, TNFα and IL-8, has been postulated (13).

HISTOPATHOLOGY. Biopsies show subcorneal or intraepidermal pustules, papillary dermal edema, and a lymphohistiocytic perivascular infiltrate with some eosinophils and neutrophils. Vasculitis and/or single cell keratinocyte necrosis may be present.

Pustular Psoriasis and Palmoplantar Pustulosis

CLINICAL FEATURES. Palmoplantar pustulosis (PPP) is characterized by pustules that are elevated slightly above the level of the epidermis and press into the dermis. In 2007 the

International Psoriasis Council proposed that PPP should be considered a separate condition from pustular psoriasis, despite the presence of common phenotypes. In a subsequent study of 80 cases, the data concerning epidemiology, clinical presentation, genetics, histopathology, and pathogenesis did not permit a clear distinction between the two conditions, suggesting that they are at least closely related. PPP appears to preferentially occur in female smokers. Based on molecular profiling of gene expression, PPP and palmoplantar pustular psoriasis are highly related diseases that appear to be distinct from psoriasis vulgaris (14).

HISTOPATHOLOGY. The pustule cavity contains many neutrophils. Smaller spongiform pustules may be present in the epidermis adjacent to the larger lesion.

Conditions to consider in the differential diagnosis:

See Table IV.1.
Acute generalized exanthematous pustulosis (AGEP)

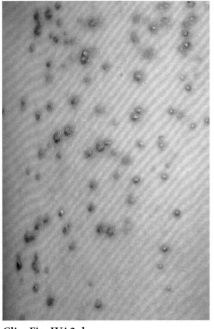

Clin. Fig. IVA2.d

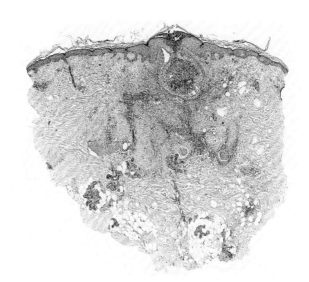

Fig. IVA2.g

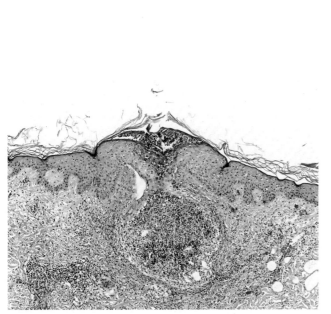

Fig. IVA2.h

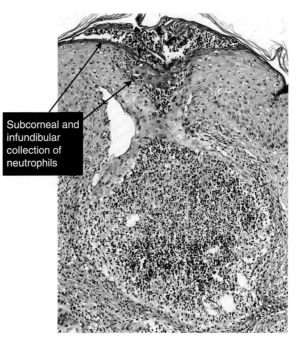

Subcorneal and infundibular collection of neutrophils

Fig. IVA.i

Clin. Fig. IVA2.d. *Folliculitis.* Multiple red papules and pustules suddenly developed in a follicular distribution on the shoulder of a 45-year-old man after taking steroids.

Fig. IVA2.g. *Folliculitis with subcorneal pustule formation, low power.* There is an intense, neutrophil-rich infiltrate which has obliterated the hair follicle. (J. Junkins-Hopkins.)

Fig. IVA2.h. *Folliculitis with subcorneal pustule formation, low power.* There is a mixed inflammatory infiltrate in the dermis around the follicle.

Fig. IVA2.i. *Folliculitis with subcorneal pustule formation, medium power.* The epidermis above the follicle shows formation of a subcorneal pustule. If only a superficial shave biopsy is taken, the biopsy resembles other entities in this subgroup and the diagnosis may be missed. (J. Junkins-Hopkins.)

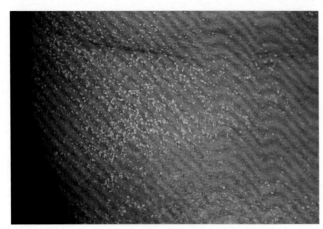

Clin. Fig. IVA2.e

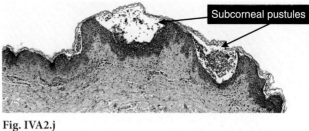

Fig. IVA2.j

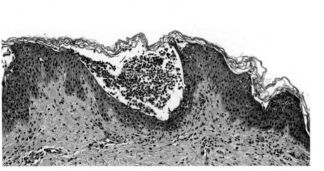

Fig. IVA2.k

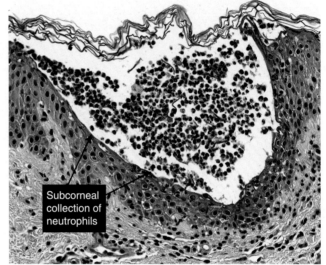

Fig. IVA2.l

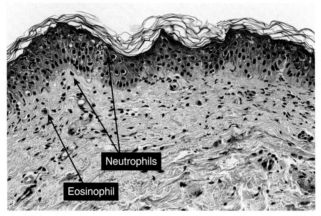

Fig. IVA2.m

Clin. Fig. IVA2.e. *Acute generalized exanthematous pustulosis (AGEP).* A 75-year-old woman suddenly developed myriads of yellow papules (pustules) after ingestion of Rhus soup, a known allergen.

Fig. IVA2.j. *Acute generalized exanthematous pustulosis (AGEP), medium power.* A subcorneal separation is seen associated with a superficial dermal infiltrate in which neutrophils are present.

Fig. IVA2.k,l. *Acute generalized exanthematous pustulosis, high power.* Neutrophils are seen in the upper epidermal layers as well as within the blister cavity. Differentiation from an early lesion of pustular psoriasis may require clinical correlation.

Fig. IVA2.m. *Acute generalized exanthematous pustulosis, high power.* Neutrophils and lymphocytes are present in the dermal infiltrate.

TABLE IV.1. Acute Generalized Exanthematous Pustulosis (AGEP), Pustular Psoriasis (von Zumbusch), Subcorneal Pustular Dermatosis (Sneddon–Wilkinson), and Bullous Impetigo Compared (11)

AGEP	Pustular Psoriasis	Subcorneal Pustular Dermatosis	Bullous Impetigo
Sterile pustules on erythematous base	Pinhead pustules in patches	Pustules coalescing in annular patterns	Small vesicles with clear yellow fluid
Fever, burning rash	Fever, chills	Oral lesions sometimes	Lymphangitis, adenopathy sometimes
Leukocytosis, eosinophilia	Leukocytosis, ESR, CRP, ASO, Ig up	May be immune dysfunction	Gram-positive cocci
Subcorneal and/or intraepithelial pustule, papillary dermal edema	Psoriasiform sometimes, spongiform pustules, papillary dermal edema	Neutrophils in pustules beneath stratum corneum	Subcorneal vesicles; spongiosis, few neutrophils, gram-positive cocci

pustular psoriasis
subcorneal pustular dermatosis (Sneddon–Wilkinson)
bullous impetigo
impetigo contagiosa
epidermis adjacent to folliculitis
impetiginized dermatitis
candidiasis
palmoplantar pustulosis
pustulosis palmaris et plantaris
IgA pemphigus
secondary syphilis
acropustulosis of infancy
transient neonatal pustular melanosis

IVA3 Sub/Intracorneal Separation, Eosinophils Predominant

There is separation in or just below the stratum corneum, with (pemphigus) or without acantholytic keratinocytes. Eosinophils are present in the epidermis, and occasionally there is eosinophilic spongiosis. The separation is associated with a dermal infiltrate that contains eosinophils. Erythema toxicum (neonatorum) is a prototypic example (15), which however is rarely biopsied.

Erythema Toxicum Neonatorum

CLINICAL SUMMARY. A benign, asymptomatic eruption affecting about 40% of term infants usually within 12 to 48 hours after birth, erythema toxicum lasts 2 to 3 days and consists of blotchy macular erythema, papules, and pustules that tend to develop at sites of pressure. The eruption is associated with blood eosinophilia.

HISTOPATHOLOGY. The macular erythema is characterized by sparse eosinophils in the upper dermis, largely in a perivascular location, and mild papillary dermal edema. The papules show an accumulation of numerous eosinophils and some neutrophils in the area of a hair follicle and the overlying epidermis. Papillary dermal edema is more intense and eosinophils more numerous. Mature pustules are subcorneal and are filled with eosinophils and occasional neutrophils. The pustules form as a result of the upward migration of eosinophils to the surface epidermis from within and around hair follicles.

DIFFERENTIAL DIAGNOSIS. The subcorneal pustules of impetigo and transient neonatal pustular melanosis are not follicular in origin and contain neutrophils rather than eosinophils. Although many eosinophils are present in the vesicles of incontinentia pigmenti, the vesicle is intraepidermal rather than subcorneal, and spongiosis is present. In addition, necrotic keratinocytes may be prominent in incontinentia pigmenti but are absent in erythema toxicum neonatorum.

Conditions to consider in the differential diagnosis:

erythema toxicum neonatorum
pemphigus foliaceus
pemphigus erythematosus
IgA pemphigus
eosinophilic pustular folliculitis
incontinentia pigmenti, vesicular
exfoliative dermatitis, drug induced
scabies

Scabies With Eosinophilic Pustulosis

An elderly patient with scabies had these unusual biopsy findings. In an appropriate setting, the differential diagnosis could include erythema toxicum neonatorum.

Acantholytic, Vesicular, and Pustular Disorders

IV

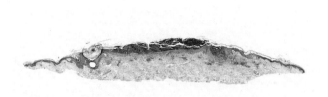

Fig. IVA3.a

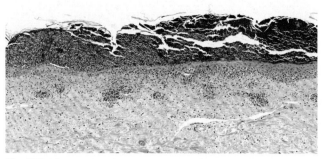

Fig. IVA3.b

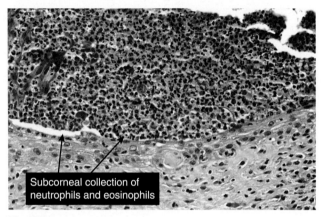

Subcorneal collection of neutrophils and eosinophils

Fig. IVA3.c

Fig. IVA3.a. *Subcorneal pustule with eosinophils.* There is a broad lesion characterized by increased cells in the stratum corneum with crust formation.

Fig. IVA3.b. *Subcorneal pustule with eosinophils.* Subcorneal pustule and a mixed cell infiltrate in the superficial dermis.

Fig. IVA3.c. *Subcorneal pustule with eosinophils.* The cells in the pustule are mostly eosinophils and also include neutrophils.

IVB INTRASPINOUS KERATINOCYTE SEPARATION, SPONGIOTIC

There are spaces within the epidermis (vesicles, bullae). There may be dyskeratosis or acantholysis, and a few eosinophils may be present in the epidermis.

1. Intraspinous Spongiosis, Scant Inflammatory Cells
2. Intraspinous Spongiosis, Lymphocytes Predominant
   2a. Intraspinous Spongiosis, Eosinophils Present
3. Intraspinous Spongiosis, Neutrophils Predominant

IVB1 Intraspinous Spongiosis, Scant Inflammatory Cells

The infiltrate in the dermis is scant, lymphocytic or eosinophilic. *Transient acantholytic dermatosis* (Grover disease [16]) and *friction blister* (17) are prototypic.

Friction Blister

CLINICAL SUMMARY. Friction blisters are caused by mechanical shearing forces, resulting in disruption to keratinocytes or cytolysis. This occurs in the normal epidermis when the structural (keratin) matrix of the keratinocyte is overwhelmed by high levels of physical agents such as friction and heat. Friction (mechanical energy applied parallel to the epidermis) leads to the shearing of keratinocytes one from another and of the keratinocytes themselves, typically at the level of the stratum spinosum, giving the characteristic clear, fluid-filled blisters. The area of the separation fills due to hydrostatic pressure with a clear transudate with a low protein level. At about 24 hours, there is high mitotic activity in the basal cells; at 48 and 120 hours, new stratum granulosum and stratum corneum, respectively, can be seen (18). Minimal friction may lead to cytolysis in subjects whose keratinocytes do not have a normal structural matrix, such as in epidermolysis bullosa.

HISTOPATHOLOGY. Usual friction blisters show evidence of initial spongiosis and then disruption of the keratinocytes in the spinous layer. In lesions of the palms or soles, the blisters remain intact for a time because of the thick stratum corneum in these sites.

Conditions to consider in the differential diagnosis:

dyskeratosis
epidermolytic hyperkeratosis
epidermolytic acanthoma

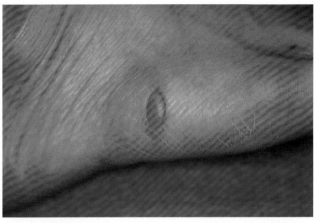

Clin. Fig. IVB1.a

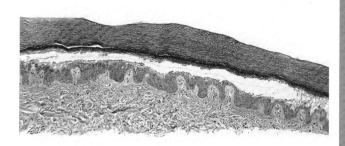

Fig. IVB1.a

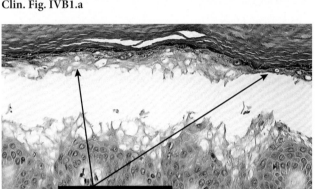
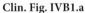

Intraepidermal
blister at various layers

Fig. IVB1.b

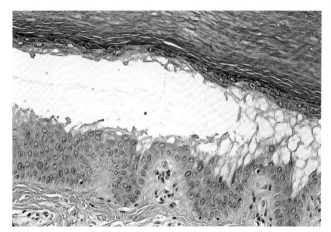

Fig. IVB1.c

Clin. Fig. IVB1.a. *Friction blister.* A blister on the foot at the site of rubbing of an ill-fitting shoe in a 56-year-old woman.

Fig. IVB1.a. *Friction blister, low power.* There is a blister in the midepidermis.

Fig. IVB1.b. *Friction blister, medium power.* The blister is formed by cytolysis of keratinocytes with spongiotic edema, but there is scant associated inflammation.

Fig. IVB1.c. *Friction blister, medium power.* There may be evidence of damage to the surface epithelium, or it may be relatively intact, especially on the palms or soles as in this example.

miliaria rubra
transient acantholytic dermatosis
bullous dermatitis of diabetes and of uremia
coma bulla
friction blisters

IVB2 Intraspinous Spongiosis, Lymphocytes Predominant

In the dermis, lymphocytes predominate. Eosinophils can be found in most examples of atopy, and in allergic contact dermatitis (ACD). The clinical manifestation of spongiotic dermatitis (a histologic pattern) is eczematous dermatitis. This is a T-cell-mediated inflammatory skin disease, where activated T cells may harm epidermal keratinocytes by direct cell–cell contact-mediated cytotoxicity or by secreted proinflammatory cytokines, accounting for at least some of the features of intercellular edema or spongiosis formation. It has been shown that activated T cells infiltrating the skin induce apoptosis of single keratinocytes, as shown *in situ*, and in the lesional skin of atopic dermatitis (AD) and ACD. Interestingly, in these studies, apoptosis of single keratinocytes was detected predominantly in suprabasal epidermal layers, concomitant with the predominant observed suprabasal spongiosis formation in these conditions. This may be due to the existence

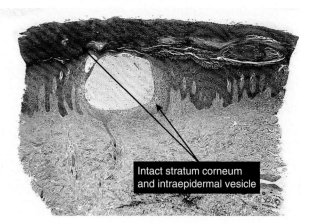

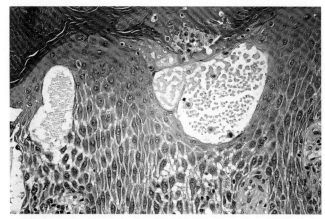

Fig. IVB2.a   Fig IVB2.b

Fig. IVB2.a. *Spongiotic dermatitis, dyshidrotic eczema, low power.* This biopsy of acral skin shows an intraepidermal vesicle and an associated superficial inflammatory infiltrate. A vesicle surrounded by spongiosis (spongiotic vesicle) is present beneath the intact acral-type stratum corneum.

Fig. IVB2.b. *Dyshidrotic eczema, high power.* There is diffuse spongiosis within the epidermis manifested by white spaces separating the keratinocytes. Several intraepidermal vesicles also form.

of antiapoptosis programs predominantly in basal keratinocytes (19). The distinction from PPP can sometimes be difficult and has been recently summarized (20).

Dyshidrotic Dermatitis/Eczema (Pompholyx)

CLINICAL SUMMARY. This entity is characterized by recurrent, severely pruritic, deep-seated vesicles (hence the name pompholyx or "bubbles") that classically involve the lateral aspects of the fingers and, in some cases, the toes. Emotional stress may exacerbate the eruption. In chronic cases, there may be more extensive involvement of the palms and soles. Although the eruption develops acutely, it may become chronic with erythema, lichenification, and fissuring. Secondary impetiginization (bacterial infection with neutrophils in the stratum corneum) is common.

HISTOPATHOLOGY. Spongiosis and intraepidermal vesiculation occur in acute lesions. There is a superficial perivascular lymphohistiocytic infiltrate with exocytosis of lymphocytes into spongiotic zones. The infiltration is usually mild. In acute lesions, the compact, thickened stratum corneum of acral skin remains intact, and the epidermal thickness is normal. With chronicity, spongiosis diminishes, acanthosis and parakeratosis predominate, and serum may be identified within the stratum corneum. Difficulty in diagnosis may occur because of the formation of vesiculopustules in older lesions.

Conditions to consider in the differential diagnosis:

spongiotic (eczematous) dermatitis (see Section IIIB.1)
atopic dermatitis
allergic contact dermatitis
photoallergic drug eruption
irritant contact dermatitis
nummular eczema
dyshidrotic dermatitis
"id" reaction
seborrheic dermatitis
stasis dermatitis
miliaria rubra
pityriasis rosea

IVB2a Intraspinous Spongiosis, Eosinophils Present

The number of eosinophils seen is variable from many in incontinentia pigmenti and pemphigus vegetans to few in AD. Eosinophilic spongiosis is a histopathologic reaction pattern that is a common and consistent finding common in certain inflammatory skin diseases, including spongiotic dermatitis, arthropod bite reactions and scabies, occasionally viral vesicular disorders, incontinentia pigmenti, and immunobullous disorders, including especially bullous pemphigoid, pemphigus, and related disorders (21). Eosinophilic spongiosis can also be encountered occasionally in a variety of other unrelated disorders, including polycythemia vera, porokeratosis, and Meyerson "inflammatory nevi." Although intraepithelial eosinophils can be found in biopsies of follicular disorders, such as Ofuji disease or eosinophilic folliculitis, the term eosinophilic spongiosis is reserved for cases with eosinophils present in spongiotic areas of the epidermis (22).

Acantholytic, Vesicular, and Pustular Disorders

IV

Acute Contact Dermatitis

Contact dermatitis (CD) is caused by a contact with environmental chemicals resulting in erythema and eczema formation. At least two distinct forms of CD can be distinguished—irritant contact dermatitis (ICD) and ACD. ICD activates innate but not adaptive inflammatory responses. It is both clinically and histopathologically a variable inflammatory condition that may be acute or chronic, depending on the causative chemical and the exposure pattern. Strong irritative chemicals such as acids, bases, and detergents immediately lead to clinical symptoms, while weak irritants may result in subtler changes. ICD leads to a rapid response, usually within minutes/hours after contact with the irritant, and is usually confined to the area of contact with the irritant. In contrast, ACD can induce widespread to systemic immune-mediated hypersensitivity reactions. ACD reactions are caused by contact with one of the >4,350 known different potential chemical sensitizers (23).

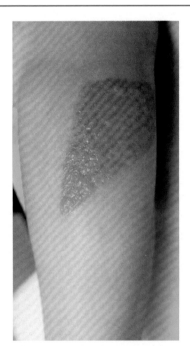

Clin. Fig. IVB2a

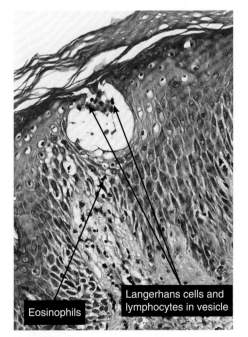

Fig IVB2a.c

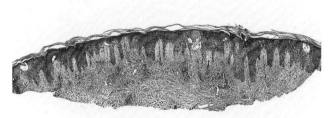

Fig. IVB2a.a

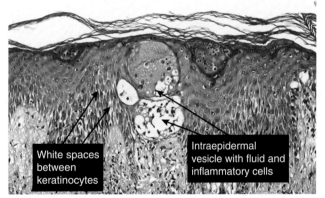

Fig. IVB2a.b

Clin. Fig. IVB2a. *Spongiotic dermatitis.* Blisters developed on an erythematous base on the forearm following exposure to plants during hiking in a 41-year-old man.

Fig. IVB2a.a. *Spongiotic dermatitis (acute contact dermatitis), low power.* In this acute lesion, the stratum corneum shows a basket-weave pattern. Intraepidermal vesicles are seen associated with a perivascular inflammatory infiltrate.

Fig. IVB2a.b,c. *Spongiotic dermatitis (acute contact dermatitis), high power.* There is diffuse spongiosis with intraepidermal vesicles. The infiltrate is mixed but contains eosinophils in the dermis, and in the spongiotic epidermis, favoring allergic contact dermatitis.

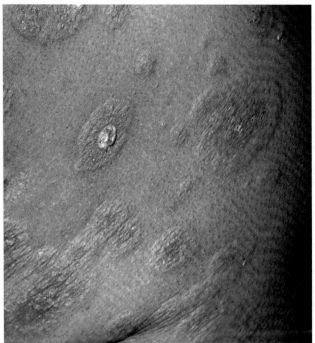

Clin. Fig. IVB2.b

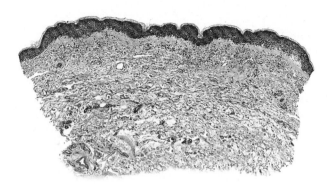

Fig. IVB2a.d

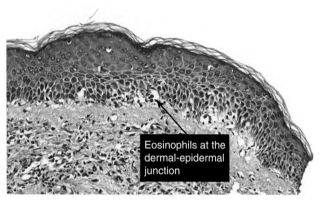

Eosinophils at the dermal-epidermal junction

Fig. IVB2a.e

Clin. Fig. IVB2.b. *Bullous pemphigoid.* Pruritic, urticarial plaques on the trunk often herald the diagnosis of this blistering disease most often seen in elderly persons.

Fig. IVB2a.d. *Bullous pemphigoid, urticarial phase, medium power.* In this example of bullous pemphigoid, it mimics an acute contact dermatitis with intraepidermal spongiosis and eosinophilic spongiosis.

Fig. IVB2a.e. *Bullous pemphigoid, urticarial phase, high power.* Eosinophils are seen accumulating at the dermal–epidermal junction and within the dermal papillae, a feature which maybe a clue to the diagnosis of pemphigoid. In many instances, if blister formation has not occurred, direct immunofluorescence may be necessary to distinguish early pemphigoid from acute contact dermatitis.

See also Section IIIB1a for discussion of histopathology. In a detailed study, it was concluded that histopathology does not reliably differentiate between ACD, ICD, and AD, but helps to exclude psoriasis, tinea, or T-cell lymphoma. The presence of numerous eosinophils somewhat favored AD. Differentiation among these conditions should be based on clinical features and results of allergy tests (24).

Bullous Pemphigoid, Urticarial Phase

See also Section IVE3.

Incontinentia Pigmenti

CLINICAL SUMMARY. Incontinentia pigmenti is a rare X-linked dominantly inherited neuroectodermal dysplasia. Males with the abnormal gene on their single X chromosome are hemizygous for this condition and hence are so severely affected that they usually die in utero. The familial form of this disorder IP2 (or classical incontinentia pigmentosa) is localized to the Xq28 region. It is due to a mutation in the IKK-gamma gene formerly called NEMO (25). While mostly a disorder of females, cases have been described in males with Klinefelter syndrome (XXY) and somatic mosaicism with a postzygotic NEMO mutation (26).

The disorder has four stages, beginning with a phase of erythema and bullae in infancy, progressing to linear, verrucous lesions which subside, leaving widely disseminated areas of irregular, spattered, or whorled pigmentation to develop. In the fourth stage, seen in adult females, subtle, faint, hypochromic, or atrophic lesions in a linear pattern are most apparent on the lower extremities. Defects of hair, nails, and teeth occur. Central nervous system manifestations in the eye and in the brain cause the most disability, and there can be other systemic involvement (27).

HISTOPATHOLOGY. The vesicles seen during the first stage arise within the epidermis and are associated with eosinophilic spongiosis, often with single dyskeratotic cells and whorls of squamous cells with central keratinization. Like the epidermis, the dermis has an infiltrate containing many eosinophils and some mononuclear cells. The combination of eosinophilic spongiosis, spongiotic vesiculation, and dyskeratotic keratinocytes is virtually pathognomonic of incontinentia pigmenti, being seen also only in Grover disease which is easily distinguishable on other grounds (22). In the second stage there is acanthosis, irregular papillomatosis, and hyperkeratosis with intraepidermal keratinization, consisting of whorls of keratinocytes and of scattered dyskeratotic cells. The basal cells are vacuolated, and there is a decrease in their melanin content. The dermis shows a mild, chronic inflammatory infiltrate intermingled with melanophages. The areas of pigmentation seen in the third stage show extensive deposits of melanin within melanophages located in the upper dermis. In the hypopigmented/atrophic stage, there is epidermal atrophy, decreased melanin in the epidermal basal layer, apoptotic bodies, and absence of the pilosebaceous units and eccrine glands.

Conditions to consider in the differential diagnosis:

spongiotic (eczematous) dermatitis
atopic dermatitis
allergic contact dermatitis
photoallergic drug eruption
bullous pemphigoid, urticarial phase
incontinentia pigmenti, vesicular stage

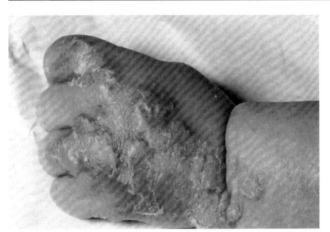

Clin. Fig. IVB2.c

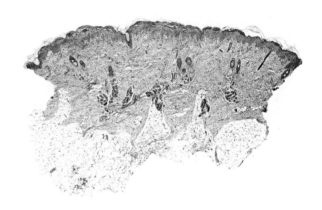

Fig. IVB2a.f

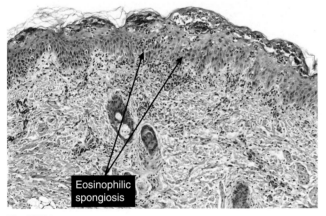

Eosinophilic spongiosis

Fig. IVB2a.g

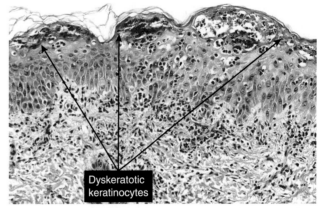

Dyskeratotic keratinocytes

Fig. IVB2a.h

Clin. Fig. IVB2.c. *Incontinentia pigmenti, verrucous stage.* A 5-month-old developed blisters followed by hyperpigmented and verrucous changes in a swirled pattern on thigh and leg. Mother and maternal grandmother had skin and dental abnormalities.

Fig. IVB2a.f,g. *Incontinentia pigmenti, low and medium power.* A vesicular stage lesion. Many eosinophils are seen in the dermis and in the focally acanthotic and spongiotic epidermis.

Fig. IVB2a.h. *Incontinentia pigmenti, high power.* Eosinophilic spongiosis and early acanthosis, with numerous dyskeratotic keratinocytes located superficially in this example.

IVB3 Intraspinous Spongiosis, Neutrophils Predominant

Neutrophils are seen in the epidermis, stratum corneum, and in the dermis. Aggregations of neutrophils in the superficial spinous layer constitute the spongiform pustules of Kogoj characteristic of psoriasis. Neutrophilic spongiosis has been less well characterized than eosinophilic spongiosis. It may be seen in a variety of conditions including psoriasis, acute generalized exanthematous pustulosis, intraepidermal blistering diseases including dermatitis herpetiformis, linear IgA bullous disease, and bullous lupus erythematosus (LE) which are all subepidermal immunobullous disorders in which neutrophils predominate in the inflammatory infiltrate, and in infections and infestations such as dermatophytosis, scabies, impetigo, and viral vesicular disorders (15).

Dermatophytosis

The presence of neutrophils in the stratum corneum, sometimes associated with layers of parakeratosis to form a "sandwich sign," constitutes clues to the presence of dermatophytes (28).

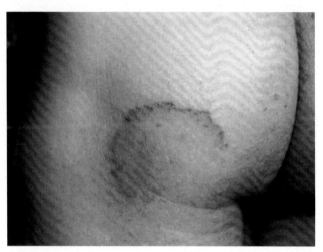

Clin. Fig. IVB3

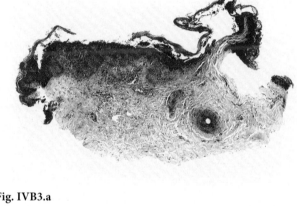

Fig. IVB3.a

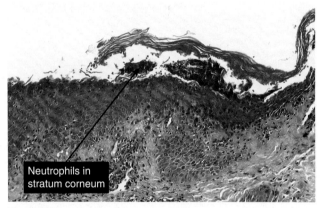

Fig. IVB3.b

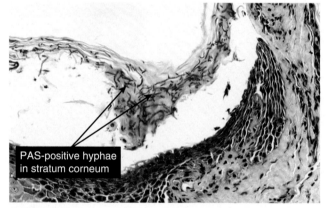

Fig. IVB3.c

Clin. Fig. IVB3. *Dermatophytosis*. A large erythematous patch showing central clearing and a polycyclic scaling border, which is quite narrow and thread like.

Fig. IVB3.a. *Dermatophytosis, low power.* There is a dense infiltrate in the dermis extending into the epidermis.

Fig. IVB3.b. *Dermatophytosis, high power.* The stratum corneum is separated and focally parakeratotic with numerous neutrophils. This pattern could mimic subcorneal pustular dermatosis or pemphigus foliaceus. Dermatophytes are often not readily identified in the H&E stain. This finding of "neutrophils in the horn" should prompt a stain for fungus.

Fig. IVB3.c. *Dermatophytosis, high power.* PAS stain reveals septate hyphae within the stratum corneum. The organisms are often much less numerous than here.

Conditions to consider in the differential diagnosis:

pustular psoriasis
Reiter syndrome
IgA pemphigus
subcorneal pustular dermatosis (Sneddon–Wilkinson)
exanthemic pustular drug eruptions
impetiginized dermatosis
dermatophytosis
rupial secondary syphilis
seborrheic dermatitis (see Section IIIB.1c)
epidermis adjacent to folliculitis
impetigo contagiosa
hydroa vacciniforme
mucocutaneous lymph node syndrome (Kawasaki disease, pustular variant)

IVC INTRASPINOUS KERATINOCYTE SEPARATION, ACANTHOLYTIC

There are spaces within the epidermis (vesicles, bullae). The process of separation is acantholysis. Keratinocytes within the spinous layer detach or separate from each other or from basal keratinocytes. There may be dyskeratosis, and a few eosinophils may be present in the epidermis. The infiltrate in the dermis is variable, composed of lymphocytes with or without eosinophils.

1. Intraspinous Acantholysis, Scant Inflammatory Cells
2. Intraspinous Acantholysis, Predominant Lymphocytes
   2a. Intraspinous Acantholysis, Eosinophils Present
3. Intraspinous Separation, Neutrophils or Mixed Cell types

IVC1 Intraspinous Acantholysis, Scant Inflammatory Cells

The infiltrate in the dermis is scant, lymphocytic or eosinophilic. *Hailey–Hailey disease* and Grover disease are prototypic.

Familial Benign Pemphigus (Hailey–Hailey Disease)

CLINICAL SUMMARY. Familial benign pemphigus is inherited as an autosomal dominant trait, with a family history obtainable in about two-thirds of the patients. It is characterized by a localized, recurrent eruption of small vesicles on an erythematous base (29). By peripheral extension, the lesions may assume a circinate configuration. The sites of predilection are the intertriginous areas, especially the axillae and the groin. Only very few instances of mucosal lesions have been reported. Mutations in ATP2Cl, encoding a calcium pump, are the cause of Hailey–Hailey disease (30,31).

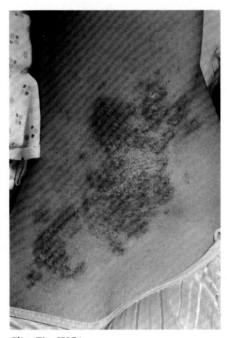

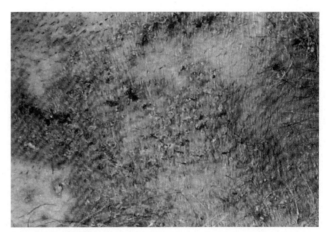

Clin. Fig. IVC1.a   **Clin. Fig. IVC1.b**

Clin. Fig. IVC1.a. *Hailey–Hailey disease.* A 39-year-old woman presented with malodorous vegetating, erythematous crusted erosions, peripheral flaccid bullae, and scattered pustules in the axillae and groin.

Clin. Fig. IVC1.b. *Hailey–Hailey disease.* The patient's 43-year-old brother has similar macerated plaques with pustules in the intertriginous areas, characteristic of this autosomal dominant disorder. (*continues*)

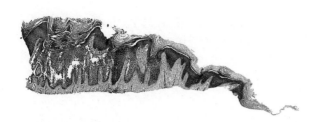

Fig. IVC1.a

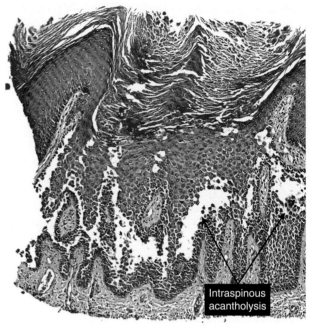

Intraspinous acantholysis

Fig. IVC1.b

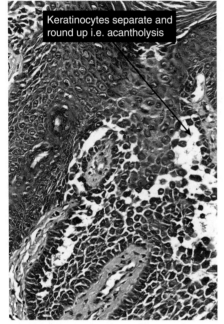

Keratinocytes separate and round up i.e. acantholysis

Fig. IVC1.c

Fig. IVC1.a. *Hailey–Hailey disease, low power.* The epidermis is hyperplastic and focally hyperkeratotic. There is diffuse intraepidermal separation of keratinocytes at all levels of the epidermis.

Fig. IVC1.b. *Hailey–Hailey disease, medium power.* The acantholysis involves the full thickness of the dermis, forming the "dilapidated brick wall." Hailey–Hailey disease may also show suprabasal acantholysis as well as dyskeratosis. The dyskeratosis is generally less prominent than what is seen in Darier disease.

Fig. IVC1.c. *Hailey–Hailey disease, high power.* High magnification of the acantholysis demonstrating separation of keratinocytes from one another, and rounding up within the blister cavity.

HISTOPATHOLOGY. Although early lesions may show small suprabasal separations, so-called lacunae, in fully developed lesions there are large separations, that is, vesicles and even bullae, in a predominantly suprabasal position. Villi, which are elongated papillae lined by a single layer of basal cells, protrude upward into the bullae, and, in some cases, narrow strands of epidermal cells proliferate downward into the dermis. Many cells of the detached stratum malpighii show loss of their intercellular bridges, so that acantholysis affects large portions of the epidermis. Individual cells and groups of cells usually are seen in large numbers in the bulla cavity. Some acantholytic cells may exhibit premature keratinization, resembling the grains of Darier disease. In spite of the extensive loss of intercellular bridges, the cells of the detached epidermis in many places are only slightly separated from one another because a few intact intercellular bridges still hold them loosely together. This quite typical feature gives the detached epidermis the appearance of a dilapidated brick wall.

Transient Acantholytic Dermatosis (Grover Disease)

CLINICAL SUMMARY. Transient acantholytic dermatosis is characterized by pruritic, discrete papules and papulovesicles on the chest, back, and thighs (32,33). In rare instances, vesicles and even bullae are seen. Most patients are middle-aged or elderly men. Although the disorder is transient in the majority of patients, lasting from 2 weeks to 3 months, it can persist for several years. Despite histologic similarity to Darier disease, Grover disease does not share an abnormality in the ATP2A2 gene (34). Lesions identical to those of Grover disease are commonly seen incidentally, for example, in melanoma or other excision specimens, and may represent a subclinical form of the disease (35). In patients on cytotoxic chemotherapy for leukemia and similar conditions, these lesions may become more prominent clinically, and histologically these, and apparently also lesions in nonspecific settings, may exhibit pronounced dysmaturation (36).

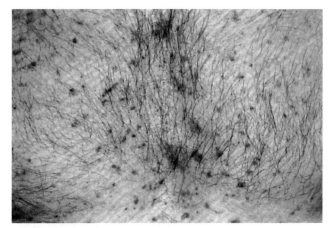

Clin. Fig. IVC1.c

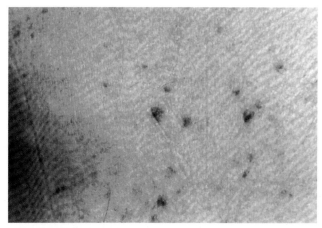

Clin. Fig. IVC1.d

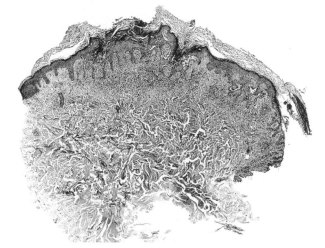

Fig. IVC1.d

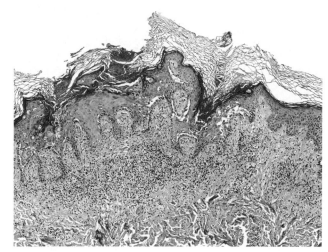

Fig. IVC1.e

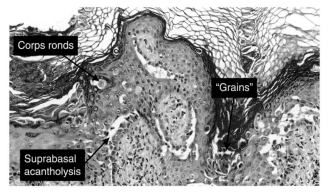

Fig. IVC1.f

Clin. Fig. IVC1.c. *Transient acantholytic dermatosis (Grover disease).* An elderly male presented with pruritic lesions on the chest and back.

Clin. Fig. IVC1.d. *Grover disease.* The lesions are discrete pruritic brown keratotic papules.

Fig. IVC1.d. *Transient acantholytic dermatosis (Grover disease), low power.* At scanning magnification, multiple foci of intraepidermal separation are seen. There is a mild superficial, dermal inflammatory infiltrate. Multiple histologic changes can be seen in these areas of intraepidermal separation, including the most common pattern seen here which mimics Darier disease, but also patterns of Hailey–Hailey disease, pemphigus vulgaris, pemphigus foliaceus, and spongiotic dermatitis.

Fig. IVC1.e. *Transient acantholytic dermatosis (Grover disease), medium power.* There is hyperkeratosis and there is an inflammatory infiltrate in the dermis.

Fig. IVC1.f. *Grover disease, Darier pattern, medium power.* There is suprabasal acantholysis with parakeratosis and corps ronds in the upper epidermal layer.

HISTOPATHOLOGY. Focal acantholysis and dyskeratosis ("focal acantholytic dyskeratosis") are present. Because these foci are small, they are sometimes found only when step sections are obtained. The acantholysis may occur in five histologic patterns, resembling Darier disease, Hailey–Hailey disease, pemphigus vulgaris, superficial pemphigus, or spongiotic dermatitis. Two or more of these patterns may be found in the same specimen. In a recent study, a number of additional patterns were described, namely cases with porokeratosis-like oblique columns of parakeratosis, lesions showing a silhouette reminiscent of a lentiginous nevus, intraepidermal vesicular lesions, lichenoid changes with basal vacuolization and dyskeratosis, and dysmature foci with keratinocyte atypia. In addition, the dermal infiltrate was quite often composed not only of lymphocytes intermingled with eosinophils, but also with neutrophils. Also, there was sometimes cytoplasmic edema of endothelial cells, and erythrocyte extravasation. In addition, involved areas were sometimes larger than 2 mm (37). The expression of Syndecan-1, a proteoglycan important for keratinocytes intercellular adhesion is markedly decreased in Grover disease, as in other acantholytic conditions such as pemphigus and herpes simplex infection (see also Section IVC1) (38).

Conditions to consider in the differential diagnosis:

  acantholytic dyskeratosis
  Darier disease
  transient acantholytic dermatosis (Grover disease)
  warty dyskeratoma (isolated keratosis follicularis)

  epidermolytic hyperkeratosis
  epidermolytic acanthoma
  Hailey–Hailey disease
  focal acantholytic dyskeratosis
  acantholytic solar keratosis
  pemphigus erythematosus
  pemphigus foliaceus
  friction blister (cytolytic blister)

IVC2 Intraspinous Acantholysis, Predominant Lymphocytes

In the dermis, lymphocytes are predominant. In erythema multiforme and related lesions there is necrosis of individual cells (apoptosis) that may become confluent. Herpes simplex and varicella-zoster are prototypic examples (39).

Herpes Simplex

Two immunologically distinct viruses can cause herpes simplex: herpes simplex virus type 1 (orofacial type) and herpes simplex virus type 2 (genital type), often referred to as HSV-1 and HSV-2, respectively (40). Primary infection with HSV-1 is usually subclinical in childhood. In about 10% of the cases, acute gingivostomatitis occurs, usually in childhood and only rarely in early adult life. HSV-2 generally is acquired venereally. Occasionally, an infant contracts HSV-2 in utero or by direct contact in the birth canal. Recurrent infections of the oral cavity, the skin, or the genitals can result either from reactivation of a latent infection or from a new infection.

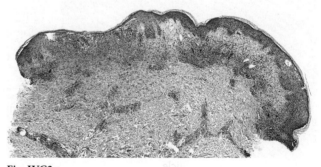

Fig. IVC2.a

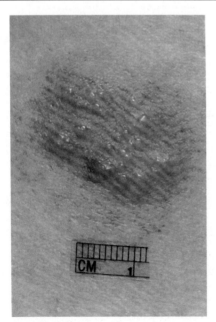

Clin. Fig. IVC2.a

Clin. Fig. IVC2.a. *Herpes simplex.* A 28-year-old woman gave a history of burning and pruritus and recurrent clusters of vesicles on an edematous erythematous base on her thigh.

Fig. IVC2.a. *Herpes simplex infection, low power.* There is diffuse epidermal spongiosis as well as intraepidermal vesicle formation. There is an associated mixed dermal inflammatory infiltrate.

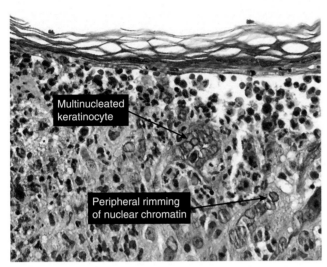

Fig. IVC2.b

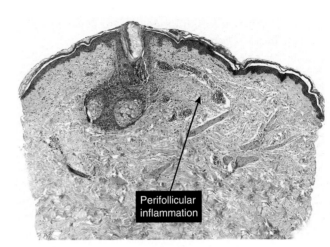

Fig. IVC2.c

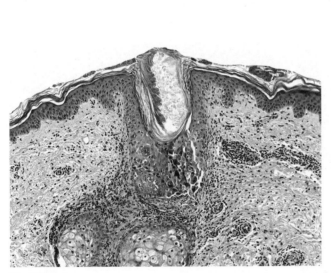

Fig. IVC2.d

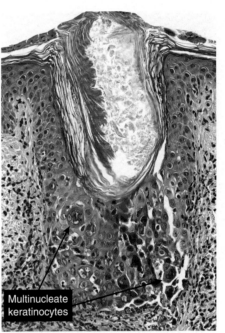

Fig. IVC2.e

Fig. IVC2.b. *Herpes simplex infection, high power.* Multiple keratinocytes of the epithelium show typical nuclear changes of herpes viral infection, including peripheral rimming and a ground glass appearance; also several multinucleated keratinocytes are present.

Fig. IVC2.c. *Follicular herpes simplex infection, low power.* Occasionally, involvement is confined to a skin appendage, such as this follicle.

Fig. IVC2.d. *Follicular herpes simplex infection, medium power.* There is a perivascular and interstitial lymphocytic infiltrate around the follicle.

Fig. IVC2.e. *Follicular herpes simplex infection, high power.* Characteristic viral cytopathic changes are seen.

Both primary and recurrent herpes simplex, in their earliest stages, show one or several groups of vesicles on an inflamed base. If located on a mucous surface, the vesicles erode quickly, whereas, if located on the skin, they may become pustular before crusting.

HISTOPATHOLOGY. Herpes simplex of the skin produces profound degeneration of keratinocytes, resulting in acantholysis. Degeneration of epidermal cells occurs in two forms: ballooning degeneration and reticular degeneration, both of which are changes typical of viral vesicles. The earliest changes include nuclear swelling of keratinocytes. With hematoxylin and eosin stains, these nuclei appear slate gray and homogeneous. Ballooning degeneration (swelling of epidermal cells) then follows.

Eosinophilic inclusion bodies are frequently observed in the centers of enlarged, round nuclei of balloon cells. Reticular degeneration is a process in which epidermal cells are distended by intracellular edema, so that cell walls rupture. Through coalescence, a multilocular vesicle results, the septa of which are formed by resistant cellular walls. In older vesicles, the cellular walls disappear and the vesicle becomes unilocular. Reticular degeneration is not specific for viral vesicles, because it also occurs in the vesicles of dermatitis. The upper dermis beneath a viral vesicle contains an inflammatory infiltrate of variable density. In some cases of herpes simplex, vascular damage is present, showing necrosis of vessel walls, microthrombi, and hemorrhage. In addition, eosinophilic inclusions may be found in endothelial cells and fibroblasts.

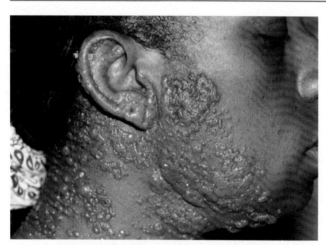

Clin. Fig. IVC2.b

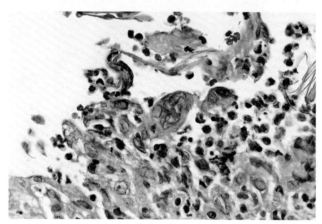

Fig. IVC2.g

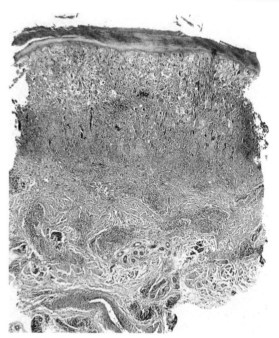

Fig. IVC2.f

Clin. Fig. IVC2.b. *Herpes zoster.* Lakes of umbilicated vesicles in a dermatomal distribution appeared in this HIV-positive middle-aged female.

Fig. IVC2.f. *Varicella-zoster infection, low power.* The epidermis shows diffuse spongiosis as well as necrosis. There is a moderately intense superficial and deep inflammatory infiltrate that may extend into the subcutaneous fat. Although varicella-zoster cannot always be distinguished from herpes simplex using histology, the infiltrate in varicella-zoster is generally more intense and extends more deeply into the dermis. Immunohistochemical staining provides specific differentiation of the two conditions.

Fig. IVC2.g. *Varicella-zoster infection, high power.* Similar to what is seen in herpes simplex infection, keratinocytes show multinucleation and the nuclei show peripheral rimming and ground glass change of the chromatin.

Varicella-Zoster Infection

Varicella-zoster virus has two distinct clinical presentations. In children, the eruption usually presents as chicken pox with generalized vesicles on an erythematous base at various stages of evolution, while in adults, painful grouped vesicles arise in a dermatomal distribution as herpes zoster, shingles (38). Persistent "herpes zoster granulomatous dermatitis" has been described up to 3 months after acute zoster dermatitis (41).

Toxic Epidermal Necrolysis, Stevens–Johnson Syndrome, and Erythema Multiforme With Intraepidermal Vesiculation

See also Section IIIH1.

In toxic epidermal necrolysis (TEN, Lyell syndrome) and Stevens–Johnson syndrome (SJS), bullous lesions of erythema multiforme, and the central portion of target lesions of erythema multiforme, there are numerous necrotic keratinocytes, with full-thickness epidermal necrosis in TEN, and a subepidermal separation to form a bulla, or to result in extensive desquamation of the necrotic epithelium. The dermal inflammatory infiltrate is sparser in TEN than in erythema multiforme and SJS. Extravasated erythrocytes are commonly found within the blister cavity. Melanophages within the papillary dermis occur in late lesions. Clinicopathologic correlation is required to distinguish among these entities.

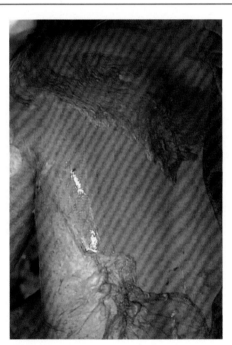

Clin. Fig. IVC2.c

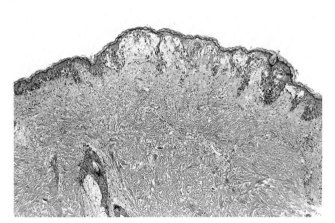

Fig. IVC2.h

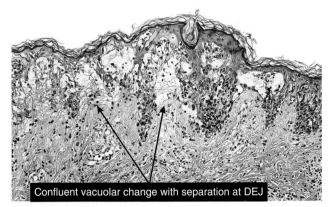

Confluent vacuolar change with separation at DEJ

Fig. IVC2.i

Clin. Fig. IVC2.c. *Toxic epidermal necrolysis.* The patient initially presented with a painful widespread erythematous rash which soon developed into sheets of peeling skin with erosions. This is a serious skin condition with a mortality of 25% to 50% and requires intensive medical care in a burn unit.

Fig. IVC2.h. *Erythema multiforme/toxic epidermal necrolysis, low power.* There is a focus of prominent epidermal spongiosis and necrosis. There is a sparse dermal infiltrate of lymphocytes.

Fig. IVC2.i. *Erythema multiforme/toxic epidermal necrolysis, medium power.* The intact, basket-weave stratum corneum portrays the acute nature of this lesion. The epidermis shows multiple zones of intraspinous separation and blister formation. (*continues*)

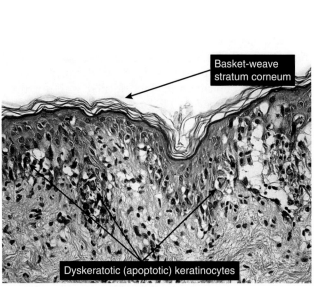

Fig. IVC2.j

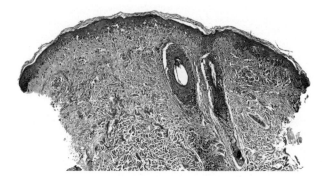

Fig. IVC2.j2

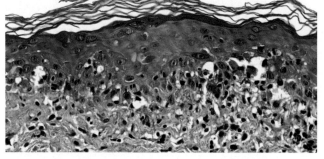

Fig. IVC2.j3

Fig. IVC2.j. *Erythema multiforme/toxic epidermal necrolysis, medium power.* At the periphery of the lesion a few lymphocytes are seen tagging the dermal–epidermal interface and are associated with vacuolar alteration, the earliest change in this process.

Fig. IVC2.j1. *Erythema multiforme.* Low power. Although not especially vesicular, this is a good additional example of erythema multiforme.

Fig. IVC2.j2. *Erythema multiforme.* Medium power.

Fig. IVC2.j3. *Erythema multiforme.* High power showing vacuolar change and numerous apoptotic keratinocytes. In TEN, the vacuolar change would become confluent and the epidermis would slough.

Paraneoplastic Pemphigus

CLINICAL SUMMARY. This condition is associated with underlying neoplasms (42), most commonly lymphoma, chronic lymphocytic leukemia, Castleman disease, thymoma, spindle cell sarcoma, and Waldenström macroglobulinemia. Patient sera recognize multiple antigens of the plakin protein family that include desmoplakin, bullous pemphigoid antigen I (BPAG1), envoplakin and periplakin, and desmogleins 1 and 3 (43). The cutaneous lesions are quite polymorphic. The most consistent clinical feature of paraneoplastic pemphigus (PNP) is the presence of intractable stomatitis mimicking SJS. Small airway occlusion, secondary to pulmonary epithelial injury can be fatal. Autoantibodies are deposited in the kidneys, bladder and muscle, resulting in a paraneoplastic multiorgan syndrome (44). The term paraneoplastic autoimmune multiorgan syndrome (PAMS) may more accurately describe the full spectrum of presentations and pathologic findings associated with this condition (45). At least 6 different clinical variants are recognized: bullous pemphigoid like, cicatricial pemphigoid like, pemphigus like, erythema multiforme like, graft-versus-host disease (GVHD) like, and lichen planus like.

HISTOPATHOLOGY. The histologic features are variable, correlating with the various clinical presentations. The lesions show a unique combination of erythema multiforme–like, lichen planus–like, pemphigus vulgaris–like, and pemphigoid-like features. The principal findings are suprabasal acantholysis as seen in pemphigus vulgaris with, in addition, basal apoptosis, in association

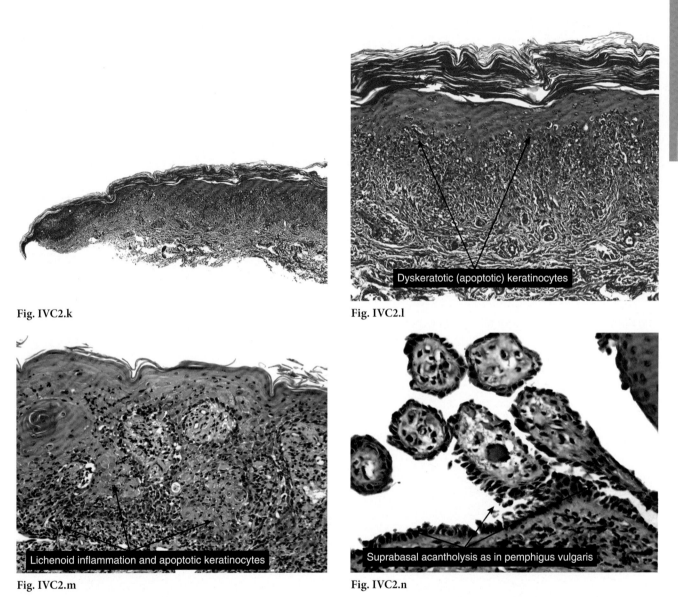

Fig. IVC2.k

Fig. IVC2.l

Dyskeratotic (apoptotic) keratinocytes

Lichenoid inflammation and apoptotic keratinocytes

Fig. IVC2.m

Suprabasal acantholysis as in pemphigus vulgaris

Fig. IVC2.n

Fig. IVC2.k. *Paraneoplastic pemphigus.* In this lesion, the pattern is predominantly lichenoid.

Fig. IVC2.l. *Paraneoplastic pemphigus.* A dense lichenoid mixed cell infiltrate with some suprabasal apoptotic cells.

Fig. IVC2.m. *Paraneoplastic pemphigus.* From another case, a mixed picture like this of lichenoid inflammation with vacuolar change and apoptotic cells in the epidermis may suggest erythema multiforme and related disorders, or other lichenoid disorders.

Fig. IVC2.n. *Paraneoplastic pemphigus.* In another area, there is suprabasal acantholysis similar to pemphigus vulgaris.

with a vacuolar interface dermatitis (erythema multiforme like) with or without lichenoid inflammation (lichen planus like). PNP may also present exclusively with lichenoid interface dermatitis in the absence of acantholysis. In pemphigoid-like lesions, a subepidermal blister is present. DIF demonstrates, in addition to keratinocyte cell surface IgG, C3 both in the intercellular space and at the dermal–epidermal junction. PNP sera also often stain other desmosome-containing tissues, such as bladder, heart, and liver, unlike the other types of pemphigus, in which only stratified squamous epithelial substrates are stained (46).

Conditions to consider in the differential diagnosis:

> erythema multiforme (with vacuolar and apoptotic changes)
> Stevens–Johnson syndrome
> toxic epidermal necrolysis (TEN, Lyell syndrome)
> herpes simplex, varicella-zoster
> hydroa vacciniforme (epidermal necrosis)
> cowpox
> hand-foot-and-mouth disease (coxsackievirus)
> orf
> paraneoplastic pemphigus

IVC2a Intraspinous Acantholysis, Eosinophils Present

The number of eosinophils seen is variable from many in incontinentia pigmenti and pemphigus vegetans to few in AD. *Pemphigus vegetans* is a prototypic example (47).

Pemphigus Vegetans

CLINICAL SUMMARY. This is an uncommon variant of pemphigus vulgaris, which historically has been divided into the Neumann type and Hallopeau type. In the Neumann type, the disease begins and ends as pemphigus vulgaris, but many of the denuded areas heal with verrucous vegetations that may contain small pustules in early stages. The Hallopeau type is relatively benign, having pustules as the primary lesions instead of bullae. Their development is followed by the formation of gradually enlarging verrucous vegetations, especially in intertriginous areas.

HISTOPATHOLOGY. In the Neumann type, the early lesions consist of bullae and denuded areas that have the same histologic picture as that of pemphigus vulgaris (see Section IVD.3). As the lesions age, however, there is formation of villi and verrucous epidermal hyperplasia. Numerous eosinophils are present within the epidermis and dermis, producing both eosinophilic spongiosis and eosinophilic pustules. Acantholysis may not be present in older lesions.

In the Hallopeau type, the early lesions consist of pustules arising on normal skin with acantholysis and formation of small clefts, many in a suprabasal position. The clefts are filled with numerous eosinophils and degenerated acantholytic epidermal cells. Early lesions may reveal more eosinophilic abscesses than in the Neumann type. The subsequent verrucous lesions are histologically identical to the Neumann type. DIF examination reveals squamous intercellular IgG (29).

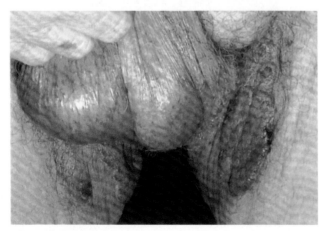

Clin. Fig. IVC2a.a

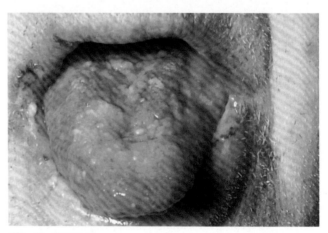

Clin. Fig. IVC2a.b

Clin. Fig. IVC2a.a. *Pemphigus vegetans.* Hallopeau type. An 80-year-old man had a 20-year history of verrucous plaques in the groin, intergluteal cleft, and parietal scalp controlled with avlosulfone.

Clin. Fig. IVC2a.b. *Pemphigus vegetans.* The oral mucous membranes, including the lips and tongue, presented with painful erosive and crusting plaques.

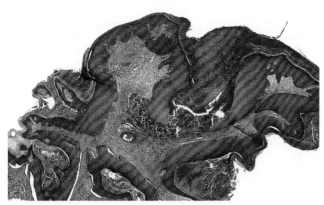

Fig. IVC2a.a

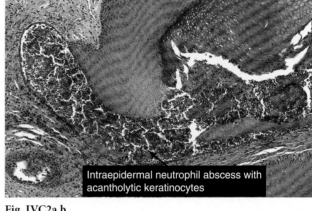

Intraepidermal neutrophil abscess with acantholytic keratinocytes

Fig. IVC2a.b

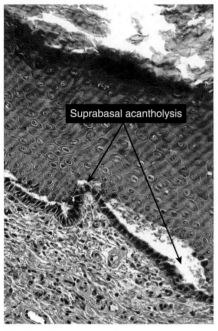

Suprabasal acantholysis

Fig. IVC2a.c

Fig. IVC2a.a. *Pemphigus vegetans, low power.* The epidermis reveals irregular acanthosis and there is a superficial and middermal inflammatory infiltrate. In most cases of pemphigus vegetans the acantholytic areas require careful inspection and may require multiple deeper levels.

Fig. IVC2a.b. *Pemphigus vegetans, medium power.* At this magnification one can identify the characteristic intraepidermal abscesses. The intraepidermal abscesses are composed in this example of neutrophils and eosinophils, associated with areas of intraspinous acantholysis.

Fig. IVC2a.c. *Pemphigus vegetans, high power.* Foci of suprabasal acantholysis, similar to those seen in pemphigus vulgaris, are also seen.

Conditions to consider in the differential diagnosis:

pemphigus vegetans
pemphigus vulgaris
incontinentia pigmenti
drug-induced pemphigus
paraneoplastic pemphigus

IVC3 **Intraspinous Separation, Neutrophils or Mixed Cell types**

Inflammatory cells in the dermis include lymphocytes and plasma cells, with or without eosinophils, neutrophils, mast cells, and histiocytes. *IgA pemphigus (IGAP)* is a prototypic example (48).

IgA Pemphigus

CLINICAL SUMMARY. This is a pruritic vesiculopustular eruption characterized by squamous intercellular IgA deposits and intraepidermal neutrophils. It occurs primarily but not exclusively in middle-aged and elderly individuals. The clinical findings are similar to those in pemphigus foliaceus or subcorneal pustular dermatosis. There are flaccid vesicles, pustules, or bullae that arise on an erythematous base and may be annular. There may be mild leukocytosis, eosinophilia, and IgA kappa paraproteinemia. Two types have been distinguished: a subcorneal pustular dermatosis-like disorder or an intraepidermal pustular eruption. DIF is positive for intercellular IgA in the upper layers of the epidermis in

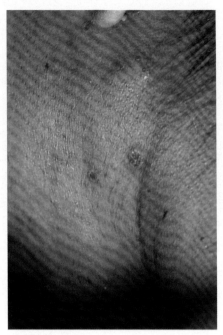

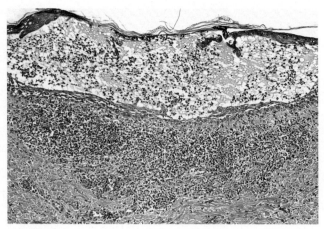

Fig. IVC3.a

Clin. Fig. IVC3. *IgA pemphigus.* A Vietnamese male suffered from recurrent pustular and crusted lesions for years.

Fig. IVC3.a. *IgA pemphigus, low power.* A subcorneal and intraepidermal blister is filled with fluid and numerous neutrophils. A few small clusters of acantholytic cells may be evident. (L. Cohen.)

Clin. Fig. IVC3

the former, and throughout the epidermis in the latter (49). Because of cases with multiple overlapping features including linear basal IgA deposition, underscoring the limitations of current classification schemes, the unifying term "IGAP spectrum" has been suggested for these conditions (50).

HISTOPATHOLOGY. Two patterns are observed that parallel the two clinical presentations. In the first, there are subcorneal neutrophilic vesicopustules or pustules with minimal acantholysis. In the second, intraepidermal vesicopustules or pustules contain small to moderate numbers of neutrophils. One case without neutrophil infiltration has been described.

IMMUNOFLUORESCENCE (IF) TESTING. DIF testing typically reveals IgA deposition in the squamous intercellular substance throughout the epidermis with increased intensity in the upper layers in some cases of the subcorneal pustular type. Complement and other immunoglobulins are usually absent. The antibodies are directed against neither the pemphigus vulgaris nor the foliaceus antigen, but bind with proteins in desmosomes (desmocollins).

Conditions to consider in the differential diagnosis:

    acantholytic solar keratosis
    acantholytic squamous cell carcinoma
    hydroa vacciniforme (epidermal necrosis)
    IgA pemphigus

IVD — SUPRABASAL KERATINOCYTE SEPARATION

There is separation between the keratinocytes of the basal layer and those of the spinous layer.

1. Suprabasal Vesicles, Scant Inflammatory Cells
2. Suprabasal Separation, Lymphocytes and Plasma Cells
3. Suprabasal Vesicles, Lymphocytes and Eosinophils.

IVD1 Suprabasal Vesicles, Scant Inflammatory Cells

The suprabasal separation may be associated with scant inflammation, and frequently with dyskeratotic or atypical keratinocytes. *Darier disease (keratosis follicularis) and warty dyskeratoma (isolated keratosis follicularis) are prototypic (51).*

Keratosis Follicularis (Darier Disease)

CLINICAL SUMMARY. In this disease, which is usually transmitted in an autosomal dominant pattern, there is a more or less extensive, persistent, slowly progressive eruption consisting of hyperkeratotic or crusted papules or verrucous lesions often showing a follicular distribution. A sarco/endoplasmic reticulum Ca2+ transport ATPase (ATP2A2) has been identified as the defective gene, emphasizing the role of extracellular Ca2+ in cell-to-cell adhesion and in epidermal differentiation (52).

The so-called seborrheic areas are the sites of predilection. The oral mucosa is involved occasionally. The nails can be affected. Special clinical variants are a hypertrophic type, a vesiculobullous type, and a linear or zosteriform type. In the hypertrophic type, widespread, markedly thickened, hyperkeratotic lesions are seen, especially in the intertriginous areas. In the vesiculobullous type, vesicles and small bullae are seen in addition to papules. In the linear or zosteriform type, usually limited to one side, there are either localized or widespread lesions that may occasionally be present at birth or may arise in infancy, childhood, or adult life. This type of lesion may represent a linear epidermal nevus with

acantholytic dyskeratosis rather than Darier disease, and the designation *acantholytic dyskeratotic epidermal nevus* has been suggested.

HISTOPATHOLOGY. The characteristic changes in Darier disease are: (1) a peculiar form of dyskeratosis resulting in the formation of corps ronds and grains, (2) suprabasal acantholysis leading to the formation of suprabasal clefts or lacunae, and (3) irregular upward proliferation into the lacunae of papillae lined with a single layer of basal cells, so-called villi. There are also papillomatosis, acanthosis, and hyperkeratosis. The dermis shows a chronic inflammatory infiltrate. In some cases,

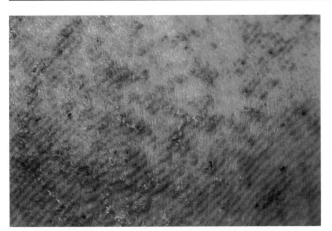

Clin. Fig. IVD1.a

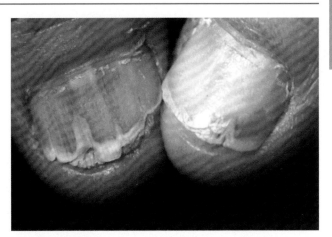

Clin. Fig. IVD1.b

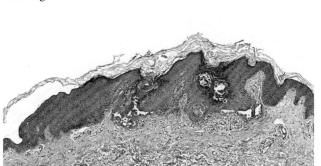

Fig. IVD1.a

Clin. Fig. IVD1.a. *Darier disease*. A 54-year-old woman with this lifelong autosomal dominant disease presented with "dirty brown" papules on the neck and trunk.

Clin. Fig. IVD1.b. *Darier disease*. The nails show characteristic changes of V-shaped nicking, linear striations, onycholysis, and subungual keratotic reaction.

Fig. IVD1.a. *Darier disease, low power*. There is mild verrucous acanthosis of the epidermis and several foci of acantholysis are seen in the lower epidermal layers.

Fig. IVD1.b. *Darier disease, medium power*. The acantholysis is suprabasal and several corps ronds are seen in the upper epidermal layers associated with a focus of parakeratosis.

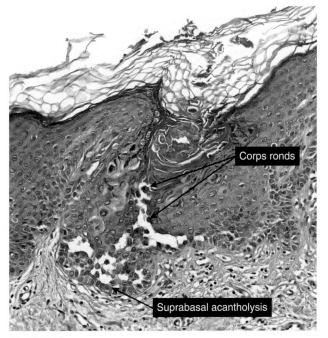

Corps ronds

Suprabasal acantholysis

Fig. IVD1.b

there is downward proliferation of epidermal cells into the dermis.

The corps ronds occur in the upper stratum malpighii, particularly in the granular and horny layers; grains are found in the horny layer and as acantholytic cells within the lacunae. Corps ronds possess a central homogeneous, basophilic, pyknotic nucleus that is surrounded by a clear halo, peripheral to which there is a shell of basophilic dyskeratotic material. The grains resemble parakeratotic cells but are somewhat larger. Their nuclei are elongated and often grain shaped and are surrounded by homogeneous dyskeratotic basophilic or eosinophilic material. The lacunae represent small, slit-like intraepidermal vesicles most commonly located directly above the basal layer, and containing acantholytic partial keratinized cells. The changes seen in particular lesions of Grover disease may be indistinguishable from Darier disease, but usually the lesions are smaller, and if multiple lesions are available from the same patient, the pattern typically varies from lesion to lesion (35).

Warty Dyskeratoma

CLINICAL SUMMARY. Warty dyskeratoma usually occurs as a solitary lesion, most commonly on the scalp, face, or neck (53). It often occurs as a slightly elevated papule or nodule with a keratotic umbilicated center, which after having reached a certain size, persists indefinitely.

HISTOPATHOLOGY. The center of the lesion is occupied by a large, cup-shaped invagination connected with the surface by a channel filled with keratinous material. The large invagination contains numerous acantholytic, dyskeratotic cells in its upper portion. The lower portion of the invagination is occupied by numerous villi, markedly elongated dermal papillae that are often lined with only a single layer of basal cells and project upward from the base of the cup-shaped invagination. Typical corps ronds can usually be seen in the thickened granular layer lining the channel at the entrance to the invagination.

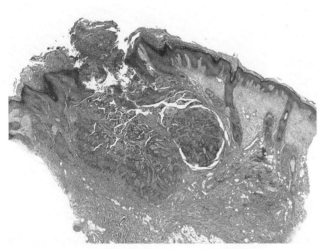

Fig. IVD1.c

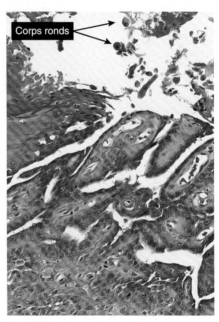

Fig. IVD1.e

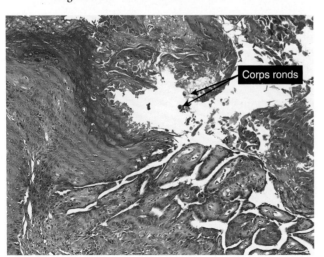

Fig. IVD1.d

Fig. IVD1.c. *Warty dyskeratoma, low power.* A solitary focus of verrucous epidermal hyperplasia with an invaginated architecture is seen in the center of this biopsy. There is a sparse dermal inflammatory infiltrate.

Fig. IVD1.d,e. *Warty dyskeratoma, high power.* There are multiple elongate finger-like projections of epithelium which show suprabasal acantholysis. There are also dyskeratotic cells and corps ronds. The pathology may be identical to Darier disease. However, the solitary nature, both clinically and histologically, allows easy differentiation between these two entities.

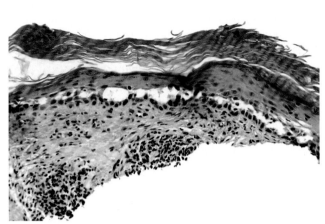

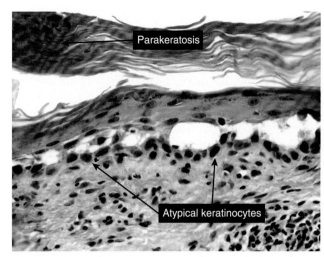

Fig. IVD2.a   **Fig. IVD2.b**

Fig. IVD2.a. *Acantholytic actinic keratosis, low power.* The epidermis shows alternating columns of hyperkeratosis and parakeratosis, with an area of separation in the lower epidermis. There is a moderately intense infiltrate in the superficial dermis.

Fig. IVD2.b. *Acantholytic actinic keratosis, high power.* Within this solar (actinic) keratosis there are foci of suprabasal acantholysis, a pattern which may mimic pemphigus vulgaris. In this keratosis, the infiltrate is composed of lymphocytes and plasma cells. The character of the infiltrate (eosinophils predominate in pemphigus vulgaris) and the presence of keratinocyte atypia aid in differentiating these two entities.

Conditions to consider in the differential diagnosis:

  transient acantholytic dermatosis (Grover)
  benign familial pemphigus (Hailey–Hailey)
  Darier disease (keratosis follicularis)
  acantholytic solar keratosis
  acantholytic squamous cell carcinoma

IVD2 | Suprabasal Separation, Lymphocytes and Plasma Cells

Suprabasal separation, associated with keratinocyte atypia, may be seen with a lymphoplasmacytic infiltrate in the dermis in an *acantholytic actinic (solar) keratosis* (54). These lesions do not appear to have any particular special relationship to acantholytic squamous cell carcinoma (55).

Acantholytic Actinic Keratosis

(**See also Section IIA.1**) Five types of actinic (solar) keratosis can be recognized histologically: hypertrophic, atrophic, bowenoid, acantholytic, and pigmented. In all types, there is random atypia of basal keratinocytes, with hyperkeratosis intermingled with areas of parakeratosis. Keratinocytes in the stratum malpighii show a loss of polarity and thus a disorderly arrangement. Some of these cells show crowding, pleomorphism, and atypicality of their nuclei, which appear large, irregular, and hyperchromatic, and some of the cells are dyskeratotic or apoptotic;

acantholytic keratoses show dyshesion of lesional cells that may simulate a glandular pattern. The acantholysis is usually suprabasal but may involve the full thickness of the epidermis.

Conditions to consider in the differential diagnosis:

  acantholytic solar keratosis (synonym)
  acantholytic squamous cell carcinoma

IVD3 | Suprabasal Vesicles, Lymphocytes and Eosinophils

There is suprabasal separation with eosinophils in the epidermis (eosinophilic spongiosis), and in the dermis. The appearance of clinical disease appears to depend on the appropriate HLA background to permit an IgG4 response to desmoglein 3, a cell surface adhesion molecule. Autoreactive T-cell responses may also be important in the pathogenesis. *Pemphigus vulgaris* is the prototype (56,57).

Pemphigus Vulgaris

CLINICAL SUMMARY. This condition develops primarily in older individuals, presenting with large and flaccid bullae. These break easily and leave denuded areas that tend to increase in size by progressive peripheral detachment of the epidermis (positive Nikolsky sign), leading in some cases to widespread cutaneous involvement. The lesions characteristically involve the oral mucosa, scalp, midface, sternum, and groin. Oral lesions are almost invariably present and are often the first manifestation of the disease. Before corticosteroids became available, the mortality of this disease was high because of fluid loss and superinfection.

HISTOPATHOLOGY. The earliest recognized change may be either eosinophilic spongiosis, or more commonly, spongiosis in the lower epidermis. Acantholysis leads first to the formation of clefts, and then to blisters in a predominantly suprabasal location, although intraepithelial separation may occasionally be higher in the stratum spinosum. The basal keratinocytes, although separated from one another through the loss of attachment to each other, remain firmly attached to the dermis like a "row of tombstones" lining the blister base. The blister roof consists of the remaining intact squamous epithelium. Within the blister cavity, there are acantholytic keratinocytes that have rounded, condensed cytoplasm about an enlarged nucleus with peripherally palisaded chromatin and enlarged nucleoli. These may reside singularly or in clusters. They may be recognized cytologically in a Tzanck preparation which is a smear taken from the underside of the roof and from the base of an early, freshly opened bulla. Acantholysis may extend into adnexal structures. There is little inflammation in the early phase of blister formation. If present, it is usually a sparse, lymphocytic perivascular infiltrate accompanied by dermal edema. If, however, eosinophilic spongiosis is apparent, numerous eosinophils may infiltrate the dermis, and as the lesions age, a mixed inflammatory cell reaction consisting of neutrophils, lymphocytes, macrophages, and eosinophils may develop. Because of the instability of the blister roof, erosion and ulceration may occur. Older blisters may also have several layers of keratinocytes at the blister base because of keratinocyte migration and proliferation, and there may be considerable downward growth of epidermal strands, giving rise to so-called villi.

IF TESTING. DIF testing is a very reliable and sensitive diagnostic test for pemphigus vulgaris, in that it demonstrates IgG in the squamous intercellular substance in 80% to 95% of cases, including early cases and those with very few lesions, and in up to 100% of cases with active disease. It remains positive, often for many years after the disease has subsided. Indirect testing is less specific than the direct test. Disease activity in pemphigus vulgaris can be correlated with antibody titers. Circulating IgG antibodies in patients with pemphigus vulgaris react with *desmogleins,* desmosomal proteins, resulting in release of plasminogen activator and activation of plasmin. This proteolytic enzyme acts on the intercellular substance and may be the primary mechanism of dyshesion. In the mucosal variant of pemphigus vulgaris, autoantibodies exclusively react with desmoglein 3 whereas patients with the mucocutaneous subtype raise antibodies against both desmoglein 3 and 1. Highly sensitive and specific ELISA have been developed for specific antibody testing (58).

Conditions to consider in the differential diagnosis:

pemphigus vulgaris
pemphigus vegetans

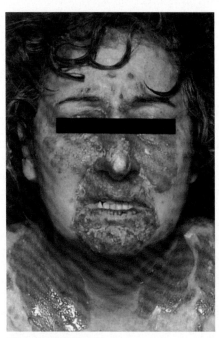

Clin. Fig. IVD3.a

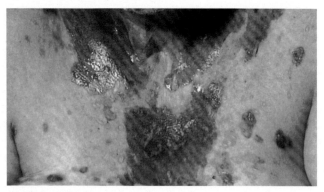

Clin. Fig. IVD3.b

Clin. Fig. IVD3.a. *Pemphigus vulgaris.* A 52-year-old woman developed mouth erosions and fragile flaccid bullae with expanding erosions and skin denudation.

Clin. Fig. IVD3.b. *Pemphigus vulgaris.* The lesions progressed over the entire body requiring Burn Unit therapy. Indirect immunofluorescence was 1:5,120 on guinea pig esophagus and 1:2,560 on monkey esophagus.

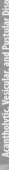

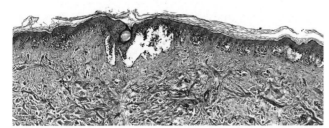

Fig. IVD3.a

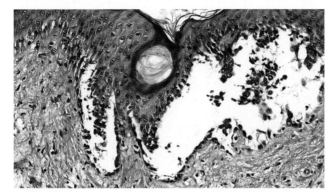

Fig. IVD3.c

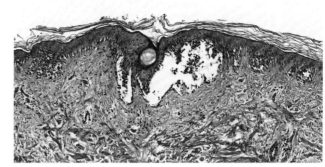

Fig. IVD3.b

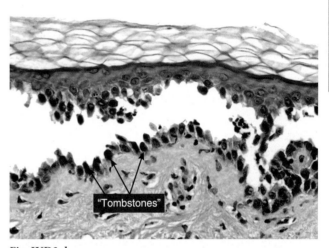

Fig. IVD3.d

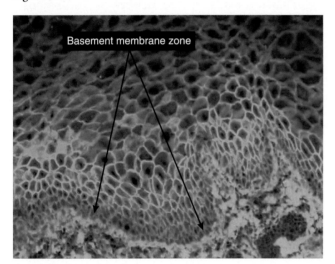
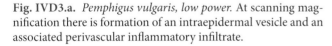

Fig. IVD3.e

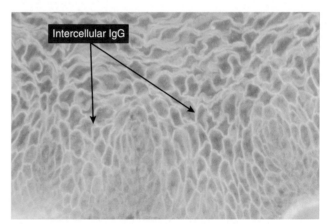

Fig. IVD3.f

Fig. IVD3.a. *Pemphigus vulgaris, low power.* At scanning magnification there is formation of an intraepidermal vesicle and an associated perivascular inflammatory infiltrate.

Fig. IVD3.b. *Pemphigus vulgaris, medium power.* There is intraspinous separation which is predominantly in the suprabasal region. The stratum corneum is intact and shows a basket-weave pattern.

Fig. IVD3.c. *Pemphigus vulgaris, medium power.* A solitary row of basal layer keratinocytes remains attached to the floor of the blister. The roof of the blister is composed of relatively intact superficial epidermal layers. The dermal infiltrate is composed of lymphocytes and eosinophils (not numerous in this case). Eosinophilic spongiosis may also be seen.

Fig. IVD3.d. *Pemphigus vulgaris, medium power.* Another example shows a characteristic single-cell "tombstone layer" of basal keratinocytes at the floor of the blister.

Fig. IVD3.e. *Pemphigus vulgaris, direct immunofluorescence, medium power.* There is cell surface (intercellular) IgG deposition. C_3 deposition is also frequently seen in pemphigus vulgaris.

Fig. IVD3.f. *Pemphigus vulgaris, indirect immunofluorescence, high power.* Using monkey esophagus as a substrate there is prominent cell surface (intercellular) staining with IgG.

IVE SUBEPIDERMAL VESICULAR DERMATITIS

A subepidermal blister refers to separation of the epidermis from the dermis. The roof of the blister is composed of an intact or (partially) necrotic epithelium.

1. Subepidermal Vesicles, Scant /No Inflammation
2. Subepidermal Vesicles, Lymphocytes Predominant
3. Subepidermal Vesicles, Eosinophils Prominent
4. Subepidermal Vesicles, Neutrophils Prominent
5. Subepidermal Vesicles, Mast Cells Prominent

IVE1 Subepidermal Vesicles, Scant /No Inflammation

The infiltrate in the dermis in most of these conditions is scant (few lymphocytes, eosinophils, neutrophils). *Porphyria cutanea tarda (PCT) and other porphyrias* are prototypic (59).

Porphyria Cutanea Tarda and Other Porphyrias

CLINICAL SUMMARY. Three forms of the dominantly inherited disorder PCT can be distinguished: sporadic, familial, and hepatoerythropoietic. In the *sporadic form*, only the hepatic activity of uroporphyrinogen decarboxylase is decreased. Almost all patients are adults, and no clinical evidence of PCT is found in other members of the patient's family. In most instances, in addition to the inherited enzymatic defect, an acquired damaging factor to liver function such as ethanol or estrogens is needed. Hepatitis C virus positivity and hemochromatosis gene mutations are also risk factors (60). In the *familial form*, in addition to the hepatic activity, the extrahepatic activity of uroporphyrinogen decarboxylase is decreased to about 50% of normal, and often, but not always, there is a family history of overt PCT. In the very rare *hepatoerythropoietic form*, the skin lesions appear in childhood, the activity of uroporphyrinogen decarboxylase in all organs is decreased to less than 10% of normal, and family studies suggest that these patients are homozygous for the causative gene.

Clinically, the sporadic form of PCT, by far the most common type of porphyria, shows blisters that arise through a combination of sun exposure and minor trauma, mainly on the dorsa of the hands but sometimes also on the face. Scarring and milia formation may result. The skin of the face and the dorsa of the hands often are thickened and sclerotic. Hypertrichosis of the face is common. In the familial and in the hepatoerythropoietic forms, the clinical picture is similar, but the changes are more pronounced. Evidence of hepatic cirrhosis with siderosis is regularly present in the sporadic form.

In *erythropoietic porphyria*, a very rare disease which typically develops during infancy or childhood, recurrent vesiculobullous eruptions in sun-exposed areas of the skin gradually result in mutilating ulcerations and scarring. In *erythropoietic protoporphyria*, the usual reaction to light is erythema and edema followed by thickening and superficial scarring of the skin. In rare instances, vesicles are present that may resemble those seen in hydroa vacciniforme. The protoporphyrin is formed in reticulocytes in the bone marrow and is then carried in circulating erythrocytes and in the plasma. In *porphyria variegata*, different members of the same family may have either cutaneous manifestations identical to those of PCT or systemic involvement analogous to acute intermittent porphyria, or both, or the condition may remain latent.

HISTOPATHOLOGY. The histologic changes in the skin lesions are the same in all six types of porphyria with cutaneous lesions. Differences are based on the severity rather than on the type of porphyria. Homogeneous, eosinophilic material is regularly observed, and bullae are present in some instances. In addition, sclerosis of the collagen is present in old lesions. In mild cases, homogeneous, pale, eosinophilic deposits are limited to the immediate vicinity of the blood vessels in the papillary dermis. These deposits are PAS positive and diastase resistant. In severely involved areas, which are most common in erythropoietic protoporphyria, the perivascular mantles of homogeneous material are wide enough in the papillary dermis to coalesce with those of adjoining capillaries. In addition, deeper blood vessels may show homogeneous material around them, and similar homogeneous material may be found occasionally around eccrine glands. In addition, the PAS-positive dermal–epidermal basement membrane zone may be thickened. In areas of sclerosis, which occur especially in PCT, the collagen bundles are thickened.

The bullae, which are most common in PCT, arise subepidermally. Some blisters are dermolytic and arise beneath the PAS-positive basement membrane zone; others form in the lamina lucida and are situated above the PAS-positive basement membrane zone. It is quite characteristic of the bullae of PCT that the dermal papillae often extend irregularly from the floor of the bulla into the bulla cavity. This phenomenon, referred to as "festooning," is explained by the rigidity of the upper dermis induced by the presence of eosinophilic material within and around the capillary walls in the papillae and the papillary dermis. The epidermis forming the roof of the blister often contains eosinophilic bodies that are elongated and sometimes segmented. These "caterpillar bodies" are PAS positive and diastase resistant. There are only a few inflammatory cells in the dermis.

Conditions to consider in the differential diagnosis:

porphyria cutanea tarda and other porphyrias
drug-induced pseudoporphyria
bullous pemphigoid, cell-poor
epidermolysis bullosa, multiple types

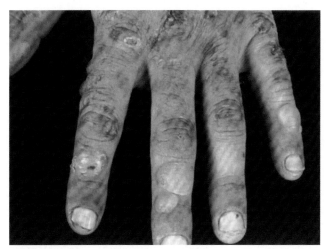

Clin. Fig. IVE.1

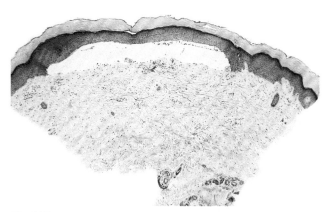

Fig. IVE1.a

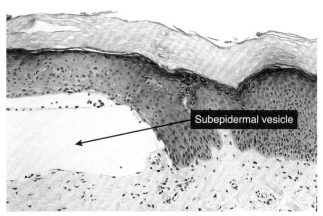

Fig. IVE1.b

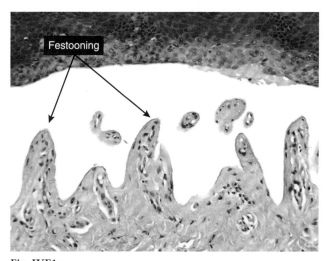

Festooning

Subepidermal vesicle

Fig. IVE1.c

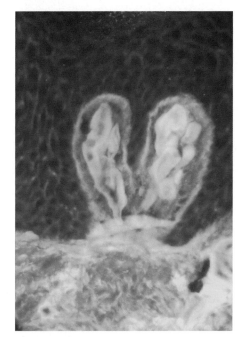

Fig. IVE1.d

Clin. Fig. IVE.1. *Porphyria cutanea tarda.* A 33-year-old man presented with intact vesicles and bullae and crusted erosions without milia on dorsal hands. His history of excessive alcohol intake and hepatitis C positivity is typical for the sporadic form of the disease.

Fig. IVE1.a. *Porphyria cutanea tarda, low power.* This biopsy of acral skin shows a subepidermal blister. There is little or no inflammation within the dermis.

Fig. IVE1.b. *Porphyria cutanea tarda, medium power.* At the edge of the blister, one can see that the roof of the blister is composed of full-thickness epidermis and the floor of the blister is composed of underlying dermis. Again, almost no inflammation is seen at the periphery of the blister.

Fig. IVE1.c. *Porphyria cutanea tarda, medium power.* At the floor of the blister, the dermal papillae tend to retain their architecture, constituting festooning. A PAS stain may reveal basement membrane thickening of the blood vessels within this dermal papilla.

Fig. IVE1.d. *Porphyria cutanea tarda, direct immunofluorescence, high power.* There is smudgy, positive staining with IgG of the blood vessels in the papillary dermis.

epidermolysis bullosa acquisita (classic)
graft-versus-host disease (GVHD), acute
acute radiation dermatitis
bullous dermatosis of diabetes
bullous dermatosis of uremia
electrical burn (polarized epidermis)
thermal burn (epidermal necrosis)
suction blister
Vibrio vulnificus septicemia (necrotic bullae)

IVE2 Subepidermal Vesicles, Lymphocytes Predominant

The epidermis is separated from the dermis, predominantly due to liquefaction of the basal cell layer. In polymorphous (polymorphic) light eruption (PMLE) and bullous dermatophytosis massive papillary dermal edema is the cause. The infiltrate in the dermis is primarily lymphocytic. *Bullous lichen planus* is an example (61).

Bullous Lichen Planus

(See also Section IIIF.1.) In lichen planus, a dense dermal infiltrate obscures the dermal–epidermal junction with vacuolar degeneration and necrosis of the basal cells. Necrotic keratinocytes, also referred to as apoptotic, colloid, hyaline, cytoid, or Civatte bodies, are present in most of the cases in the lower epidermis and especially in the papillary dermis. Because of this disruption of the dermal–epidermal junction, small areas of artifactual separation between the epidermis and the dermis, known as Max-Josef spaces, are occasionally seen. In some instances, the separation occurs *in vivo* and subepidermal blisters form (*vesicular or bullous lichen planus*). These vesicles form as a result of extensive damage to the basal cells. In bullous lichen planus, the blisters are limited to areas of lichen planus, while in lichen planus pemphigoides, blisters are seen in sites independent of the lesions of lichen planus (62).

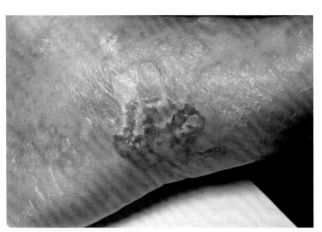

Clin. Fig. IVE2.a

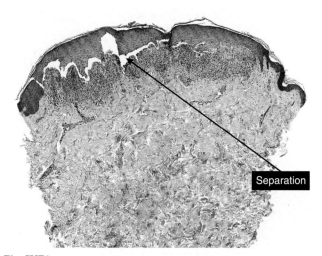

Fig. IVE2.a

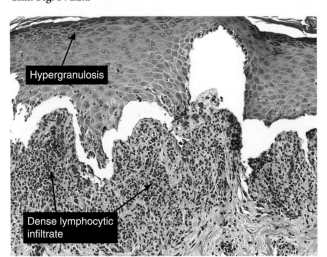

Fig. IVE2.b

Clin. Fig. IVE2.a. *Bullous lichen planus.* A 93-year-old woman with a history of hypertrophic lichen planus presented with a sudden eruption of hemorrhagic ruptured bullae on a background of violaceous plaques on the soles of her feet. The eruption was treated successfully with a short course of systemic steroids.

Fig. IVE2.a. *Bullous lichen planus, low power.* There is a band-like inflammatory infiltrate which obscures the dermal–epidermal interface. Inflammation is not seen within the deep dermis.

Fig. IVE2.b. *Bullous lichen planus, medium power.* The epidermis shows irregular acanthosis, hypergranulosis, and a thickened orthokeratotic scale. The epidermis has separated from the underlying dermis forming a subepidermal cleft. There is an intense band-like infiltrate composed predominantly of lymphocytes.

Polymorphous (Polymorphic) Light Eruption

CLINICAL SUMMARY. This is a commonly occurring, transient, intermittent, sunlight-induced eruption of non-scarring, erythematous, itchy papules, plaques, or vesicles of exposed skin, most severe in spring and summer and commonest in young women (63). Attacks develop during sunny vacations and summer weather, often persisting or recurring, sometimes with gradual reduction in severity, from spring until fall. They typically follow around 15 minutes to a few hours of sun exposure, and last for hours, days, or rarely weeks.

HISTOPATHOLOGY. This may vary, but usually there is variable epidermal spongiosis and dermal, perivascular, predominantly mononuclear cell infiltration with papillary dermal edema, which in older lesions may extend into the deeper dermis and may be so severe as to occasionally result in an apparent subepidermal blister. This finding is not unique to PMLE, being also occasionally seen in acute lupus and some discoid lupus lesions, and in dermatomyositis. The cells of the infiltrate are usually T lymphocytes, but occasionally eosinophils and neutrophils are present as well.

According to Pincus et al., the differential diagnosis of a lesion that has a perivascular lymphocytic infiltrate with papillary dermal edema should include PMLE, lupus, dermatomyositis, dermatophytosis, "dermal" CD and an arthropod reaction, and occasionally lichen sclerosus (LS) and perniosis as well. Reliable histopathologic clues favoring a diagnosis of lupus over PMLE include significant vacuolar change with necrotic keratinocytes, the presence of dermal mucin deposition, a periadnexal infiltrate, and CD123+ plasmacytoid dendritic cells in clusters amidst the dermal lymphocytic infiltrates (64).

The distinction between PMLE and tumid LE can be problematic. Both are characterized clinically by erythematous papules and plaques on sun-exposed skin. By histology, both have a superficial to deep perivascular lymphocytic infiltrate. While dermal mucin is a key feature of tumid LE, it has also been found to be common in PMLE (65). In addition, papillary dermal edema, a key feature of PMLE, can also be seen in lupus (66).

Bullous Dermatophytosis

Tinea pedis may present as scaling erythematous plaques in a "moccasin" distribution, as interdigital

Acantholytic, Vesicular, and Pustular Disorders — IV

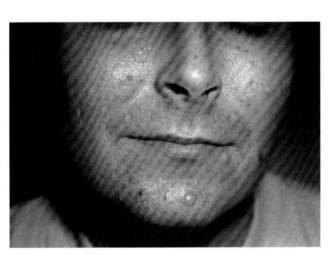

Clin. Fig. IVE2.b

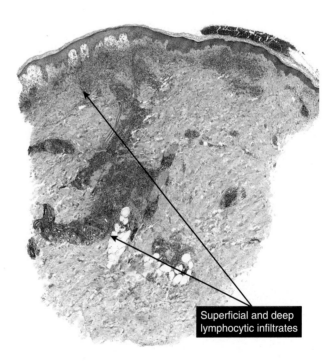

Superficial and deep
lymphocytic infiltrates

Fig. IVE2.c

Clin. Fig. IVE2.b. *Polymorphous light eruption.* Pruritic papules and vesicles developed on an intermittent basis several hours after sun exposure.

Fig. IVE2.c. *Polymorphous light eruption, low power.* There is both intraepidermal spongiosis as well as edema of the papillary dermis. There is an associated superficial and deep inflammatory infiltrate. The papillary dermal edema is frequently more intense, a helpful feature in making a diagnosis at low power. (*continues*)

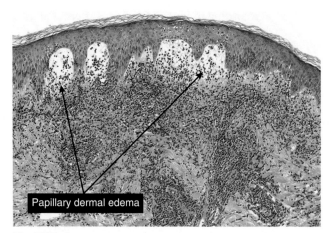

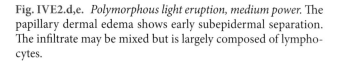

Fig. IVE2.d

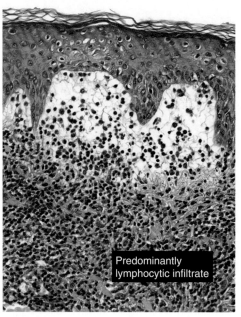

Fig. IVE2.d,e. *Polymorphous light eruption, medium power.* The papillary dermal edema shows early subepidermal separation. The infiltrate may be mixed but is largely composed of lymphocytes.

Fig. IVE2.e

scaling, or occasionally as a vesiculobullous eruption (67). Bullous tinea pedis is most commonly caused by Trichophyton and other species including *Epidermophyton floccosum* and *T. rubrum*. The differential diagnosis for a bullous dermatophyte infection includes dyshidrotic eczema, bullous impetigo, fixed drug eruption, a pox or herpesvirus infection, or an autoimmune bullous dermatosis. Although DIF should help to identify the latter, false-positive reactions have been reported, including in bullous dermatophyte infections.

See also Section IVB3.

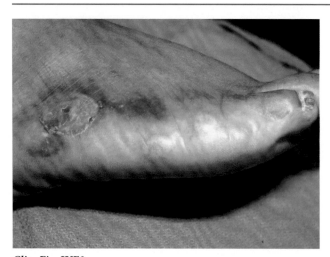

Clin. Fig. IVE2.c

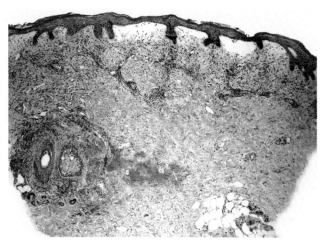

Fig. IVE2.f

Clin. Fig. IVE2.c. *Bullous tinea pedis.* Note denuded bulla, two intact bullae, and thickened toe nail. KOH preparation confirmed diagnosis.

Fig. IVE2.f. *Bullous tinea corporis, low and medium power.* In addition to the marked papillary dermal edema, the epidermis shows spongiosis and parakeratosis. The infiltrate is mixed, containing neutrophils, eosinophils, and mononuclear cells.

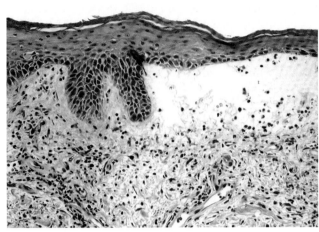

Fig. IVE2.g

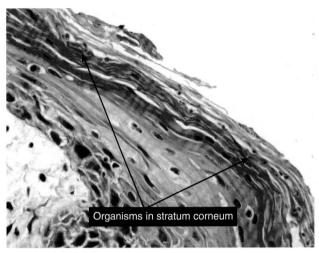

Organisms in stratum corneum

Fig. IVE2.h

Fig. IVE2.g. *Bullous tinea corporis, low power.* There is marked papillary dermal edema, which is sometimes reminiscent of polymorphous light eruption. In addition, there is a moderately intense perivascular, periadnexal, and interstitial inflammatory infiltrate.

Fig. IVE2.h. *Bullous tinea corporis, high power.* Slightly basophilic dermatophyte organisms are seen in the stratum corneum on this hematoxylin and eosin-stained section.

Bullous Lichen Sclerosus et Atrophicus

See also Section IIIC3.

CLINICAL SUMMARY. Bullous LS may be genital or extragenital, and is characterized by flaccid bullae that may be hemorrhagic. These lead to ulcerations and erosions that eventually heal and form the characteristic white sclerotic plaques (68).

HISTOPATHOLOGY. Bulla formation may occur through two mechanisms. Firstly, the vacuolar dermatitis can lead to liquefaction degeneration of the basal layer disrupting the stability of the basement membrane zone. Second, edema of the papillary dermis may disrupt and weaken the collagen fibers supporting the attachment of the epidermis to the dermis (66).

Conditions to consider in the differential diagnosis:

bullous lichen planus (more often histologic than clinical)
erythema multiforme
fixed drug eruption
lichen sclerosus et atrophicus

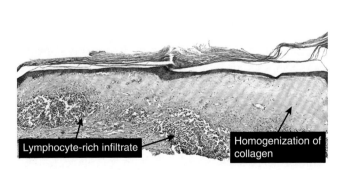

Lymphocyte-rich infiltrate

Homogenization of collagen

Fig. IVE2.i

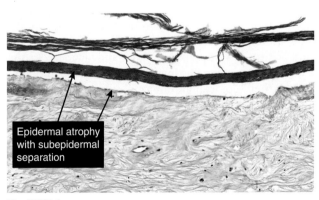

Epidermal atrophy with subepidermal separation

Fig. IVE2.j

Fig. IVE2.i. *Lichen sclerosus et atrophicus, low power.* The epidermis is atrophic and has lost the rete ridge architecture. The stratum corneum is thickened and orthokeratotic. There is pallor and homogenization of the expanded papillary dermis. Beneath the homogenized papillary dermis, there is a predominantly lymphocytic infiltrate which extends into the superficial reticular dermis.

Fig. IVE2.j. *Lichen sclerosus et atrophicus, medium power.* Early subepidermal separation is seen.

bullous erythematosus, mononuclear type
graft-versus-host disease
polymorphous light eruption
bullous dermatophytosis
epidermolysis bullosa acquisita (usually neutrophils)

IVE3 Subepidermal Vesicles, Eosinophils Prominent

The subepidermal blister is associated with dermal infiltrate rich in eosinophils. Eosinophils may extend into the overlying epidermis. *Bullous pemphigoid* is a prototypic example (69).

Bullous Pemphigoid

CLINICAL SUMMARY. First described by Lever in 1953 (70), bullous pemphigoid affects primarily elderly patients with large tense bullae arising on an urticarial erythematous base or on nonerythematous skin. The course is chronic and benign. In contrast to pemphigus, the Nikolsky sign is negative. The lesions involve the trunk, the extremities, and the intertriginous areas, with the oral mucosa involved in about one-third of the cases. Bullous pemphigoid may start as a nonspecific eruption suggestive of urticaria or dermatitis, and can persist for weeks or months.

HISTOPATHOLOGY. In early lesions, papillary dermal edema in combination with a variably cell-poor or cell-rich perivascular lymphocytic and eosinophilic infiltrate is present. The cell-poor pattern is observed when blisters develop on relatively normal skin and the cell-rich pattern when the blisters arise on erythematous skin. In the cell-poor pattern, there is usually scant perivascular lymphocytic inflammation with few eosinophils, some scattered throughout the dermis and others near the epidermis. In the cell-rich pattern, eosinophilic dermal abscesses may develop with numerous perivascular and interstitial eosinophils intermingled with lymphocytes and neutrophils in the papillary and deeper dermis. Eosinophilic spongiosis may occur. The blister arises at the dermal–epidermal junction, although epithelial migration and regeneration may result in an intraepidermal location in older blisters. Similar to pemphigus vegetans, a pseudoepitheliomatous hyperplasia of the epidermis, subepidermal bullae, and accumulations of eosinophils and lymphocytes may be seen.

IF TESTING. DIF testing of perilesional skin has shown linear C3 deposition at the dermal–epidermal junction in virtually all of cases and IgG in most. IIF studies reveal circulating anti–basement membrane zone IgG antibodies in most cases, with IgA and IgM in a minority. No correlation exists between the antibody titer and the clinical severity of the disease. The IgG is located within the lamina lucida, where it binds specifically most often to the noncollagenous domain NC16A of a transmembrane protein, collagen XVII (COL17, BP180), which is a type II transmembrane protein that spans the lamina lucida and projects into the lamina densa of the epidermal basement membrane zone (71). Autoantibodies against this protein are seen not only in bullous pemphigoid, but also in pemphigoid gestationis (PG), mucous membrane pemphigoid, linear IgA disease, lichen planus pemphigoides, and pemphigoid nodularis (72). The majority of bullous pemphigoid sera contain, in addition to IgG reactivity, IgA antibodies to BP180, and often also to another antigen BP230 (39). Specimens submitted for DIF examination may also be examined by the salt-split (direct salt-split) skin technique. When this technique is used in pemphigoid, IgG is present on the roof of the blister.

"Serration pattern analysis" by routine DIF showing "linear n-serration" or "linear u-serration" patterns of immunodepositions along the basement membrane zone can be used to help distinguish among bullous dermatoses. The u-serration pattern supports the diagnosis of epidermolysis bullosa acquisita (EBA) or of bullous lupus and represents immunoglobulin depositions in upstanding arms ("grass") of the sublamina densa zone between the rootlets of basal keratinocytes. In most other bullous dermatoses, as in bullous pemphigoid, the antigens are located in the lamina lucida or above, so the immune deposits follow the rootlets of the basal keratinocytes showing the n-serration pattern (73).

Bullous Drug Eruption

The blister in a bullous drug eruption is typically the result of intense papillary dermal edema, stretching the papillary dermis and forming an impression of a separation of the epidermis from the dermis. Generalized bullous fixed drug eruption is different and can mimic TEN (74).

Pemphigoid Gestationis (Herpes Gestationis)

CLINICAL SUMMARY. PG is a self-limiting, autoimmune subepidermal bullous dermatosis of pregnancy resulting from the production of antiplacental antibodies that cross-react with the same proteins in skin. The main antigen of PG is collagen XVII (BP180), present in both skin and placenta, which is exposed to the maternal immune system through an abnormal expression of MHC class II molecules in the placenta (75). Lesions usually develop during the second or third trimester. Lesions typically develop around the umbilicus and the extremities and can spread to other parts of the body.

HISTOPATHOLOGY. The appearances are exactly similar to those in bullous pemphigoid.

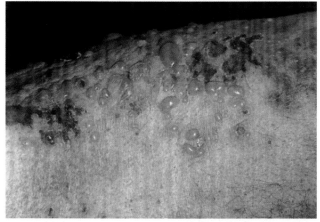

Clin. Fig. IVE3

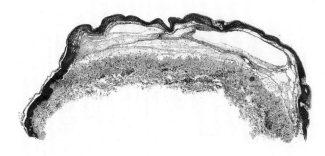

Fig. IVE3.a

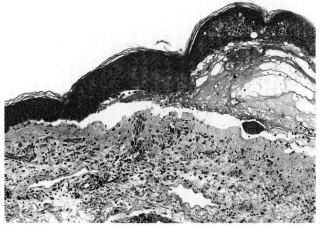

Fig. IVE3.b

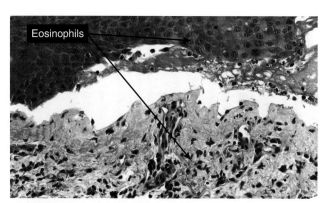

Eosinophils

Fig. IVE3.c

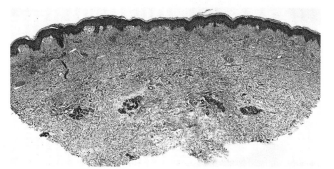

Fig. IVE3.d

Clin. Fig. IVE3. *Bullous pemphigoid.* An elderly man presented with multiple tense bullae on an erythematous base and erosions, distributed primarily on the medial thighs and trunk.

Fig. IVE3.a. *Bullous pemphigoid, low power.* At scanning magnification there is a subepidermal blister with an associated superficial inflammatory infiltrate.

Fig. IVE3.b. *Bullous pemphigoid, medium power.* The blister contains inflammatory cells and there is an associated superficial dermal inflammatory infiltrate.

Fig. IVE3.c. *Bullous pemphigoid, high power.* At the edge of the blister eosinophils are seen within the blister and in the papillary dermis.

Fig. IVE3.d. *Bullous pemphigoid, low power.* In an early lesion, areas of subepidermal separation can be seen at scanning power, and there is an inflammatory infiltrate in the dermis.

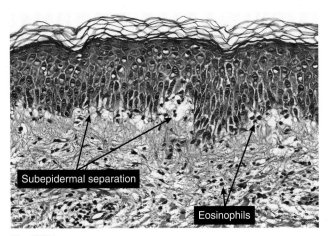

Fig. IVE3.e

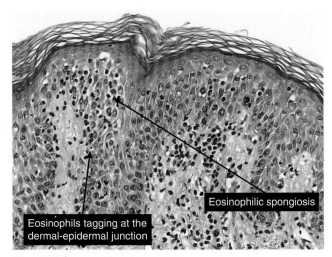

Fig. IVE3.f

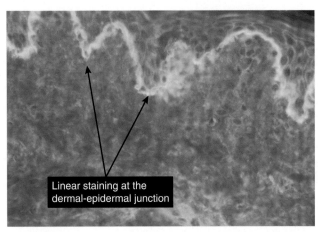

Fig. IVE3.g

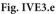

Fig. IVE3.h

Fig. IVE3.e. *Bullous pemphigoid, medium power.* In these early lesions, eosinophils are seen within the papillary dermis and focally extending into the overlying epidermis.

Fig. IVE3.f. *Bullous pemphigoid, medium power.* Eosinophilic spongiosis is a common finding in pemphigoid where numerous eosinophils extend into the overlying spongiotic epidermis.

Fig. IVE3.g. *Bullous pemphigoid, medium power.* Direct immunofluorescence reveals linear staining of C_3 at the basement membrane zone. Other immune reactants including IgG, IgA, and IgM may also be detected. C_3 is the most common reactant, followed by IgG.

Fig. IVE3.h. *Bullous pemphigoid, high power.* Indirect immunofluorescence using monkey esophagus as the substrate and patient's serum as the test sample. Linear staining of IgG is seen at the basement membrane zone.

IF TESTING. DIF findings are similar to those in bullous pemphigoid, with deposition of C3 along the interface in 100% of cases, and of IgG in 25% to 50%. ELISA testing can be helpful in establishing the diagnosis.

Conditions to consider in the differential diagnosis:
bullous pemphigoid
cicatricial pemphigoid
bullous drug eruption
herpes gestationis

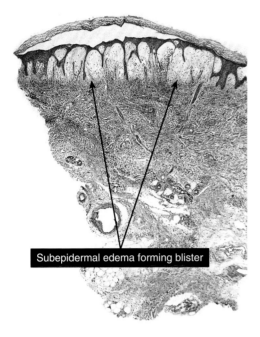

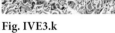

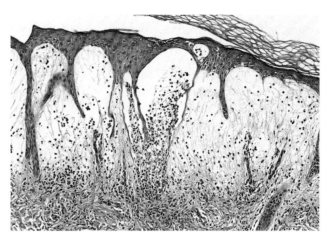

Fig. IVE3.i　　　　　　　　　　**Fig. IVE3.j**

Fig. IVE3.i. *Bullous drug eruption, low power.* There is marked edema of the papillary dermis forming a subepidermal blister. This is associated with a superficial and deep inflammatory infiltrate.

Fig. IVE3.j. *Bullous drug eruption, medium power.* The subepidermal separation is associated with a mixed inflammatory infiltrate which contains eosinophils. Eosinophilic spongiosis, however, is less common than in pemphigoid. Stretched fibers can be seen spanning the gap between the dermis and the epidermis, indicating that there is not a "true" separation. However, immunofluorescence may still be necessary for definitive diagnosis.

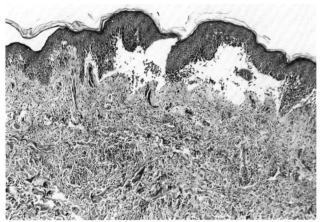

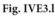

Fig. IVE3.k　　　　　　　　　　**Fig. IVE3.l**

Fig. IVE3.k. *Pemphigoid gestationis, low power.* There is subepidermal blister formation and a superficial predominantly perivascular infiltrate.

Fig. IVE3.l. *Pemphigoid gestationis, medium power.* The subepidermal blister shows eosinophils within the blister cavity at the dermal–epidermal interface and within the epidermal layer. Scattered dyskeratotic cells may also be present. The histology is generally indistinguishable from that of bullous pemphigoid.

bullous insect bite reaction
bullous scabies
dermatitis herpetiformis (certain old bullae)

IVE4 Subepidermal Vesicles, Neutrophils Prominent

A neutrophilic infiltrate is seen often in dermal papillae at the dermal–epidermal junction adjacent to the subepidermal blister, or in the blister. *Dermatitis herpetiformis* is a prototypic example (76,77).

Dermatitis Herpetiformis (Duhring Disease)

CLINICAL SUMMARY. This is an intensely pruritic, chronic recurrent dermatitis that has a slight male predilection. The lesions usually develop in young to middle-aged adults as symmetrically grouped papulovesicles, vesicles, or crusts on erythematous bases. Oral lesions are absent. The elbows, knees, buttocks, scapula, and scalp are commonly involved. Most patients have asymptomatic gluten-sensitive enteropathy, and the pathogenesis appears to involve the development in susceptible individuals of IgA antibodies that cross-react between antigenically similar molecules in the skin and intestine (78). There is an increased but low risk of lymphoma.

HISTOPATHOLOGY. The typical histologic features are best observed in erythematous skin adjacent to early blisters. In these zones, neutrophils accumulate at the tips of dermal papillae. With an increase in size to microabscesses, a significant admixture of eosinophils may be noted. As the neutrophilic or mixed microabscesses form, a separation develops between the tips of the dermal papillae and the overlying epidermis, so that early blisters are multiloculated. The presence of fibrin in the papillae may give them a bluish appearance. Within 1 to 2 days, the rete ridges lose their attachment to the dermis, and the blisters then become unilocular and clinically apparent. At this time, the characteristic papillary microabscesses may be observed at the blister periphery. The dermis beneath the papillae may have a relatively intense inflammatory infiltrate of lymphocytes, neutrophils, and some eosinophils. Apoptotic keratinocytes may be noted above the papillary microabscesses.

IF TESTING. Granular deposits of IgA are found alone or in combination with other immune reactants within the dermal papillae in both lesional and nonlesional skin in most cases. A fibrillar pattern has also been described (79). Early in the course of the disease, IgA deposits may be absent, and repeat DIF is necessary. False-negative results may occur when blistered or inflamed skin is

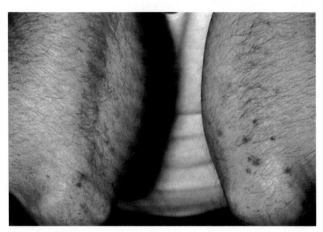

Clin. Fig. IVE4.a

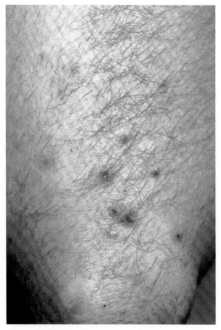

Clin. Fig. IVE4.b

Clin. Fig. IVE4.a. *Dermatitis herpetiformis.* A 27-year-old man developed pruritic symmetrically grouped vesicles on an erythematous base on the elbows and knees. (W. Witmer.)

Clin. Fig. IVE4.b. *Dermatitis herpetiformis.* Single and grouped discrete vesicles which later responded to avlosulfone and a gluten-free diet. (W. Witmer.)

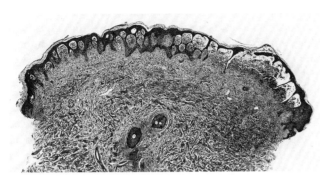

Fig. IVE4.a

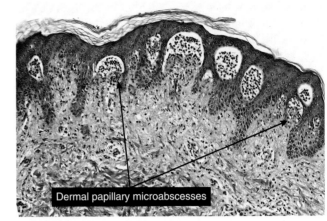

Dermal papillary microabscesses

Fig. IVE4.b

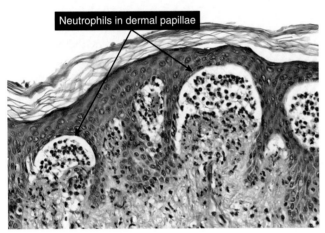

Neutrophils in dermal papillae

Fig. IVE4.c

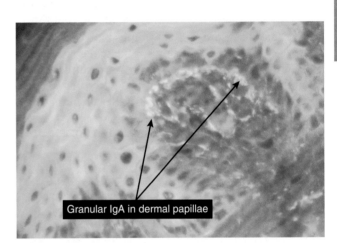

Granular IgA in dermal papillae

Fig. IVE4.d

Fig. IVE4.a. *Dermatitis herpetiformis, low power.* At scanning magnification there is subepidermal blister formation associated with a superficial inflammatory infiltrate.

Fig. IVE4.b. *Dermatitis herpetiformis, medium power.* There are numerous papillary dermal microabscesses which are seen adjacent to the subepidermal blisters. Within the dermis there is a mild mixed inflammatory infiltrate.

Fig. IVE4.c. *Dermatitis herpetiformis, high power.* The papillary dermal abscesses are composed almost entirely of neutrophils.

Fig. IVE4.d. *Dermatitis herpetiformis, high power, direct immunofluorescence.* Granular deposition of IgA is seen in dermal papillae, concentrated at the dermal–epidermal junction.

evaluated. Circulating IgA antibodies that react against reticulin, smooth muscle endomysium, the dietary antigen gluten, bovine serum albumin, and *b*-lactoglobin may be present. Using monkey or pig gut as substrate, IIF has been used to detect antiendomysial antibodies. The immune precipitates contain epidermal transglutaminase, an enzyme closely related to tissue transglutaminase, which appears to be a source of autoantibodies in celiac disease (53). Sensitive and specific commercial ELISA systems for IgA reactivity against epidermal and tissue transglutaminase are available (39).

Linear IgA Bullous Dermatosis

CLINICAL SUMMARY. Two relatively definitive clinical phenotypes of linear IgA bullous dermatosis (LABD) are based on patient age and clinical features (80). These are adult linear IgA dermatosis and childhood linear IgA dermatosis (chronic bullous disease of childhood) (81). Other cases may be associated with drug therapy at any age. In the adult type, vesicles and bullae are present, which are less symmetrical and less pruritic than those in dermatitis herpetiformis but are distributed in similar locations.

Ocular and oral lesions may be present in up to 50% of cases. It is not infrequent for adult-type LABD to be associated with drug therapy. Vancomycin, lithium, diclofenac, captopril, and somatostatin have been associated with such presentations. Histologically, the changes are identical to LABD in most cases. In some cases, there is an associated lymphoeosinophilic infiltrate in combination with an interface neutrophilic infiltration.

The childhood type of LABD, originally known as chronic bullous disease of childhood, is a unique disorder that presents in prepubertal, often preschool children, and rarely in infancy. Vesicles or bullae develop on an erythematous or normal base, occasionally giving rise to a so-called "string of pearls," a characteristic lesion in which peripheral vesicles develop on a polycyclic plaque. They involve the buttocks, lower abdomen, and genitalia, and characteristically have a perioral distribution on the face. Oral lesions may occur. The disorder usually remits by age 6 to 8.

HISTOPATHOLOGY. The features are similar if not identical to dermatitis herpetiformis. According to some, there is a lesser tendency for papillary microabscess formation and a greater tendency for uniform neutrophil infiltration along the entire dermal–epidermal junction and rete in inflamed skin. DIF reveals linear IgA along the basement membrane zone in perilesional skin in 100% of cases. If IgG as well as IgA is present, the differential diagnosis with bullous pemphigoid may be difficult or impossible (linear IgA/IgG dermatosis). In the great majority of patients, serum IgA autoantibodies target the cell-derived soluble ectodomain of BP180, LAD-1 (39). The antibodies are deposited principally within the lamina lucida and less commonly beneath the lamina densa. The histologic and immunofluorescent features of childhood LABD are similar to those of the adult-type disease.

Bullous Lupus Erythematosus

CLINICAL SUMMARY. Vesicles and bullae may develop in patients with systemic LE (82). In contrast to dermatitis herpetiformis, they are nonpruritic and neither symmetrical nor do they have a predilection for extensor surfaces of arms, elbows, or scalp. The lesions may be photodistributed. These patients rarely have classic lesions of discoid,

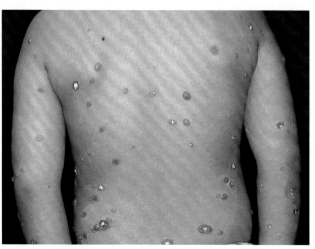

Clin. Fig. IVE4.c

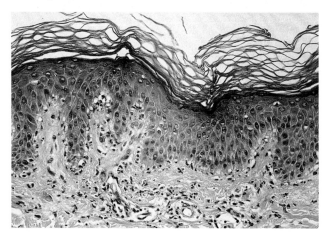

Fig. IVE4.f

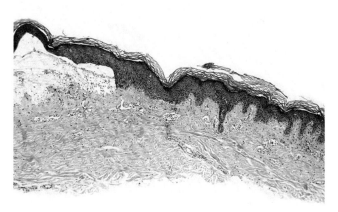

Fig. IVE4.e

Clin. Fig. IVE4.c. Childhood linear IgA bullous dermatosis (chronic bullous disease of childhood). A 4-year-old girl developed multiple tense blisters on the entire body with "string of pearls" appearance, suddenly developed 5 days ago.

Fig. IVE4.e. *Linear IgA bullous dermatosis, low power.* There is a subepidermal blister associated with a superficial inflammatory infiltrate.

Fig. IVE4.f. *Linear IgA bullous dermatosis, medium power.* At the edge of the blister, where the dermal–epidermal junction is intact, inflammatory cells are seen tagging along the basal cell layer.

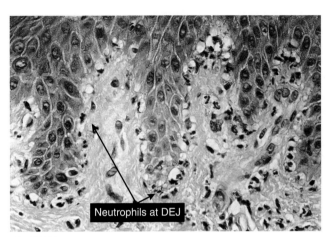

Neutrophils at DEJ

Fig. IVE4.g

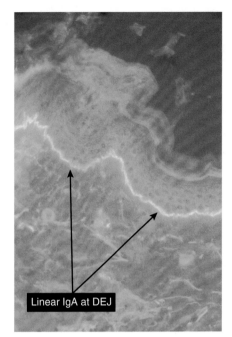

Linear IgA at DEJ

Fig. IVE4.h

Fig. IVE4.g. *Linear IgA bullous dermatosis, high power.* At high magnification, one can see that the inflammatory cells are neutrophils and they are seen not only at the tips of papillae (as is seen in dermatitis herpetiformis), but they are also quite prominent along the tips of the rete ridges, a feature which may help distinguish linear IgA disease from dermatitis herpetiformis.

Fig. IVE4.h. *Linear IgA bullous dermatosis, direct immunofluorescence, high power.* IgA is deposited in a linear fashion at the dermal–epidermal junction. Other immune reactants may be seen less commonly and intensely than IgA.

systemic, or subacute cutaneous LE when they develop blisters.

HISTOPATHOLOGY. Three histologic patterns have been identified in such lesions. The first is striking basal layer vacuolization with subsequent blister formation. The second is vasculitis with subepidermal blister and pustule formation. The third and most common is a dermatitis herpetiformis–like histologic pattern. Approximately 25% of cases are said to have a small-vessel, neutrophil-rich leukocytoclastic vasculitis beneath the blister. Histologic features more routinely identified with LE are not present, other than the presence of dermal mucin and hyaluronic acid in the dermis. By IF, IgG and C3 deposits are demonstrated at the epidermal basement membrane zone. The pattern may be linear or "granular band like." A salt-split skin preparation using patient serum reveals localization to the split floor as in EBA. Antibodies to type VII collagen may be present. Immunoelectron microscopic examination reveals electron-dense deposits of IgG at the lower edge of the basal lamina and immediately subjacent dermis in an identical location to the antibody in EBA.

Epidermolysis Bullosa Acquisita

CLINICAL FEATURES. EBA is an acquired blistering skin disorder. Classically, this was a diagnostic term for the adult onset of a disease with clinical lesions resembling epidermolysis bullosa dystrophica, resulting in scarring and milia formation, a negative family history of epidermolysis bullosa dystrophica, and exclusion of other bullous diseases. Subsequently a subset of cases resembling bullous pemphigoid was described, with a lesser tendency to scarring (83).

HISTOPATHOLOGY. The bullous pemphigoid-like ("inflammatory") form is the most common presentation of EBA. There is a subepidermal blister with a predominantly lymphocytic and neutrophilic cellular response. Eosinophils are variably present. In the classic form, the blisters are noninflammatory and result in scarring. In both forms, there is typically deposition of C3 and IgG, sometimes with IgM and IgA along the dermal–epidermal junction. Deposition of C3 alone, and also of multiple immunoglobulins, tends to favor EBA. The deposits are located beneath the lamina densa in the anchoring

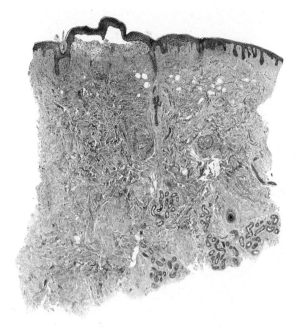

Fig. IVE4.i

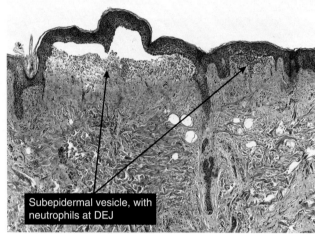

Subepidermal vesicle, with neutrophils at DEJ

Fig. IVE4.j

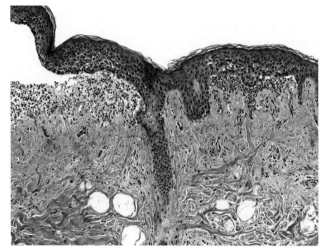

Fig. IVE4.k

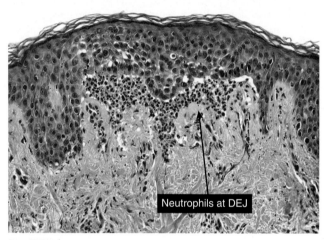

Neutrophils at DEJ

Fig. IVE4.l

Fig. IVE4.i. *Bullous lupus erythematosus, medium power.* There is a large subepidermal bulla containing inflammatory cells.

Fig. IVE4.j. *Bullous lupus erythematosus, high power.* There is an early lesion adjacent to the larger vesicle.

Fig. IVE4.k,l. *Bullous lupus erythematosus, high power.* The inflammatory cells in the lesions are mostly neutrophils.

fibril zone, and the autoimmune response is directed at type VII collagen (COL7), which was first recognized as a 290-kD autoantigen. This location differs from that of immune deposits in bullous pemphigoid, which are located in the lamina lucida. The location of the deposits can be demonstrated by the salt-split skin technique (84), and also by recognition of the "linear u pattern" of deposition (71).

Conditions to consider in the differential diagnosis:
dermatitis herpetiformis
bullous lupus erythematosus, neutrophilic type
bullous vasculitis
linear IgA dermatosis (adult, childhood, drug associated)
epidermolysis bullosa acquisita (inflammatory)
vesiculopustular eruption of hepatobiliary disease
toxic shock syndrome

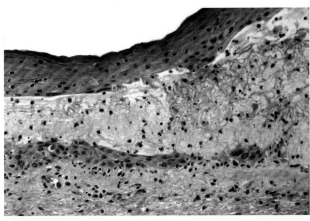

Fig. IVE4.m

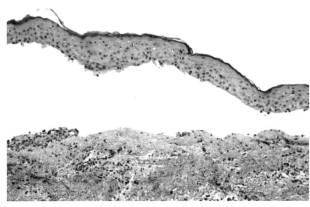

Fig. IVE4.n

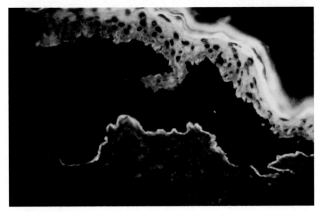

Fig. IVE4.o

Fig. IVE4.m. *Epidermolysis bullosa acquisita.* Inflammatory type: Some neutrophils and eosinophils are in the blister cavity and the superficial dermis. The blister is partly re-epithelialized. (Wu H, Allan AE, and Harrist TJ) (Reprinted with permission from Elder DE. *Lever's Histopathology of the Skin.* 11th ed. Philadelphia, PA: Wolters Kluwer Health; 2015.)

Fig. IVE4.n. *Epidermolysis bullosa acquisita.* Noninflammatory type with a subepidermal blister. (Wu H, Allan AE, and Harrist TJ) (Reprinted with permission from Elder DE. *Lever's Histopathology of the Skin.* 11th ed. Philadelphia, PA: Wolters Kluwer Health; 2015.)

Fig. IVE4.o. *Epidermolysis bullosa acquisita.* Salt-split direct immunofluorescence reveals linear deposition of IgG in the blister base. (Wu H, Allan AE, and Harrist TJ) (Reprinted with permission from Elder DE. *Lever's Histopathology of the Skin.* 11th ed. Philadelphia, PA: Wolters Kluwer Health; 2015.)

IVE5 Subepidermal Vesicles, Mast Cells Prominent

The epidermis is separated from the dermis. There is an infiltrate in the superficial dermis composed almost entirely of mast cells, with or without a few eosinophils. This may be associated with separation of the epidermis from the dermis. *Bullous mastocytosis* is the only example (85,86).

Bullous Mastocytosis

CLINICAL SUMMARY. Vesicles or bullae may be seen in all of the types of cutaneous mastocytosis (urticaria pigmentosa) except telangiectasia macularis eruptiva perstans. The maculopapular type, which is the most common type, may be seen in children or adults and consists usually of dozens or even hundreds of brown lesions that urticate on stroking (Darier sign); the multinodular type exhibits multiple brown nodules or plaques, and, on stroking, shows urtication and occasionally blister formation. The nodular type seen almost exclusively in infants, is characterized by a usually solitary, large cutaneous

nodule, which on stroking often shows not only urtication but also large bullae. The diffuse erythrodermic type always starts in early infancy and shows generalized

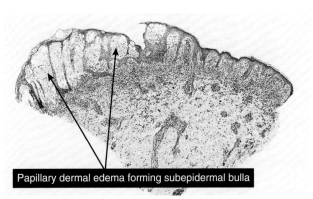

Papillary dermal edema forming subepidermal bulla

Fig. IVE5.a

Fig. IVE5.a. *Bullous mastocytosis, low power.* There is subepidermal blister formation associated with a moderately intense infiltrate involving the superficial and middermis. (*continues*)

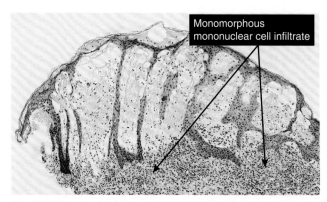

Fig. IVE5.b

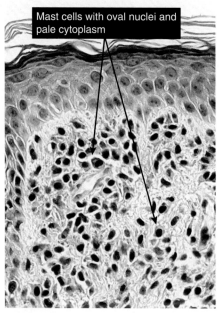

Fig. IVE5.c

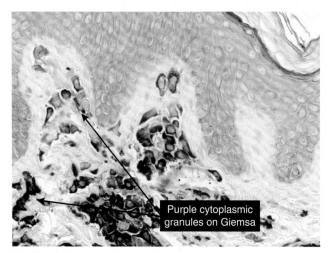

Fig. IVE5.d

Fig. IVE5.b. *Bullous mastocytosis, medium power.* The subepidermal blister is associated with a diffuse, interstitial mononuclear cell infiltrate.

Fig. IVE5.c. *Bullous mastocytosis, high power.* The infiltrate is composed almost entirely of mast cells with small uniform oval nuclei. There are scattered eosinophils.

Fig. IVE5.d. *Bullous mastocytosis, high power.* Giemsa stain metachromatically stains the granules of mast cells purple. C-Kit immunostaining is a specific and reliable marker for mast cells.

brownish red, soft infiltration of the skin, with urtication on stroking. Multiple blisters may form during the first 2 years of life on stroking and also spontaneously. If bullae are a predominant clinical feature, the term *bullous mastocytosis* has been applied.

HISTOPATHOLOGY. The bullae that may occur in infants with multiple or solitary nodules or with the diffuse erythrodermic type arise subepidermally. Because of regeneration of the epidermis at the base of the bulla, older bullae may be located intraepidermally. The bullous cavity often contains mast cells as well as eosinophils.

References

1. Bystryn JC, Rudolph JL. Pemphigus. *Lancet* 2005;366:61–73.
2. Stanley JR, Amagai M. Pemphigus, bullous impetigo, and the staphylococcal scalded-skin syndrome. *N Engl J Med* 2006; 355(17):1800–1810. Review.
3. Brenner S, Bialy-Golan A, Ruocco V. Drug-induced pemphigus. *Clin Dermatol* 1998;16:393–397.
4. Hans-Filho G, Aoki V, Bittner NRH, et al. Fogo selvagem: endemic pemphigus foliaceus. *An Bras Dermatol* 2018;93(5): 638–650.
5. James KA, Culton DA, Diaz LA. Diagnosis and clinical features of pemphigus foliaceus. *Dermatol Clin* 2011;29(3):405–412, viii. Review.
6. Amagai M, Kormai A, Hashimoto T, et al. Usefulness of enzyme-linked immunosorbent assay (ELISA) using recombinant desmogleins 1 and 3 for serodiagnosis of pemphigus. *Br J Dermatol* 1999;140:351–357.
7. Wick MR. Bullous, pseudobullous, & pustular dermatoses. *Semin Diagn Pathol* 2017;34(3):250–260.
8. Dagan R. Impetigo in childhood: changing epidemiology and new treatments. *Pediatr Ann* 1993;22:235–240.
9. Leung AKC, Barankin B, Leong KF. Staphylococcal-scalded skin syndrome: evaluation, diagnosis, and management. *World J Pediatr* 2018;14(2):116–120.
10. Elias PM, Fritsch P, Epstein EH Jr. Staphylococcal scalded skin syndrome (review). *Arch Dermatol* 1977;113:207–219.
11. Bukowski M, Wladyka B, Dubin G. Exfoliative toxins of Staphylococcus aureus. *Toxins (Basel)* 2010;2(5):1148–1165.
12. Sideroff A, Halevy S, Bavinck J, et al. Acute generalized exanthematous pustulosis (AGEP)—a clinical reaction pattern. *J Cutan Pathol* 2001;28:113–119.

13. Feldmeyer L, Heidemeyer K, Yawalkar N. Acute generalized exanthematous pustulosis: pathogenesis, genetic background, clinical variants and therapy. *Int J Mol Sci* 2016;17(8):E1214.

14. Bissonnette R, Suárez-Fariñas M, Li X, et al. Based on molecular profiling of gene expression, palmoplantar pustulosis and palmoplantar pustular psoriasis are highly related diseases that appear to be distinct from psoriasis vulgaris. *PLoS One* 2016; 11(5):e0155215.

15. Freeman RG, Spiller R, Knox JM. Histopathology of erythema toxicum neonatorum. *Arch Dermatol* 1960;82:586–589.

16. Lacarrubba F, Boscaglia S, Nasca MR, et al. Grover's disease: dermoscopy, reflectance confocal microscopy and histopathological correlation. *Dermatol Pract Concept* 2017;7(3):51–54.

17. Cruickshank CN. The microanatomy of the epidermis in relation to trauma. *J Tissue Viability* 2006;16(2):16–19.

18. Knapik JJ, Reynolds KL, Duplantis KL, et al. Friction blisters. Pathophysiology, prevention and treatment. *Sports Med* 1995; 20(3):136–147. Review.

19. Armbruster N, Trautmann A, Bröcker EB, et al. Suprabasal spongiosis in acute eczematous dermatitis: cFLIP maintains resistance of basal keratinocytes to T-cell-mediated apoptosis. *J Invest Dermatol* 2009;129(7):1696–1702.

20. Masuda-Kuroki K, Murakami M, Kishibe M, et al. Diagnostic histopathological features distinguishing palmoplantar pustulosis from pompholyx. *J Dermatol* 2019;46(5):399–408.

21. Crotty C, Pittelkow M, Muller SA. Eosinophilic spongiosis: a clinicopathologic review of seventy-one cases. *J Am Acad Dermatol* 1983;8(3):337–343.

22. Machado-Pinto J, McCalmont TH, Golitz LE. Eosinophilic and neutrophilic spongiosis: clues to the diagnosis of immunobullous diseases and other inflammatory disorders. *Semin Cutan Med Surg* 1996;15(4):308–316.

23. Esser PR, Martin SF. Pathomechanisms of contact sensitization. *Curr Allergy Asthma Rep* 2017;17(12):83.

24. Frings VG, Böer-Auer A, Breuer K. Histomorphology and immunophenotype of eczematous skin lesions revisited-skin biopsies are not reliable in differentiating allergic contact dermatitis, irritant contact dermatitis, and atopic dermatitis. *Am J Dermatopathol* 2018;40(1):7–16.

25. The International Incontinentia Pigmenti Consortium: genomic rearrangement in NEMO impairs NF-KappaB activation and is a cause of incontinentia pigmenti. *Nature* 2000;405:466–472.

26. Pacheco TR, Levy M, Collyer JC, et al. Incontinentia pigmenti in male patients. *J Am Acad Dermatol* 2006;55(2):251–255.

27. Greene-Roethke C. Incontinentia pigmenti: a summary review of this rare ectodermal dysplasia with neurologic manifestations, including treatment protocols. *J Pediatr Health Care* 2017;31(6):e45–e52.

28. Gottlieb GJ, Ackerman AB. The "sandwich sign" of dermatophytosis. *Am J Dermatopathol* 1986;8(4):347–350.

29. Ikeda S, Welsh EA, Peluso AM, et al. Localization of the gene whose mutations underlie Hailey-Hailey disease to chromosome 3q. *Hum Mol Genet* 1994;(7):1147–1150.

30. Hu Z, Bonifas JM, Beech J, et al. Mutations in ATP2Cl, encoding a calcium pump, cause Hailey-Hailey disease. *Nat Genet* 2000; 24:61–65.

31. Nellen RG, Steijlen PM, van Steensel MA, et al; European Professional Contributors. Mendelian disorders of cornification caused by defects in intracellular calcium pumps: mutation update and database for variants in ATP2A2 and ATP2C1 associated with Darier disease and Hailey-Hailey disease. *Hum Mutat* 2017;38(4):343–356.

32. Grover RW. Transient acantholytic dermatosis. *Arch Dermatol* 1970;101:426–434.

33. Chalet M, Grover R, Ackerman AB. Transient acantholytic dermatosis. *Arch Dermatol* 1977;113:431–435.

34. Powell J, Sakuntabhai A, James M, et al. Grover's disease, despite histological similarity to Darier's disease, does not share an abnormality in the ATP2A2 gene. *Br J Dermatol* 2000;143(3):658.

35. DiMaio DJ, Cohen PR. Incidental focal acantholytic dyskeratosis. *J Am Acad Dermatol* 1998;38(2 Pt 1):243–247.

36. Aljarbou OZ, Asgari M, Al-Saidi N, et al. Grover disease with epidermal dysmaturation pattern: a common histopathologic finding. *Am J Dermatopathol* 2018;40(9):642–646.

37. Fernández-Figueras MT, Puig L, Cannata P, et al. Grover disease: a reappraisal of histopathological diagnostic criteria in 120 cases. *Am J Dermatopathol* 2010;32(6):541–549.

38. Bayer-Garner I, Dilday B, Sanderson R, et al. Acantholysis and spongiosis are associated with loss of Syndecan-1 expression. *J Cutan Pathol* 2001;28:135–139.

39. Blank H, Haines H. Viral diseases of the skin, 1975: a 25-year perspective. *J Invest Dermatol* 1976;67:169–176.

40. Hoyt B, Bhawan J. Histological spectrum of cutaneous herpes infections. *Am J Dermatopathol* 2014;36(8):609–619.

41. Ferenczi K, Rosenberg AS, McCalmont TH, et al. Herpes zoster granulomatous dermatitis: histopathologic findings in a case series. *J Cutan Pathol* 2015;42(10):739–745.

42. Anhalt GJ, Kim SC, Stanley JR, et al. Paraneoplastic pemphigus: an autoimmune mucocutaneous disease associated with neoplasia. *N Engl J Med* 1990;323:1729–1735.

43. Zhu X, Zhang B. Paraneoplastic pemphigus. *J Dermatol* 2007; 34(8):503–511. Review.

44. Nguyen VT, Ndoye A, Bassler KD, et al. Classification, clinical manifestations, and immunopathological mechanisms of the epithelial variant of paraneoplastic autoimmune multiorgan syndrome: a reappraisal of paraneoplastic pemphigus. *Arch Dermatol* 2001;137(2):193–206.

45. Frew JW, Murrell DF. Paraneoplastic pemphigus (paraneoplastic autoimmune multiorgan syndrome): clinical presentations and pathogenesis. *Dermatol Clin* 2011;29(3):419–425.

46. Mihai S, Sitaru C. Immunopathology and molecular diagnosis of autoimmune bullous diseases. *J Cell Mol Med* 2007;11(3):462–481. Review.

47. Ahmed AR, Blose DA. Pemphigus vegetans, Neumann type and Hallopeau type. *Int J Dermatol* 1984;23:135–141.

48. Beutner EH, Chorzelski TP, Wilson RM, et al. IgA pemphigus foliaceus. *J Am Acad Dermatol* 1989;20:89–97.

49. Tsuruta D, Ishii N, Hamada T, et al. IgA pemphigus. *Clin Dermatol* 2011;29(4):437–442.

50. Geller S, Gat A, Zeeli T, et al. The expanding spectrum of IgA pemphigus: a case report and review of the literature. *Br J Dermatol* 2014;171(3):650–656.

51. Gottlieb SK, Lutzner MA. Darier's disease. *Arch Dermatol* 1973;107:225–230.

52. Hovnanian A. Darier's disease: from dyskeratosis to endoplasmic reticulum calcium ATPase deficiency. *Biochem Biophys Res Commun* 2004;322:1237–1244.

53. Kaddu S, Dong H, Mayer G, et al. Warty dyskeratoma–"follicular dyskeratoma": analysis of clinicopathologic features of a distinctive follicular adnexal neoplasm. *J Am Acad Dermatol* 2002;47(3):423–428.

54. Carapeto FJ, García-Pérez A. Acantholytic keratosis. *Dermatologica* 1974;148:233–239.

55. Ogawa T, Kiuru M, Konia TH, et al. Acantholytic squamous cell carcinoma is usually associated with hair follicles, not acantholytic actinic keratosis, and is not "high risk": diagnosis, management, and clinical outcomes in a series of 115 cases. *J Am Acad Dermatol* 2017;76(2):327–333.

56. Hertl M. Humoral and cellular autoimmunity in autoimmune bullous skin disorders. *Int Arch Allergy Immunol* 2000;122:91–100.

57. Kridin K. Pemphigus group: overview, epidemiology, mortality, and comorbidities. *Immunol Res* 2018;66(2):255–270.

58. Schmidt E, Zillikens D. Modern diagnosis of autoimmune blistering skin diseases. *Autoimmun Rev* 2010;10(2):84–89.

59. Handler NS, Handler MZ, Stephany MP, et al. Porphyria cutanea tarda: an intriguing genetic disease and marker. *Int J Dermatol* 2017;56(6):e106–e117.

60. Rossmann-Ringdahl I, Olsson R. Porphyria cutanea tarda in a Swedish population: risk factors and complications. *Acta Derm Venereol* 2005;85(4):337–341.

61. Liakopoulou A, Rallis E. Bullous lichen planus—a review. *J Dermatol Case Rep* 2017;11(1):1–4.

62. Anand D, Bernardin R, Rubin AI. Blisters and plaques on the extremities. What is your diagnosis? Lichen planus pemphigoides. *Int J Dermatol* 2011;50(2):147–149.

63. Hawk JLM. Cutaneous photobiology. In: Rook A, Ebling FJG, Champion RH, Burton JL, eds. *Textbook of Dermatology*. 5th ed. Oxford: Blackwell Scientific Publications; 1991:849.

64. Pincus LB, LeBoit PE, Goddard DS, et al. Marked papillary dermal edema—an unreliable discriminator between polymorphous light eruption and lupus erythematosus or dermatomyositis. *J Cutan Pathol* 2010;37(4):416–425.

65. Vincent JG, Chan MP. Specificity of dermal mucin in the diagnosis of lupus erythematosus: comparison with other dermatitides and normal skin. *J Cutan Pathol* 2015;42(10):722–729.

66. Pincus LB, LeBoit PE, Goddard DS, et al. Marked papillary dermal edema—an unreliable discriminator between polymorphous light eruption and lupus erythematosus or dermatomyositis. *J Cutan Pathol* 2010;37(4):416–425.

67. Miller DD, Bhawan J. Bullous tinea pedis with direct immunofluorescence positivity: when is a positive result not autoimmune bullous disease? *Am J Dermatopathol* 2013;35(5):587–594.

68. Sauder MB, Linzon-Smith J, Beecker J. Extragenital bullous lichen sclerosus. *J Am Acad Dermatol* 2014;71(5):981–984.

69. Eng AM, Moncada B. Bullous pemphigoid and dermatitis herpetiformis: histologic differentiation. *Arch Dermatol* 1974;110:51.

70. Lever WF. Pemphigus. *Medicine (Baltimore)* 1953;32:1–123.

71. Ujiie H, Shibaki A, Nishie W, et al. What's new in bullous pemphigoid. *J Dermatol* 2010;37(3):194–204. Review.

72. Powell AM, Sakuma-Oyama Y, Oyama N, et al. Collagen XVII/BP180: a collagenous transmembrane protein and component of the dermoepidermal anchoring complex. *Clin Exp Dermatol* 2005;30:682–687.

73. Terra JB, Meijer JM, Jonkman MF, et al. The n- vs. u-serration is a learnable criterion to differentiate pemphigoid from epidermolysis bullosa acquisita in direct immunofluorescence serration pattern analysis. *Br J Dermatol* 2013;169(1):100–105.

74. Cho YT, Lin JW, Chen YC, et al. Generalized bullous fixed drug eruption is distinct from Stevens-Johnson syndrome/toxic epidermal necrolysis by immunohistopathological features. *J Am Acad Dermatol* 2014;70(3):539–548.

75. Semkova K, Black M. Pemphigoid gestationis: current insights into pathogenesis and treatment. *Eur J Obstet Gynecol Reprod Biol* 2009;145(2):138–144. Review.

76. MacVicar DN, Graham JH, Burgoon CF Jr. Dermatitis herpetiformis, erythema multiforme and bullous pemphigoid: a comparative histopathological and histochemical study. *J Invest Dermatol* 1963;41:289–300.

77. Karpati S. Dermatitis herpetiformis: close to unravelling a disease. *J Dermatol Sci* 2004;34:83–90.

78. Nicolas ME, Krause PK, Gibson LE, et al. Dermatitis herpetiformis. *Int J Dermatol* 2003;42:588–600.

79. Ko CJ, Colegio OR, Moss JE, et al. Fibrillar IgA deposition in dermatitis herpetiformis—an underreported pattern with potential clinical significance. *J Cutan Pathol* 2010;37(4):475–477.

80. Smith SB, Harrist TJ, Murphy GF, et al. Linear IgA bullous dermatosis v. dermatitis herpetiformis. *Arch Dermatol* 1984;120:324–328.

81. Wojnarowska F, Whitehead P, Leigh IM, et al. Identification of the target antigen in chronic bullous disease of childhood and linear IgA disease of adults. *Br J Dermatol* 1991;124:157–162.

82. Tsuchida T, Furue M, Kashiwado T, et al. Bullous systemic lupus erythematosus with cutaneous mucinosis and leukocytoclastic vasculitis. *J Am Acad Dermatol* 1994;31:387–390.

83. Gammon WR, Briggaman RA, Woodley DT, et al. Epidermolysis bullosa acquisita—a pemphigoid-like disease. *J Am Acad Dermatol* 1984;11(5 Pt 1):820–832.

84. Iwata H, Vorobyev A, Koga H, et al. Meta-analysis of the clinical and immunopathological characteristics and treatment outcomes in epidermolysis bullosa acquisita patients. *Orphanet J Rare Dis* 2018;13(1):153.

85. Orkin M, Good RA, Clawson CC, et al. Bullous mastocytosis. *Arch Dermatol* 1970;101:547–564.

86. Avshalumov K, Pichardo R, Jorizzo JL, et al. Bullous mastocytosis: report of a patient and a brief review of the literature. *Am J Dermatopathol* 2008;30(5):455–457.

Perivascular, Diffuse, and Granulomatous Infiltrates of the Reticular Dermis

V

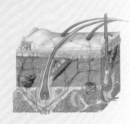

The dermis serves as a reaction site for a variety of inflammatory, infiltrative, and desmoplastic processes. These include infiltrations of a variety of cells (lymphocytes, histiocytes, eosinophils, plasma cells, melanocytes, etc.); perivascular and vascular reactions; infiltration with organisms and foreign bodies; and proliferations of dermal fibers and precursors of dermal fibers as reactions to a variety of stimuli.

SUPERFICIAL AND DEEP PERIVASCULAR INFILTRATES WITHOUT VASCULITIS

In some of the diseases considered here, the infiltrates are predominantly in the upper reticular dermis (urticarial eruptions), while others are both superficial and deep (gyrate erythemas). Most of these also involve the superficial plexus. A few diseases are mainly deep (some examples of lupus erythematosus [LE], scleroderma).

1. Perivascular Infiltrates, Lymphocytes Predominant
2. Perivascular infiltrates, Neutrophils Predominant
3. Perivascular Infiltrates, Lymphocytes and Eosinophils
4. Perivascular Infiltrates, With Plasma Cells
5. Perivascular Infiltrates, Mixed Cell Types

VA1 Perivascular Infiltrates, Lymphocytes Predominant

In the dermis there is no vasculitis, only perivascular collections of lymphocytes as the predominant cell. Erythema annulare centrifugum (EAC) is prototypic (1,2).

Erythema Annulare Centrifugum

CLINICAL SUMMARY. Also known as gyrate erythema, this disorder represents a hypersensitivity reaction manifesting as arcuate and polycyclic areas of erythema. The condition has been categorized into superficial and deep variants (2). The deep form is characterized clinically by annular areas of palpable erythema with central clearing and absence of surface changes. The superficial variant differs only by the presence of a characteristic trailing scale, a delicate annular rim of scale that trails behind the advancing edge of erythema. Small vesicles may occur. The lesions may attain considerable size (up to 10 cm across) over a period of several weeks, may be mildly pruritic, and have a predilection for the trunk and proximal extremities. EAC can be considered a reactive phenomenon, and has been associated with a variety of disparate conditions including pregnancy, surgical procedures, breast cancer, lymphoma, leukemia, herpes zoster, medication reactions, as well as others. Most cases resolve spontaneously within 6 weeks; however, the condition may persist for years.

HISTOPATHOLOGY. In the classic deep or indurated type, a perivascular lymphocytic infiltrate characterized by a tightly cuffed "coat-sleeve–like" pattern is present in the middle and lower portions of the dermis. In the superficial variant, there is a superficial perivascular tightly cuffed lymphohistiocytic infiltrate with endothelial cell swelling and focal extravasation of erythrocytes in the papillary dermis, and focal epidermal spongiosis and parakeratosis can be seen. Erythema chronicum migrans (ECM) is an important differential, but often presents with plasma cells or mixed cells as well as lymphocytes and is therefore discussed also in Sections VA4 and VA5.

Erythema Chronicum Migrans

See discussion in Section VA5.

Tumid Lupus Erythematosus

The dermal form of LE without surface/epithelial changes is known as tumid LE. Clinically, affected patients display

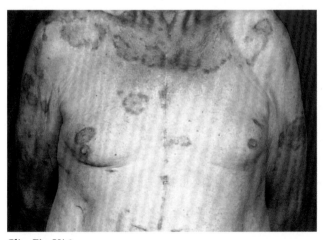

Clin. Fig. VA1.a

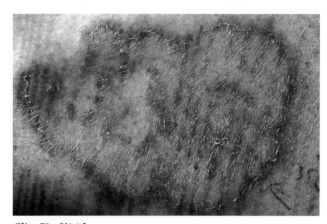

Clin. Fig. VA1.b

Clin. Fig. VA1.a. *Erythema annulare centrifugum.* Multiple annular lesions developed on the trunk of a middle-aged man.

Clin. Fig. VA1.b. *Erythema annulare centrifugum.* An annular area of palpable erythema with central clearing and a delicate annular rim of scale trailing behind the advancing edge of the erythema.

V Perivascular, Diffuse, and Granulomatous Infiltrates of the Reticular Dermis

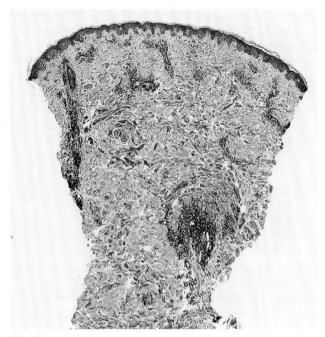

Fig. VA1.a

Fig. VA1.a. *Erythema annulare centrifugum, low power.* A tight cuff of small round cells surrounds the vessels of the superficial and middermal plexuses.

Fig. VA1.b. *Erythema annulare centrifugum, medium power.* The vessels at the center of the infiltrates show no evidence of damage other than slight endothelial cell swelling.

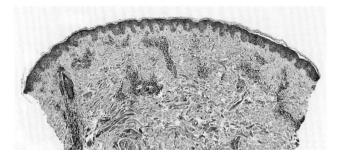

Fig. VA1.b

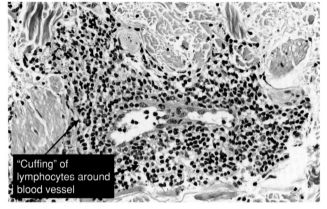

"Cuffing" of lymphocytes around blood vessel

Fig. VA1.c

Fig. VA1.c. *Erythema annulare centrifugum, high power.* The infiltrate is composed almost entirely of mature small lymphocytes.

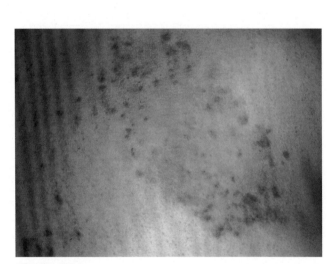

Clin. Fig. VA1.c

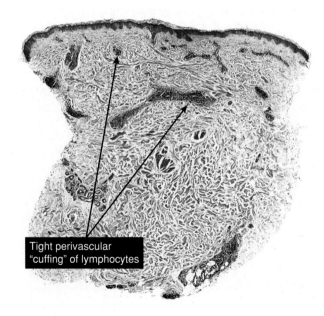

Tight perivascular "cuffing" of lymphocytes

Fig. VA1.d

Clin. Fig. VA1.c. *Erythema chronicum migrans.* Note the central bite area and expanding border of erythema in a confirmed case of Lyme disease.

Fig. VA1.d. *Erythema chronicum migrans, low power.* Similar to EAC, there is a tight cuff of small cells around the vessels of the superficial and deep dermal plexuses.

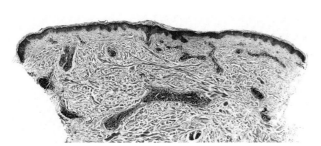

Fig. VA1.e

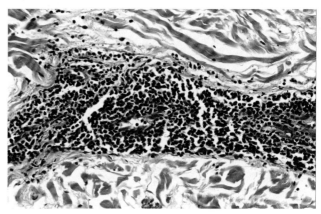

Fig. VA1.f

Fig. VA1.e. *Erythema chronicum migrans, medium power.* The infiltrate surrounds vessels quite tightly, without a significant interstitial infiltrate.

Fig. VA1.f. *Erythema chronicum migrans, high power.* Although plasma cells are usually present, in some instances, as here, the infiltrate is composed almost entirely of mature small lymphocytes.

indurated papules, plaques, and nodules without hyperkeratosis, atrophy, or ulceration of the surface. Histologically, superficial and deep dermal perivascular, interstitial, and periappendageal lymphoplasmacytic infiltrates associated with stromal mucin deposits are observed (3,4).

Conditions to consider in the differential diagnosis:

pityriasis lichenoides et varioliformis acuta (PLEVA)
stasis dermatitis
acne rosacea

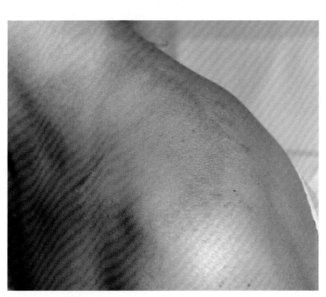

Clin. Fig. VA1.d

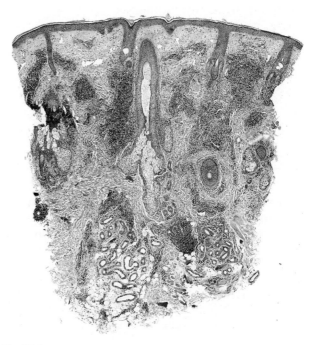

Fig. VA1.g

Clin. Fig. VA1.d. *Tumid lupus.* This is a deeper and more nodular form of lupus that presents with little to no scale. Some consider it a variant of subacute cutaneous lupus.

Fig. VA1.g. *"Tumid" lupus erythematosus, low power.* A dense lymphocytic infiltrate is present around the vessels of the superficial, mid, and deep dermal plexuses, and around adnexal structures. (*continues*)

V Perivascular, Diffuse, and Granulomatous Infiltrates of the Reticular Dermis

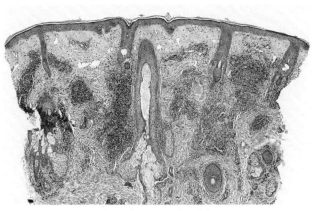

Fig. VA1.h

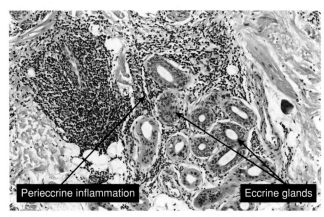

Perieccrine inflammation   Eccrine glands

Fig. VA1.i

Fig. VA1.h. *"Tumid" lupus erythematosus, medium power.* In contrast to EAC and ECM, the cuff of small lymphocytes appears less tight around the vessels of the superficial, mid, and deep dermal plexuses, because there is also an interstitial component to the infiltrate.

Fig. VA1.i. *"Tumid" lupus erythematosus, high power.* Although plasma cells are usually present, the infiltrate is often as here composed almost entirely of mature small lymphocytes. Involvement of skin appendages (sweat glands) is a clue to the diagnosis of lupus, and also the presence of stromal mucin.

---

discoid lupus erythematosus (DLE)
polymorphous light eruption
deep gyrate erythemas
    erythema annulare centrifigum
    erythema chronicum migrans
Jessner lymphocytic infiltrate
reticulated erythematous mucinosis (REM)
perioral dermatitis
papular acrodermatitis (Gianotti–Crosti)
leprosy, indeterminant
    "tumid" lupus erythematosus
perniosis (chilblains)

VA2 | **Perivascular Infiltrates, Neutrophils Predominant**

In this pattern, neutrophils are seen in perivascular or perivascular and diffuse patterns in the dermis. Edema is prominent in some instances. Sweet syndrome can present as a perivascular infiltrate, but is more often nodular and is therefore discussed in Section VC2. Neutrophil-rich urticaria may present as a predominantly neutrophilic infiltrate, but eosinophils are usually also present (see Section VA3). The other conditions listed are mostly infections. Biopsies from the periphery of a lesion may appear perivascular, but the fully developed center of these lesions will consist of diffuse infiltrates (Section VA3).

Cellulitis

See discussion in Section VC2.

Conditions to consider in the differential diagnosis:

acute febrile neutrophilic dermatosis (Sweet)
erysipelas
necrotizing fasciitis

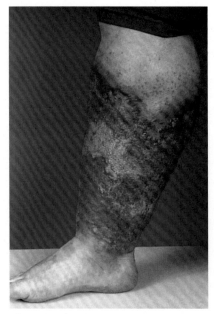

Clin. Fig. VA.2

Clin. Fig. VA.2. *Cellulitis.* This middle-aged female was admitted with septic shock secondary to her cellulitis. She had marked erythema and bullous changes and rapidly improved on IV antibiotics.

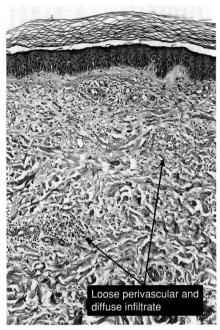

Fig. VA2.a

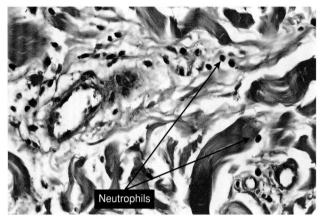

Fig. VA2.b

Fig. VA2.a. *Cellulitis, low power.* There is edema and a patchy infiltrate in the reticular dermis, appearing at this magnification to be mainly perivascular.

Fig. VA2.b. *Cellulitis, high power.* The cells about the vessels are mainly neutrophils. In other areas, the infiltrate appears more diffuse (see VC2).

pyoderma gangrenosum (early)
ecthyma gangrenosum
neutrophil-rich urticaria
solar urticaria
rheumatoid arthritis
neutrophilic dermatosis of the dorsal hands
other neutrophilic dermatoses
    Behçet disease
    Bowel bypass syndrome (Bowel-associated dermatosis–arthritis syndrome)
    erythema elevatum diutinum

VA3   Perivascular Infiltrates, Lymphocytes and Eosinophils

Lymphocytes and eosinophils are mixed in the infiltrate. Lymphocytes are always seen, eosinophil numbers may vary being greatest in bite reactions and often (though variable and sometimes very few) in eosinophilic fasciitis. Papular urticaria is a prototypic example (5).

Papular Urticaria

CLINICAL SUMMARY. Also known as lichen urticatus, this condition is the result of hypersensitivity to bites from certain insects, especially mosquitoes, fleas, and bedbugs. One observes edematous papules and papulovesicles,

which, because of severe itching, usually are excoriated. The eruption is more common in children than in adults, and, if caused by mosquitoes, is limited to the summer months.

HISTOPATHOLOGY. The stratum malpighii shows intercellular and intracellular edema and occasionally a spongiotic vesicle. A predominantly lymphocytic infiltrate is present around the vessels of the dermis, often extending into the lower dermis and containing a significant admixture of eosinophils. In a study of 30 cases, mild acanthosis, mild spongiosis, exocytosis of lymphocytes, mild subepidermal edema, extravasation of erythrocytes, a superficial and deep mixed inflammatory cell infiltrate of moderate density, and interstitial eosinophils were present in >50%. The changes may be difficult to distinguish from an actual arthropod assault (bite or sting) (6).

Urticaria

CLINICAL SUMMARY. Urticaria is characterized by the presence of abrupt onset, transient and recurrent wheals, which are raised erythematous and edematous areas of skin that are often pruritic. When large wheals occur and the edema extends to the subcutaneous or submucosal tissues, the process is referred to as angioedema. Acute episodes of urticaria generally last only

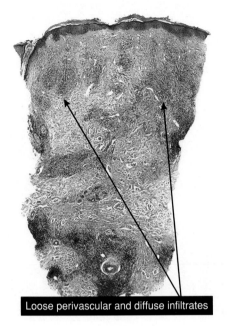

Loose perivascular and diffuse infiltrates

Fig. VA3.a

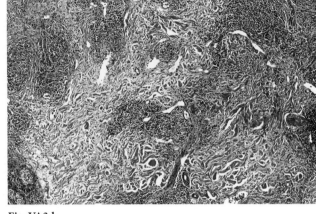

Fig. VA3.b

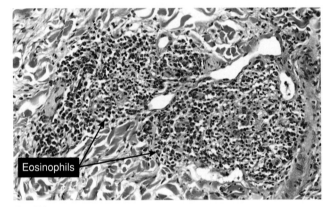

Eosinophils

Fig. VA3.c

Fig. VA3.a. *Papular urticaria/arthropod bite, low power.* A dense perivascular infiltrate of lymphocytes and eosinophils, more conspicuous than in many instances of typical "papular urticaria."

Fig. VA3.b. *Papular urticaria/arthropod bite, medium power.* The infiltrate shows both a perivascular and interstitial pattern.

Fig. VA3.c. *Papular urticaria/arthropod bite, high power.* The infiltrate is composed primarily of lymphocytes, with a striking component of eosinophils. Plasma cells may also be present in some cases.

---

several hours. When episodes of urticaria last up to 24 hours and recur over a period of at least 6 to 8 weeks, the condition is considered chronic urticaria. The various causes of urticaria include soluble antigens in foods, drugs, insect venom; contact allergens; physical stimuli such as pressure, vibration, solar radiation, cold temperature; occult infections and malignancies; and some hereditary syndromes, but in many cases the cause remains undetermined.

HISTOPATHOLOGY. In acute urticaria the prominent feature is interstitial dermal edema, with dilated lymphatics and venules with endothelial swelling, and a paucity of inflammatory cells. In chronic urticaria interstitial dermal edema and a perivascular and interstitial mixed cell infiltrate with variable numbers of lymphocytes, eosinophils, and neutrophils are present. In a

review of 58 cases, two distinctive patterns were observed, namely lymphocyte and neutrophil predominant. The former was characterized by a perivascular location, while the latter was associated with an interstitial location and a denser infiltrate. Eosinophils were also commonly present (7).

Pruritic Urticarial Papules and Plaques of Pregnancy

CLINICAL SUMMARY. Pruritic urticarial papules and plaques of pregnancy (PUPPP) is a fairly common entity that has a predilection for primigravidas in the third trimester of pregnancy (8). It can also occur directly postpartum. PUPPP is associated with excessive maternal weight gain and multiple gestation pregnancies (e.g., triplets). The rash usually starts on the abdomen and is composed of intensely pruritic erythematous urticarial

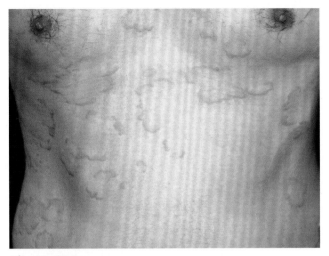

Clin. Fig. VA3.a

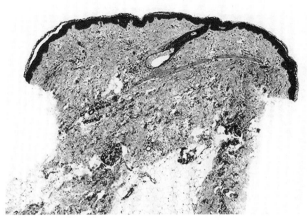

Fig. VA3.d

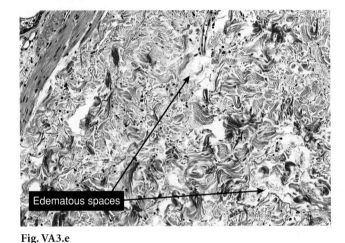

Edematous spaces

Fig. VA3.e

Eosinophils

Fig. VA3.f

Clin. Fig. VA3.a. *Urticaria.* Edematous plaques with central clearing and geographic configuration in a 39-year-old man are typical of urticaria.

Fig. VA3.d. *Urticaria, low power.* A patchy perivascular infiltrate of lymphocytes and eosinophils, which could be seen in "papular urticaria" or in idiopathic urticaria.

Fig. VA3.e. *Urticaria, medium power.* There is sparse dermal infiltrate with edema.

Fig. VA3.f. *Urticaria, high power.* The infiltrate includes mostly eosinophils and neutrophils. This density of infiltrate is compatible with chronic urticaria.

papules, which may be surmounted by vesicles. The proximal parts of the extremities are also affected. There is no increased incidence of the rash in subsequent pregnancies. Typically, lesions begin within striae distensae, and sparing of the umbilical area is a characteristic finding (as opposed to pemphigoid gestationis). The rash usually involutes spontaneously after delivery. Fetal outcome appears to be unaffected. The skin of the newborn child is unaffected (9).

HISTOPATHOLOGY. Microscopic findings most commonly show a superficial and middermal perivascular lymphohistiocytic infiltrate with variable numbers of eosinophils and neutrophils together with edema of the superficial dermis. Epidermal involvement is variable and consists of focal spongiosis with exocytosis, parakeratosis, and mild acanthosis.

Conditions to consider in the differential diagnosis:

urticaria/angioedema
pruritic urticarial papules and plaques of pregnancy (PUPPP)
prurigo simplex
papular urticaria
morbilliform drug eruption
photoallergic reaction

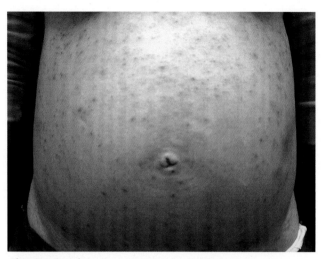

Clin. Fig. VA3.b

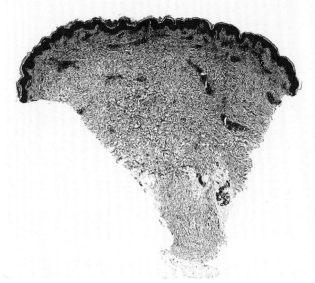

Fig. VA3.g

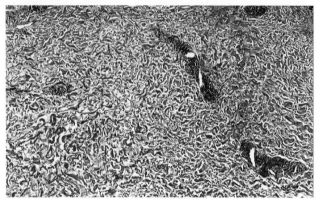

Fig. VA3.h

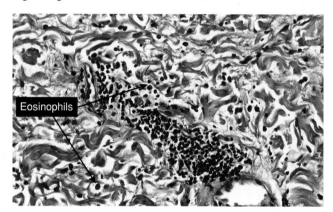

Eosinophils

Fig. VA3.i

Clin. Fig. VA3.b. *Pruritic and urticarial papules and plaques of pregnancy (PUPPP).* A rash starting on the abdomen and composed of intensely pruritic erythematous urticarial papules in a 33-year-old 31 weeks' pregnant woman with duration of 7 days.

Fig. VA3.g. *Pruritic and urticarial papules and plaques of pregnancy (PUPPP), low power.* There is a tight perivascular infiltrate of lymphocytes and eosinophils about the superficial and midplexuses.

Fig. VA3.h. *PUPPP, medium power.* As in usual urticaria, there is dermal edema separating collagen fibers, and lymphatic channels are dilated.

Fig. VA3.i. *PUPPP, high power.* The perivascular and interstitial infiltrate includes lymphocytes and eosinophils, which may not be numerous as in this case.

---

eosinophilic fasciitis/scleroderma
angiolymphoid hyperplasia with eosinophilia (ALHE)
insect bite reaction

VA4 | Perivascular Infiltrates, With Plasma Cells

In addition to lymphocytes, plasma cells are found in the dermal infiltrate. Secondary syphilis is a prototypic example (10).

Secondary Syphilis

Secondary syphilis results from the hematogenous dissemination of *Treponema pallidum*, resulting in widespread clinical signs accompanied by constitutional symptoms inclusive of fever, malaise, and generalized lymphadenopathy. A generalized eruption occurs, comprising brown-red macules and papules, and, rarely, pustules. Lesions may be follicular, annular, or serpiginous. Other skin findings include alopecia and condylomata lata, the latter comprising broad, raised, gray, confluent papular lesions arising in anogenital areas, and mucous patches composed of multiple shallow, painless ulcers. Scaling macules or papules on the palms and soles are a characteristic feature, and this is also known as a "copper penny" rash.

HISTOPATHOLOGY. The two fundamental pathologic changes in syphilis are (1) swelling and proliferation of endothelial cells and (2) a predominantly perivascular infiltrate composed of lymphoid cells and often plasma cells. However, plasma cells and endothelial swelling are not invariably present. Frank necrotizing vasculitis is distinctly unusual. In late secondary and tertiary syphilis, there are also granulomatous infiltrates of epithelioid histiocytes and giant cells.

Biopsies generally reveal psoriasiform hyperplasia of the epidermis with spongiosis and basilar vacuolar alteration, exocytosis of lymphocytes, spongiform pustulation, and parakeratosis. The parakeratosis may be patchy or broad, with or without intracorneal neutrophilic abscesses. Scattered necrotic keratinocytes may be observed. Ulceration is not usual except in lues maligna. The dermal changes include marked papillary dermal edema and a perivascular and/or periadnexal and often lichenoid infiltrate that may be lymphocyte predominant, lymphohistiocytic, histiocytic predominant, or frankly granulomatous and is of greatest intensity in the papillary dermis and extends as loose perivascular aggregates into the reticular dermis. In a few cases, atypical-appearing nuclei may be present and may suggest the possibility of lymphoma.

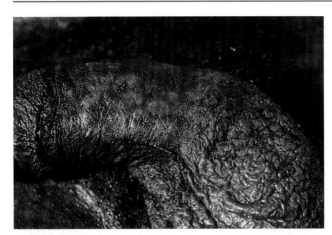

Clin. Fig. VA4.a

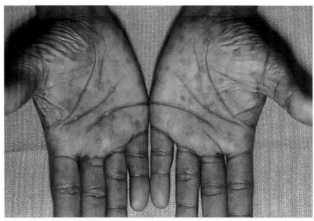

Clin. Fig. VA4.b

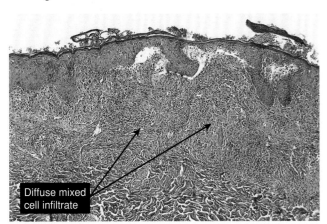

Fig. VA4.a

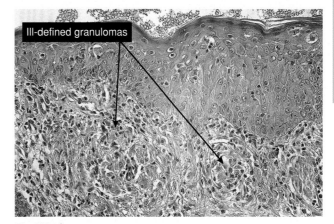

Fig. VA4.b

Clin. Fig. VA4.a. *Secondary syphilis.* This HIV-positive male presented with annular papules on his penis.

Clin. Fig. VA4.b. *Secondary syphilis.* Brown-red macules were present on his palms. RPR was positive.

Fig. VA4.a. *Secondary syphilis, low power.* There is irregular hyperplasia of the epidermis, with hyperkeratosis. In the dermis, there is a perivascular to diffuse infiltrate of mixed cell types.

Fig. VA4.b. *Secondary syphilis, medium power.* Epidermal changes include spongiosis and basilar vacuolar alteration, exocytosis of lymphocytes, and parakeratosis. A perivascular to mixed infiltrate is present in the dermis. (*continues*)

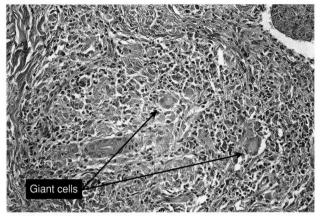

Fig. VA4.c

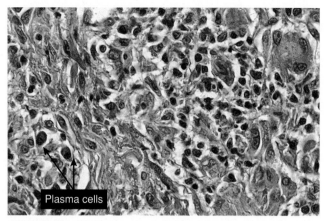

Fig. VA4.d

Fig. VA4.c. *Secondary syphilis, high power.* The cells in the dermis include lymphocytes and prominent plasma cells, as a well as a few histiocytes and giant cells in this example, forming ill-defined noncaseating granulomas.

Fig. VA4.d. *Secondary syphilis, high power.* A mixed infiltrate of lymphocytes, histiocytes, plasma cells, often also including neutrophils and eosinophils is present.

Neutrophils are not infrequent and may permeate the eccrine coil to produce a neutrophilic eccrine hidradenitis. Granulomatous inflammation develops after a few months. In a systematic study, features that should raise the possibility of secondary syphilis included endothelial swelling, interstitial inflammation, irregular acanthosis, elongated rete ridges, the presence of vacuolar interface dermatitis with a lymphocyte in nearly every vacuole, lymphocytes with visible cytoplasm, and plasma cells (11).

A silver stain is positive for spirochetes in about a third of the cases. Silver stains can be difficult to interpret because of high background. Additionally, positive results do not necessarily indicate the presence of *T. pallidum* as a silver stain is not specific for this organism. Immunohistochemistry using antibodies directed against Treponema Pallidum Antigen have been shown to be more sensitive than silver stains and reflect a new standard for adjunct histologic testing. Polymerase chain reaction (PCR) analysis is another technique which is valuable for the detection of *T. pallidum* (12–14). The organisms are seen in the epidermis, follicular epithelium, and blood vessels. Lesions of condylomata lata show all of the aforementioned changes, but with more florid epithelial hyperplasia and intraepithelial microabscess formation.

Tertiary Syphilis

See Clin. Fig. VA4.c.

Morphea (See Description in VF)

See Figs. VA4.e–g.

Conditions to consider in the differential diagnosis:

 erythema chronicum migrans
 acne rosacea
 perioral dermatitis
 scleroderma/morphea
 secondary syphilis
 Kaposi sarcoma, early lesions

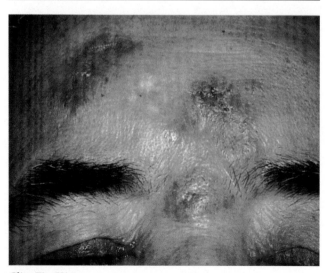

Clin. Fig. VA4.c

Clin. Fig. VA4.c. *Tertiary syphilis.* A bartender with positive syphilis serology presented with gummatous lesions characterized by subcutaneous swellings and ulceration.

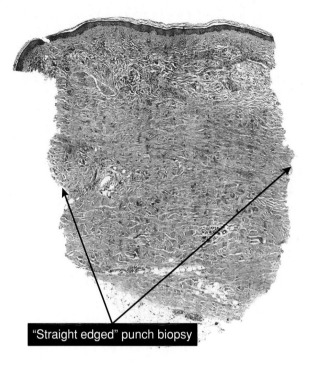

Fig. VA4.e

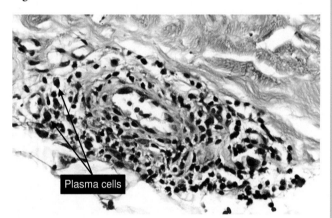

Diminished peri-eccrine fat

Fig. VA4.f

"Straight edged" punch biopsy

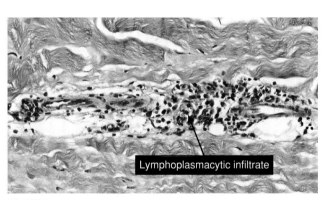

Lymphoplasmacytic infiltrate

Fig. VA4.g

Plasma cells

Fig. VA4.h

V   Perivascular, Diffuse, and Granulomatous Infiltrates of the Reticular Dermis

Fig. VA4.e. *Morphea, low power.* Scanning magnification reveals a perieccrine infiltrate associated with sclerosis of the lower portion of the reticular dermis. The eccrine glands appear "trapped" within the sclerotic collagen. In the inflammatory stage of morphea, sclerosis, although usually detectable as here, may not be as prominent as it is in later stages of the disease.

Fig. VA4.f. *Morphea, medium power.* The collagen bundles are thickened and there is loss of perieccrine adipose tissue.

Fig. VA4.g,h. *Morphea, high power.* The infiltrate usually includes plasma cells as well as lymphocytes, and is frequently present at the dermal–subcutaneous junction.

VA5 Perivascular Infiltrates, Mixed Cell Types

In addition to lymphocytes, plasma cells and eosinophils are found in the dermal infiltrate. ECM is a prototypic example (15).

Erythema Chronicum Migrans

CLINICAL SUMMARY. ECM is the distinctive cutaneous manifestation of stage I Lyme disease and represents the site of primary tick inoculation. The lesion starts as an area of scaly erythema or a distinct red papule within 3 to 30 days after the tick bite, before spreading centrifugally with central clearing after a few weeks, occasionally reaching a diameter of 25 cm. Average lesional duration is a few weeks but in some cases, lesions may persist for as long as 12 months. The lesions may be solitary or multiple, the latter reflecting hematogenous dissemination of the spirochete, which may be accompanied by fever, fatigue, headaches, cough, and arthralgias (16).

HISTOPATHOLOGY. An intense superficial and deep angiocentric, neurotropic, and eccrinotropic infiltrate predominated by lymphocytes with a variable admixture of plasma cells and eosinophils is the principal histopathology. Plasma cells have been identified most frequently in the peripheries of lesions of ECM, whereas eosinophils are identified in the centers of the lesions. Not infrequently, these florid dermal alterations are accompanied by eczematous epithelial alterations, and interstitial infiltration of the reticular dermis with a concomitant incipient sclerosing reaction. A Warthin–Starry stain may be positive, especially if taken from the advancing border of the lesion. The changes may be subtle; based on the variable histopathologic finding, it is important to consider ECM in the differential diagnosis of a skin biopsy specimen from any expanding annular erythematous lesion (16).

Conditions to consider in the differential diagnosis:

secondary syphilis
erythema chronicum migrans
arthropod assault reaction
erythema annulare centrifigum

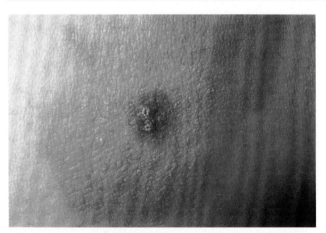

Clin. Fig. VA5

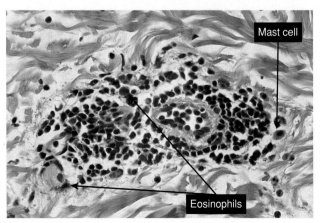

Fig. VA5.b

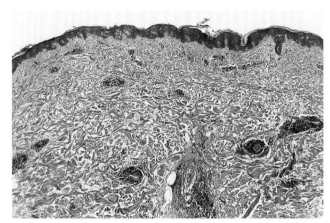

Fig. VA5.a

Clin. Fig. VA5. *Erythema chronicum migrans.* A 17-year-old female presented with an expanding annular erythematous patch and a central violaceous papule on the posterior calf. Her Lyme titer was positive and she responded to antibiotic treatment.

Fig. VA5.a. *Erythema chronicum migrans, low power.* There is a tight cuff of small round cells about the vessels of the superficial and middermal plexuses.

Fig. VA5.b. *Erythema chronicum migrans, high power.* Lymphocytes, eosinophils, and mast cells (and often plasma cells) are present in the perivascular infiltrate.

VB VASCULITIS AND VASCULOPATHIES

True vasculitis is defined by eosinophilic degeneration of the vessel wall ("fibrinoid necrosis"), infiltration of the vessel wall by neutrophils, with neutrophils, nuclear dust, and extravasated red cells in the vessel walls and adjacent dermis. Some of the conditions mentioned here lack these prototypic findings, and may be termed "vasculopathies" (e.g., Degos disease).

1. Vascular Damage, Scant Inflammatory Cells
2. Vasculitis, Lymphocytes Predominant
3. Vasculitis, Neutrophils Prominent
4. Vasculitis, Mixed Cell Types and/or Granulomas
5. Thrombotic and Other Microangiopathies

VB1 Vascular Damage, Scant Inflammatory Cells

Although there is significant vascular damage, there is little early inflammatory response. Degos syndrome is an example (17).

Degos Syndrome

CLINICAL SUMMARY. The clinical manifestations include crops of asymptomatic, slightly raised, yellowish red papules that gradually develop an atrophic porcelain-white center. These papules tend to affect the trunk and proximal extremities. Degos initially described a cutaneointestinal syndrome, in which distinct skin findings ("drops of porcelain") were associated with recurrent attacks of abdominal pain that often ended in death from intestinal perforations. He chose the name *malignant atrophic papulosis* (MAP) to emphasize the serious clinical course of the disease. It is nowadays believed that MAP is a clinicopathologic reaction pattern that can be associated with a number of conditions that are not always lethal. Lesions similar if not identical to MAP have been noted, in particular, in connective tissue diseases such as LE, dermatomyositis, and progressive systemic sclerosis, in atrophie blanche, and in Creutzfeldt–Jakob disease. Some lesions remain confined to the skin ("benign atrophic papulosis"). On dermoscopy, a telangiectatic rim can be seen at the periphery of lesions, which can help differentiate this entity from other skin disorders (18).

HISTOPATHOLOGY. Although the pathogenesis of Degos syndrome is poorly understood, a thrombotic vasculopathy is a characteristic associated finding. A typical lesion shows a wedge-shaped area of altered dermis covered by atrophic epidermis with slight hyperkeratosis. Dermal alterations may include frank necrosis, but more common are edema, extensive mucin deposition, and slight sclerosis. There may be a sparse perivascular lymphocytic infiltrate but the vessel walls are not inflamed. Typically, vascular damage is noted in the vessels at the base of the "cone of necrobiosis." This damage may be limited to endothelial swelling, but more characteristically, intravascular fibrin thrombi may be noted,

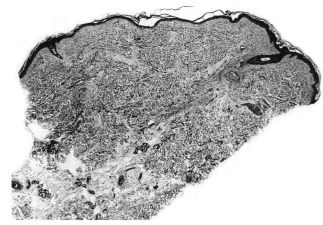

Fig. VB1.a

Fig. VB1.a. *Degos lesion, low power.* Atrophic epidermis overlies a wedge-shaped area of altered dermis. (R. Barnhill and K. Busam.)

Fig. VB1.b. *Degos lesion, medium power.* Within the wedge, there is interstitial degeneration of collagen, and interstitial mucin deposition. (R. Barnhill and K. Busam.) (*continues*)

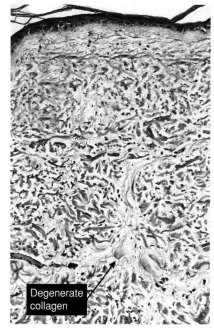

Degenerate collagen

Fig. VB1.b

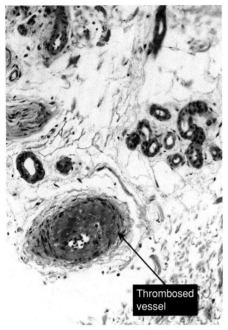

Fig. VB1.c

Fig. VB1.c. *Degos lesion, high power.* At the base of the lesion, there is a thrombosed vessel with a thickened wall. This lesion occurred in a patient with dermatomyositis. (R. Barnhill and K. Busam.)

suggesting that the dermal and epidermal changes result from ischemia.

Conditions to consider in the differential diagnosis:

Degos syndrome (malignant atrophic papulosis)
atrophie blanche

VB2 Vasculitis, Lymphocytes Predominant

The term "lymphocytic vasculitis" is controversial, but there are some conditions in which perivascular and intramural lymphocytes may be associated with some degree of vessel wall damage, not usually including frank fibrinoid necrosis. Most of these conditions are discussed elsewhere as "perivascular lymphocytic infiltrates." In angiocentric lymphomas, the cells infiltrating the vessel walls are neoplastic, but the process may be mistaken for an inflammatory reaction. *Pernio* (perniosis) is a prototypic inflammatory example (19).

Pernio

CLINICAL SUMMARY. Pernio or chilblains usually consists of tender or painful, raised, violaceous plaques on the fingers or toes. Occasionally it is found at a more proximal portion of an extremity in a deeper location in the skin or subcutis. Pernio is caused in susceptible individuals by prolonged exposure to cold above the freezing point, especially in damp climates. It is important to distinguish idiopathic chilblains from chilblains in LE or those associated with other autoimmune disease. However, there is considerable overlap in the histopathology.

HISTOPATHOLOGY. In pernio, intense edema of the papillary dermis is observed. A marked perivascular mononuclear cell infiltrate is seen in the upper dermis but sparing the edematous papillary dermis. The blood vessels are said to show a diffuse "fluffy" edema of their walls. The mononuclear infiltrate of the vascular walls is consistent with a lymphocytic vasculitis. The perivascular infiltrate can extend throughout the dermis into the subcutaneous fat. When comparing histology between idiopathic pernio and chilblains associated with autoimmune disease, it has been suggested that perieccrine distribution of lymphocytes is seen more with idiopathic pernio (20).

Pityriasis Lichenoides

Pityriasis lichenoides is an uncommon cutaneous eruption usually classified in two forms that differ in severity. Simultaneous appearance of the two types and transitions between them often occur, suggesting that they are variants of the same disease. Both present as usually nonpruritic and painful self-healing lesions occurring in crops and affecting mainly young adults and occasionally children.

The milder form, pityriasis lichenoides chronica, is characterized by recurrent crops of brown-red papules, 4 to 10 mm in size, mainly on the trunk and extremities, that are covered with a scale and generally involute within 3 to 6 weeks with postinflammatory pigmentary changes. The more severe form, pityriasis lichenoides et varioliformis acuta (PLEVA), also referred to as Mucha–Habermann disease, consists of a fairly extensive eruption, present mainly on the trunk and proximal extremities, and characterized by erythematous papules that develop into papulonecrotic, occasionally hemorrhagic or vesiculopustular lesions that resolve within a few weeks, usually with little or no scarring. Although the individual lesions follow an acute course, the disorder is chronic, extending over several months or even years with development of new lesions and variable periods of remission (21).

HISTOPATHOLOGY. In pityriasis lichenoides chronica, there is a superficial perivascular and lichenoid infiltrate composed of lymphocytes that extend into the epidermis, where there is vacuolar alteration of the basal layer, mild spongiosis, a few necrotic keratinocytes, and confluent parakeratosis. Melanophages and small numbers of extravasated erythrocytes are commonly seen in the

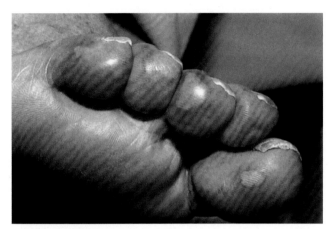

Clin. Fig. VB2.a

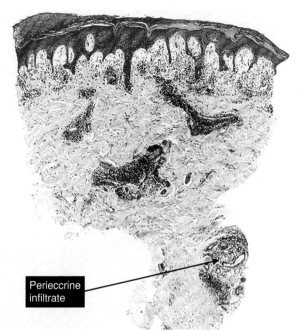

Fig. VB2.a

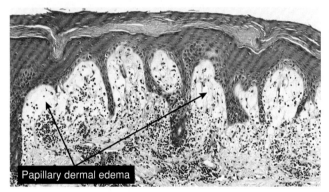

Fig. VB2.b

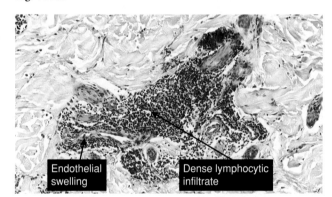

Fig. VB2.c

Clin. Fig. VB2.a. *Pernio.* A 62-year-old male presented tender, edematous, erythematous macules and plaques with a hint of bullous change after spending a considerable time out in the cold. Lesions improved with avoidance and protection from the cold.

Fig. VB2.a. *Pernio, low power.* There is edema of the papillary dermis, with a superficial and deep perivascular and interstitial infiltrate.

Fig. VB2.b. *Pernio, medium power.* The infiltrate tends to be localized about and within the walls of vessels of the superficial plexus. Papillary dermal edema may be mild or pronounced, as seen here.

Fig. VB2.c. *Pernio, high power.* The vessel walls are edematous and are infiltrated by lymphocytes.

papillary dermis. In PLEVA, there is a perivascular and dense band-like predominantly lymphocytic infiltrate in the papillary dermis that extends into the reticular dermis in a wedge-shaped pattern. The infiltrate obscures the dermal–epidermal junction with pronounced vacuolar alteration of the basal layer, marked exocytosis of lymphocytes and erythrocytes, and intercellular and intracellular edema leading to variable degree of epidermal necrosis. Ultimately, erosion or ulceration may occur. The overlying cornified layer shows parakeratosis and a scaly crust with neutrophils in the more severe cases. Variable degrees of papillary dermal edema, endothelial swelling,

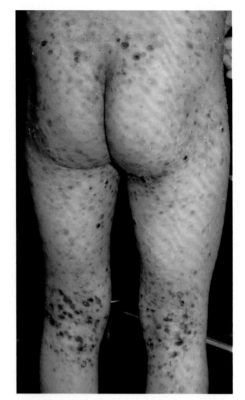

Clin. Fig. VB2.b

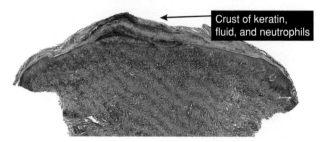

Crust of keratin, fluid, and neutrophils

Fig. VB2.e

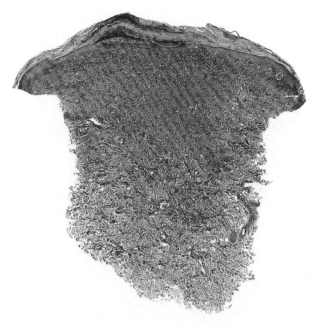

Fig. VB2.d

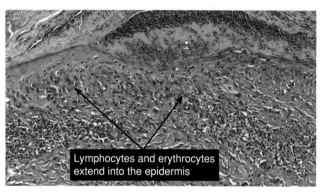

Lymphocytes and erythrocytes extend into the epidermis

Fig. VB2.f

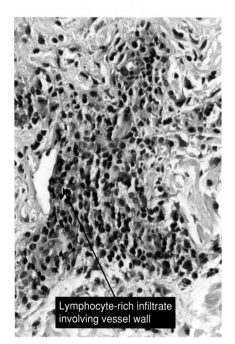

Lymphocyte-rich infiltrate involving vessel wall

Fig. VB2.g

Clin. Fig. VB2.b. *Pityriasis lichenoides et varioliformis acuta (PLEVA).* An extensive eruption, mainly on the trunk and proximal extremities, with erythematous papules that develop into papulonecrotic, occasionally hemorrhagic or vesiculopustular lesions.

Fig. VB2.d. *Pityriasis lichenoides et varioliformis acuta (PLEVA), low power.* There is a dense perivascular, predominantly lymphocytic infiltrate in the papillary dermis and extending into the reticular dermis in a wedge-shaped pattern.

Fig. VB2.e. *PLEVA, medium power.* The infiltrate obscures the dermal–epidermal junction and there is a surface crust with neutrophils.

Fig. VB2.f. *PLEVA, high power.* There is parakeratosis, with vacuolar alteration of the basal layer, exocytosis of lymphocytes and erythrocytes into the epidermis.

Fig. VB2.g. *PLEVA, high power.* Vessel walls are obscured by a dense lymphocytic infiltrate, often with endothelial swelling, and extravasated erythrocytes are seen in the majority of cases. However, there is no true vessel wall necrosis.

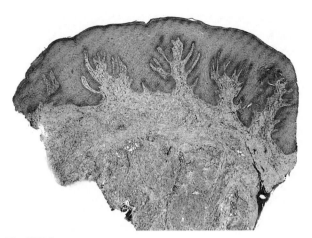

Fig. VB2.h

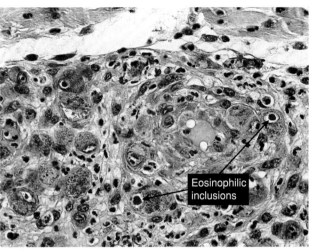

Fig. VB2.i

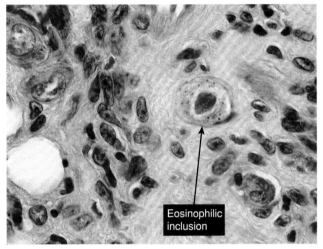

Fig. VB2.j

Fig. VB2.h. *Cytomegalovirus infection of endothelial cells, low power.* A biopsy of an oral lesion in a patient with AIDS shows a perivascular and diffuse infiltrate composed mainly of lymphocytes with a few plasma cells.

Fig. VB2.i. *Cytomegalovirus, medium power.* Endothelial cells are markedly swollen, and some contain inclusions (intranuclear and/or cytoplasmic).

Fig. VB2.j. *Cytomegalovirus, high power.* A fibroblast contains a characteristic large eosinophilic intranuclear inclusion body.

and extravasated erythrocytes are seen. Severe vascular damage is rarely found except in a severe febrile ulceronecrotic variant of PLEVA where lymphocytic vasculitis with leukocytoclasis may be seen.

Cytomegalovirus Infection

The relationship between infection and vasculitis is a debatable topic. A causative role has been documented only for few pathogens, while others may be better considered as trigger factors for vasculitis (22).

Erythema Chronicum Migrans

See also Section VA5.
See Figs. VB2.k,l.

Conditions to consider in the differential diagnosis:

"lymphocytic vasculitis"
    lupus erythematosus
    lymphomatoid papulosis
    pityriasis lichenoides et varioliformis acuta (PLEVA)
    pityriasis lichenoides chronica
    purpura pigmentosa chronica
    morbilliform viral infections
    Lyme disease
    perniosis (chilblains)
angiocentric mycosis fungoides
angiocentric T-cell lymphoma/lymphomatoid granulomatosis
cytomegalovirus inclusion disease
Behçet syndrome

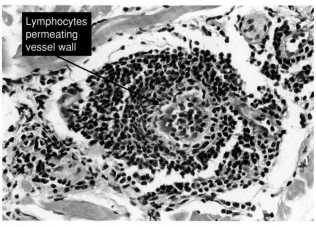

Lymphocytes permeating vessel wall

Fig. VB2.l

Fig. VB2.k

Fig. VB2.k. *Erythema chronicum migrans, low power.* A tight perivascular cuff of lymphocytes about the superficial and mid dermal vessels.

Fig. VB2.l. *Erythema chronicum migrans, high power.* In this example, the lymphocytes diffusely infiltrate the vessel wall. However, there is no vessel wall necrosis (see VB3).

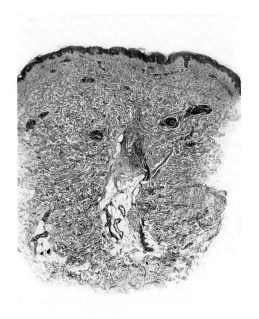

VB3 | Vasculitis, Neutrophils Prominent

Neutrophils are prominent in the infiltrate, with fibrinoid necrosis and nuclear dust; eosinophils and lymphocytes are also found. Polyarteritis nodosa (PAN) is prototypic (23).

Polyarteritis Nodosa and Microscopic Polyangiitis

CLINICAL SUMMARY. *Classic PAN* is a systemic vasculitic disorder in which large arteries are involved and in which ischemic glomerular lesions are common but glomerulonephritis is rare. *Microscopic PAN*, also termed *microscopic polyangiitis* (MPA), refers to a systemic small-vessel vasculitis primarily affecting arterioles and capillaries that is typically associated with focal necrotizing glomerulonephritis with crescents. The majority of patients with MPA are anti-MPO (p-ANCA, i.e., perinuclear anti-neutrophil cytoplasmic antibody) positive. Some cases of vasculitis present with an *overlapping syndrome* affecting both small and medium-sized arteries.

The majority of patients with MPA are male and over 50 years of age. Prodromal symptoms include fever, myalgias, arthralgias, and sore throat. The most common clinical feature is renal disease manifesting as microhematuria, proteinuria, or acute oliguric renal failure. Although in classic PAN cutaneous involvement is rare, 30% to 40% of patients with MPA exhibit skin changes. With cutaneous PAN, the initial signs include livido reticularis, tender subcutaneous nodules, and ulcerations. Purpura, petechiae, and necrosis can be seen. The legs are most

commonly affected (24). With MPA, the most common clinical sign is palpable purpura on the legs. MPA can also present with ulcers, cutaneous necrosis, splinter hemorrhages, and vesicles (25).

HISTOPATHOLOGY. The characteristic lesion of classic PAN is a panarteritis involving medium-sized and small arteries. Even though in classic PAN the arteries show the characteristic changes in many visceral sites, affected skin often shows only small-vessel disease, and arterial involvement is typically focal. The changes affecting cutaneous small vessels are usually those of a necrotizing leukocytoclastic vasculitis (LCV). If there is a clinical presentation of cutaneous nodules, panarteritis similar to visceral lesions is usually detected. In classic PAN, the lesions typically are in different stages of development (i.e., fresh and old). Early lesions show degeneration of the arterial wall with deposition of fibrinoid material, and partial to complete destruction of the external and internal elastic laminae. An infiltrate present within and around the arterial wall is composed largely of neutrophils showing evidence of leukocytoclasia, although it often contains eosinophils. At a later stage, intimal proliferation and thrombosis lead to complete occlusion of the lumen with subsequent ischemia and possibly ulceration. The infiltrate also may contain lymphocytes, histiocytes, and some plasma cells. In the healing stage, there is fibroblastic proliferation extending into the perivascular area. The small vessels of the middle and upper dermis often exhibit a nonspecific lymphocytic perivascular infiltrate.

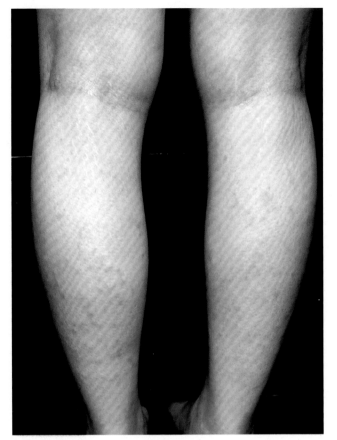

Clin. Fig. VB3.a

Fig. VB3.a

Artery with damage and surrounding inflammation

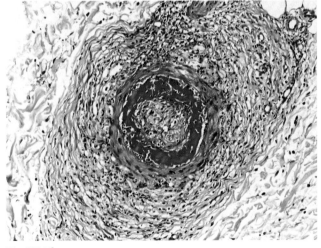

Fig. VB3.b

Clin. Fig. VB3.a. *Polyarteritis nodosa.* A 27-year-old woman with an 8-month history of tender nodules in the lower legs with livedo reticularis pattern, arthralgia of knee, and ankle joints and positive c-ANCA.

Fig. VB3.a. *Polyarteritis nodosa, low power.* A biopsy from the patient of Clin. Fig. VB3.a contains a thick-walled vessel in the deep dermis and subcutis with a surrounding inflammatory infiltrate.

Fig. VB3.b. *Polyarteritis nodosa, high power.* There are areas of eosinophilic change ("fibrinoid necrosis"), with neutrophilic infiltration, in the wall of a large vessel (small muscular artery).

Neutrophilic Small-Vessel Vasculitis (Leukocytoclastic Vasculitis)

CLINICAL SUMMARY. Many different disease processes can be accompanied by small-vessel vasculitis with predominantly neutrophilic infiltrates. The clinical and histologic manifestations are thus fairly nonspecific. The majority of cases are idiopathic but associated diseases to be considered range from conditions limited to the skin such as most cases of drug-induced vasculitis to systemic conditions such as infections including hepatitis C, malignancies, Henoch–Schönlein purpura, connective tissue diseases, or ANCA-associated disorders (26), which include MPA, granulomatosis with polyangiitis (GPA, formerly known as Wegener granulomatosis), and eosinophilic granulomatosis with polyangiitis (EGPA, formerly Churg–Strauss disease) (27).

Standardized names, definitions, and descriptions were promulgated in 2018 for cutaneous components of systemic vasculitides (e.g., cutaneous IgA vasculitis as a component of systemic IgA vasculitis), skin-limited variants of systemic vasculitides (e.g., skin-limited IgA vasculitis, drug-induced skin-limited ANCA-associated vasculitis), and cutaneous single organ vasculitides that have no systemic counterparts (e.g., nodular vasculitis).

HISTOPATHOLOGY. Neutrophilic small-vessel vasculitis is a reaction pattern of small dermal vessels, almost exclusively postcapillary venules, characterized by a combination of vascular damage and an infiltrate composed largely of neutrophils. Because there is often fragmentation of nuclei (karyorrhexis or leukocytoclasis), the term *LCV* is frequently used. Depending on its severity, this process may be subtle and limited to the superficial dermis or be pandermal and florid and associated with necrosis and ulceration. If edema is prominent, a subepidermal blister may form. If the neutrophilic infiltrate is dense and there is pustule formation, the term pustular vasculitis may be applied. In a typical case of LCV, the dermal vessels show swelling of the endothelial cells and deposits of strongly eosinophilic strands of fibrin within and around

their walls. The deposits of fibrin and the marked edema together give the vessel walls a "smudgy" appearance referred to as fibrinoid degeneration. The cellular infiltrate is present predominantly around the dermal blood vessels or within the vascular walls, so that the outline of the blood vessels may appear indistinct. The infiltrate consists mainly of neutrophils and of varying numbers of eosinophils and mononuclear cells. The infiltrate also is scattered throughout the upper dermis in association with fibrin deposits between and within collagen bundles. Extravasation of erythrocytes is commonly present. The appearance of the reaction pattern depends on the stage at which the biopsy is taken. In older lesions, the number of neutrophils may be decreased and the number of mononuclear cells increased so that mononuclear cells may predominate and a designation of a lymphocytic or even granulomatous vasculitis or vascular reaction might be made.

In the ANCA-associated vasculitides, the presence of ANCA is a defining feature. MPA in the skin represents vasculitis of small vessels with few or no immune deposits. There is an association with ANCAs, but no granulomatous inflammation in any organ. There is often involvement of subcutaneous vessels, including arteries. GPA involves cutaneous vasculitis indistinguishable from that in MPA, but in addition there are interstitial dermal granulomas, with palisaded epithelioid macrophages and giant

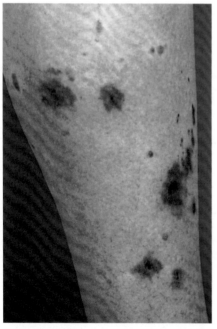

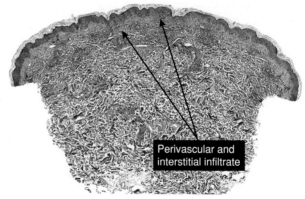

Clin. Fig. VB3.b   Fig. VB3.c

Clin. Fig. VB3.b. *Leukocytoclastic vasculitis.* Hemorrhagic purpuric papules and plaques on the lower leg in a middle-aged female were felt to be secondary to a nonsteroidal anti-inflammatory drug (NSAID).

Fig. VB3.c. *Leukocytoclastic vasculitis (LCV), low power.* Although LCV is often confined to the superficial plexus, deeper small vessels including frequently those in the middermis, are often involved, as in this example.

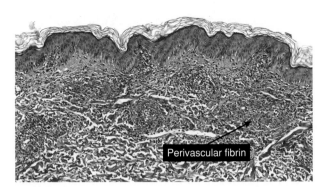

Fig. VB3.d

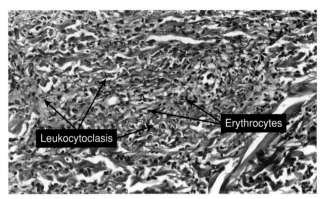

Fig. VB3.e

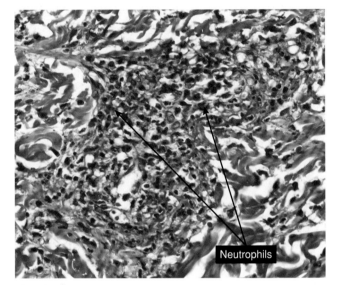

Fig. VB3.f

Fig. VB3.d. *Leukocytoclastic vasculitis, medium power.* The neutrophil-rich infiltrate is angiocentric with a less-intense interstitial component.

Fig. VB3.e,f. *Leukocytoclastic vasculitis, high power.* There is fibrinoid necrosis of vessel walls, with neutrophilic infiltration and leukocytoclasia around the involved vessels.

cells. Some lesions may present as interstitial granulomatous dermatitis (IGD). Eosinophils and eosinophilia are not prominent. EGPA has cutaneous vasculitis and granulomatous inflammation, as in GPA, but also has prominent eosinophils and there is a history of asthma (29).

Erythema Elevatum Diutinum

CLINICAL SUMMARY. This rare condition is characterized by persistent, initially red to violaceous and later brown to yellow papules, nodules, and plaques. The lesions are typically distributed symmetrically on the extensor surfaces of the extremities. They are initially soft and then evolve into fibrous nodules. Erythema elevatum diutinum (EED) may be a reaction pattern rather than a distinct disease.

HISTOPATHOLOGY. In the early stages there is nonspecific LCV. In later stages, granulation tissue and fibrosis develop with a diffuse mixed cell infiltrate with a predominance of neutrophils. Granulomas are occasionally present. The capillaries may have deposits of fibrinoid material or

fibrous thickening. Fully developed lesions may be indistinguishable from neutrophilic dermatoses, Behçet disease, or a neutrophilic drug reaction. In old, fibrotic lesions there are spindle cells and collagen bundles often parallel to the skin surface, or concentrically arranged around vessels, with vertically arranged capillaries similar to a scar.

Conditions to consider in the differential diagnosis:

Small-vessel leukocytoclastic vasculitis
neutrophilic dermatoses
    Sweet syndrome
    granuloma faciale
    bowel-associated dermatosis–arthrosis syndrome
septic/embolic lesions of gonococcemia/meningococcemia
Rocky Mountain spotted fever (Rickettsia rickettsii)
polyarteritis nodosa
erythema elevatum diutinum
Behçet syndrome
papulonecrotic tuberculid

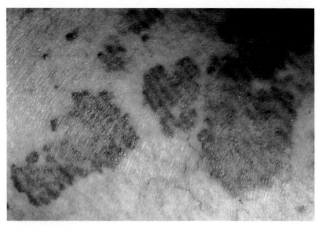

Clin. Fig. VB3.c

Clin. Fig. VB3.c. *Erythema elevatum diutinum.* Brownish-yellow annular plaques with an infiltrated border developed on the extensor surface of the lower extremity. No monoclonal or polyclonal gammopathy was detected. (S. Binnick.)

<hr />

VB4 | Vasculitis, Mixed Cell Types and/or Granulomas

Histiocytes and giant cells are a part of the infiltrate. Lymphocytes and eosinophils can also be found depending on the diagnosis. Giant cell arteritis is a true inflammation of the artery wall (true arteritis), although there is no fibrinoid necrosis. Most cases of giant cell arteritis involve vessels of the subcutis. EGPA is prototypic of a granulomatous arteritis (29).

Eosinophilic Granulomatosis With Polyangiitis

CLINICAL SUMMARY. EGPA (previously termed Churg–Strauss syndrome) is a systemic disease occurring in asthmatic patients characterized by vasculitis, eosinophilic infiltration of multiple organs, and peripheral eosinophilia. There is considerable overlap of this disease process with other systemic vasculitides, and with other inflammatory disorders exhibiting eosinophils, such as eosinophilic pneumonitis. The internal organs most commonly involved are the lungs, the gastrointestinal tract, and, less commonly, the peripheral nerves and the heart. In contrast to PAN, renal failure is rare. A slightly broader definition of EGPA has been proposed requiring asthma, blood hypereosinophilia, and systemic vasculitis involving two or more extrapulmonary organs.

Two types of cutaneous lesions may occur: (1) hemorrhagic lesions similar to Henoch–Schönlein purpura varying from petechiae to extensive ecchymoses, often with areas of erythema and sometimes with necrotic ulcers, and (2) cutaneous–subcutaneous nodules. The extremities are the most common sites of skin lesions, but the trunk may also be involved and some cases are generalized. ANCA

tests obtained during an active phase of the disease contain p-ANCA in the majority of cases. There is also a limited form, in which the lesions are confined to the conjunctiva, the skin, and subcutaneous tissue.

HISTOPATHOLOGY. The areas of cutaneous hemorrhage typically have changes of LCV. Eosinophils may be conspicuous. In some instances, the dermis shows a granulomatous reaction composed predominantly of radially arranged histiocytes and, frequently, multinucleated giant cells centered around degenerated collagen fibers. The central portions of the granulomas contain not only degenerated collagen fibers but also dense aggregates of disintegrated cells, particularly eosinophils. These granulomas have been referred to as Churg–Strauss granulomas. However, they are not always present and similar findings can also be observed in other disease processes, such as connective tissue diseases (rheumatoid arthritis [RA] and LE), Wegener granulomatosis, PAN, lymphoproliferative disorders, subacute bacterial endocarditis, chronic active hepatitis, and inflammatory bowel disease. The granulomas in the subcutaneous tissue may attain considerable size through expansion and confluence, thus giving rise to the clinically apparent cutaneous–subcutaneous nodules. They are embedded in a diffuse inflammatory exudate rich in eosinophils. Similar changes have also been observed in other diseases, such as PAN.

Papulonecrotic Tuberculid

Papulonecrotic tuberculid (PNT) is said to be a hypersensitivity reaction to *Mycobacterium tuberculosis* (MTB). However, some reports indicate that organisms are demonstrable by PCR, and it is possible that some cases at least may represent cutaneous tuberculosis (28).

On microscopy, necrosis and epithelioid granulomas are common, with an infiltrate of mostly lymphocytes, and occasionally eosinophils. Some cases have been associated with vasculitis, which might be more consistent with an "id" reaction (i.e., a dermatitis developing later at skin locations distant from an initial inflammatory or infectious site) (29). Lesions usually improve on treatment for MTB.

Conditions to consider in the differential diagnosis:

eosinophilic granulomatosis with polyangiitis (EGPA)
granulomatosis with polyangiitis (GPA)
giant cell arteritis (temporal arteritis)
erythema chronicum migrans
erythema nodosum leprosum
some insect bite reactions
"secondary vasculitis" at the base of ulcers of diverse etiology
Behçet syndrome
palisaded and neutrophilic granulomatosis
interstitial granulomatous dermatitis

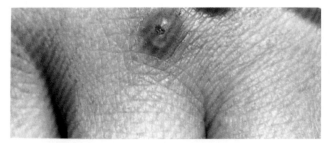

Clin. Fig. VB.4

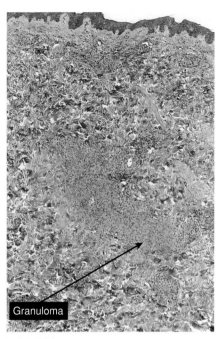

Fig. VB4.a

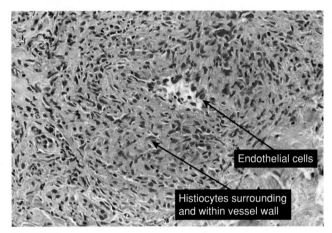

Fig. VB4.b

Clin. Fig. VB.4. *Granulomatous vasculitis.* This inflammatory nodule histologically showed evidence of a granulomatous vasculitis.

Fig. VB4.a. *Granulomatous vasculitis, low power.* There is a perivascular granulomatous infiltrate of histiocytes and lymphocytes in the reticular dermis. (R. Barnhill and K. Busam.)

Fig. VB4.b. *Granulomatous vasculitis, medium power.* The wall of a middermal vessel is damaged. The differential diagnosis for this lesion could include several of the conditions listed below in the differential diagnosis of this condition. Most cases of EGPA would likely have a more prominent component of eosinophils in the inflammatory infiltrate. (R. Barnhill and K. Busam.)

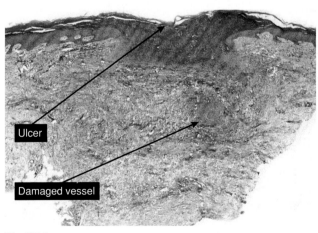

Fig. VB4.c

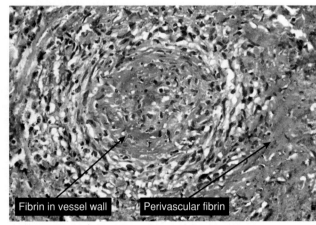

Fig. VB4.d

Fig. VB4.c. *Papulonecrotic tuberculid, low power.* Wedge-shaped infarction of the dermis and epidermis, caused by vasculitis. (S. Lucas.)

Fig. VB4.d. *Papulonecrotic tuberculid, high power.* Necrotizing vasculitis of a dermal artery, with surrounding granulomatous inflammation. (S. Lucas.)

VB5 Thrombotic and Other Microangiopathies

The dermal vessels contain fibrin, red cells and platelet thrombi, and/or eosinophilic protein precipitates. Coagulopathies of diverse etiologies may have similar histologic features (see Section IIIG). Calciphylaxis is a microangiopathy that appears to be caused by calcification of the media of small arteries, followed by fibroplasia affecting the intima and occluding the lumen (30).

Calciphylaxis

See also discussion in VIIIC8.

CLINICAL SUMMARY. Calciphylaxis is a life-threatening condition in which there is progressive calcification of small and medium-sized vessels of the subcutis with thickening of the intima by fibrosis and subsequent vascular compromise resulting in ischemia and necrosis. It most frequently arises in the setting of hyperparathyroidism associated with chronic renal failure, and is often, but not always, associated with an elevated serum calcium/phosphate product. Hypercoagulability is also an important association (31). Clinically, the lesions present as a panniculitis or vasculitis. Bullae, ulcerations, or a livedo reticularis–like eruption can be present. Lesions usually occur over areas with high fat content such as the abdomen, thighs, calves, and buttocks. The digits, breasts, tongue, and penis can also be affected. Early lesions appear as subcutaneous nodules or violaceous plaques. Later lesions with black central necrosis are seen. A biopsy from the center of an eschar will usually show characteristic changes (32).

HISTOPATHOLOGY. The histologic changes in calciphylaxis include calcium deposits in the subcutis, chiefly within the walls of small and medium-sized arteries. These deposits can be associated with endovascular fibrosis, thrombosis, or global calcific obliteration. Calcification can also be identified within the soft tissues. Changes similar to LCV are also commonly present. The vascular lesions result in ischemic and/or gangrenous necrosis of the subcutaneous fat and overlying skin.

Livedo Reticularis

Conditions to consider in the differential diagnosis:

septicemia
disseminated intravascular coagulation
thrombotic thrombocytopenic purpura
purpura fulminans
warfarin necrosis
lupus anticoagulant
amyloidosis
porphyria cutanea tarda and other porphyrias

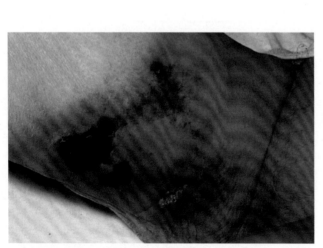

Clin. Fig. VB5.a

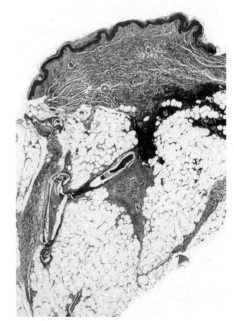

Fig. VB5.a

Clin. Fig. VB5.a. *Calciphylaxis.* This elderly female with end-stage renal disease and elevated parathyroid hormone level developed widespread induration of the lower extremities which led to purpuric and necrotic ulcerations.

Fig. VB5.a. *Calciphylaxis, low power.* Associated with fat necrosis and hemorrhage, there is a vessel in the subcutis with a calcified and thickened wall.

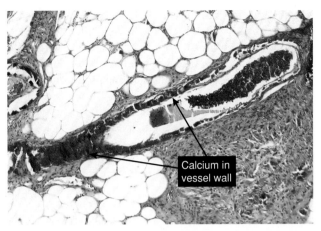

Fig. VB5.b

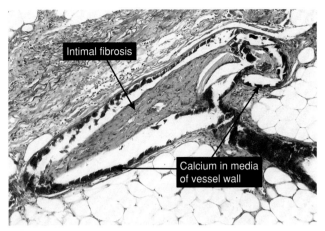

Fig. VB5.c

Fig. VB5.b. *Calciphylaxis, medium power.* There is necrosis of fat adjacent to the abnormal vessel. Necrosis is often much more extensive than in this example, and often involves the dermis.

Fig. VB5.c. *Calciphylaxis, high power.* The calcification affects the media of this small artery. In the same vessel, the intima is thickened by delicate fibroplasia, greatly compromising the lumen. The intimal fibrosis has retracted from the stiffened calcified wall due to fixation artifact.

calciphylaxis

thrombophlebitis and superficial migratory thrombophlebitis

Lucio reaction

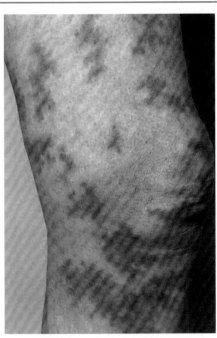

Clin. Fig. VB5.b

Clin. Fig. VB5.b. *Livedo reticularis.* Persistent red-blue mottling of the skin in a net-like pattern is a nonspecific sign of sluggish blood flow that may occur in association with a vasculitis or a vasculopathy in several different contexts, such as infection, atrophie blanche, cholesterol emboli, and connective tissue disease. A biopsy from a white area may show a thick-walled vessel with the lumen occluded by a thrombus.

 VC ## DIFFUSE INFILTRATES OF THE RETICULAR DERMIS

Diffuse infiltrates of the reticular dermis may show some relation to vessels or to skin appendages, or may be randomly distributed in the reticular dermis.

1. Diffuse Infiltrates, Lymphocytes Predominant
2. Diffuse Infiltrates, Neutrophils Predominant
3. Diffuse Infiltrates, "Histiocytoid" Cells Predominant
4. Diffuse Infiltrates, Plasma Cells Prominent
5. Diffuse Infiltrates, Mast Cells Predominant
6. Diffuse Infiltrates, Eosinophils Predominant
7. Diffuse Infiltrates, Mixed Cell Types
8. Diffuse Infiltrates, Pigment Cells
9. Diffuse Infiltrates, Extensive Necrosis

VC1 Diffuse Infiltrates, Lymphocytes Predominant

Lymphocytes are seen almost to the exclusion of other cell types. Jessner lymphocytic infiltration is prototypic (33).

Jessner Lymphocytic Infiltration of the Skin

CLINICAL SUMMARY. This poorly understood entity is characterized by asymptomatic papules or well-demarcated, slightly infiltrated red plaques, which may develop central clearing. In contrast to lesions of chronic LE, the surface shows no follicular plugging or atrophy. The eruption may be precipitated or aggravated by sunlight. Lesions arise most often on the face, but may also involve the neck and upper trunk. Affected patients are usually middle-aged men and women. Variable numbers of lesions (one to many) often persist for several months or years. They may disappear without sequelae, or recur at previously involved sites or elsewhere. As a historical note, this condition is one of those termed the "Five L's" by Lever, namely: Lupus erythematosus, lymphocytic Lymphoma, Lymphocytoma cutis, polymorphous Light eruption of the plaque type, and Lymphocytic infiltration of the skin of Jessner. In a detailed clinicopathologic study, it was concluded that Jessner lymphocytic infiltrate and tumid LE have more similarities than differences. The differential diagnosis between them was found to rely mostly on clinical features, with facial lesions, especially on the nose predominating for women with tumid lupus, and annular lesions predominantly on the back for Jessner, and also on immunopathologic features (a positive lupus band test result for lupus). The features do not have high specificity (34).

Clin. Fig. VC1.a

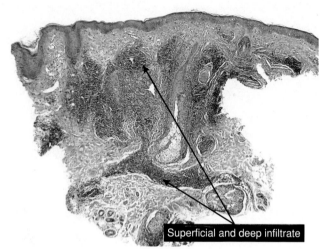

Superficial and deep infiltrate

Fig. VC1.a

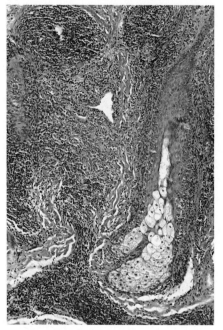

Fig. VC1.b

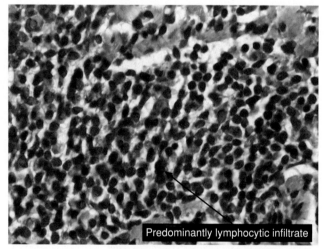

Predominantly lymphocytic infiltrate

Fig. VC1.c

Clin. Fig. VC1.a. *Jessner lymphocytic infiltrate.* Typical infiltrated red plaques with central clearing are seen on the forehead.

Fig. VC1.a. *Jessner lymphocytic infiltration, low power.* A dense perivascular and interstitial infiltrate extends through the full thickness of the dermis.

Fig. VC1.b. *Jessner lymphocytic infiltration, medium power.* The infiltrate is partly perivascular but mainly diffuse.

Fig. VC1.c. *Jessner lymphocytic infiltration, high power.* The lesional cells are mature small lymphocytes.

HISTOPATHOLOGY. The epidermis may be normal but often appears slightly flattened. In the dermis, there are moderately dense perivascular and diffuse infiltrates composed of small, mature lymphocytes admixed with occasional histiocytes and plasma cells. The infiltrate may extend around folliculosebaceous units and into subcutaneous adipose tissue.

Leukemia Cutis
See also Section VIB9.

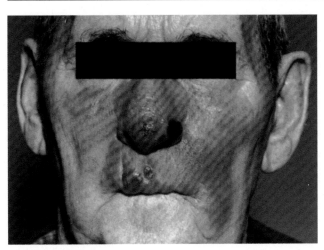

Clin. Fig. VC1.b

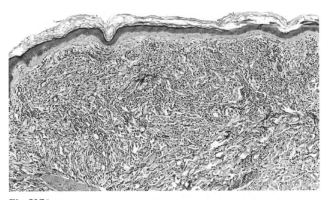

Fig. VC1.e

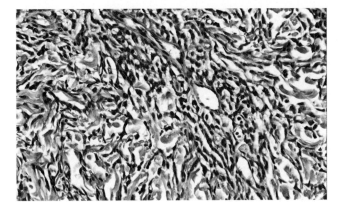

Fig. VC1.g

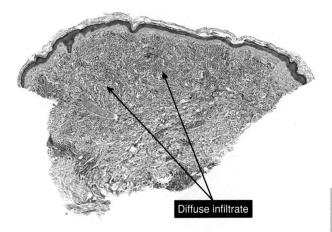

Diffuse infiltrate

Fig. VC1.d

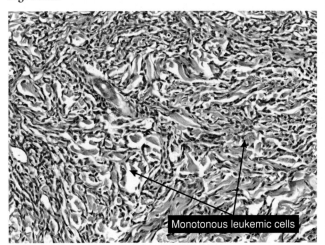

Monotonous leukemic cells

Fig. VC1.f

Clin. Fig. VC1.b. *Leukemia cutis.* An elderly man with chronic lymphocytic leukemia developed recurrent ulcerated nodules on an infiltrated violaceous plaque. Local radiation therapy was successful.

Fig. VC1.d. *Leukemia cutis, low power.* In this example of acute myelogenous leukemia, there is a dense diffuse infiltrate in the reticular dermis.

Fig. VC1.e. *Leukemia cutis, medium power.* The infiltrate shows little tendency to perivascular or periadnexal orientation. There is no epidermal involvement.

Fig. VC1.f. *Leukemia cutis, high power.* The lesional cells tend to dissect between collagen bundles.

Fig. VC1.g. *Leukemia cutis, high power.* The lesional cells have ovoid or indented nuclei and an appreciable amount of eosinophilic cytoplasm, consistent with acute myelogenous leukemia. Phenotyping should be done on blood or bone marrow if possible.

V Perivascular, Diffuse, and Granulomatous Infiltrates of the Reticular Dermis

Conditions to consider in the differential diagnosis:

> Jessner lymphocytic infiltrate
> leukemia cutis (lymphocytic lymphoma, CLL)
> cutaneous lymphoid hyperplasia/lymphocytoma cutis
> lymphoma cutis

VC2 Diffuse Infiltrates, Neutrophils Predominant

Neutrophils are the main infiltrating cells although lymphocytes can be found. Sweet syndrome is prototypic (35). Erysipelas is another good example (36).

Acute Febrile Neutrophilic Dermatosis (Sweet Syndrome)

CLINICAL SUMMARY. Two constant features are required for the diagnosis of Sweet syndrome: the clinical presentation of abrupt onset of painful or tender erythematous papules, plaques, or nodules, and the histologic finding of a dense, predominantly neutrophilic dermal infiltrate. Minor or variable features include associations with inflammatory diseases such as chronic autoimmune disorders, infections, with hemoproliferative disorders or solid malignant tumors, or with pregnancy, fever >38°C, abnormal laboratory values at presentation, including elevations of ESR and CRP, leukocytosis and eosinophilia, and also (albeit retrospectively), an excellent response to treatment with systemic corticosteroids or potassium iodide (37).

HISTOPATHOLOGY. There is a dense perivascular infiltrate composed largely of neutrophils, often with leukocytoclasia. In addition, there are mononuclear cells, such as lymphocytes and histiocytes, and occasional eosinophils. The inflammatory cells typically assume a band-like distribution throughout the papillary dermis. The density of the infiltrate varies and may be limited in a small proportion of cases. There is usually vasodilation and swelling of endothelium with moderate erythrocyte extravasation. Prominent edema of the upper dermis in some instances may result in subepidermal blister formation. Extensive vascular damage is not a feature of Sweet syndrome. The histologic appearance varies depending on the stage of the process. In later stages, lymphocytes and histiocytes may predominate. It is important to realize that the composition and distribution of the infiltrate are not specific enough to histologically rule out an infectious process.

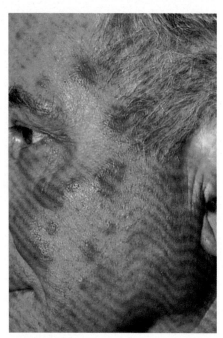

Clin. Fig. VC2

Clin. Fig. VC2. *Sweet syndrome.* A middle-aged man experienced the acute onset of fever and erythematous plaques on the face. (Photo by William K. Witmer.)

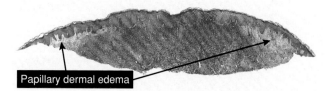

Papillary dermal edema

Fig. VC2.a

Fig. VC2.a. *Sweet syndrome, low power.* There is edema of the upper dermis and a diffuse cellular infiltrate in the reticular dermis.

Fig. VC2.b. *Sweet syndrome, medium power.* The infiltrate may involve the epidermis.

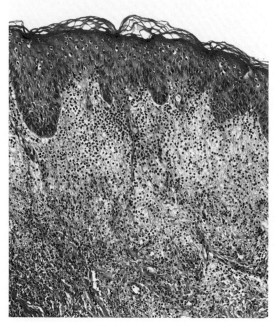

Fig. VC2.b

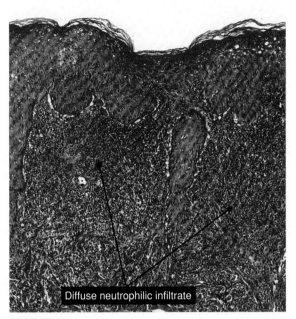

Fig. VC2.c

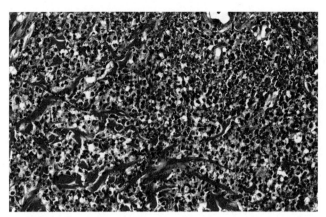

Fig. VC2.d

Fig. VC2.c. *Sweet syndrome, medium power.* The infiltrate is composed almost entirely of neutrophils. Diagnostic changes of leukocytoclastic vasculitis are not observed.

Fig. VC2.d. *Sweet syndrome, high power.* The neutrophilic infiltrate is variable, but often very dense, as in this example. Leukocytoclasia is prominent.

Neutrophilic Dermatosis of the Dorsal Hands

CLINICAL SUMMARY. Neutrophilic dermatosis of the dorsal hands is an entity in the family of neutrophilic dermatoses which also includes Sweet syndrome, pyoderma gangrenosum, and rheumatoid neutrophilic dermatosis (38,39). These patients present with an eruption that is limited to the dorsal aspect of the hands. The lesions begin as tender plaques and nodules with edema and pustules and a violaceous rim. The pustules may become quite large and some lesions may ulcerate. There is preferential involvement for the radial aspect of the hand. Neutrophilic dermatosis of the dorsal hands most commonly occurs in women (76%) and in adults (mean age of 62 years). There may be an accompanying fever. Unlike classic Sweet syndrome, neutrophilic dermatosis of the dorsal hands is generally not associated with an underlying systemic disease or malignancy.

HISTOPATHOLOGY. Biopsies of neutrophilic dermatosis of the dorsal hands reveal a dense neutrophilic infiltrate throughout the dermis which is abscess like. There may be dermal edema and leukocytoclasia. Some cases have shown vasculitis and fibrinoid necrosis of small vascular channels, however, in many cases the blood vessels are unaltered (40). This histopathology can be indistinguishable from Sweet syndrome and pyoderma gangrenosum making clinical–pathologic correlation paramount. One must always exclude the possibility of an infectious process by the use of special stains for organisms as well as tissue culture.

Erysipelas

CLINICAL SUMMARY. Erysipelas is an acute superficial cellulitis of the skin caused by group A streptococci. It is characterized by a well-demarcated, slightly indurated, dusky red area with an advancing, palpable border. In some patients, erysipelas has a tendency to recur periodically in the same areas. In the early antibiotic era, the incidence of erysipelas appeared to be on the decline and most cases occurred on the face. More recently, however, there appears to have been an increase in the incidence, and facial sites are now less common whereas erysipelas of the legs is predominant. Obesity has been found to be an independent risk factor for local complications of erysipelas, including hemorrhage, bullous lesions, abscesses, and necrosis (41).

HISTOPATHOLOGY. In the dermis there is marked edema and dilatation of the lymphatics and capillaries. There is a diffuse infiltrate, composed chiefly of neutrophils, that extends throughout the dermis and occasionally into the subcutaneous fat. It is loosely arranged around dilated blood and lymph vessels. If sections are stained with the Giemsa or Gram stain, streptococci may be found in the tissue and within lymphatics. In cases of recurring erysipelas, the lymph vessels of the dermis and subcutaneous tissue show fibrotic thickening of their walls with partial or complete occlusion of the lumen. Erysipelas and cellulitis must be distinguished from Sweet-like eruptions and vice versa. This distinction cannot always be made on histologic grounds alone—correlations with culture and clinical findings are essential.

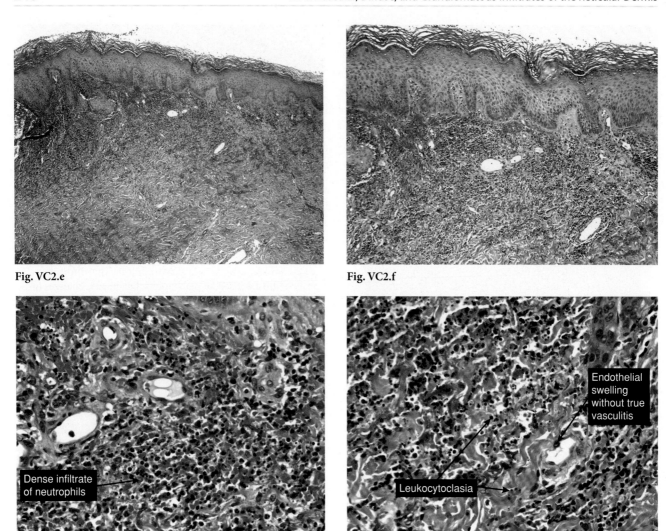

Fig. VC2.e

Fig. VC2.f

Fig. VC2.g

Fig. VC2.h

Fig. VC2.e. *Neutrophilic dermatosis of the dorsal hands, low magnification.* There is a dense inflammatory infiltrate in the upper and midreticular dermis.

Fig. VC2.f. *Neutrophilic dermatosis of the dorsal hands, medium power.* The infiltrate in the dermis is diffuse and sometimes associated with dermal hemorrhage. The overlying epidermis may show edema or ulceration.

Fig. VC2.g. *Neutrophilic dermatosis of the dorsal hands, high power.* The infiltrate is composed predominantly of neutrophils. In this case, leukocytoclastic vasculitis is not seen, although vasculitis has been described in some cases of this entity.

Fig. VC2.h. *Neutrophilic dermatosis of the dorsal hands, high power.* The neutrophilic infiltrate is frequently associated with prominent leukocytoclasia.

Conditions to consider in the differential diagnosis:

acute neutrophilic dermatosis (Sweet syndrome)
erythema elevatum diutinum
rheumatoid neutrophilic dermatosis
infectious abscess from bacteria, mycobacteria, or fungi
neutrophilic dermatosis of the dorsal hands
granuloma faciale
cutaneous reaction to cytokines especially G-CSF

bowel-associated dermatosis–arthritis syndrome (BADAS)
erysipelas
cellulitis
pyoderma gangrenosum
dermis adjacent to folliculitis
abscess
Behçet syndrome
halogenoderma

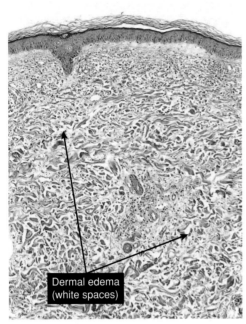

Fig. VC2.i

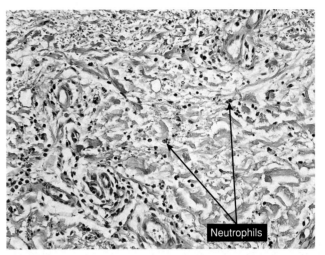

Fig. VC2.j

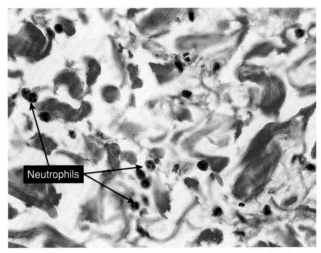

Fig. VC2.k

Fig. VC2.i. *Cellulitis, low power.* The dermis is edematous and there is a patchy infiltrate in the reticular dermis.

Fig. VC2.j. *Cellulitis, medium power.* The infiltrate is partly perivascular, but also diffuse.

Fig. VC2.k. *Cellulitis, high power.* Most of the cells in the infiltrate are neutrophils. There is no necrosis, and bacteria are frequently not demonstrable in the dermis.

VC3 Diffuse Infiltrates, "Histiocytoid" Cells Predominant

Histiocytes or histiocytoid cells are found in great numbers in the dermal infiltrate. Some may be foamy; others may contain organisms. The leukemic cells of myeloid leukemia may be easily mistaken for histiocytes and may have histiocytic differentiation (myelomonocytic leukemia). Lepromatous leprosy (LL) is a good example (42).

Lepromatous Leprosy

LL initially has cutaneous and mucosal lesions, with neural changes occurring later. The lesions usually are numerous and are symmetrically arranged. There are three clinical types: macular, infiltrative–nodular, and diffuse. In the macular type, numerous ill-defined, confluent, either hypopigmented or erythematous macules are observed. They are frequently slightly infiltrated. The infiltrative–nodular type, the classical and most common variety,

may develop from the macular type or arise as such. It is characterized by papules, nodules, and diffuse infiltrates that are often dull red. Involvement of the eyebrows and forehead often results in a leonine facies, with a loss of lateral eyebrows and eyelashes. The lesions themselves are not notably hypoesthetic, although, through involvement of the large peripheral nerves, disturbances of sensation and nerve paralyses develop. The nerves that are most commonly involved are the ulnar, radial, and common peroneal nerves. The diffuse type of leprosy, called Lucio leprosy, most common in Mexico and Central America, shows diffuse infiltration of the skin without nodules. This infiltration may be quite inconspicuous except for the alopecia of the eyebrows and eyelashes it produces. Acral, symmetric anesthesia is generally present. Rarely, LL can present as a single lesion, rather than as multiple lesions.

HISTOPATHOLOGY. In the usual macular or infiltrative–nodular lesions, there is an extensive cellular infiltrate

V Perivascular, Diffuse, and Granulomatous Infiltrates of the Reticular Dermis

that is almost invariably separated from the flattened epidermis by a narrow grenz zone of normal collagen. The infiltrate causes destruction of the cutaneous appendages and extends into the subcutaneous fat. In florid early lesions, the macrophages have abundant eosinophilic cytoplasm and contain a mixed population of solid and fragmented bacilli. There is no macrophage activation to form epithelioid cell granulomas. Lymphocyte infiltration is not prominent, but there may be many plasma cells. In time, and with antimycobacterial chemotherapy, degenerate bacilli accumulate in the macrophages constituting the so-called lepra cells or Virchow cells which then have foamy or vacuolated cytoplasm. The Wade-Fite stain reveals that the bacilli are fragmented or granular and, especially in very chronic lesions, disposed in large basophilic clumps called globi. In LL, in contrast to tuberculoid leprosy, the nerves in the skin may contain considerable numbers of leprosy bacilli, but remain well-preserved for a long time and slowly become fibrotic. The histopathology of Lucio (diffuse) leprosy is similar, but with a characteristic heavy bacillation of the small blood vessels in the skin.

It has been stated that: "histopathologic diagnosis of leprosy is impossible without exact clinical data, such as anamnesis (origin or travels to endemic countries; contact with leprosy patients; household leprosy cases); number, distribution, and type of the lesions; presence or absence of anesthesia; therapies; and other pertinent signs and symptoms (e.g., of type 1 or type 2 reaction). The final diagnosis and classification of a leprosy patient in a referral center should always be formulated on a detailed clinical–pathologic correlation" (43).

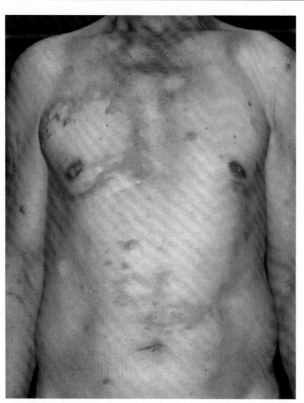

Clin. Fig. VC3.a

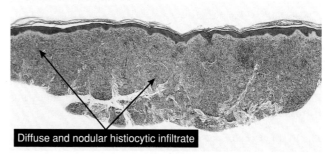

Diffuse and nodular histiocytic infiltrate

Fig. VC3.a

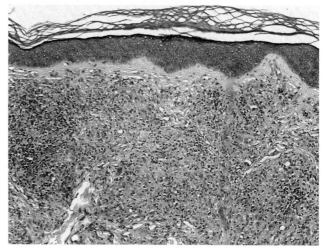

Fig. VC3.b

Clin. Fig. VC3.a. *Borderline lepromatous leprosy.* A 66-year-old man with a 4-month history of infiltrative nodular type, characterized by papules, nodules, and diffuse geographic plaques that are dull red. The lesions progressed into lepromatous leprosy later.

Fig. VC3.a. *Lepromatous leprosy, low power.* There is a diffuse to nodular infiltrate, nearly obliterating the architecture of the dermis.

Fig. VC3.b. *Lepromatous leprosy, medium power.* The infiltrate is composed of large histiocytes as well as small lymphocytes.

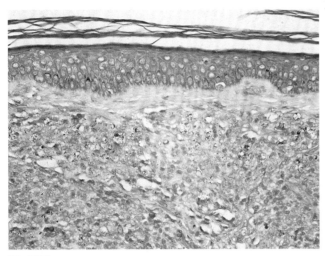

Fig. VC3.c

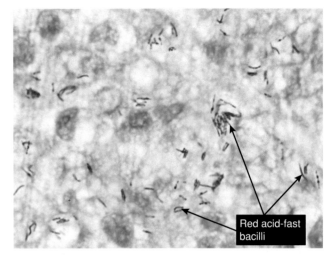

Red acid-fast bacilli

Fig. VC3.d

Fig. VC3.c. *Lepromatous leprosy, medium power, Fite stain.* Even at this magnification, the presence of acid-fast organisms can be appreciated.

Fig. VC3.d. *Lepromatous leprosy, high power, Fite stain.* The organisms are arranged in clumps within the cytoplasm of the histiocytes.

Langerhans Cell Histiocytosis (Histiocytosis X)

Langerhans cell histiocytosis (LCH) or histiocytosis X is characterized by a proliferation of dendritic or Langerhans histiocytes (44,45). If LCH occurs during the first year of life, it is usually characterized by significant, potentially fatal visceral involvement and classified as acute disseminated LCH (Letterer–Siwe disease). If LCH develops during early childhood, the disease is manifested predominantly by osseous lesions with less extensive visceral involvement and known as chronic multifocal LCH or Hand–Schüller–Christian disease. In older children and adults, LCH is usually of the chronic focal type, often presenting one or few bone lesions known as eosinophilic granuloma. Cutaneous lesions are very commonly encountered in Letterer–Siwe disease and occur occasionally

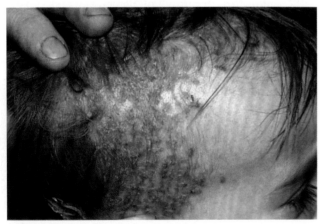

Clin. Fig. VC3.b

Clin. Fig. VC3.b. *Langerhans cell histiocytosis.* An 18-month-old boy with a persistent scalp eruption characterized by closely set brownish papules covered with scales and crust required hospital admission for chemotherapy. A similar eruption was present in the diaper area.

Fig. VC3.e. *Langerhans cell histiocytosis, low power.* There is a diffuse infiltrate in the dermis, close to the epidermis. (*continues*)

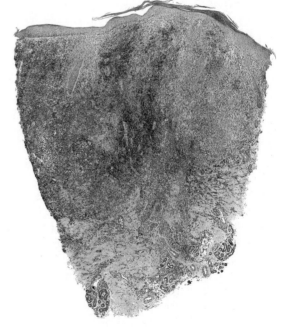

Fig. VC3.e

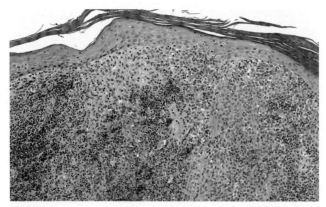

Fig. VC3.f

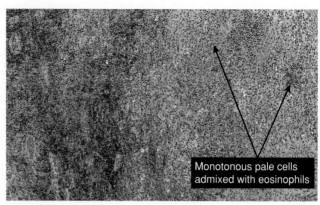

Monotonous pale cells admixed with eosinophils

Fig. VC3.g

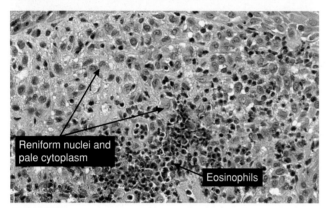

Reniform nuclei and pale cytoplasm

Eosinophils

Fig. VC3.h

Fig. VC3.f,g. *Langerhans cell histiocytosis, medium power.* There are many pale-staining monotonous large cells as well as many eosinophils. The lesional cells are focally epidermotropic.

Fig. VC3.h. *Langerhans cell histiocytosis, high power.* The lesional cells are large with abundant pink cytoplasm and reniform nuclei. There is an admixture of inflammatory cells including occasional eosinophils.

in the two other forms. The cutaneous lesions usually consist of petechiae and papules. In some cases, there are numerous closely set, brownish papules covered with scales or crusts, involving particularly the scalp, face, and trunk. The clinical course and the prognosis of LCH are difficult to predict. BRAF V600E mutations are present in about half of the cases (48).

HISTOPATHOLOGY. The key to diagnosis is identifying the typical Langerhans cell in the appropriate surroundings. The cell has a distinct folded or lobulated, often kidney-shaped nucleus. Nucleoli are not prominent, and the slightly eosinophilic cytoplasm is unremarkable. A typical clinical and light microscopic picture leads to a presumptive diagnosis; confirmation by typical S-100 staining produces a diagnosis; a definite diagnosis requires either a positive CD1a or preferably a langerin (CD207) stain, or electron microscopic demonstration of Birbeck granules (48). Although three kinds of histologic reactions have been described in LCH histiocytosis—proliferative, granulomatous, and xanthomatous—only the first two are commonly seen. In general, the proliferative reaction with its almost purely histiocytic infiltrate is typical of acute disseminated LCH and a granulomatous reaction is usually present with chronic focal or multifocal LCH, as the name *eosinophilic granuloma* suggests. Xanthomatous lesions

in the skin are decidedly rare. The proliferative reaction is characterized by the presence of an extensive infiltrate of histiocytes. The infiltrate usually lies close to or involves the epidermis, resulting in ulceration and crusting.

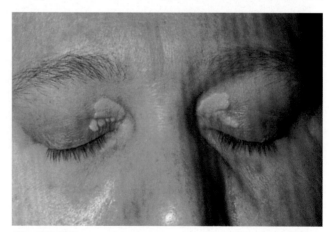

Clin. Fig. VC3.c

Clin. Fig. VC3.c. *Xanthelasma.* Most often no underlying lipid abnormalities are present when patients present with these typical yellowish plaques on the eyelids.

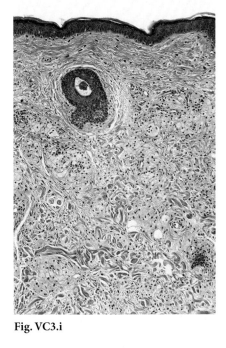

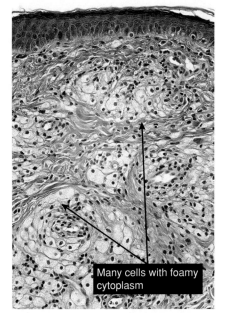

Many cells with foamy cytoplasm

Fig. VC3.i   **Fig. VC3.j**

Fig. VC3.i. *Xanthelasma, low power.* There is a diffuse infiltrate of pale-staining cells in the dermis.

Fig. VC3.j. *Xanthelasma, high power.* The lesional cells are large with abundant foamy cytoplasm. There is no admixture of inflammatory cells.

Inflammatory cells are also present, most often lymphocytes but also eosinophils. The granulomatous reaction has extensive aggregates of histiocytes often extending deep into the dermis, with variable eosinophils, multinucleated giant cells, neutrophils, and lymphoid cells, and plasma cells may be present.

Xanthelasma

Conditions to consider in the differential diagnosis:

xanthelasma, xanthomas (usually nodular)
atypical mycobacteria
    Mycobacterium avium-intracellulare (MAI)
deep fungus infection
cryptococcosis
histoplasmosis
paraffinoma
silicone granuloma
talc and starch granuloma
annular elastolytic giant cell granuloma (actinc granuloma)
lepromatous leprosy
histoid leprosy
cutaneous leishmaniasis
rhinoscleroma (Klebsiella rhinoscleromatis)
histiocytosis X
leukemia cutis (myeloid, myelomonocytic)
anaplastic large cell lymphoma (Ki-1)
reticulohistiocytic granuloma
malakoplakia

VC4 | Diffuse Infiltrates, Plasma Cells Prominent

Plasma cells are found in the diffuse dermal infiltrate, though they may not be the predominant cell. Secondary syphilis may be predominantly perivascular and has been discussed as such in VA4. Other examples of this condition may present as a diffuse infiltrate.

Secondary Syphilis

CLINICAL SUMMARY. The characteristic rash of secondary syphilis may begin with prodromal fever and malaise, and appear as a pruritic maculopapular rash, evolving initially from macules to small reddish-brown papules with minor scaling later. There may be target lesions (46).

HISTOPATHOLOGY. The skin biopsy will likely manifest psoriasiform lichenoid dermatitis with plasma cells. Anti-*T. pallidum* antibody can be used to confirm the presence of spirochetes.

Conditions to consider in the differential diagnosis:

insect bite reaction
plasmacytoma, myeloma
circumorificial plasmacytosis
Zoon balanitis
syphilis, secondary or tertiary
yaws, primary or secondary
acne keloidalis nuchae

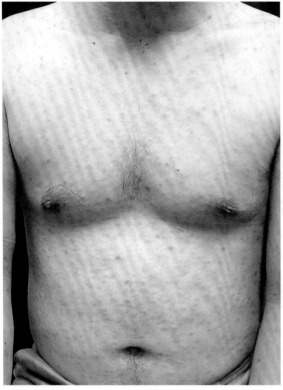

Clin. Fig. VC4

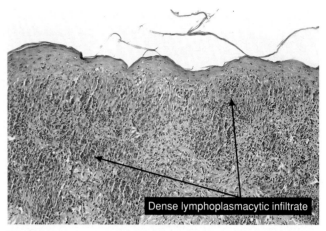

Fig. VC4.b

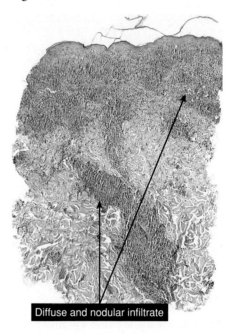

Fig. VC4.a

Clin. Fig. VC4. *Secondary syphilis.* A 30-year-old man with AIDS developed an asymptomatic generalized rash with a 1-month history of well-demarcated erythematous scaly papules.

Fig. VC4.a. *Secondary syphilis, low power.* There is a dense diffuse and perivascular infiltrate in the superficial and deep dermis.

Fig. VC4.b. *Secondary syphilis, medium power.* In this example, the infiltrate is band like in architecture and is composed mostly of plasma cells and lymphocytes.

VC5 Diffuse Infiltrates, Mast Cells Predominant

Mast cells compose almost the entire dermal infiltrate. There may be an admixture of eosinophils. *Urticaria pigmentosa (UP)* is the prototype (see Sections IIIA2, IVE4, VIB10).

Urticaria Pigmentosa

There are three recognized subforms of cutaneous mastocytosis, namely maculopapular cutaneous mastocytosis/ urticaria pigmentosa (MPCM/UP), diffuse cutaneous mastocytosis (DCM), and mastocytoma of skin. In the MPCM subform, skin lesions are typically brownish to reddish oval or round macules and papules, but in some cases large plaques or nodules can coexist or may predominate. MPCM can be divided into two variants, monomorphic and polymorphic. In the latter, the skin lesions are heterogeneous and have different shapes and sizes, but are generally larger than those from the monomorphic variant. The monomorphic MPCM variant is more commonly seen in adult-onset mastocytosis, in which the skin involvement usually coexists with systemic mastocytosis (SM) (47).

Conditions to consider in the differential diagnosis:

urticaria pigmentosa (nodular or diffuse)
mastocytoma

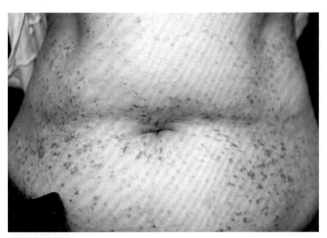

Clin. Fig. VC.5

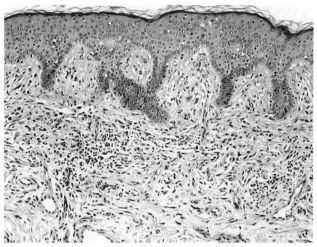

Fig. VC5.a

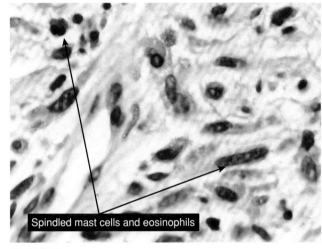

Spindled mast cells and eosinophils

Fig. VC5.b

Metachromatic granules
(different color)

Fig. VC5.c

Clin. Fig. VC.5. *Urticaria pigmentosa.* A "monomorphous" pattern of red-brown oval to round macules and papules in a 56-year-old woman with a 2-year history.

Fig. VC5.a. *Urticaria pigmentosa, medium power.* There is a diffuse cellular infiltrate in the papillary and upper reticular dermis.

Fig. VC5.b. *Urticaria pigmentosa, high power.* The lesion cells have amphophilic cytoplasm with cytoplasmic granules, and a slightly eccentrically placed oval to round nucleus.

Fig. VC5.c. *Urticaria pigmentosa, high power.* The granules stain in a metachromatic (different color) manner with Giemsa (or toluidine blue). Staining for c-kit (CD117) will also provide presumptive identification as mast cells.

VC6 | Diffuse Infiltrates, Eosinophils Predominant

Eosinophils are prominent although not the only infiltrating cell. Lymphocytes are also found, and plasma cells may also be present. Eosinophilic cellulitis is a good example (48).

Eosinophilic Cellulitis (Wells Syndrome)

CLINICAL SUMMARY. This rare dermatosis presents as a sudden eruption of a variable number of bright erythematous patches, which over a period of a few days expand into indurated erythematous plaques that may be painful. The overlying epidermis may produce vesicles or small blisters. The disease, if untreated, may persist for a few weeks or months and may be recurrent, however the prognosis is generally good (49). Associated or provoking stimuli may include insect bites and cutaneous parasitosis, cutaneous viral infections and drug reactions, leukemic and myeloproliferative disorders, and atopic dermatitis and fungal infections. The patients are usually adults.

Peripheral blood eosinophilia is usually present. The clinical appearance may mimic bacterial cellulitis (50).

HISTOPATHOLOGY. Early lesions demonstrate diffuse but dense dermal infiltrates of eosinophils; eosinophil degranulation is prominent. Infiltrates generally extend throughout the dermis and may involve the subcutaneous tissue or occasionally the underlying muscle. Where the epidermis is substantially involved, multilocular spongiotic intraepidermal vesicles develop, but blistering is usually of subepidermal type. Eosinophils are found in the epidermis. Older lesions show more extensive eosinophil degranulation; the granular material aggregates focally around collagen fibers, forming the characteristic "flame figures." These foci may develop a palisade of macrophages and sometimes giant cells. In florid lesions, necrobiosis may develop within the palisading histiocytic reaction.

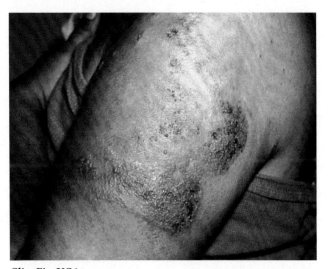

Clin. Fig. VC6.a

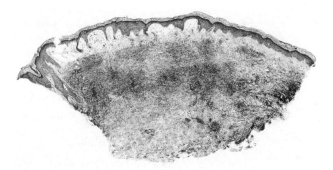

Fig. VC6.a

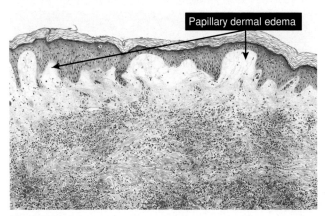

Fig. VC6.b

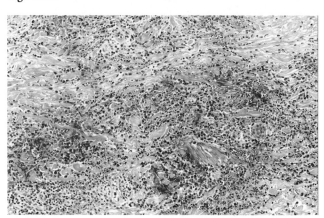

Fig. VC6.c

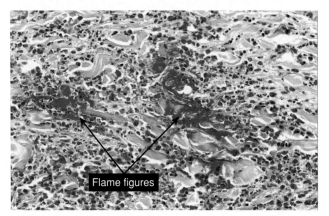

Fig. VC6.d

Clin. Fig. VC6.a. *Wells Syndrome.* A middle-aged female presented with an erythematous, indurated plaque with vesiculation at the borders. Peripheral blood eosinophilia was present.

Fig. VC6.a. *Eosinophilic cellulitis (Wells), low power.* Striking "flame figures" are present in the reticular dermis.

Fig. VC6.b. *Eosinophilic cellulitis (Wells), low power.* There is intense subepidermal edema.

Fig. VC6.c. *Eosinophilic cellulitis (Wells), medium power.* Numerous eosinophils are present in the dermis at the edge of the flame figure.

Fig. VC6.d. *Eosinophilic cellulitis (Wells), high power.* The flame figure is composed of eosinophil granules.

Tick Bite

In the United States, it is said that at least 11 species of ticks are vectors of pathogens of public health importance. As reviewed by Gleim et al. (51), two species (*Amblyomma americanum* and *Ixodes scapularis*) are responsible for the transmission of most known pathogens. For example, *A. americanum* transmits the causative agents of human monocytic ehrlichiosis (HME), *Ehrlichia ewingii* ehrlichiosis, Panola Mountain ehrlichiosis, tularemia, southern tick–associated rash illness (STARI), and the heartland virus. Additionally, *I. scapularis* transmits the causative agents of Lyme disease, *Borrelia miyamotoi* relapsing fever, human granulocytic anaplasmosis (HGA), and babesiosis. Other tick-borne diseases

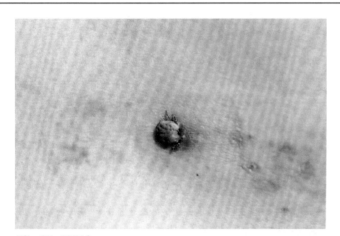

Clin. Fig. VC6.b

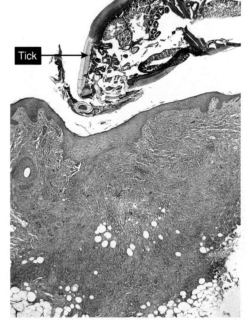

Fig. VC6.e

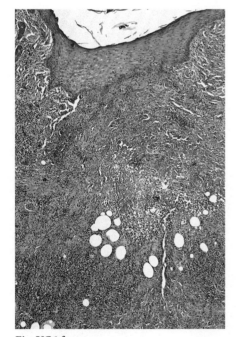

Fig. VC6.f

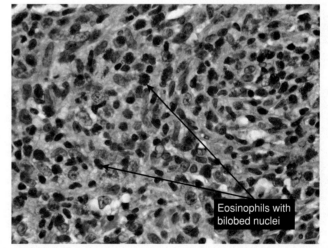

Fig. VC6.g

Clin. Fig. VC6.b. *Insect bite.* A punch biopsy was used to remove the engorged tick embedded in an edematous erythematous papule on the lower back.

Fig. VC6.e. *Tick bite, low power.* A tick is seen above a re-epithelializing wound.

Fig. VC6.f. *Tick bite, medium power.* There is a diffuse mixed cellular infiltrate with eosinophils in the dermis.

Fig. VC6.g. *Tick bite, high power.* The infiltrate includes many eosinophils as well as lymphocytes and plasma cells.

Perivascular, Diffuse, and Granulomatous Infiltrates of the Reticular Dermis

V

of importance, particularly in the South east, include Rocky Mountain spotted fever (RMSF) and *Rickettsia parkeri* rickettsiosis.

Conditions to consider in the differential diagnosis:

eosinophilic cellulitis (Wells syndrome)
arthropod assault reaction
granuloma faciale

VC7 Diffuse Infiltrates, Mixed Cell Types

The diffuse infiltrate contains plasma cells, lymphocytes, histiocytes, and a variety of acute inflammatory cells. Leishmaniasis is a good example (52).

Cutaneous Leishmaniasis

CLINICAL SUMMARY. Leishmaniasis is transmitted by a number of different strains of the protozoan parasite Leishmania. Cutaneous leishmaniasis (CL) occurs initially as single or multiple erythematous papules on exposed areas of the body, weeks to months after the bite of an infected sandfly. The papules may enlarge to form indurated nodules, which frequently ulcerate to form a central crater. CL can be placed along a clinical and immuno-pathologic spectrum in which the clinical features depend on the response of the host to the parasite. At one pole of the spectrum is the localized form (LCL), characterized by the occurrence of one or a few lesions with very few para-sites and a well-developed immunologic response. These cases generally respond very well to treatment. At the other pole is the diffuse form (DCL), characterized by multiple lesions, large numbers of parasites, absence of immunologic response, and a poor response to treatment. More than 90% of CL cases can be placed in the localized end of the spectrum. There are intermediate forms called mucocutaneous, verrucous, or relapse CL which taken together account for about 8% of CL in the Americas. Diffuse cases are extremely rare. They are characterized by plaque-like or nodular lesions that can be localized in a single area of the body in the early stages and then extend

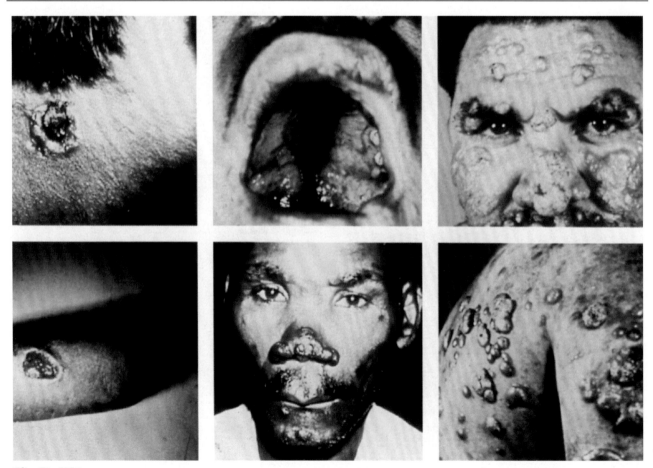

Clin. Fig. VC7.a

Clin. Fig. VC7.a. *Spectrum of American cutaneous leishmaniasis.* **Left** panels: localized cutaneous leishman-iasis. **Middle** panels: mucocutaneous leishmaniasis (espundia). **Right** panels: diffuse cutaneous leishmaniasis. (J. Convit.)

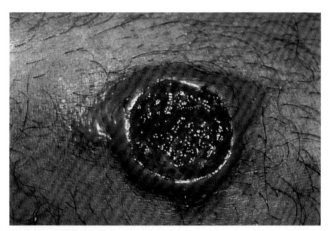

Clin. Fig. VC7.b

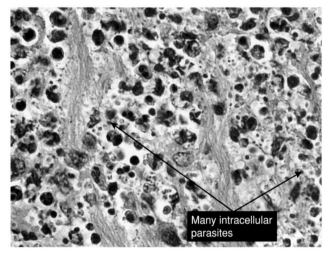

Many intracellular
parasites

Fig. VC7.b

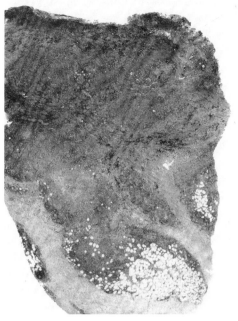

Fig. VC7.a

Clin. Fig. VC7.b. *American cutaneous leishmaniasis.* Lesion of localized cutaneous leishmaniasis presenting as an indurated nodule with an ulcerated crateriform center. (J. Convit.)

Fig. VC7.a. *Localized cutaneous leishmaniasis, low power.* A diffuse infiltrate extends into the subcutis. The epidermis is ulcerated.

Fig. VC7.b. *Localized cutaneous leishmaniasis, high power.* The infiltrate is mixed, with many plasma cells and neutrophils but with histiocytes predominating. In this stage, many organisms are seen within the histiocytes.

until they cover most of the skin and start to slowly compromise nasal, buccal, and laryngeal mucous tissue. Clinically, these lesions can be confused with LL or cutaneous lymphomas.

HISTOPATHOLOGY. Early lesions of LCL are characterized by a macrophagic infiltrate with a slight tendency to epithelioid differentiation (related to time of evolution), with associated infiltration by lymphoid cells. In this stage there are variably abundant parasites inside macrophages, facilitating diagnosis both through direct lesional touch smears and in biopsy sections. In the intermediate or late stages most lesions are ulcerated. In the few lesions that are not ulcerated the morphology is characterized by a tuberculoid-type granuloma with prominent lymphoid infiltration. When the lesions are ulcerated, they show a subacute or chronic mixed cell reaction provoked by secondary infection. The latter may present with macrophagic infiltrates, formation of small abscesses, necrotic areas, plasma cell infiltrates, and proliferation of small

vessels. In this stage, parasites in lesions become increasingly difficult to find. The histopathology of acute lesions is usually characterized by epithelial loss, but in chronic lesions there can be a variable degree of epithelial hypertrophy.

The microscopic morphology of diffuse CL is a macrophagic infiltrate with sparse lymphocytes and with enormous numbers of parasites inside macrophages.

Conditions to consider in the differential diagnosis:

> B-Cell cutaneous lymphoid hyperplasia
> > pseudolymphoma
> > lymphocytoma cutis
> syphilis, primary, secondary, or tertiary
> acrodermatitis chronica atrophicans
> cutaneous reactions to cytokines
> chronic actinic dermatitis (actinic reticuloid)
> rhinosporidiosis
> rhinoscleroma
> histoplasmosis

dermal hematopoiesis (extramedullary hematopoiesis)
cutaneous leishmaniasis
granuloma inguinale
granuloma gluteale infantum

VC8 | Diffuse Infiltrates, Pigment Cells

The diffuse infiltrate contains bipolar, cuboidal or dendritic cells with brown cytoplasmic pigment. Nevus of Ota is a well-known example (53).

Nevi of Ota and Ito and Dermal Melanocyte Hamartoma

CLINICAL SUMMARY. The *nevus of Ota* presents as a usually unilateral discoloration of the face composed of blue and brown, partially confluent macular lesions. The periorbital region, temple, forehead, malar area, and nose are usually involved, giving rise to the term nevus fuscocaeruleus ophthalmomaxillaris. There is frequently also a patchy blue discoloration of the sclera of the ipsilateral eye and occasionally also of the conjunctiva, cornea, and retina. In some instances, the oral and nasal mucosae are similarly affected. In a few cases, the lesions of the nevus of Ota are bilateral rather than unilateral. The involved areas of the skin show a brown to slate-blue even or mottled discoloration, usually without any infiltration. Occasionally,

some areas are slightly raised, and sometimes discrete nodules of highly variable size up to a few centimeters and having the appearance of blue nevi are found within the lesion. The *nevus of Ito* has a similar clinical appearance but differs by its location in the supraclavicular, scapular, and deltoid regions. It may occur alone or in association with an ipsilateral or bilateral nevus of Ota. In the *dermal melanocyte hamartoma*, a single, very extensive area of gray-blue pigmentation may be present from the time of birth. The involvement may be nearly generalized, or there may be several coalescing blue macules that gradually extend within a circumscribed area from childhood.

HISTOPATHOLOGY. The noninfiltrated areas of the nevus of Ota, as well as the nevus of Ito and the dermal melanocyte hamartoma, contain elongated, dendritic melanocytes scattered among the collagen bundles. Although most of the fusiform melanocytes lie in the upper third of the reticular dermis, they may also occur in the papillary layer, and may extend as far down as the subcutaneous tissue. Melanophages are uncommon. Slightly raised and infiltrated areas show a larger number of elongated, dendritic melanocytes than do noninfiltrated areas, thus approaching the histologic picture of a blue nevus, and nodular areas are indistinguishable histologically from a blue nevus. Malignant changes in lesions of nevus of Ota have been reported in a handful of cases. The

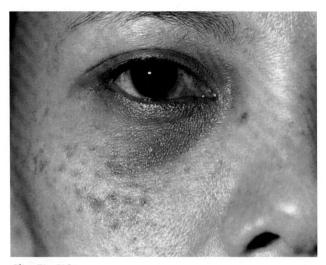

Clin. Fig. VC8

Clin. Fig. VC8. *Nevus of Ota.* Mottled and even colored slate-blue discoloration with scleral involvement in the typical location of the periorbital area.

Fig. VC8.a. *Nevus of Ota, low power.* The melanocytic infiltrate is easily missed at scanning magnification. There is no melanocytic proliferation in the epidermis. Small areas of brown pigment are seen within the upper epidermis.

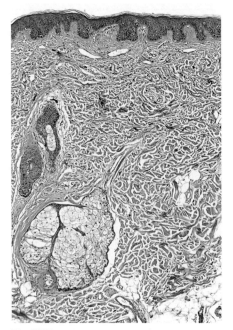

Fig. VC8.a

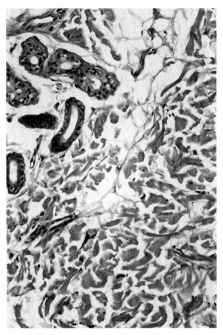

Fig. VC8.b

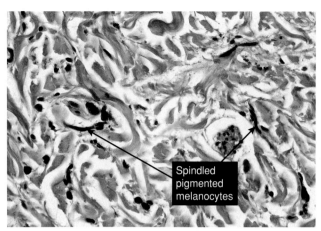

Fig. VC8.c

Spindled pigmented melanocytes

Fig. VC8.b. *Nevus of Ota, medium power.* Pigmented cells are present between otherwise normal reticular dermis collagen bundles.

Fig. VC8.c. *Nevus of Ota, high power.* The lesional cells are elongated dendritic–spindle-shaped heavily pigmented melanocytes.

histologic appearance of the tumors is typically that of a malignant or cellular blue nevus. Rarely, a primary melanoma of the choroid, iris, orbit, or brain may develop in patients with a nevus of Ota involving an eye. These melanomas typically share the same driver mutation as the nevus, often GNAQ or GNA11, and also have alterations in genes related to tumor progression, such as BAP1 loss or inactivating mutation (54).

Conditions to consider in the differential diagnosis:

Mongolian spot
nevus of Ota, nevus of Ito
dermal melanocytic hamartoma
acquired dermal melanocytosis

VC9 Diffuse Infiltrates, Extensive Necrosis

Vascular and dermal necroses are found secondary to vascular occlusion, or to destruction by organisms. Gangrenous ischemic necrosis is a good example (55).

Gangrenous Ischemic Necrosis

CLINICAL SUMMARY. Gangrenous necrosis is usually seen in the distal extremity as a consequence of peripheral vascular disease, most often related to atherosclerosis. The onset is usually in old age. Diabetics are at especial risk, and tend to present at a younger age, with severe disease, which is more likely to be complicated by infection. In chronic ischemia, there may be evidence of atrophy, with thin, shiny skin and loss of skin appendages, or there may be hypertrophic changes with hyperkeratosis and thickening

of the nails. The latter changes are especially likely when there is associated venous stasis. When an extremity or a digit becomes necrotic, there may be initial pallor or duskiness, depending on the degree of occlusion and/or stasis. Ultimately, the affected portion will become black. If an ulcer develops, it is likely to become infected, often with the development of osteomyelitis of the underlying digit.

HISTOPATHOLOGY. There may be evidence of chronic ischemia in the form of atrophy of skin, appendages, and muscle fibers. The early changes of acute ischemia, which may be seen at the edges of areas of infarction, include basal vacuolar change, coagulation necrosis of surface keratinocytes beginning superficially, and necrosis of appendages especially the metabolically active sweat glands. In established infarcts, the architecture may be evident as a ghostly outline, with loss of cell nuclei, but with some preservation of cell shape and connective tissue matrix. At the edge of the infarct, there is an inflammatory zone of neutrophils, with leukocytoclasia in the ischemic area itself. There may be occlusive thrombi in small and sometimes large vessels. In general, changes of severe atherosclerosis are confined to proximal vessels, which are not present in amputation specimens from the distal extremity.

Conditions to consider in the differential diagnosis:

gangrenous ischemic necrosis
tertiary syphilis (gummatous necrosis)
tuberculosis (caseous necrosis)
sporotrichosis

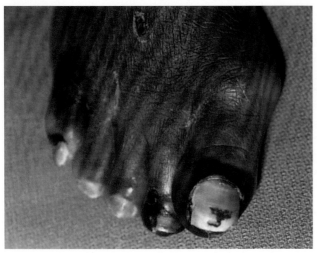

Clin. Fig. VC9

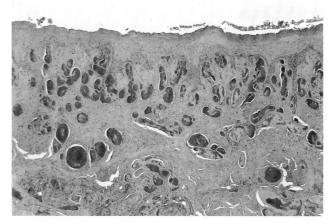

Fig. VC9

Clin. Fig. VC9. *Gangrene.* Severe peripheral vascular disease in a patient with a long-standing history of insulin dependent diabetes mellitus led to cold feet with dusky and black patches of necrosis.

Fig. VC9. *Gangrene, low power.* Full-thickness coagulation necrosis of skin with loss of nuclear and fine cytologic detail is evident even at scanning magnification. The dermal vessels are acutely congested.

---

deep fungus infections
atypical mycobacterial infections
infarcts
vasculitis and deep vasculitis
thrombi and deep thrombi
calciphylaxis
warfarin necrosis

VD — DIFFUSE OR NODULAR INFILTRATES OF THE RETICULAR DERMIS WITH EPIDERMAL PROLIFERATION

Ill-defined nodules or diffuse infiltrates of inflammatory cells, usually including lymphocytes, plasma cells, and neutrophils, are present in the dermis, and the epidermis is irregularly thickened.

1. Epidermal Proliferation With Mixed Cellular Infiltrates

VD1 Epidermal Proliferation With Mixed Cellular Infiltrates

There is a dermal inflammatory infiltrate composed of a variable mixture of lymphocytes, plasma cells, eosinophils, neutrophils, and histiocytes. There may be central necrosis forming an abscess, and there may be ill-defined or well-defined granulomas. The overlying epidermis is irregularly hyperplastic, with tongues of epithelium penetrating into the dermis. The epithelium in general shows

evidence of good maturation from a well-defined basal layer to a thickened stratum corneum. Eruptions that may be associated with ingestion of halogens are good examples (56), as are the deep fungal infections such as blastomycosis (57).

North American Blastomycosis

CLINICAL SUMMARY. North American blastomycosis, caused by *Blastomyces dermatitidis,* occurs in three forms: primary cutaneous inoculation blastomycosis, pulmonary blastomycosis, and systemic blastomycosis. Primary cutaneous inoculation blastomycosis is very rare and occurs almost exclusively as a laboratory or autopsy room infection. It starts at the site of injury on a hand or wrist as an indurated, ulcerated, chancriform solitary lesion. Lymphangitis and lymphadenitis may develop in the affected arm. Small nodules may be present along the involved lymph vessel. Spontaneous healing takes place within few weeks or months.

Pulmonary blastomycosis, the usual route of acquisition of the infection, may be asymptomatic or may produce mild to moderately severe, acute pulmonary signs, such as fever, chest pain, cough, and hemoptysis. The pulmonary lesions either resolve or progress to chronic pulmonary blastomycosis with cavity formation.

In systemic blastomycosis, the lungs are the primary site of infection. Granulomatous and suppurative lesions may occur in many different organs, but, aside from the lungs, they are most commonly found in the skin, followed by the bones, the male genital system, the oral and nasal mucosa, and the central nervous system. Cutaneous lesions are very common in systemic blastomycosis, occurring in about 70% of the patients. They may be solitary or numerous. They occur in two types, either as verrucous lesions, the more common type, or as ulcerative lesions. Verrucous lesions show central healing with scarring and a slowly advancing, raised, verrucous border that is beset by a large number of pustules or small, crusted abscesses. These lesions can clinically resemble basal cell carcinoma, squamous cell carcinoma, and keratoacanthoma. Ulcerative lesions begin as pustules and rapidly develop into ulcers with a granulating base. In addition, subcutaneous abscesses may occur; they usually develop as an extension of bone lesions.

HISTOPATHOLOGY. In primary cutaneous inoculation blastomycosis, the primary lesion shows at first a nonspecific inflammatory infiltrate without epithelioid or giant cells. Numerous organisms, many in a budding state, are present. After a few weeks occasional giant cells may be seen, and later on the primary lesion may show the verrucous histologic pattern usually seen in skin lesions of

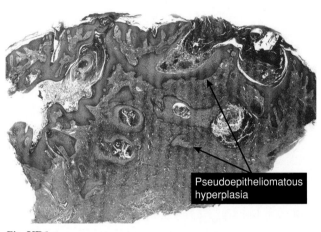

Fig. VD1.a

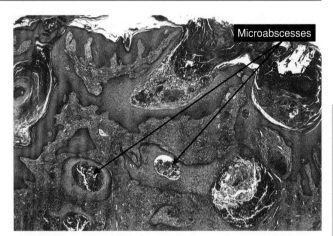

Fig. VD1.b

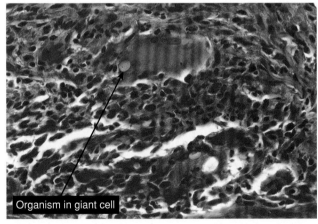

Fig. VD1.c

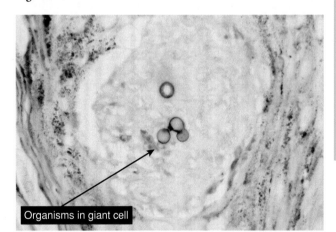

Fig. VD1.d

Fig. VD1.a. *North American blastomycosis, low power.* There is pseudoepitheliomatous hyperplasia of squamous epithelium, extending down into the reticular dermis in relation to a dense, diffuse infiltrate.

Fig. VD1.b. *North American blastomycosis, medium power.* Microabscesses are present within the epithelial tongues.

Fig. VD1.c. *North American blastomycosis, high power.* The inflammatory infiltrate is mixed, with neutrophils predominating, but with an admixture of lymphocytes, plasma cells, and giant cells. One of the latter contains an organism, which can be visualized as a circular defect in its cytoplasm.

Fig. VD1.d. *North American blastomycosis, high power, silver stain for fungi.* The silver stain or a PAS stain highlights the organisms, which are thick-walled spores 8 to 15 mm in diameter. One of the organisms demonstrates broad-based budding.

systemic blastomycosis. In the verrucous lesions of systemic blastomycosis, in a biopsy taken from the active border, there is considerable downward proliferation of the epidermis, often amounting to pseudoepitheliomatous hyperplasia. This can resemble a squamous cell carcinoma. Intraepidermal abscesses often are present. Occasionally, multinucleated giant cells are completely enclosed by the proliferating epidermis. There is a polymorphous dermal infiltrate dominated by neutrophils which often form small abscesses. Multinucleated giant cells are scattered throughout the dermis, with only occasional ill-formed granulomas. The spores of *B. dermatitidis* are found in histologic sections often only after a diligent search, usually in clusters of neutrophils or within giant cells. The spores have a thick wall, which gives them a double-contoured appearance. They measure 8 to 15 μm in diameter (average, 10 μm). In immunocompromised hosts, many organisms can be seen in tissue sections with minimal inflammation. Classically, multinucleate yeast forms with broad-based buds are seen.

Deep Fungal Infections—General

HISTOPATHOLOGY. Histologic reactions in deep cutaneous fungal infections, including primary cutaneous aspergillosis, chromomycoses, pheohyphomycosis, pheomycetoma, rhinosporidiosis, and lobomycosis, typically consist of a mixed dermal infiltrate that is often associated with pseudoepitheliomatous hyperplasia and occasionally with dermal fibrosis. Incidental cutaneous infections by fungi that usually primarily involve other organs, such as blastomycosis or coccidioidomycosis, typically show a pattern similar to that seen with the deep primary cutaneous fungi: a mixed dermal infiltrate with multinucleated giant cells associated with pseudoepitheliomatous hyperplasia (58). A similar reaction pattern of pseudoepitheliomatous hyperplasia is seen in eruptions associated with halogen ingestion—bromoderma, fluoroderma, iododerma.

A few organisms, such as *Histoplasma* and *Loboa loboi*, are more likely to be associated with epidermal thinning than with hyperplasia, and other systemic fungal infections, such as disseminated candidiasis with its microabscess formation, cryptococcosis with its gelatinous and granulomatous reaction patterns, or zygomycosis and aspergillosis with their tendency for vascular invasion and infarction, show special tissue reaction patterns.

Conditions to consider in the differential diagnosis:

> squamous cell carcinoma
> pseudoepitheliomatous hyperplasia
> halogenodermas
> deep fungal infections
> > North American blastomycosis
> > paracoccidioidomycosis
> > chromoblastomycosis

> > coccidioidomycosis
> > rhinosporidiosis
> > protothecosis
> > verrucous cutaneous leishmaniasis
> > North American blastomycosis
> verrucous lupus vulgaris
> tuberculosis verrucosa cutis
> Mycobacterium marinum
> granuloma inguinale (Calymmatobacterium granulomatis)
> pyoderma vegetans
> verruciform xanthoma
> verrucose sarcoidosis
> granuloma gluteale infantum
> verrucous lupus erythematosus
> hypertrophic lichen planus
> keratoacanthoma

VE NODULAR INFLAMMATORY INFILTRATES OF THE RETICULAR DERMIS—GRANULOMAS, ABSCESSES, AND ULCERS

A granuloma may be defined as a localized collection of histiocytes, which may have abundant cytoplasm and confluent borders ("epithelioid histiocytes"), often with Langhans-type giant cells. Granulomas may be associated with necrosis or may palisade around areas of necrobiosis, may be mixed with other inflammatory cells, may include foreign-body giant cells, and may contain ingested foreign material or pathogens (acid-fast bacilli, fungi). An abscess is a localized area of suppurative necrosis, containing abundant neutrophils mixed with necrotic debris, and usually surrounded by a reaction of granulation tissue and fibrosis.

1. Epithelioid Cell Granulomas Without Necrosis
2. Epithelioid Cell Granulomas With Necrosis
3. Palisading Granulomas
4. Mixed Cell Granulomas
5. Inflammatory Nodules With Prominent Eosinophils
6. Inflammatory Nodules With Mixed Cell Type
7. Inflammatory Nodules With Necrosis and Neutrophils (Abscesses)
8. Inflammatory Nodules With Prominent Necrosis
9. Chronic Ulcers and Sinuses Involving the Reticular Dermis

VE1 Epithelioid Cell Granulomas Without Necrosis

Large epithelioid histiocytes are common in the infiltrate as well as giant cells. The infiltrate may also contain a few plasma cells as well as lymphocytes. Sarcoidosis is prototypic (59).

Sarcoidosis

CLINICAL SUMMARY. Sarcoidosis is a systemic granulo-matous disease of undetermined etiology. A distinction is made between the rare subacute, transient type of sarcoidosis and the usual chronic, persistent type. In subacute, transient sarcoidosis, which subsides in almost all patients within a few months without sequelae, cutaneous manifestations other than erythema nodosum do not occur.

In chronic, persistent sarcoidosis, cutaneous lesions are quite common and may be the only manifestation. The most common type of cutaneous lesion consists of brown-red or purple papules and plaques. Through central clearing, annual or circinate lesions may result. When the papules or plaques are situated on the nose, cheeks, and ears, the term *lupus pernio* is applied. Rare manifestations of sarcoidosis include the lichenoid form, in which small, papular lesions are found, as well as the very rare erythrodermic, ichthyosiform, atrophic, ulcerating, verrucous, angiolupoid, hypopigmented, and alopecic forms. Subcutaneous nodules of sarcoidosis are infrequent.

HISTOPATHOLOGY. Like lesions in other organs, the cutaneous lesions of chronic, persistent sarcoidosis are characterized by the presence of circumscribed granulomas of epithelioid cells, so-called epithelioid cell tubercles showing little or no necrosis. Occasionally, a slight degree of necrosis showing eosinophilic staining is found in the center of some of the granulomas. Classically, sarcoid has been associated with only a sparse lymphocytic infiltrate, particularly at the margins of the epithelioid cell granulomas. Because of this sparse infiltrate of lymphocytes, the granulomas have been referred to as "naked" tubercles. However, lymphocytic infiltrates in sarcoid may occasionally be dense, as in tuberculosis.

In typical lesions of sarcoidosis of the skin, the well-demarcated islands of epithelioid cells contain only few, if any, giant cells, usually of the Langhans type (with their nuclei arranged at the periphery of the cytoplasm). A moderate number of giant cells can be found in old lesions. These may contain asteroid bodies or Schaumann bodies, which are star-shaped eosinophilic structures or round/oval, laminated, partly calcified blue structures, respectively. Neither of the two bodies is specific for sarcoidosis.

The papules, plaques, and lupus pernio–type lesions have variously sized aggregates of epithelioid cells scattered irregularly through the dermis with occasional extension into the subcutaneous tissue. In the erythrodermic form, the infiltrate shows rather small granulomas of epithelioid cells in the upper dermis intermingled with numerous lymphocytes and rare giant cells. Typical epithelioid cell tubercles are found in the ichthyosiform lesions. Verrucous sarcoid shows prominent acanthosis and hyperkeratosis.

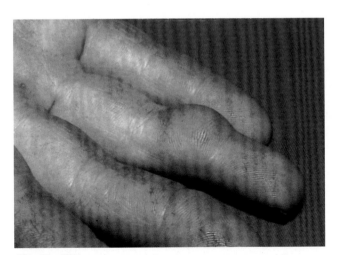

Clin. Fig. VE1

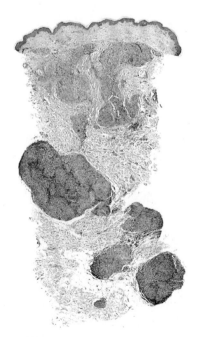

Fig. VE1.a

Clin. Fig. VE1. *Sarcoidosis.* A 39-year-old male with pulmonary sarcoidosis developed several fleshy subcutaneous nodules on his palmar digits. The lesions resolved with intralesional steroids.

Fig. VE1.a. *Sarcoidosis, low power.* A multinodular infiltrate diffusely involves the superficial and deep reticular dermis. (*continues*)

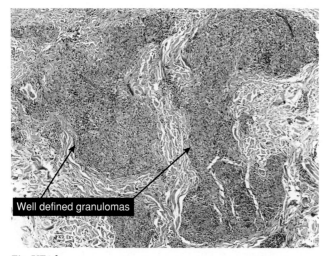

Fig. VE1.b

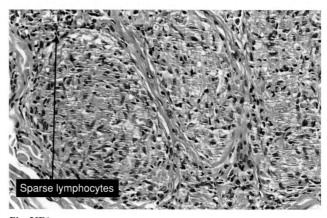

Fig. VE1.c

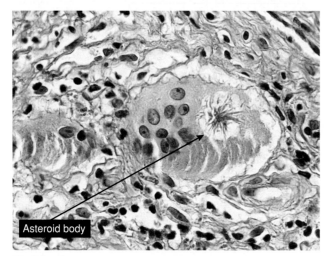

Fig. VE1.d

Fig. VE1.b. *Sarcoidosis, medium power.* The nodules are granulomas composed of epithelioid histiocytes, with relatively sparse surrounding lymphocytes.

Fig. VE1.c. *Sarcoidosis, medium power.* The granulomas contain epithelioid histiocytes, occasional giant cells, and they are generally noncaseating.

Fig. VE1.d. *Sarcoidosis, high power.* A giant cell contains a prominent asteroid body. Although characteristic, these are not diagnostic of sarcoidosis.

Subcutaneous sarcoidosis (also known as Darier–Roussy sarcoidosis) is a form of sarcoidosis where the granulomatous infiltrates are limited to the subcutaneous adipose tissue (60).

In the common form of tuberculosis of the skin, lupus vulgaris, epidermal involvement is often a feature, and there is often a more prominent lymphocytic infiltrate between the granulomas.

Lupus Vulgaris

The granulomas of lupus vulgaris, which is a form of cutaneous tuberculosis due to hematogenous spread, are usually nonnecrotizing (see also Section VE2).

Conditions to consider in the differential diagnosis:

sarcoidosis (lupus pernio and other types)
granulomatous granuloma annulare
foreign-body granulomas
syphilis, secondary or tertiary
granulomatous rosacea
cheilitis granulomatosa (Miescher–Melkersson–Rosenthal)
tuberculoid leprosy
tuberculosis
    lupus vulgaris
    lichen scrofulosorum
Crohn disease
allergic granulomatous reactions to chemical agents
silica, zirconium, aluminum, beryllium (may have necrosis)
collagen implant granuloma
granulomatous mycosis fungoides
chronic cutaneous leishmaniasis

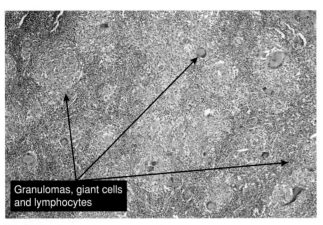

Fig. VE1.e

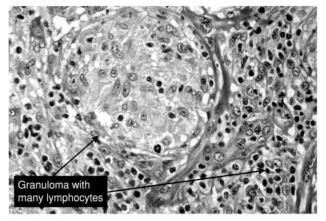

Fig. VE1.f

Fig. VE1.e. *Lupus vulgaris, low power.* Near-confluent nonnecrotizing granulomas in the dermis. The lymphocytic infiltrate is more intense than in sarcoidosis. (S. Lucas.)

Fig. VE1.f. *Lupus vulgaris, high power.* Same lesion as Fig. VE1.e, showing an epithelioid cell granuloma and interstitial lymphocytes. (S. Lucas.)

VE2 Epithelioid Cell Granulomas With Necrosis

The presence of necrosis in an epithelioid cell granuloma of the skin strongly suggests cutaneous tuberculosis except in lesions of the face. Further, some cutaneous tuberculous eruptions do not contain prominent necrosis. However, tuberculosis is prototypic of necrotizing granulomas (61).

Tuberculosis

CLINICAL SUMMARY. Infection of the skin and subcutis by *MTB* occurs by three routes: (1) by direct inoculation into the skin (causing a primary chancre, or tuberculosis verrucosa cutis, or tuberculosis cutis orificialis lesions); (2) by hematogenous spread from an internal lesion (causing lupus vulgaris, miliary tuberculosis, and tuberculous gumma lesions); and (3) from an underlying tuberculous lymph node by direct extension (causing scrofuloderma). In clinical practice, many cases do not readily fit into these clinical and histologic categories. The necrotic granuloma is typical of tuberculosis and other mycobacterial infections, but it is not specific.

HISTOPATHOLOGY. In *lupus vulgaris*, tuberculoid granulomas composed of epithelioid cells and giant cells are present. Caseation necrosis within the tubercles is slight or may be absent. The giant cells usually are of the Langhans type, with peripheral arrangement of the nuclei, but some can be of the foreign-body type. There is an associated infiltrate of lymphocytes, which are sometimes more prominent that the granulomatous component. There is destruction of the cutaneous appendages.

In areas of healing, extensive fibrosis may be present. Tubercle bacilli may be difficult to demonstrate. In *miliary tuberculosis*, the center of the papular lesions is necrotic constituting a microabscess containing neutrophils, cellular debris, and numerous tubercle bacilli, surrounded by a zone of macrophages with occasional giant cells. In *scrofuloderma*, the center of the lesion usually exhibits nonspecific acute inflammatory changes, but in the deeper portions and at the periphery of the lesion, there are tuberculoid granulomas with considerable necrosis and inflammation. *Tuberculosis verrucosa cutis* represents inoculation infection in an individual with prior immunity. There is epithelial hyperkeratosis and acanthosis, and in the dermis there are epithelioid cell granulomas with necrosis. The lesions of *tuberculosis cutis orificialis* are shallow ulcers with a granulating base occurring near mucosal orifices due to spread by direct contamination from an internal lesion that is excreting bacilli. In most instances, tuberculoid granulomas with pronounced necrosis are found deep in the dermis. Tubercle bacilli are usually readily demonstrated in the sections, even when the histologic appearance is nonspecific. In a *tuberculous gumma*, most of the lesion is caseation necrosis with a rim of epithelioid cells and giant cells. Acid-fast bacilli are scant.

Secondary changes in the epidermis are common, and are most pronounced in tuberculosis verrucosa cutis. The epidermis may undergo atrophy and subsequent destruction, causing ulceration, or it may become hyperplastic, showing acanthosis, hyperkeratosis, and papillomatosis. At the margins of ulcers, pseudoepitheliomatous hyperplasia often exists. In rare instances, squamous cell carcinoma supervenes.

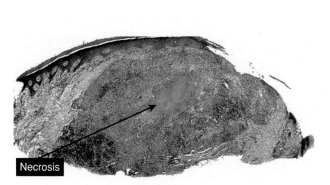

Fig. VE2.a

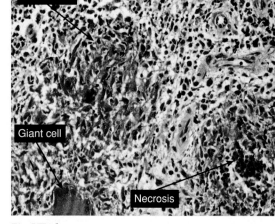

Fig. VE2.b

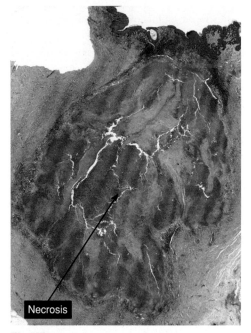

Fig. VE2.c

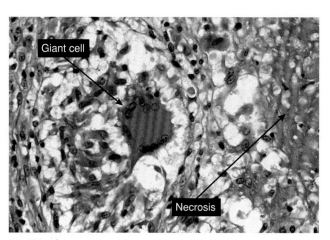

Fig. VE2.d

Fig. VE2.a. *Inoculation tuberculosis, low power.* A prosector's wart from inoculation of a finger from an infected cadaver. There is central caseation necrosis with dense surrounding macrophages and lymphocytes. (S. Lucas.)

Fig. VE2.b. *Inoculation tuberculosis, medium power.* An epithelioid cell granuloma at left, a Langhans giant cell at left lower, and a granuloma with central necrosis and acute inflammation. Occasional acid-fast bacilli were observed in this case. (S. Lucas.)

Fig. VE2.c. *Tuberculous gumma, low power.* A tuberculoma-like appearance with extensive caseation necrosis in the dermis, with a surrounding cellular infiltrate. (S. Lucas.)

Fig. VE2.d. *Tuberculous gumma, high power.* The edge of the necrosis (right) with histiocytes, lymphocytes, and a Langhans giant cell at left of the image.

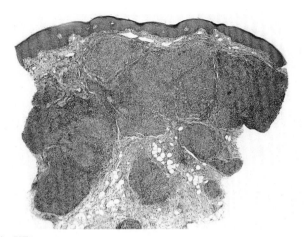

Fig. VE2.e

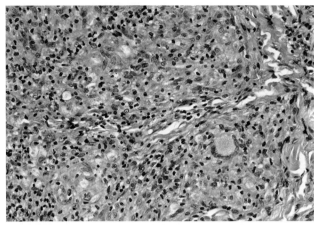

Fig. VE2.f

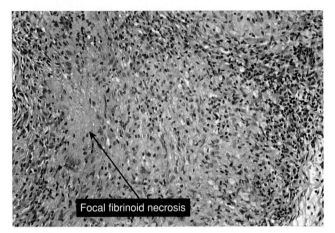

Fig. VE2.g

Fig. VE2.e. *Tuberculoid leprosy, low power.* The reticular dermis is replaced by epithelioid cell granulomas. The epidermis is not much involved.

Fig. VE2.f. *Tuberculoid leprosy, medium power.* The granulomas are admixed with lymphocytes.

Fig. VE2.g. *Tuberculoid leprosy, high power.* There is focal fibrinoid necrosis, as may be seen in an upgrading delayed-type hypersensitivity (type 1) reaction.

(In Fig. VE2.g image: Focal fibrinoid necrosis)

Tuberculoid Leprosy

(See also Section VC3)
    See Figs. VE2.e–g.

Lupus Miliaris Disseminatus Facei

CLINICAL SUMMARY. Although now considered a variant of rosacea, lupus miliaris disseminatus faciei has its own distinct clinical presentation. Characteristic lesions are discrete papules—single papules or small groups of flesh-colored or mildly erythematous papules—involving the face but specifically involving the eyelids and upper lip, areas where rosacea lesions are uncommon, and lacking the erythema and telangiectasia of rosacea. The lesions are the size of a millet seed or half a rice grain. The etiology is unclear and some have speculated that it is caused by a foreign-body reaction to hair follicles and their decomposition products (62).

HISTOPATHOLOGY. Biopsy specimens sectioned through the central portion of a papular lesion demonstrate one of the most highly characteristic patterns of cutaneous histopathology. Surrounding a usually large area of caseous necrosis, aggregates of epithelioid histiocytes and occasional multinucleate giant cells form a substantial "tubercle." There are sparse lymphoid infiltrates peripheral to the granulomas.

Conditions to consider in the differential diagnosis:

tuberculosis
    tuberculosis verrucosa cutis
    miliary tuberculosis
    lupus vulgaris (necrosis usually slight or absent)
nontuberculosis mycobacteria (e.g., M. ulcerans)
type 1 reaction in tuberculoid leprosy
lupus miliaris disseminatus facei
granulomatous rosacea
tertiary syphilis
epithelioid sarcoma
cryptococcosis
histoplasmosis

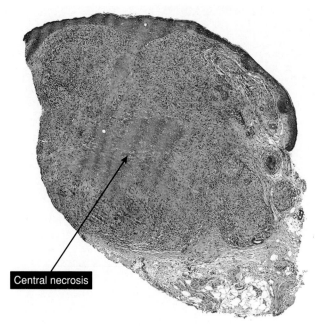

Central necrosis

Fig. VE2.h

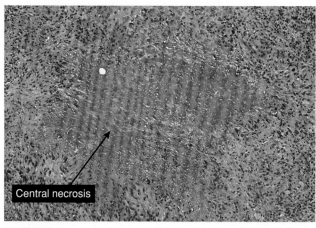

Central necrosis

Fig. VE2.i

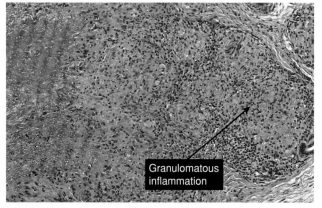

Granulomatous inflammation

Fig. VE2.j

Fig. VE2.h. *Lupus miliaris disseminatus facei, low power.* A papular lesion characterized by a dense lymphohistiocytic infiltrate with a conspicuous area of caseous necrosis.

Fig. VE2.i. *Lupus miliaris disseminatus facei, medium power.* The caseous necrosis characteristic of this condition is not indicative of mycobacterial or other infection.

Fig. VE2.j. *Lupus miliaris disseminatus facei, medium power.* Granulomatous inflammation surrounds the necrosis.

VE3   Palisading Granulomas

There are foci of altered collagen ("necrobiosis") surrounded by histiocytes, and lymphocytes. Histiocytic giant cells are also seen in the infiltrate. The lesions of epithelioid sarcoma are associated with true tumor necrosis, but may superficially resemble rheumatoid nodules (RNs). Granuloma annulare is the prototype (63).

Granuloma Annulare

CLINICAL SUMMARY. The lesions of granuloma annulare consist of small, firm, asymptomatic papules that are flesh colored or pale red and are often grouped in a ring-like or circinate fashion, found most commonly on the hands and feet. Though chronic, they subside after a number of years. Unusual variants of granuloma annulare include (1) a generalized form, consisting of hundreds of papules that are either discrete or confluent but only rarely show an annular arrangement; (2) perforating granuloma annulare, with umbilicated lesions that may be local or generalized; (3) erythematous granuloma annulare, showing large, slightly infiltrated erythematous patches, with a palpable border, on which scattered papules may subsequently arise; and (4) subcutaneous granuloma annulare, in which subcutaneous nodules similar to RNs occur, especially in children, either alone or in association with intradermal lesions.

HISTOPATHOLOGY. Histologically, granuloma annulare is characterized by an infiltrate of histiocytes and lymphocytes, which may be present in an interstitial pattern without organization, or in a well-developed palisade completely surrounding areas with prominent mucin. Patterns between these two extremes occur. Although degenerated collagen and small quantities of fibrin may be present, it is the increased mucin (hyaluronic acid) that is the hallmark of granuloma annulare (though it may be absent from some lesions, especially those that lack good palisading). The increased mucin is usually apparent on routinely stained sections as faint blue material with a stringy and finely granular appearance. Stains such as colloidal iron and alcian blue can be used to highlight it. Plasma cells are present rarely, and a sparse to moderately dense infiltrate of eosinophils can occur. Multinucleated histiocytes are present more often than not, but they are usually few and often subtle. They can occasionally be

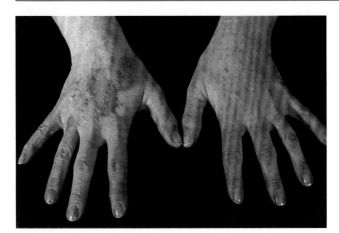

Clin. Fig. VE3.a

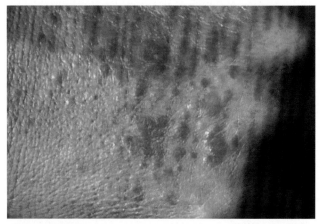

Clin. Fig. VE3.b

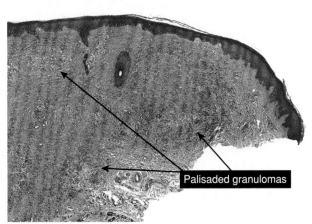

Fig. VE3.a

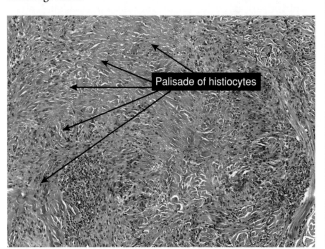

Palisade of histiocytes

Fig. VE3.b

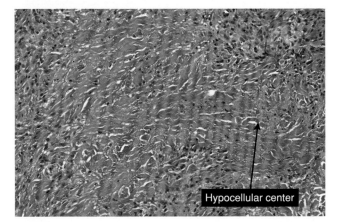

Hypocellular center

Fig. VE3.c

Clin. Fig. VE3.a. *Granuloma annulare.* A middle-aged female with generalized granuloma annulare presents a typical annular plaque on her dorsal right hand.

Clin. Fig. VE3.b. *Granuloma annulare.* Multiple orangish papules of granuloma annulare on the left dorsal hand in the same patient.

Fig. VE3.a. *Granuloma annulare, low power.* There are ill-defined areas of pallor in the reticular dermis, surrounded by a somewhat palisaded infiltrate.

Fig. VE3.b. *Granuloma annulare, medium power.* Histiocytes and lymphocytes are arranged around the areas of mucin deposition and collagen alteration.

Fig. VE3.c. *Granuloma annulare, high power.* The hypocellular center of the palisaded granuloma may show mucinous ground substance.

seen to have engulfed short, thick, blue-gray elastic fibers. On rare occasions in granuloma annulare, there are granulomas resembling those of sarcoidosis ("granulomatous granuloma annulare"). In perforating granuloma annulare, at least part of the palisading granulomatous process is located very superficially and is associated with disruption of the epidermis. The nodules of subcutaneous granuloma annulare usually show large foci of palisaded histiocytes surrounding areas of degenerated collagen and prominent mucin with a pale appearance.

Necrobiosis Lipoidica

CLINICAL SUMMARY. Most patients with necrobiosis lipoidica have or will have diabetes, abnormal glucose tolerance, or a family history of diabetes, although of all patients with diabetes, less than 1% develop necrobiosis lipoidica (also known as "necrobiosis lipoidica diabeticorum"). The lesions present as one or several sharply but irregularly demarcated patches or plaques often with central telangiectases, usually on the shins, elsewhere on the lower extremities, or occasionally elsewhere (64,65).

HISTOPATHOLOGY. The epidermis may be normal, atrophic, or hyperkeratotic, or ulcerated. Usually the entire thickness of the dermis or its lower two-thirds is affected by variable degrees of granulomatous inflammation, degeneration of collagen, and sclerosis. Giant cells are usually of the Langhans or foreign-body type occasionally with Touton cells or asteroid bodies. There may or may not be histiocytes arranged in a palisade, which may tend to be somewhat horizontally oriented and vaguely tiered. Histiocytes may encircle altered connective tissue, particularly degenerated collagen, referred to as "necrobiosis," and differing from normal collagen tinctorially by having a paler grayer hue and structurally by appearing more fragmented and more haphazardly arranged, or more compact. Increased mucin is usually inapparent or just subtle, in contrast to granuloma annulare. Other findings include a sparse to moderately dense, primarily perivascular lymphocytic infiltrate, plasma cells in the deep dermis in some biopsies, involvement of the upper subcutis with thickened fibrous septa, and lipids in foamy histiocytes or in cholesterol clefts. Older lesions show telangiectases superficially. Blood vessels, particularly in the middle and lower dermis, often exhibit thickening of their walls with PAS-positive, diastase-resistant material and proliferation of their endothelial cells. The process may lead to partial and rarely to complete occlusion of the lumen.

DIFFERENTIAL DIAGNOSIS. Although it is true that histologic distinction between necrobiosis lipoidica and granuloma annulare may be difficult or impossible, usually it can be accomplished by using the following criteria: (1) Necrobiosis lipoidica rarely involves just one focus of the dermis or predominantly the upper half of the dermis,

whereas granuloma annulare commonly does. (2) Histiocytes in palisades that completely encircle altered connective tissue are more common in granuloma annulare, whereas histiocytes in linear array that are horizontally oriented in a somewhat tiered fashion are more typical of necrobiosis lipoidica. (3) Abundant mucin is typical of granuloma annulare and distinctly uncommon in necrobiosis lipoidica. (4) Necrobiosis lipoidica often shows dermal sclerosis and thickened subcutaneous septa, whereas granuloma annulare does not (the sclerosis often produces a straight edge to the sides of a punch biopsy, in contrast to the inward retraction and/or more irregular edge seen in biopsies without sclerosis). Other features that are more characteristic of necrobiosis lipoidica include more numerous giant cells, more pronounced vascular changes such as thickened blood vessel walls, and prominent plasma cells in the deep dermis, and occasionally extensive deposits of lipids or nodular lymphocytic infiltrates in the deep dermis or subcutis.

Necrobiotic Xanthogranuloma With Paraproteinemia

CLINICAL SUMMARY. A rare disorder, necrobiotic xanthogranuloma with paraproteinemia presents with large, often yellow, indurated plaques with atrophy, telangiectasia, and occasionally also ulceration (66). The most common location is periorbital, and the thorax is also commonly involved. In most patients, serum protein electrophoresis shows an IgG monoclonal gammopathy that usually consists of kappa light chains. Bone marrow examination may reveal multiple myeloma. The skin lesions of necrobiotic xanthogranuloma are reactive and are not associated with monoclonal plasma cells or multiple myeloma (67). Treatment directed at the underlying plasma cell dyscrasia can be beneficial (68).

HISTOPATHOLOGY. Granulomatous masses are present either as focal aggregates or as large, intersecting bands occupying the dermis and subcutaneous tissue. The intervening tissue separating the granulomas shows extensive necrobiosis. The granulomas contain histiocytes, foam cells, and often also an admixture of inflammatory cells, often arranged as lymphoid follicles. A distinctive feature is the presence of numerous large giant cells, both of the Touton type with a peripheral rim of foamy cytoplasm and of the foreign-body type. Aggregates of cholesterol clefts are also common.

Rheumatoid Nodules

CLINICAL SUMMARY. RNs vary in size from a few millimeters to 5 cm and may be solitary or numerous. They occur in patients with RA, particularly over extensor surfaces (69), and rarely in extracutaneous sites. *Pseudorheumatoid nodule* refers to nodules in the subcutis that mimic RN histologically but that develop in the absence of RA (or systemic LE). The subsequent development of RA

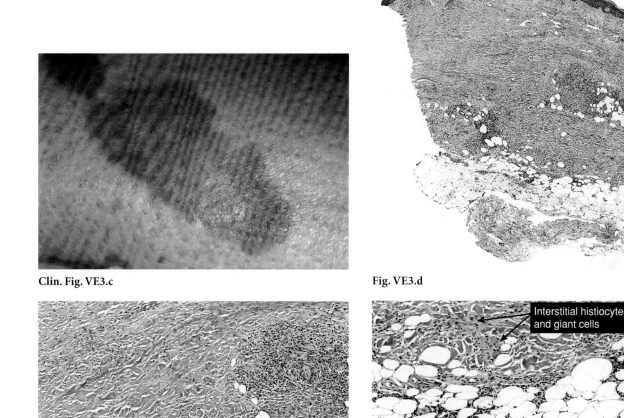

Clin. Fig. VE3.c

Fig. VE3.d

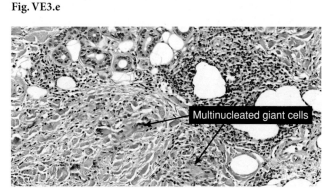

Fig. VE3.e

Fig. VE3.f

Interstitial histiocytes and giant cells

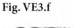

Multinucleated giant cells

Fig. VE3.g

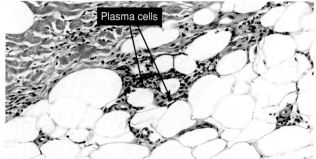

Plasma cells

Fig. VE3.h

Clin. Fig. VE3.c. *Necrobiosis lipoidica.* A solitary plaque of the anterior tibial region shows a pink-brown color, atrophy, and telangiectasia. (W. Witmer.)

Fig. VE3.d. *Necrobiosis lipoidica, low power.* The presence of fibrosis can be identified because of the straight edges of the biopsy. The infiltrate involves the full thickness of the dermis and is arranged in a tier-like fashion.

Fig. VE3.e. *Necrobiosis lipoidica, medium power.* Histiocytes and lymphocytes on the left surround degenerated collagen. Compared to the normal collagen, the degenerated collagen has a more compact appearance and appears more gray-blue than pink.

Fig. VE3.f–h. *Necrobiosis lipoidica, high power.* Ill-defined epithelioid granulomas in the deep dermis and lymphocytes and plasma cells at the dermal–subcutaneous junction are features that favor necrobiosis lipoidica over granuloma annulare.

occurs infrequently in adults and rarely, if ever, in children. These nodules have been considered to represent a subcutaneous variant of granuloma annulare. Modern pharmacologic treatment for RA has only limited effect on RN, despite being efficaceous for other manifestations of the disease (70).

HISTOPATHOLOGY. RNs occur in the subcutis and lower dermis and have one or several areas of fibrinoid degeneration of collagen that stain homogeneously red. Nuclear fragments and basophilic material may be present, but mucin is almost always minimal or absent. These areas are surrounded by histiocytes in a palisaded arrangement, often with scattered foreign-body giant cells. In the surrounding stroma, there is a proliferation of blood vessels, with fibrosis and a fairly sparse infiltrate of other inflammatory cells including predominantly lymphocytes and a few neutrophils, but also mast cells, plasma cells, and eosinophils occasionally.

Palisaded Neutrophilic and Granulomatous Dermatitis

Interstitial granulomatous dermatitis
Interstitial granulomatous drug reaction
Reactive granulomatous dermatitis

CLINICAL SUMMARY. Palisaded neutrophilic and granulomatous dermatitis (PNGD) is an inflammatory reactive process in the skin that is generally associated with underlying immune-mediated systemic disease (71,72). Clinically, the patients present with papules, plaques, and linear band-like lesions. The lesions favor the extremities

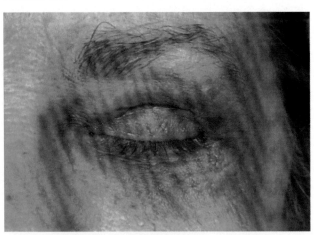

Clin. Fig. VE3.d

Clin. Fig. VE3.d. *Necrobiotic xanthogranuloma.* A 65-year-old woman developed asymmetric periorbital induration with violaceous color change.

Fig. VE3.i. *Necrobiotic xanthogranuloma, low power.* A diffuse infiltrate spans the dermis and subcutaneous tissue.

Fig. VE3.j. *Necrobiotic xanthogranuloma, medium power.* The infiltrate is vaguely granulomatous, with intersecting bands of acellular necrosis and cellular infiltrates which are present either as focal aggregates or as large, intersecting bands occupying the dermis and subcutaneous tissue.

Fig. VE3.k. *Necrobiotic xanthogranuloma, high power.* The granulomatous infiltrate contains histiocytes, foam cells, and an admixture of lymphocytes and plasma cells, with numerous large giant cells of the Touton type with a peripheral rim of foamy cytoplasm, or of foreign-body type.

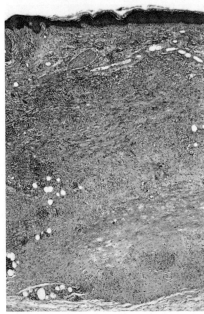

Fig. VE3.i

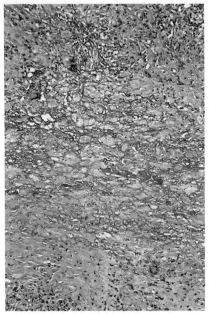

Fig. VE3.j

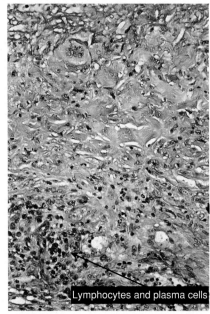

Lymphocytes and plasma cells

Fig. VE3.k

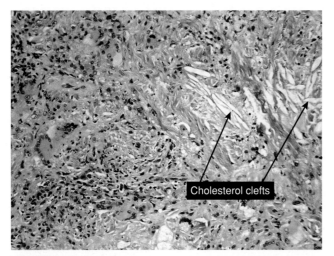

Fig. VE3.l

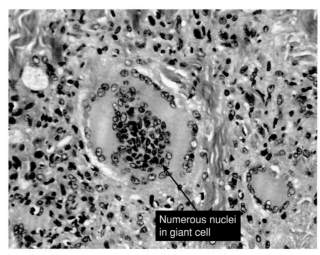

Fig. VE3.m

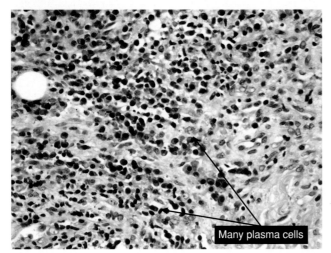

Fig. VE3.n

Fig. VE3.l. *Necrobiotic xanthogranuloma, high power.* Amidst the granulomatous inflammation there are cholesterol clefts.

Fig. VE3.m. *Necrobiotic xanthogranuloma, high power.* Necrobiotic xanthogranuloma contains numerous multinucleated giant cells. Some of them are quite large with many nuclei.

Fig. VE3.n. *Necrobiotic xanthogranuloma, high power.* The mononuclear cell infiltrate is rich in plasma cells.

especially the extensor surfaces. The papules may have a central crust, umbilication, or ulceration. They may be asymptomatic or painful. Seventy-four percent of the reported cases have occurred in women and PNGD generally occurs in middle-aged adults. It has been associated with the following underlying systemic diseases: RA, systemic LE, GPA and EGPA syndromes, Takayasu aortitis, sarcoidosis, and lymphoproliferative disorders (73). It has also been induced by medications, including allopurinol (74). There are overlapping clinical and histopathologic findings with an entity called IGD. This entity also occurs in patients with a history of arthritis and/or arthralgias and characteristically has linear plaques in intertriginous and extremity areas that have been described as the "rope sign." Another condition, "interstitial granulomatous drug reaction" (IGDR) has also been distinguished. Because of clinical and histologic overlap among these entities, the term "reactive granulomatous dermatitis" (RGD) has been proposed to encompass the group of cutaneous

reactive eruptions hitherto classified as PNGD, IGD, or IGDR (75).

HISTOPATHOLOGY. Early lesions of PNGD may have intense neutrophilic inflammation, karyorrhectic debris, and frank LCV. As the lesions evolve, there are piecemeal areas of collagen degeneration and palisades of histiocytes and small granulomas, eventually accompanied by areas of fibrosis. The presence of vasculitis is felt to distinguish PNGD from IGD (81). There are areas of neutrophilic inflammation with leukocytoclastic debris and prominent basophilia surrounded by poorly defined palisaded histiocytic inflammation. The inflammatory infiltrate is mixed with neutrophils, eosinophils, and mononuclear cells. In IGD, similarly, there may be an interstitial and/or palisaded histiocytic infiltrate with collagen alteration. Neutrophilic inflammation with vasculitis, leukocytoclasia, and basophilic debris are much less intense. As noted above PNGD and IGD may have overlapping histologic features.

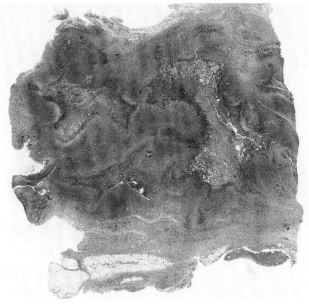

Fig. VE3.o

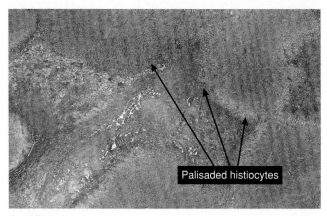

Fig. VE3.p

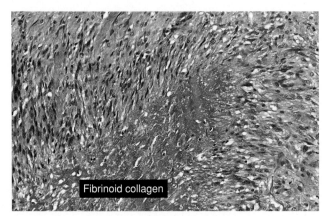

Fig. VE3.q

Fig. VE3.o. *Rheumatoid nodule, low power.* There are patches of hypocellular collagen surrounded by a cellular infiltrate in the reticular dermis.

Fig. VE3.p. *Rheumatoid nodule, medium power.* The patches are areas of degenerated acellular collagen.

Fig. VE3.q. *Rheumatoid nodule, high power.* The fibrinoid hypocellular areas are surrounded by histiocytes in a palisaded arrangement.

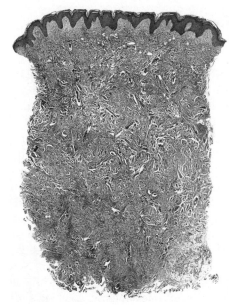

Fig. VE3.r

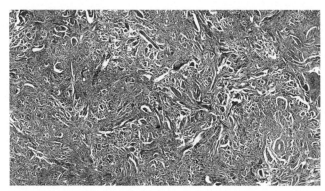

Fig. VE3.s

Fig. VE3.r. *Palisaded neutrophilic and granulomatous dermatitis, low power.* In the dermis, there is edema associated with a diffuse infiltrate which is both perivascular and interstitial.

Fig. VE3.s. *Palisaded neutrophilic and granulomatous dermatitis, medium power.* Characteristically one sees granular basophilic material within the reticular dermis associated with a mixed inflammatory infiltrate.

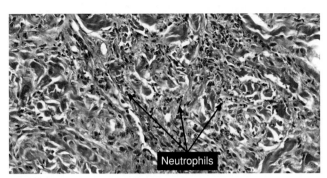

Fig. VE3.t

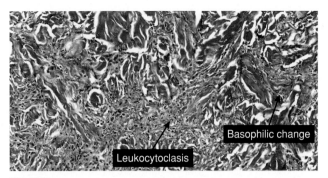

Fig. VE3.u

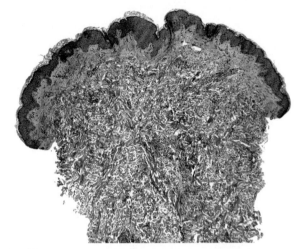

Fig. VE3.v

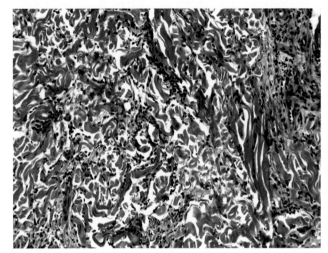

Fig. VE3.w

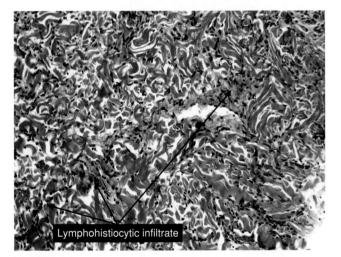

Fig. VE3.x

Fig. VE3.t,u. *Palisaded neutrophilic and granulomatous dermatitis, high power.* In some areas, neutrophils predominate in the infiltrate and may show vasculitis. In these images, one also sees the characteristic basophilic material. Eosinophils are also present.

Fig. VE3.v. *Interstitial granulomatous dermatitis, low power.* There is a superficial and deep perivascular and interstitial infiltrate without involvement of the epidermis.

Fig. VE3.w. *Interstitial granulomatous dermatitis, high power.* The lymphohistiocytic infiltrate shows a predominately interstitial pattern which resembles early granuloma annulare.

Fig. VE3.x. *Interstitial granulomatous dermatitis, high power.* The infiltrate is predominantly lymphohistiocytic. Collagen bundles are separated by edema. Vasculitis is not seen.

Conditions to consider in the differential diagnosis (Table V.1):

granuloma annulare
rheumatoid nodule
necrobiosis lipoidica
subcutaneous granuloma annulare
leukocytoclastic vasculitis

granuloma annulare–like medication reactions
interstitial granulomatous dermatitis (IGD)
necrobiotic xanthogranuloma with paraproteinemia
annular elastolytic giant cell granuloma (actinc granuloma)
rheumatoid nodule
epithelioid sarcoma
occasional examples of deep fungus infections

V Perivascular, Diffuse, and Granulomatous Infiltrates of the Reticular Dermis

TABLE V.1. Comparison of Palisading Granulomas

	Granuloma Annulare	Necrobiosis Lipoidica	Rheumatoid Nodule	PNGD/IGDR/RGD	NXG
Location in tissue	Dermis commonly, subcutaneous variant exists	Dermis	Lower dermis and subcutaneous fat	Dermis	Dermis
Typical clinical description	Closely set papules in an annular configuration on the dorsum of the extremities	Waxy yellow patches and plaques with surrounding erythema on the shins. The center of the plaques are atrophic with telangiectasia	Subcutaneous nodules over joints	Symmetrical papules on the extremities	Firm plaques and nodules periorbitally and on the trunk and extremities with atrophy and telangiectasia
Key histologic feature	Palisaded granulomas surrounding degenerated collagen, interstitial pattern possible	Palisaded granulomatous dermatitis in a layered arrangement, parallel to the overlying epidermis. Plasma cells are present	Palisaded granulomatous dermatitis surrounding large areas of fibrin	Varies by age of lesion, but neutrophils are prominent. Can resemble GA or NL	Palisaded granulomatous dermatitis with cholesterol clefts. Touton and foreign-body giant cells can be present
Presence of mucin	Yes	No	No	No	No
Associated disorders	Considered to be a reaction pattern to many entities including trauma and infections	Diabetes mellitus	Rheumatoid arthritis	Many, including systemic lupus erythematosus, rheumatoid arthritis, inflammatory bowel disease, and infections	IgG paraproteinemia, lymphoproliferative disorders, plasma cell dyscrasias

PNGD, palisaded neutrophilic and granulomatous dermatitis; IGDR, interstitial granulomatous drug reaction; RGD, reactive granulomatous dermatitis; NXG, necrobiotic xanthogranuloma with paraproteinemia; GA, granuloma annulare; NL, necrobiosis lipoidica.

279

VE4 Mixed Cell Granulomas

Lymphocytes and plasma cells are present in addition to epithelioid histiocytes, which may form loose clusters, and giant cells, which may be quite inconspicuous. In many of these granulomatous infiltrates, organisms are found. Keratin granuloma is the most common mixed granuloma. Flakes of keratin may be appreciated as fibers, often gray rather than pink, in the cytoplasm of giant cells. Foreign-body reactions may present as mixed cell granulomas (76).

Foreign-Body Reactions

CLINICAL SUMMARY. Foreign substances, when injected or implanted accidentally into the skin, can produce a focal, nonallergic foreign-body reaction, or in persons specifically sensitized to them, a focal allergic response. In addition, certain substances formed within the body may produce a nonallergic foreign-body reaction when deposited in the dermis or the subcutaneous tissue. Such endogenous foreign-body reactions are produced,

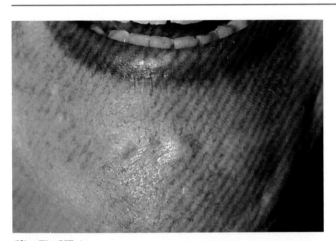
Clin. Fig. VE.4

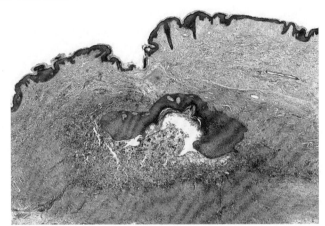
Fig. VE4.a

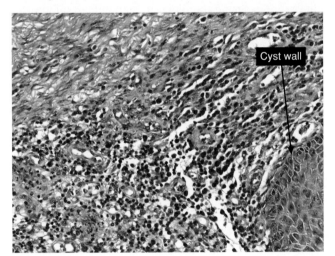
Fig. VE4.b

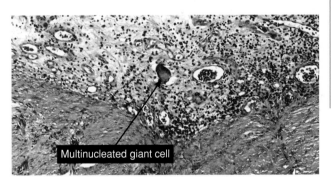
Fig. VE4.c

Clin. Fig. VE.4. *Foreign-body reaction.* Silicone injections for wrinkles led to whitish firm tender nodules.

Fig. VE4.a,b. *Foreign-body granuloma in ruptured epidermal cyst, low power.* Foreign-body granuloma in ruptured epidermal cyst is commonly submitted for histologic examination, often with the designation of "infected cyst" or "abscess," however the inflammation is a reaction to interstitial keratin and the lesions are sterile. Remnants of a cyst are present adjacent to a mixed cell inflammatory infiltrate. Flakes of keratin from the cyst appear to elicit the inflammatory response.

Fig. VE4.c. *Ruptured epidermal cyst, high power.* The inflammatory reaction contains a mixed cell granulomatous infiltrate including lymphocytes, plasma cells, some neutrophils, and giant cells. In lesions where a remnant cyst is not identified, the diagnosis can often be made by searching for keratin flakes in the cytoplasm of giant cells. These flakes are often gray in color, rather than pink.

for instance, by urates in gout and by keratinous material in pilomatricoma, as well as in ruptured epidermoid and trichilemmal cysts.

HISTOPATHOLOGY. A *nonallergic* foreign-body reaction typically shows a granulomatous response with histiocytes and giant cells around the foreign material. Often, some of the giant cells are of the foreign-body type, in which the nuclei are in haphazard array. In addition, lymphocytes are usually present, as may be plasma cells and neutrophils, constituting a mixed cell granuloma. Frequently, some of the foreign material is seen within macrophages and giant cells, a finding that of course is of great diagnostic value. The most common cause of a foreign-body granuloma is rupture of a hair follicle or follicular cyst, and sometimes only the cyst content, rather than residual cyst wall, is identifiable. Exogenous substances producing nonallergic foreign-body reactions are, for instance, silk and nylon sutures, wood, paraffin and other oily substances, silicone gel, talc, surgical glove starch powder, and cactus spines. Some of these substances—nylon sutures, wood, talc, surgical glove starch powder, and sea urchin spines—are doubly refractile on polarizing examination. Double refraction often is very helpful in localizing foreign substances.

An *allergic* granulomatous reaction to a foreign body typically shows a sarcoidal or tuberculoid pattern consisting of epithelioid cells with or without giant cells. Phagocytosis of the foreign substance is slight or absent. Substances that in sensitized persons produce an allergic granulomatous reaction are, for instance, zirconium, beryllium, and certain dyes used in tattoos. Some substances that at first act as foreign material may later on, after sensitization has occurred, act as allergens, as in the case of sea urchin spines and silica.

Conditions to consider in the differential diagnosis:

> keratin granuloma
> > ruptured cyst
> > folliculitis
>
> foreign-body granulomas
> sporotrichosis
> persistent arthropod bite
> syphilis, secondary and tertiary
> cryptococcosis
> candidal granuloma
> nontuberculosis mycobacteria
> cat-scratch disease
> North American blastomycosis
> South American blastomycosis
> chromomycosis
> pheohyphomycosis
> coccidioidomycosis

VE5 Inflammatory Nodules With Prominent Eosinophils

The nodular dermal infiltrates contain many eosinophils often admixed with lymphocytes. Angiolymphoid hyperplasia is a good example (77).

Angiolymphoid Hyperplasia With Eosinophilia

Epithelioid Hemangioma

Kimura Disease

CLINICAL SUMMARY. Lesions of angiolymphoid hyperplasia with eosinophilia (ALHE) may arise superficially in the dermis, or in the subcutaneous or deeper tissues. Superficial lesions, which have been referred to as pseudopyogenic granuloma or epithelioid hemangioma (78), present often in young to middle-aged women with pruritic papules and plaques often at or around the external ear or elsewhere in the head and neck. Lesions of subcutaneous and deeper tissues typically present as a solitary, slowly growing, firm, subcutaneous swelling up to 10 cm in size usually in the head and neck region with some predilection for the pre- or postauricular sites. Blood eosinophilia and modest enlargement of neighboring lymph nodes and salivary tissue may occur. The conditions are chronic, but serious complications do not occur. Synonymous or related terms for ALHE have included inflammatory angiomatous nodule, pseudopyogenic granuloma, eosinophilic granuloma of soft tissue, eosinophilic lymphofolliculosis, eosinophilic hyperplastic lymphogranuloma, epithelioid hemangioma, epithelioid hemangioendothelioma, histiocytoid hemangioma, and angioblastic lymphoid hyperplasia.

When ALHE was first described in Western Europe, similarities to *Kimura disease* as reported in the Far East were noted. However, more recently most authorities emphasize differences between the two entities. Angiolymphoid hyperplasia and Kimura disease occur most commonly in the head and neck region in adults and both share the histologic features of extensive lymphoid proliferation, tissue eosinophilia, and evidence of vascular hyperplasia. Kimura disease, however, demonstrates a wider age span with male predominance and a tendency for more extensive lesions to occur, often with involvement of salivary tissue and lymph nodes and at sites distant from the head and neck region.

HISTOPATHOLOGY. The main components of the pathology are: (1) Proliferation of small to medium-sized blood vessels often showing a lobular architecture and lined by greatly enlarged (epithelioid) endothelial cells; (2) A perivascular inflammatory cell infiltrate composed mainly of lymphocytes and eosinophils; (3) Nodular areas of lymphocytic infiltrate occurring with or without follicle formation; and (4) Inflammatory vascular occlusive changes in medium-sized arteries associated with endothelial cell proliferation.

In superficial lesions there is variable vascular hyperplasia that can include areas in which the proliferation is almost angiomatous. A distinctive feature is the "cobblestone" or "hobnail" appearance of enlarged endothelial cells that project into the lumina of some vessels. These cells lack atypia or mitotic activity. Affected vessels often contain endothelial cells with intracytoplasmic vacuoles, the so-called "histiocytoid hemangioma" pattern. In subcutaneous lesions the inflammatory cell infiltrate is usually more massive, with a central, poorly circumscribed nodule that replaces the fat. The nodule is composed of confluent sheets of small lymphocytes and eosinophils in which a network of poorly canalized thick-walled capillaries is embedded. Satellite smaller islands of lymphoid cells with lymphoid follicles usually surround the central nodule. Commonly, there is involvement of medium- to large-sized arteries, with infiltration of the vessel wall by inflammatory cells and occlusion of the lumen.

Histologic differences between ALHE and Kimura disease include the lesser degree of exuberant vascular hyperplasia lacking prominent eosinophilic endothelial cells and the absence of uncanalized blood vessels in Kimura disease. Other points of difference are eosinophilic abscesses and marked fibrosis around the lesions in Kimura disease and the absence of lesions centered around damaged arteries. There is an important association between Kimura disease and nephrotic syndrome.

Scabetic Nodule

The clinical features of scabies, caused by the mite *Sarcoptes scabei*, include a pruritic rash which tends to occur in

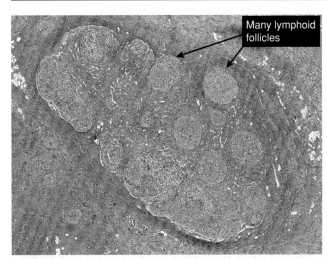

Fig. VE5.a

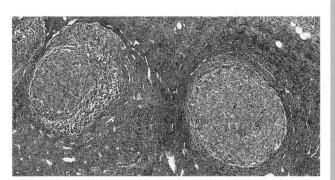

Fig. VE5.b

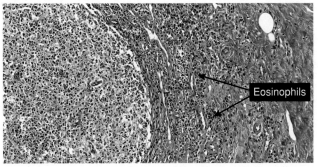

Fig. VE5.c

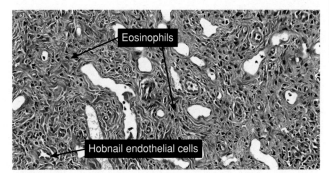

Fig. VE5.d

Fig. VE5.a. *Kimura disease, low power.* A nodular cluster of lymphoid follicles in the deep dermis and subcutaneous tissue.

Fig. VE5.b. *Kimura disease, medium power.* The follicles are surrounded by fibrosis and separated by a meshwork of prominent small vessels.

Fig. VE5.c. *Kimura disease, medium power.* Eosinophils are often abundant.

Fig. VE5.d. *Kimura disease, high power.* The endothelial cells lining the small vessels are swollen and may protrude into the lumen, imparting a cobblestone appearance.

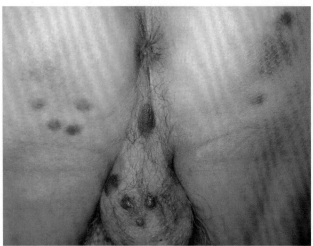

Clin. Fig. VE5

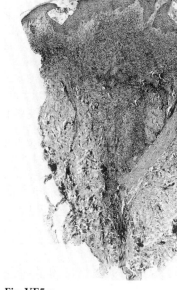

Fig. VE5.e

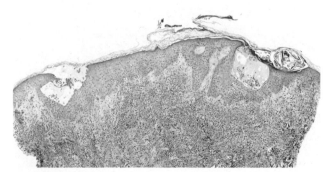

Fig. VE5.f

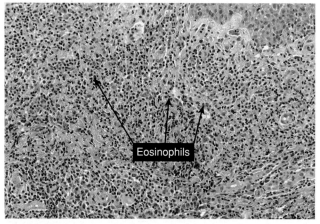

Fig. VE5.g

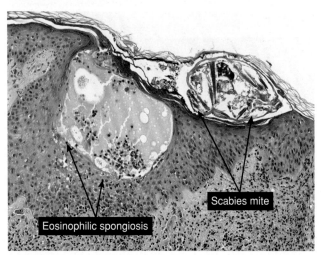

Fig. VE5.h

Clin. Fig. VE5. *Scabetic nodules.* Erythematous nodules in the genital and intertriginous areas of a 70-year-old man.

Fig. VE5.e. *Scabies infestation, low power.* A dense infiltrate in the reticular dermis. If mites are not appreciated in the epidermis, the diagnosis of scabies may be missed.

Fig. VE5.f, g. *Scabies infestation, low and high power.* In the dermis, eosinophils are a conspicuous component of the inflammatory infiltrate.

Fig. VE5.h. *Scabies infestation, high power.* Spongiosis as well as eosinophilic spongiosis may be seen in the epidermis. A scabies mite is present in the stratum corneum.

skin folds. Burrows caused by movement of the causative mites may be seen. There are often changes secondary to scratching and infection. The findings overlap with those of other skin conditions, and pathognomonic features may not be present or easily demonstrable. Skin scrapings for scabies are prone to false negatives (79). "Persistent nodules in scabies" or "nodular scabies" seem to represent a prolonged response of immune cells to mite antigens (80).

Conditions to consider in the differential diagnosis:

> angiolymphoid hyperplasia with eosinophils
> Kimura disease
> scabetic nodule
> arthropod assault reaction (e.g., insect or spider etc. bite or sting)

VE6 | Inflammatory Nodules With Mixed Cell Types

There is a variety of cells in the infiltrate, including neutrophils, histiocytes, plasma cells, giant cells, and lymphocytes. Sporotrichosis is a good example (81).

Sporotrichosis

CLINICAL SUMMARY. Clinical sporotrichosis usually occurs as one of two primary cutaneous forms, either the fixed cutaneous or the lymphocutaneous form. Both result from direct inoculation at a site of minor trauma. Systemic sporotrichosis is rare and more commonly follows pulmonary infection in association with immunosuppression. The lymphocutaneous form of sporotrichosis starts with a painless papule that grows into an ulcer, usually on a finger or hand. Subsequently, a chain of asymptomatic nodules appears along the lymph vessel draining the area, in a pattern of "lymphangitic" or "sporotrichoid" spread. These lymphatic nodules may undergo suppuration with subsequent ulceration. In the fixed cutaneous form, a solitary plaque or occasionally a group of lesions is seen, most commonly on an arm or the face. It may show superficial crusting or a verrucous surface. There is no tendency toward lymphatic spread.

HISTOPATHOLOGY. Early lesions of primary cutaneous sporotrichosis usually show a nonspecific inflammatory infiltrate composed of neutrophils, lymphoid cells, plasma cells, and histiocytes. In an older lesion with an elevated border or a verrucous appearance, small abscesses are often found in the hyperplastic epidermis, and the dermis contains small abscesses and granulomas often associated with asteroid bodies and scattered through a lymphoplasmacytic infiltrate with eosinophils and giant cells. Later, through coalescence, a characteristic arrangement of the infiltrate in three zones may develop. These include a central "suppurative" zone

composed of neutrophils; a "tuberculoid" zone with epithelioid cells and multinucleated histiocytes; and peripherally, a "round cell" zone of lymphoid cells and plasma cells.

The nodules of sporotrichosis at first show scattered granulomas within an inflammatory infiltrate, predominantly in the deep dermis and subcutaneous fat. These enlarge and coalesce to form irregularly shaped suppurative granulomata, and eventually a large abscess surrounded by zones of histiocytes and lymphocytes as described for primary lesions.

In many instances, it is not possible to recognize the causative organisms of *S. schenckii* in tissue sections. Immunohistochemical staining may increase the yield. In a recent study of 119 samples of confirmed cutaneous sporotrichosis, the fungus was not seen in 65% of the specimens. The authors note that histopathologic changes related to older lesions or to a more developed immune response were directly associated with absence of the organism (81). If present, the spores of *Sporotrichum schenckii* appear as round to oval bodies 4 to 6 mm in diameter that stain more strongly at the periphery than in the center. Single or occasionally multiple buds are present. In some instances, small, cigar-shaped bodies up to 8 mm long are also present. Asteroid bodies in sporotrichosis consist of a central spore 5 to 10 mm in diameter surrounded by radiating elongations of a homogeneous eosinophilic material, known as the Splendore–Hoeppli phenomenon and thought to represent deposition of antigen–antibody complexes and host debris.

Atypical Mycobacteria

CLINICAL SUMMARY. Among the nontuberculosis, nonleprosy mycobacterial infections of the skin, important species include *Mycobacterium marinum* and the rapidly growing mycobacteria: *M. fortuitum, M. abscessus,* and *M. chelonae* (82). Unlike *M. tuberculosis,* which is transmitted from person to person, nontuberculosis mycobacteria are abundant in nature, in soil and water, and contact is frequent in most zones of the world.

These skin infections may be acquired by direct inoculation into the skin or by hematogenous spread from a visceral focus. Increased use of immunosuppression in medicine (e.g., for transplantation and cancer chemotherapy) and the pandemic of HIV/AIDS have resulted in many more mycobacterial skin infections. The cell-mediated immune system is a major defense against such organisms and is affected or destroyed during the course of these immunosuppressive conditions. The clinical and histopathologic patterns are also altered, with organisms being found in greater density than in immunocompetent persons.

HISTOPATHOLOGY. The histopathologic picture in nontuberculosis mycobacterioses is just as variable as the clinical picture and may present nonspecific acute and

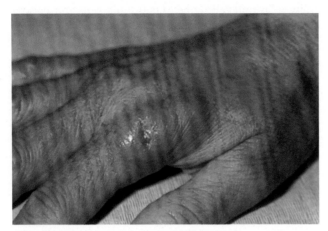

Clin. Fig. VE6.a

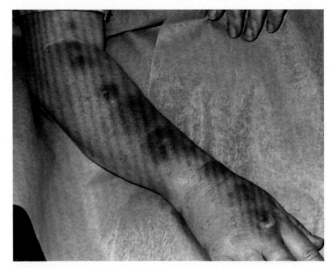

Clin. Fig. VE6.b

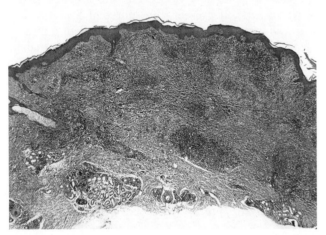

Fig. VE6.a

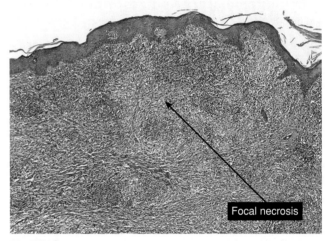

Fig. VE6.b

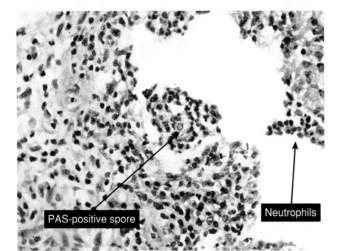

Fig. VE6.c

Clin. Fig. VE6.a. *Sporotrichosis.* An ulcerated nodule developed after the area was pricked by a rose bush.

Clin. Fig. VE6.b. *Sporotrichosis.* Subsequently nodules along the draining lymph vessels appeared (a "sporotrichoid" pattern of spread).

Fig. VE6.a. *Sporotrichosis, low power.* A patchy to diffuse infiltrate spanning the dermis.

Fig. VE6.b. *Sporotrichosis, medium power.* Focal areas of necrosis can be appreciated within the infiltrate, which in some areas is granulomatous.

Fig. VE6.c. *Sporotrichosis, high power.* PAS stain. A rare small spore is identified in the area of inflammation.

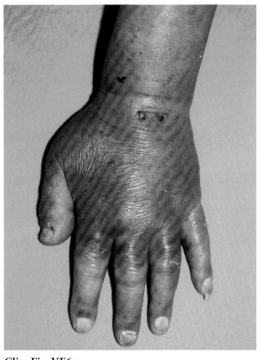

Clin. Fig. VE6.c

Clin. Fig. VE6.c. *Mycobacterium chelonae infection.* A 72-year-old man developed painful swelling and erythema of his hand after being injured on the proximal thumb nail fold by a rusty iron rod while farming (defects are biopsy and culture sites).

Fig. VE6.d. *Atypical mycobacteria.* There is an ill-defined cellular lesion in the dermis.

Fig. VE6.e. *Atypical mycobacteria.* The inflammatory infiltrate constituting the lesion is comprised of a mixed population of cells including neutrophils (which may predominate in some cases), plasma cells, histiocytes, and giant cells.

Fig. VE6.f. *Atypical mycobacteria.* Some foamy histiocytes are present in the infiltrate. These may predominate in some lesions with a high load of organisms.

Fig. VE6.g. *Atypical mycobacteria.* Acid-fast bacilli are often readily demonstrable, usually within the cytoplasm of histiocytes.

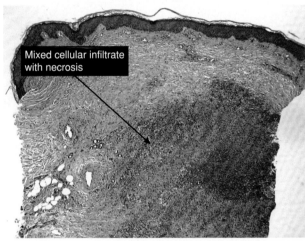

Mixed cellular infiltrate with necrosis

Fig. VE6.d

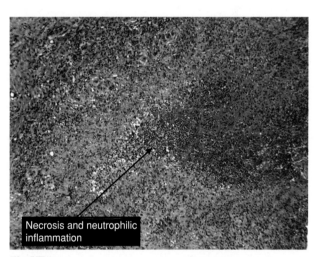

Necrosis and neutrophilic inflammation

Fig. VE6.e

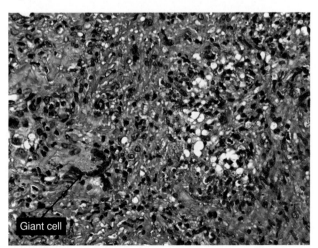

Giant cell

Fig. VE6.f

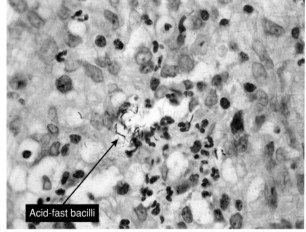

Acid-fast bacilli

Fig. VE6.g

V · Perivascular, Diffuse, and Granulomatous Infiltrates of the Reticular Dermis

chronic inflammation, suppuration and abscess formation, or tuberculoid granulomas with or without caseation (83). In some instances, both tissue reactions occur concurrently. The presence or absence of acid-fast bacilli depends on the tissue reaction. In suppurative lesions, numerous acid-fast bacilli often can be found.

Conditions to consider in the differential diagnosis:

> chronic bacterial infections
> keratin granuloma
> > ruptured cyst
> > folliculitis
> sporotrichosis
> rhinoscleroma (Klebsiella rhinoscleromatis)
> atypical mycobacteria

> Mycobacterium avium-intracellulare
> > Mycobacterium marinum
> > Mycobacterium abscessus
> nocardiosis
> lobomycosis
> protothecosis

VE7 Inflammatory Nodules With Necrosis and Neutrophils (Abscesses)

Inflammatory nodules characterized by central suppurative necrosis, with neutrophils adjacent to the necrosis, and often with granulation tissue, mixed inflammatory cells including epithelioid histiocytes and giant cells, and fibrosis at the periphery. Botryomycosis is prototypic (84).

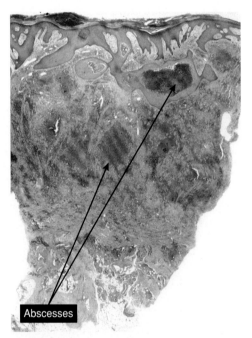

Fig. VE7.a

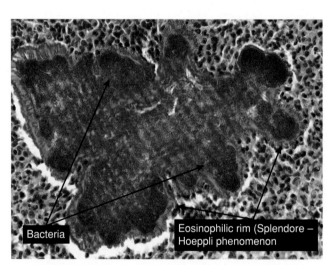

Fig. VE7.b

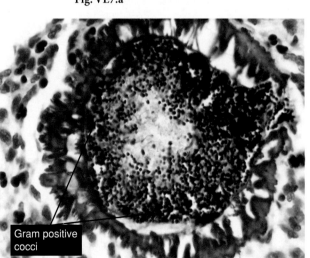

Fig. VE7.c

Fig. VE7.a. *Botryomycosis, low power.* There is pseudoepitheliomatous hyperplasia of the epidermis, and there are small abscesses in the dermis. (S. Lucas.)

Fig. VE7.b. *Botryomycosis, medium power.* An abscess within which is a basophilic bacterial colony with a surrounding eosinophilic Splendore–Hoeppli phenomenon. (S. Lucas.)

Fig. VE7.c. *Botryomycosis, high power.* A staphylococcal lesion showing gram-positive cocci (centrally they are degenerate and nonstaining). (S. Lucas.)

Botryomycosis

CLINICAL SUMMARY. Botryomycosis is a chronic suppurative infection of skin (and other organs such as lungs and meninges) in which pyogenic bacteria form granules similar to those seen in mycetoma. Most patients have no known immune defect. The skin lesions are local nodules, ulcers, or sinuses communicating with deep abscesses. They occur mainly on the extremities.

HISTOPATHOLOGY. The dermal inflammation is predominantly that of neutrophilic abscesses with surrounding granulation tissue and fibrosis. Within the abscesses are granules (grains) shaped like a bunch of grapes, hence the name of the disease. The grains, which may range up to 2 mm in diameter, are composed of closely aggregated nonfilamentous bacteria with a peripheral, radial deposition of intensely eosinophilic material—a Splendore–Hoeppli (HS) reaction. The bacteria are usually *Staphylococcus aureus,* but streptococci and certain gram-negative bacilli such as *Proteus, Pseudomonas,* and *E. coli* are sometimes found. The overlying epithelium often exhibits pseudoepitheliomatous hyperplasia. Transepithelial elimination of grains may be observed.

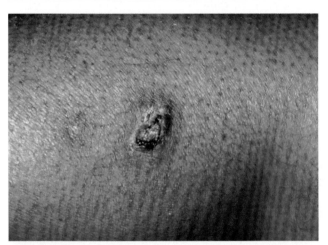

Clin. Fig. VE7

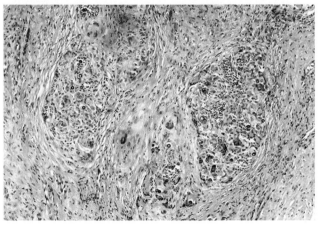

Fig. VE7.e

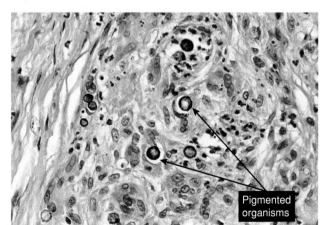

Ulceration and dense vaguely nodular infiltrates

Fig. VE7.d

Pigmented organisms

Fig. VE7.f

Clin. Fig. VE7. *Chromoblastomycosis.* Skin biopsy in the center of this ulcerated, crusted plaque revealed the characteristic, dark brown spores.

Fig. VE7.d. *Chromoblastomycosis, low power.* An ulcerated epidermis overlies a mixed cell inflammatory infiltrate in the dermis.

Fig. VE7.e. *Chromoblastomycosis, medium power.* The infiltrate includes lymphocytes and epithelioid cells with giant cells but without well-formed epithelioid cell granulomas.

Fig. VE7.f. *Chromoblastomycosis, high power.* The organisms appear as dark brown, thick-walled, ovoid, or spheric spores lying within giant cells as well as free in the tissue.

Chromoblastomycosis

CLINICAL SUMMARY. Chromoblastomycosis is a slowly progressive cutaneous mycosis caused by pigmented (dematiaceous) fungi that occur as round, nonbudding forms in tissue sections. In as much as budding is absent, the designation chromoblastomycosis is somewhat inappropriate. The causative fungi are saprophytes that can be found growing in soil, decaying vegetation, or rotten wood in subtropical and tropical countries. The primary lesion is thought to develop as a result of traumatic implantation of the fungus into the skin. The lesions are most common on the lower extremities and consist of verrucous papules, nodules, and plaques that may itch. The most common cause of chromoblastomycosis is *Fonsecea pedrosoi* (85).

HISTOPATHOLOGY. The cutaneous type of chromoblastomycosis resembles North American blastomycosis in histologic appearance with a lichenoid granulomatous inflammatory pattern, with pseudoepitheliomatous epidermal hyperplasia and an extensive dermal infiltrate composed of many epithelioid histiocytes, as well as multinucleated giant cells, small abscesses with clusters of neutrophils, and variable numbers of lymphocytes, plasma cells, and eosinophils. Tuberculoid formations may be present, but caseation necrosis is absent. The causative organisms are found within giant cells as well as free in the tissue, especially in the abscesses. They appear as conspicuous, dark brown, thick-walled, ovoid or spheric spores varying in size from 6 to 12 µm and lying either singly or in chains or clusters. In a study of 27 cases of chromoblastomycosis from Brazil, sclerotic bodies were noted in 92.5% of cases (86). Fontana staining and the use of unstained and destained sections can be helpful in identifying the causative organism (87).

Conditions to consider in the differential diagnosis:

> acute or chronic bacterial abscesses
> deep fungal infections
>> phaeohyphomycotic cyst
>> North American blastomycosis
>> chromoblastomycosis
>> cutaneous alternariosis
>> paracoccidioidomycosis
>> coccidioidomycosis
>> sporotrichosis
> atypical mycobacteria
> botryomycosis
> actinomycosis
> nocardiosis
> cat scratch disease
> erythema nodosum leprosum (Type 2 leprosy reaction)
> scrofuloderma
> tuberculous gumma
> protothecosis

VE8   Inflammatory Nodules With Prominent Necrosis

Necrosis is a striking feature along with variable but sometimes sparse infiltrates of inflammatory cells that may include plasma cells, epithelioid histiocytes, neutrophils, lymphocytes, and hemorrhage. Organisms may be demonstrable. Aspergillosis is prototypic (88).

Aspergillosis

CLINICAL SUMMARY. Cutaneous aspergillosis may occur as a primary infection or may be secondary to disseminated aspergillosis. The lesions of primary cutaneous aspergillosis are usually found at an intravenous infusion site. One observes either one or several macules, papules, plaques, or hemorrhagic bullae, which may rapidly progress into necrotic ulcers that are covered by a heavy black eschar. Death often results from secondary systemic dissemination of the aspergillosis. Primary cutaneous infection has been seen in patients with AIDS. In addition, *Aspergillus* may colonize burn or surgical wounds and subsequently invade viable tissue; in these cases, the prognosis is generally good. Secondary cutaneous aspergillosis, usually associated with invasive lung disease, shows multiple scattered lesions as a result of embolic, hematogenous spread, and has a poor prognosis.

HISTOPATHOLOGY. Unlike most deep cutaneous fungal infections, cutaneous aspergillosis is not characteristically associated with pseudoepitheliomatous epidermal hyperplasia. In the more serious primary forms and in the secondary disseminated form, numerous *Aspergillus* hyphae are seen in the dermis with hematoxylin-eosin–stained sections, or with PAS or silver methenamine staining. The 2- to 4-µm hyphae are often arranged in a radiate fashion, are septate, and branch at an acute angle. Hyphae characteristically invade blood vessels giving rise to areas of ischemic necrosis with very little inflammation in some instances. In other cases, there may be an acute inflammatory reaction with polymorphonuclear leukocytes in addition to lymphocytes and histiocytes. In patients with primary cutaneous or subcutaneous aspergillosis who are otherwise in good health, the number of hyphae present is relatively small, and there may be a well-developed granulomatous reaction.

Conditions to consider in the differential diagnosis:

> tertiary syphilis
> tertiary yaws
> aspergillosis
> zygomycosis (mucormycosis)
> tuberculosis
> atypical mycobacteria
> infarcts
> deep vasculitis
> deep thrombi

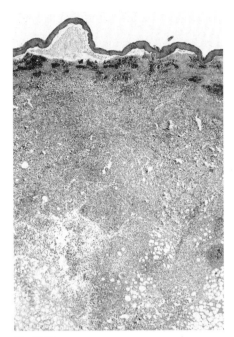

Fig. VE8.a

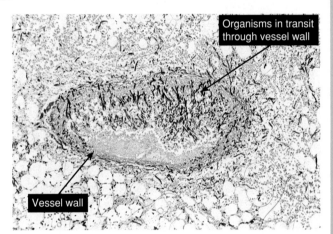

Fig. VE8.b

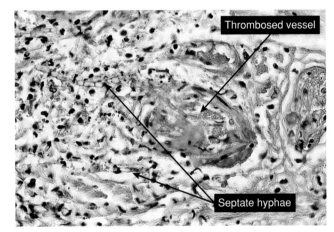

Fig. VE8.c

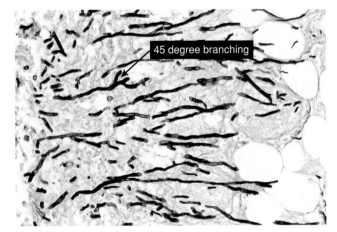

Fig. VE8.d

Fig. VE8.e

Fig. VE8.a. *Cutaneous aspergillosis, low power.* There is an extensive dermal inflammatory infiltrate throughout most of the field, with a less cellular area of necrosis at the lower left of the image. The epidermis has separated due to ischemic changes of basal keratinocytes.

Fig. VE8.b. *Cutaneous aspergillosis, medium power.* At the periphery of the necrotic area (lower left), there is an inflammatory infiltrate in the viable dermis. Both areas are extensively infiltrated by fungal hyphae.

Fig. VE8.c. *Cutaneous aspergillosis, high power.* A thrombosed vessel surrounded by acute inflammatory cells, with fungal hyphae of Aspergillus organisms in typical pose spanning the vessel wall.

Fig. VE8.d. *Cutaneous aspergillosis, medium power, silver stain for fungi.* Black stained fungal hyphae in the vessel lumen, wall, and surrounding tissue.

Fig. VE8.e. *Cutaneous aspergillosis, high power, silver stain for fungi.* The hyphae are narrow, fairly uniform, septate, and tend to branch at acute angles.

V   Perivascular, Diffuse, and Granulomatous Infiltrates of the Reticular Dermis

calciphylaxis
frostbite
necrobiotic xanthogranuloma with paraproteinemia
gangrenous ischemic necrosis
epithelioid sarcoma

VE9 Chronic Ulcers and Sinuses Involving the Reticular Dermis

A chronic ulcer is characterized by central suppurative necrosis, with neutrophils adjacent to the necrosis, and often with granulation tissue, fibrosis, and reactive epithelium at the periphery. A sinus extends deeper into the dermis than most ulcers, in a serpentine fashion. A fistula is an abnormal communication between two epithelial-lined surfaces. The histologic architecture of fistulas and sinuses is similar to that of chronic ulcers. Chancroid is a good example of a chronic ulcer (89).

Chancroid

CLINICAL SUMMARY. Chancroid, caused by *Haemophilus ducreyi*, is a sexually transmitted disease leading to one or several ulcers, chiefly in the genital region. The ulcers exhibit little if any induration and often have undermined borders. They are usually tender. Inguinal lymphadenitis, either unilateral or bilateral, is common and, unless treated, often results in an inguinal abscess.

HISTOPATHOLOGY. The histologic changes beneath the ulcer are sufficiently distinct to permit a presumptive diagnosis of chancroid in many instances. The lesion consists of three zones overlying each other and shows characteristic vascular changes. The surface zone at the floor of the ulcer is rather narrow and consists of neutrophils, fibrin, erythrocytes, and necrotic tissue. The next zone is fairly wide and contains many newly formed

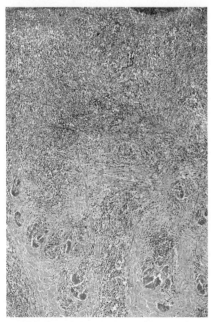

Clin. Fig. VE9.a

Clin. Fig. VE9.a. *Chancroid.* Multiple, painful, nonindurated ulcers require investigation for this venereal disease.

Fig. VE9.a. *Chancroid, low power.* Cutaneous ulcer with the characteristic three-zone pattern of inflammation—a superficial acute inflammatory exudate, a midzone of granulation tissue, and a deep zone of plasma cells and lymphocytes. (S. Lucas.)

Fig. VE9.b. *Chancroid, medium power.* The superficial necrotic zone and underlying granulation tissue. (S. Lucas.)

Fig. VE9.c. *Chancroid, high power.* A Giemsa stained image from the superficial necrotic zone, containing bacilli lying in parallel chains. (S. Lucas, courtesy of A. Freinkel.)

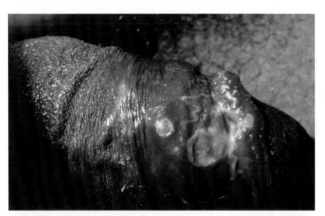

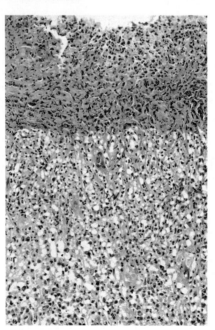

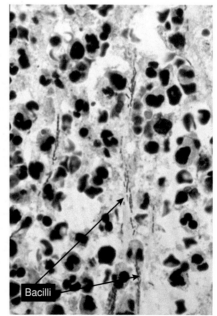

Bacilli

Fig. VE9.a   **Fig. VE9.b**   **Fig. VE9.c**

blood vessels showing marked proliferation of their endothelial cells. As a result of the endothelial proliferation, the lumina of the vessels are often occluded, leading to thrombosis. In addition, there are degenerative changes in the walls of the vessels. The deep zone is composed of a dense infiltrate of plasma cells and lymphoid cells. Demonstration of bacilli in tissue sections stained with Giemsa stain or Gram stain is occasionally possible. The bacilli are most apt to be found between the cells of the surface zone. *H. ducreyi* is a fine, short, gram-negative coccobacillus, measuring about 1.5 by 0.2 μm, often arranged in parallel chains.

Pyoderma Gangrenosum

CLINICAL SUMMARY. The lesions begin as tender papulopustules or as folliculitis that eventually may ulcerate. In the fully developed stage, the lesions have a raised, undermined border, which has a dusky purple hue. Pyoderma gangrenosum may occur as an isolated cutaneous phenomenon or may be a cutaneous manifestation associated with various systemic disease processes, such as inflammatory bowel disease, connective tissue diseases, and lymphoproliferative lesions. Trauma is a common inciting factor, with surgical incisions being a frequently reported instigator.

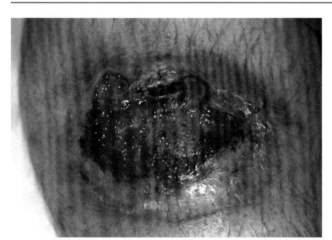

Clin. Fig. VE9.b

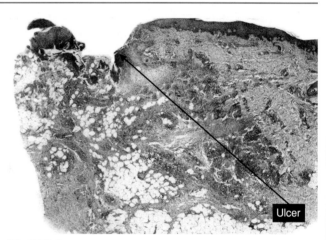

Ulcer

Fig. VE9.d

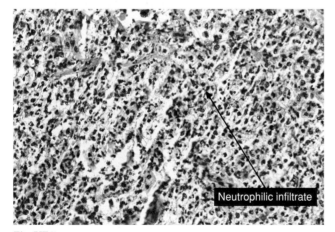

Neutrophilic infiltrate

Fig. VE9.e

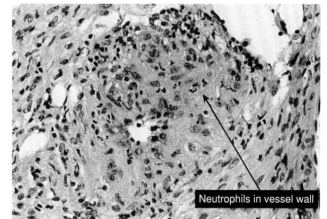

Neutrophils in vessel wall

Fig. VE9.f

Clin. Fig. VE9.b. *Pyoderma gangrenosum.* A 25-year-old man with ulcerative colitis developed a fluctuant calf nodule which broke down into a painful enlarging ulcer with purple-red undermined borders.

Fig. VE9.d. *Pyoderma gangrenosum, low power.* A punched-out ulcer with an undermined edge extending deeply into the dermis.

Fig. VE9.e. *Pyoderma gangrenosum, medium power.* The ulcer base is lined by an intense infiltrate of neutrophils.

Fig. VE9.f. *Pyoderma gangrenosum, high power.* Neutrophils are present in a vessel walls without true vasculitis, which requires fibrinoid necrosis. Necrotizing vasculitis that may be seen at the surface of acute ulcers may be secondary to the ulcer, and should not necessarily be considered pathogenic.

Commonly the lesions are located on the legs, breast, and abdomen, and peristomal areas may also occur. Pyoderma gangrenosum often heals with a cribiform scar (90,91).

HISTOPATHOLOGY. The histologic findings are nonspecific and the diagnosis is primarily clinical. Most authors studying early lesions have reported a primarily neutrophilic infiltrate, which frequently involves follicular structures, but is often also diffuse, and may overlap with a Sweet reaction. Others, however, have stated that the lesions begin with a lymphocytic reaction. Degrees of vessel involvement range from none to fibrinoid necrosis.

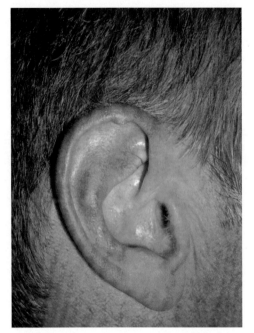

Clin. Fig. VE9.c

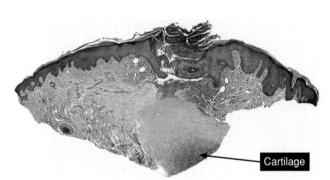

Fig. VE9.g

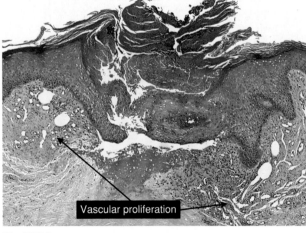

Fig. VE9.h

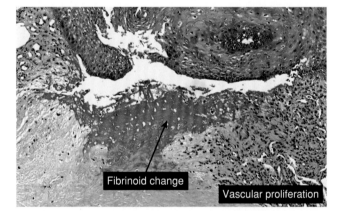

Fig. VE9.i

Clin. Fig. VE9.c. *Chondrodermatitis nodularis helicis.* This tender, crusted nodule on the superior helix requires biopsy to distinguish from skin carcinoma.

Fig. VE9.g. *Chondrodermatitis nodularis helicis.* Hyperkeratosis and a hyperplastic epithelium are associated with a focal ulcer and an inflammatory reaction that extends to the cartilage of the ear.

Fig. VE9.h. *Chondrodermatitis nodularis helicis.* Beneath the focal ulcer there is a characteristic zone of eosinophilic degeneration of collagen extending to the cartilage.

Fig. VE9.i. *Chondrodermatitis nodularis helicis.* Around the zone of eosinophilic degeneration, there is a proliferation of small mature vascular channels with inflammatory cells.

In the majority of lesions, a neutrophilic infiltrate is present with some, but limited, vascular damage. Outright vasculitis has been reported and has led to speculations about its possible role in the etiology of pyoderma gangrenosum. Focal vasculitis is often observed in fully developed lesions, but appears secondary to the inflammatory process. The infiltrate tends to be deeper and more extensive than that in classic Sweet syndrome. Fully developed lesions exhibit ulceration, necrosis, and a mixed inflammatory cell infiltrate. The pattern of breakdown of tissue that results from these processes has been termed "pathergy." Involvement of the deep reticular dermis and subcutis may exhibit primarily mononuclear cell and granulomatous inflammatory reactions. The key histologic differential diagnosis is that of an infectious process.

Chondrodermatitis Nodularis Helicis

The etiology of chondrodermatitis nodularis helicis (CNH) is unknown, but may involve local ischemia. Clinically the lesion presents as a solitary firm pink to pearly gray crusted nodule, about 4 to 6 mm in size. The nodule usually enlarges rapidly to a maximum size and remains stable. Biopsy is often indicated; the differential diagnosis includes actinic keratosis, basal cell carcinoma, keratoacanthoma, and squamous cell carcinoma (92).

Conditions to consider in the differential diagnosis:

> pyoderma gangrenosum
> ecthyma gangrenosum
> deep fungal infection
> > North American blastomycosis
> > eumycetoma
> tuberculosis cutis orificialis
> enterocutaneous fistula
> chondrodermatitis nodularis helicis
> ecthyma
> papulonecrotic tuberculid
> Buruli ulcer (M. ulcerans)
> chancroid (Haemophilus ducreyi)
> granuloma inguinale (Calymmatobacterium granulomatis)
> lymphogranuloma venereum (Chlamydia trachomatis)
> follicular occlusion disorder
> > pilonidal sinus
> > hidradenitis suppurativa
> > acne conglobata
> > perifolliculitis capitis abscedens et suffodiens (dissecting cellulitis of the scalp)
> Anthrax (Bacillus anthracis)
> Tularemia (Francisella tularensis)
> cutaneous leishmaniasis
> necrotizing sialometaplasia of hard palate
> eosinophilic ulcer of the tongue

VF DERMAL MATRIX FIBER DISORDERS

The dermis serves as a reaction site for a variety of inflammatory, infiltrative, and desmoplastic processes. These may include accumulations or deficiencies of dermal fibrous and nonfibrous matrix constituents as reactions to a variety of stimuli.

1. Fiber Disorders, Collagen Increased
2. Fiber Disorders, Collagen Reduced
3. Fiber Disorders, Elastin Increased or Prominent
4. Fiber Disorders, Elastin Reduced
5. Fiber Disorders, Perforating

VF1 Fiber Disorders, Collagen Increased

Dermal collagen is increased with production at the dermal–subcutaneous interface. Inflammation is seen at this site. The inflammatory cells are lymphocytes, plasma cells, and eosinophils. Fibroblasts in some instances are increased. Scleroderma is the prototype (93).

Scleroderma

CLINICAL SUMMARY. Scleroderma is a connective tissue disorder characterized by thickening and fibrosis of the skin. Two types of scleroderma exist: circumscribed scleroderma (*morphea*) and systemic scleroderma (*progressive systemic sclerosis*). In morphea, the lesions usually are limited to the skin and to the subcutaneous tissue beneath the cutaneous lesions. Morphea may be divided according to morphology and distribution of lesions into six types: guttate, plaque, linear, segmental, subcutaneous, and generalized. The underlying cause of morphea is unknown, but its development is thought to require a predisposition and a trigger from the environment. Known triggers include trauma, radiation, medications, and infections. Autoimmunity is also suspected to play a role (94).

Lesions of the plaque type, the most common, are indurated, with a smooth surface, and an ivory color with a violaceous border in growing lesions, the so-called lilac ring. Guttate lesions are small and superficial. Linear lesions may have the configuration of a saber-cut (*coup de sabre*). Segmental morphea occurs on one side of the face, resulting in hemiatrophy. In subcutaneous morphea (morphea profunda) the involved skin is thickened and bound to the underlying fascia and muscle. Generalized morphea comprises very extensive cases showing a combination of several of the five types just described.

In systemic scleroderma, visceral lesions are present in addition to involvement of the skin and the subcutaneous tissue, leading to death in some patients. The indurated lesions of the skin are not sharply demarcated or "circumscribed," as in morphea. Facial changes include a mask-like expressionless face, and tightening of the skin around the mouth associated with radial folds. There may be diffuse hyperpigmentation, mainly in diffuse systemic scleroderma. The hands show nonpitting edema involving the dorsa of the fingers, hands, and forearms. Gradually the fingers become tapered, the skin becomes hard, and flexion contractures form. These changes, referred to as acrosclerosis, are associated with Raynaud phenomenon. Macular telangiectasias on the face and hands, calcinosis cutis on the extremities, and ulcerations, especially on the tips of the fingers, over the knuckles, and on the lower extremities, occur predominantly in acrosclerosis.

Systemic sclerosis with limited scleroderma, known as CREST syndrome is a variant of acrosclerosis that consists of several or all of the following manifestations: Calcinosis cutis, Raynaud phenomenon, involvement of the Esophagus with dysphagia, Sclerodactyly, and Telangiectases. Death from visceral lesions is rather infrequent in the CREST syndrome.

Multiple autoantibodies, many directed against intranuclear antigens such as anticentromere (ACA, anti-CENP-B), anti-topoisomerase I (anti-topo I), anti-RNA polymerase I/III, and anti-Th/To, are present in patients with scleroderma; there is controversy as to whether and to what extent these may be pathogenic (95). There are associations between the presence of specific autoantibodies and the phenotypic expression of disease as well as clinical outcome in scleroderma (96).

HISTOPATHOLOGY. The different types of morphea cannot be differentiated histologically. Early inflammatory and late sclerotic stages can be distinguished. In the early inflammatory stage, particularly at the active violaceous border, the reticular dermis collagen bundles are thickened and there is a moderately intense interstitial and perivascular inflammatory infiltrate, which is predominantly lymphocytic admixed with plasma cells. A much more pronounced inflammatory infiltrate often involves the subcutaneous fat and extends upward toward the eccrine glands. Trabeculae subdividing the subcutaneous fat are thickened by an inflammatory infiltrate and deposition of new collagen. Large areas of subcutaneous fat are replaced by newly formed collagen composed of fine, wavy fibers. Vascular changes in the early inflammatory stage may consist of endothelial swelling and edema of the walls of the vessels.

In the late sclerotic stage, as seen in the center of old lesions, the inflammatory infiltrate has disappeared almost completely, except in some areas of the subcutis. The epidermis is normal. The collagen bundles in the reticular dermis often appear thickened, closely packed, hypocellular, and hypereosinophilic. In the papillary dermis, homogeneous collagen may replace the normal loosely arranged fibers. The eccrine glands are atrophic, have few or no adipocytes surrounding them, and are surrounded by newly formed collagen. Few blood vessels are seen within the sclerotic collagen; they often have a fibrotic wall

and a narrowed lumen. Hair follicles and sebaceous glands are absent. The fascia and striated muscles underlying lesions of morphea may be affected in the linear, segmental, subcutaneous, and generalized types, showing fibrosis and sclerosis similar to that seen in subcutaneous tissue. The muscle fibers appear vacuolated and separated from one another by edema and focal collections of inflammatory cells.

The histologic appearance of the skin lesions in systemic scleroderma is similar to that of morphea so that their histologic differentiation is not possible. However, in early lesions of systemic scleroderma the inflammatory reaction is less pronounced than in morphea. The vascular changes in early lesions are slight, as in morphea. In contrast, in the late stage, systemic scleroderma shows more pronounced vascular changes than morphea, particularly in the subcutis. These changes include a paucity of blood vessels, thickening and hyalinization of their walls, and narrowing of the lumen. Even in late lesions, the epidermis usually appears normal. Aggregates of calcium may also be seen in the late stage within areas of sclerotic, homogeneous collagen of the subcutaneous tissue.

Some patients have coexistent changes of morphea and lichen sclerosis. In a large study, compared with the incidence in the general population, lichen sclerosus was 18-fold more frequent in patients with localized scleroderma (morphea) (97).

Radiation Dermatitis

CLINICAL SUMMARY. Early or acute radiation dermatitis develops after large doses of x-rays or radium. Erythema develops within about a week, and may heal with desquamation and pigmentation. If the dose was high enough, painful blisters may develop at the site of erythema. In that case, healing usually takes place with atrophy, telangiectasia, and irregular hyperpigmentation. Subsequent to very large doses ulceration occurs, generally within 2 months. Such an ulcer may heal ultimately with severe atrophic scarring, or it may not heal.

Late (chronic) radiation dermatitis occurs from a few months to many years after the administration of fractional doses of x-rays or radium. The skin shows atrophy, telangiectasia, and irregular hyper- and hypopigmentation. Ulceration, as well as foci of hyperkeratosis, may be seen within the areas of atrophy. Squamous cell carcinomas or basal cell carcinomas may develop. Minimally invasive procedures are becoming more common and pathologists should consider fluoroscopy-induced chronic radiation dermatitis when such histologic features are identified. Usually a history of radiation exposure is not provided. Characteristic sites of involvement include the axilla, scapula, and midback. Lesions can develop days to years after exposure. The clinical appearance is that of an atrophic plaque that can have ulceration and telangiectasia (98).

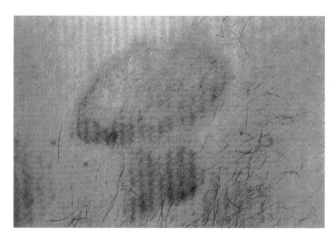

Clin. Fig. VF1.a

Fig. VF1.a

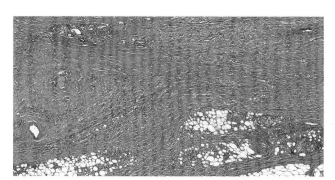

Fig. VF1.b

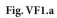
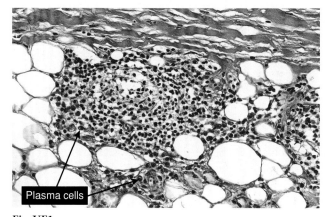

Fig. VF1.c

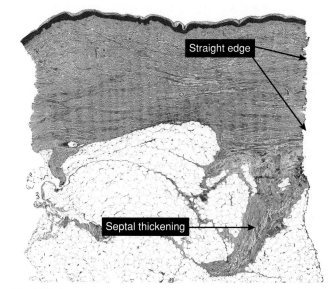

Fig. VF1.d

Clin. Fig. VF1.a. *Morphea.* Asymptomatic, indurated depressed plaques with white-appearing sclerotic centers are seen on the back of an otherwise healthy elderly male.

Fig. VF1.a. *Morphea, low power.* A late inflammatory lesion, with a patchy interstitial and perivascular inflammatory infiltrate, and partial sclerosis of dermal collagen.

Fig. VF1.b. *Morphea, medium power.* The infiltrate tends to be especially pronounced at the dermal–subcutaneous junction.

Fig. VF1.c. *Morphea, high power.* Lymphocytes and plasma cells are admixed in the infiltrate.

Fig. VF1.d. *Morphea, low power.* A late sclerotic lesion. The presence of dermal sclerosis is indicated by the straight sides of the punch biopsy. (*continues*)

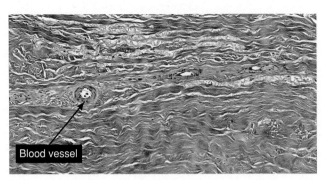

Fig. VF1.e

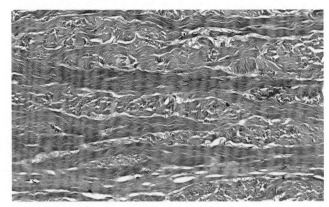

Fig. VF1.f

Fig. VF1.e. *Morphea, medium power.* Skin appendages are lost within the sclerotic reticular dermis.

Fig. VF1.f. *Morphea, high power.* The collagen bundles in the reticular dermis appear thickened, closely packed, hypocellular, and hypereosinophilic. Blood vessels are few within the sclerotic collagen.

HISTOPATHOLOGY. In early radiation dermatitis, there is intracellular edema of the epidermis with pyknosis of the nuclei of epidermal and adnexal cells. An inflammatory infiltrate is present throughout the dermis and may permeate the epidermis. Some of the blood vessels are dilated, whereas others, especially large ones in the deep dermis, show edema of their walls, endothelial proliferation, and even thrombosis. The collagen bundles are edematous. In cases with blisters, the degenerated epidermis is detached from the dermis, and there may be ulceration, with necrosis and neutrophilic infiltration.

In subacute radiation dermatitis (weeks to a few months after exposure), there is an interface dermatitis, which can include prominent satellite cell necrosis, that can resemble graft-versus-host disease (99).

In late radiation dermatitis, the epidermis is irregular, with variable atrophy and hyperplasia, often with hyperkeratosis. The cells of the stratum malpighii may be disorderly, with individual cell keratinization, and some of the nuclei may be atypical. The epidermis may also show irregular downward growth and may even grow around telangiectatic vessels, nearly enclosing them. In the dermis, the collagen bundles are swollen and often hyalinized. Large, bizarre, stellate "radiation fibroblasts" may be found, with nuclei that are enlarged, irregular, and hyperchromatic. This "radiation atypia" differs from that seen in neoplasms because the cellularity is low and the atypical nuclei are scattered among other, less atypical cells. Thus, the atypia is "random" rather than "uniform." Also, there is typically no mitotic activity. Blood vessels in the deep dermis often show fibrous thickening of their walls, nearly or entirely occluding the lumen. Some of the vessels show thrombosis and recanalization. In contrast, the vessels of the upper dermis may be telangiectatic, and there may be lymphedema in the subepidermal region. Hair structures and sebaceous glands are absent, but the sweat glands usually are preserved at least in part, except in areas of severe injury.

Nephrogenic Systemic Fibrosis

CLINICAL SUMMARY. Nephrogenic systemic fibrosis (NSF) was initially recognized in 1997, described in 2000, and was called nephrogenic fibrosing dermopathy in 2001. The name was subsequently changed to NSF to reflect the systemic involvement of the disease. Development of NSF is linked to the use of gadolinium-containing magnetic resonance imaging contrast agents in patients with renal dysfunction (100). Early lesions develop with erythema, edema, and indurated plaques of the trunk or extremities. There are large poorly defined plaques with irregular borders that become firm and indurated. The induration can become severe and disabling. The thickened fibrotic skin which develops eventually can lead to joint contractures and immobility. Early on there is edema and indurated plaques in the skin that can demonstrate polygonal, reticular, or amoeboid shapes. Papules and nodules have also been reported. Lesions are often located in a symmetric and bilateral distribution. The extremities are commonly affected. Yellow scleral plaques can also occur. The pathogenesis of NSF relates to increased collagen deposition and fibrosis that affects multiple organ systems including the lungs and heart. Skeletal muscle, the kidney, testes, and dura have also been affected. Development of NSF has been linked to decreased renal function (acute and chronic) and proinflammatory events such as surgical procedures (101). It clinically has overlap features with scleroderma and scleromyxedema. However, the patients lack antibodies to Scl-70 and they also lack the paraproteinemia that is associated with scleromyxedema. Judicious use of gadolinium-containing agents has led to reduction in the incidence of NSF (102).

HISTOPATHOLOGY. The histopathologic findings are essentially indistinguishable from those seen in scleromyxedema (103). There is a proliferation of spindled cells within the dermis and occasionally extending into the

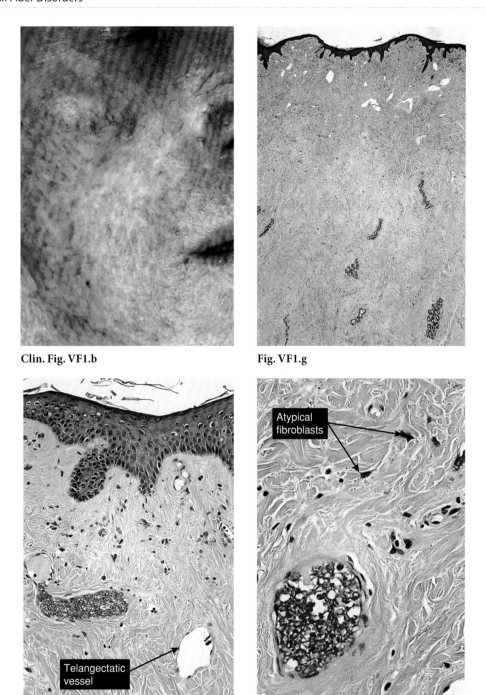

Clin. Fig. VF1.b

Fig. VF1.g

Fig. VF1.h

Fig. VF1.i

Clin. Fig. VF1.b. *Radiation dermatitis.* Chronic radiation changes of atrophy, hypopigmentation, hyperpigmentation, and telangiectases developed many years after radiation therapy for acne.

Fig. VF1.g. *Late radiation dermatitis, low power.* The dermal collagen is homogenized, telangiectatic vessels are apparent, and there are irregular down-growths of the epidermis. Adnexal structures are markedly diminished.

Fig. VF1.h. *Late radiation dermatitis, medium power.* Stellate fibroblasts are prominent in the sclerotic collagen.

Fig. VF1.i. *Late radiation dermatitis, high power.* Randomly scattered fibroblasts exhibit nuclear enlarged and hyperchromatic nuclei. There are no mitoses, and there is no contiguous proliferation of the atypical cells.

subcutaneous tissue. The epidermis is unaffected. The degree of cellularity and mucin deposition is variable depending on the age of the lesion. Calcification and osseous metaplasia may occur in long-standing lesions. Characteristically, the spindle cells are positive with antibodies to CD34 and procollagen I. Early lesions show collagen bundles with edema and varying amounts of mucin. Elastic fibers are increased. Later lesions show thickened collagen bundles and there are smaller clefts between collagen bundles, but the clefts are maintained (104,105). Since these findings are indistinguishable from scleromyxedema, that diagnosis must be differentiated based on clinical findings. Scleroderma and scleredema fail to reveal the spindle cell hypercellularity as one sees in NSF.

Regressing Melanoma

Melanomas may clinical undergo partial (or rarely, complete) regression with appearance of a gray area within the lesion that may progressively adopt the normal skin morphology. Histologic changes are characteristic (106).

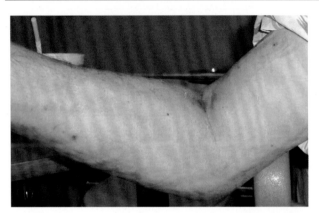

Clin. Fig. VF1.c

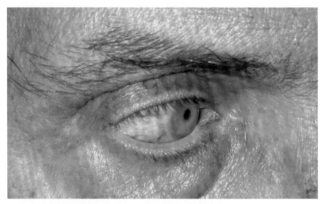

Clin. Fig. VF1.d

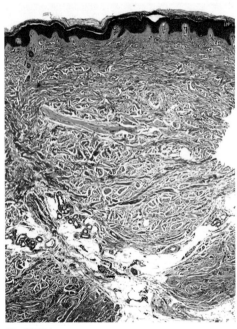

Fig. VF1.j

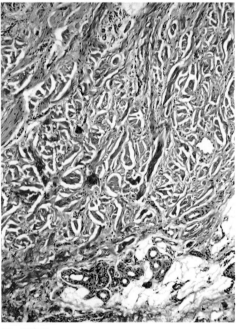

Fig. VF1.k

Clin. Fig. VF1.c. *Nephrogenic fibrosing dermopathy.* Skin tightening led to decreased range of motion.

Clin. Fig. VF1.d. *Nephrogenic fibrosing dermopathy.* Yellow plaque in sclera is a characteristic finding.

Fig. VF1.j. *Nephrogenic fibrosing dermopathy, low power.* Scanning magnification reveals subtle increased cellularity within the reticular dermis. This may be seen either in the upper or lower reticular dermis, and it may extend into the subcutaneous septa.

Fig. VF1.k. *Nephrogenic fibrosing dermopathy, medium power.* There is an increased number of spindled cells within the reticular dermis.

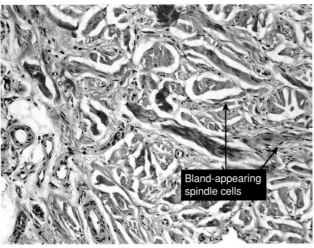

Fig. VF1.l

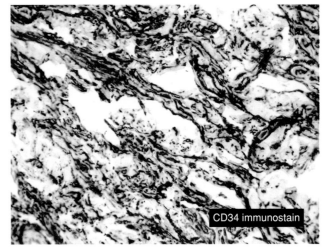

Fig. VF1.m

Fig. VF1.l. *Nephrogenic fibrosing dermopathy, high power.* The spindle cells in nephrogenic fibrosing dermopathy are bland in appearance and resemble fibroblasts.

Fig. VF1.m. *Nephrogenic fibrosing dermopathy, high power, CD34 immunoperoxidase stain.* The spindle cells are strongly and diffusely positive with CD34.

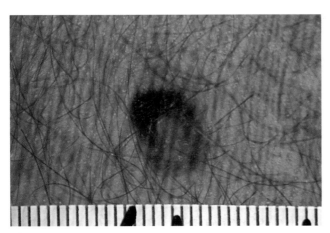

Clin. Fig. VF1.e

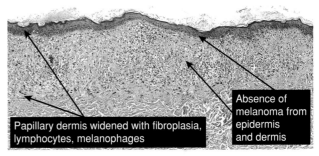

Fig. VF1.n

Clin. Fig. VF1.e. *Regressing melanoma.* The gray- to skin-colored area in the center of this asymmetrical variegated pigmented plaque is an area of partial regression. Note the lack of symmetry in this lesion compared to benign nevi including halo nevi.

Fig. VF1.n. *Regression within a melanoma, low power.* In the right half of the image, there is a tumor in the dermis composed of large cells. In the left half, the papillary dermis is widened by fibroplasia which represents an area of regression of a portion of the radial growth phase of the tumor.

Fig. VF1.o. *Regression within a melanoma, medium power.* Regression in melanoma is characterized by an expanded papillary dermis which shows delicate fibroplasia as well as edema. There is an increased number of small mature vascular channels, a lymphocytic infiltrate, and pigment-laden macrophages.

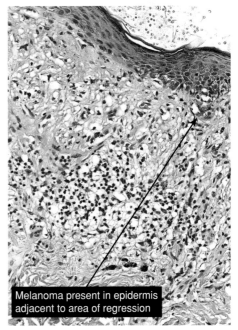

Fig. VF1.o

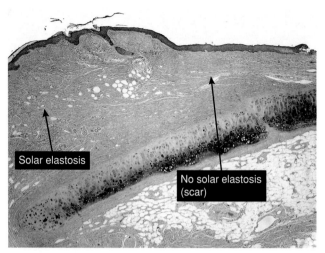

Fig. VF1.p

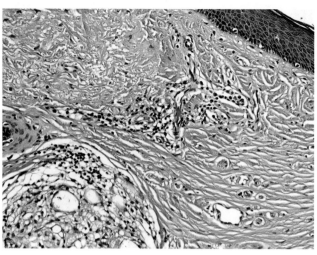

Fig. VF1.q

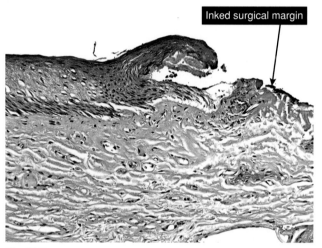

Fig. VF1.r

Fig. VF1.p. *Surgical scar.* At scanning magnification, the scar at the scene presents as a relatively subtle alteration of dermal collagen above the cartilage in this section from the ear. To the left of the image, the native actinically-damaged skin is seen, with a gray color imparted by actinic elastosis.

Fig. VF1.q. *Surgical scar.* The boundary between the scar to the right of the figure and the native skin with actinic elastosis to the left, with a region of lymphocytic and histiocytic inflammation with foamy histiocytes (an area of fat necrosis) to the bottom left of the field. Inflammation is often minimal and subtle in a mature scar like this one.

Fig. VF1.r. *Surgical scar.* At the edge of the scar, it extends to an inked resection margin. If this is a re-excision for neoplasm at this site, the procedure is inadequate because the scar extends to the margin of the excision specimen. In this case, the scar was related to an old procedure.

Superficial Scar (e.g., Biopsy Site Reaction)

It is important to recognize a scar in the dermis, because this can be a clue to a prior biopsy for example of a neoplasm at the site.

Conditions to consider in the differential diagnosis:

scar, keloid
scleroderma/morphea
sclerodermoid graft versus host disease
scleromyxedema
scleredema
nephrogenic fibrosing dermopathy
phytonadione-induced pseudoscleroderma
necrobiosis lipoidica
eosinophilic fasciitis
radiation fibrosis
regressing lesion (melanoma, other tumors)
fibromatosis

acrodermatitis chronica atrophicans
facial hemiatrophy
chronic lymphedema
necrobiosis lipoidica
acro-osteolysis
scleroderma

VF2   Fiber Disorders, Collagen Reduced

Collagen may be reduced focally or diffusely as part of an inborn error of collagen fiber metabolism, or as an acquired phenomenon. Focal dermal hypoplasia is a prototypic example (107).

Focal Dermal Hypoplasia (Goltz Syndrome)

CLINICAL SUMMARY. Focal dermal hypoplasia, or Goltz syndrome, is an X-linked dominant syndrome lethal in homozygous males. Therefore, the syndrome occurs largely in females. It is caused by mutations in the PORCN gene located on chromosome Xp11.23. This gene encodes an O-acyltransferase that affects Wnt signaling proteins required for fibroblast proliferation and osteogenesis. The cutaneous manifestations include widely distributed linear areas of hypoplasia of the skin resembling striae distensae; soft, yellow nodules, often in linear arrangement; and large ulcers due to congenital absence of skin that gradually heal with atrophy. The skin lesions often follow Blaschko lines. The presence of fine, parallel, vertical striations in the metaphysis of long bones on radiography, referred to as osteopathia striata, is a reliable diagnostic marker of Goltz syndrome. Ocular and dental malformations can also occur (108).

HISTOPATHOLOGY. The linear areas of hypoplasia of the skin show a marked diminution in the thickness of the dermis, the collagen being present as thin fibers not united into bundles. The soft, yellow nodules represent accumulations of fat that largely replace the dermis, so that the subcutaneous fat extends upward to the epidermis in some areas. Thin fibers of collagen and even some bundles of collagen resembling those of normal dermis may be located between the subepidermal adipose tissue and the subcutaneous fat.

Conditions to consider in the differential diagnosis:

Ehlers–Danlos syndrome
Marfan syndrome
penicillamine-induced atrophy
striae distensae
aplasia cutis
focal dermal hypoplasia (Goltz)
atrophoderma (Pasini and Pierini)
relapsing polychondritis (type II collagen degeneration of cartilage)

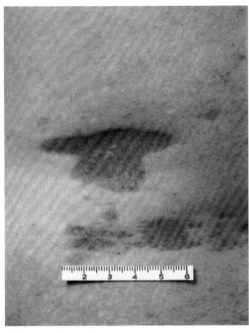

Clin. Fig. VF2

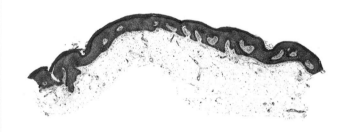

Fig. VF2.a

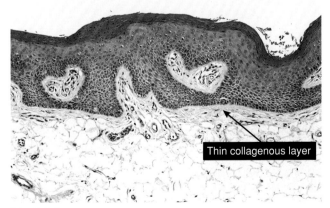

Thin collagenous layer

Fig. VF2.b

Clin. Fig. VF2. *Atrophoderma.* Sharply demarcated brown plaques with cliff-drop borders on the trunk are typical.

Fig. VF2.a. *Focal dermal hypoplasia syndrome (Goltz), low power.* The dermis is essentially absent. The epidermis in this example shows reactive changes.

Fig. VF2.b. *Focal dermal hypoplasia syndrome (Goltz), medium power.* Lobules of the subcutaneous fat extend up to the basal layer of the epidermis, partially separated only by a few wisps of collagen.

VF3 | Fiber Disorders, Elastin Increased or Prominent

Abnormal elastic fibers are increased focally in the dermis and may become calcified as in pseudoxanthoma elasticum, or there is diffuse elastosis in the superficial reticular dermis of sun-exposed skin. Pseudoxanthoma elasticum is a good example (109).

Pseudoxanthoma Elasticum

In this disorder, genetically abnormal elastic fibers with a tendency toward calcification occur in the skin and

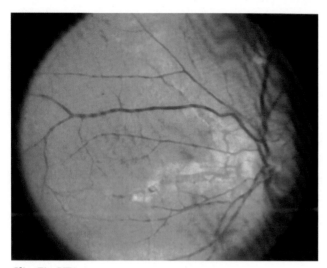

Clin. Fig. VF3.a

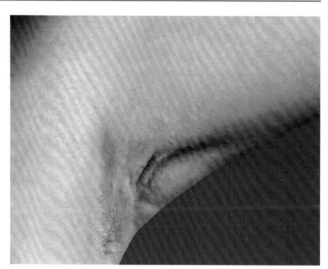

Clin. Fig. VF3.b

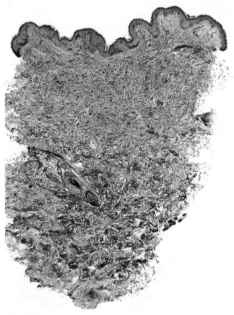

Fig. VF3.a

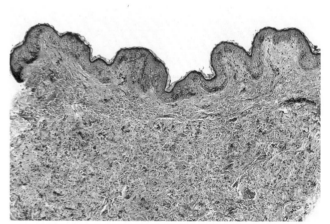

Fig. VF3.b

Clin. Fig. VF3.a. *Pseudoxanthoma elasticum.* An ophthalmologist detected angioid streaks in the retina of a middle-aged woman.

Clin. Fig. VF3.b. *Pseudoxanthoma elasticum.* Referral to dermatology confirmed the diagnosis of PXE with multiple yellowish waxy papules present in her axillae as shown here as well as in her antecubital fossae and neck region.

Fig. VF3.a. *Pseudoxanthoma elasticum, low power.* In this example, there is little calcification. The architecture of the reticular dermis appears subtly altered at scanning magnification.

Fig. VF3.b. *Pseudoxanthoma elasticum, medium power.* The collagen fibers are not arranged in their normal interlacing pattern.

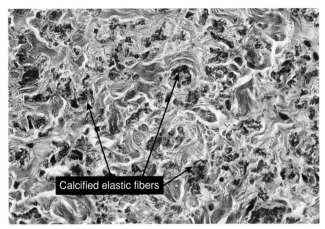

Fig. VF3.c

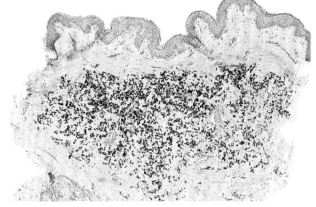

Fig. VF3.d

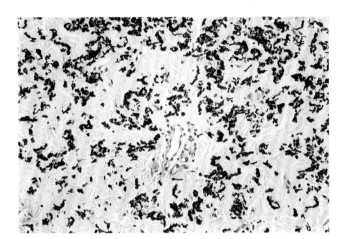

Fig. VF3.e

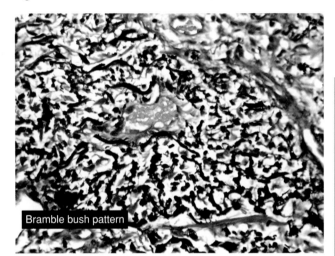

Fig. VF3.f

Fig. VF3.c. *Pseudoxanthoma elasticum, high power.* At this power, the abnormal fibers, here staining a bright pink color, can be appreciated.

Fig. VF3.d. *Pseudoxanthoma elasticum, low power.* An elastic stain reveals the tangle of abnormal elastic fibers in the dermis.

Fig. VF3.e. *Pseudoxanthoma elasticum, medium power.* The fibers are abnormally short, swollen, and irregularly clumped.

Fig. VF3.f. *Pseudoxanthoma elasticum, high power.* In penicillamine-induced pseudoxanthoma elasticum, the elastic fibers are coarse and fragmented with a "bramble-bush" appearance. (Verhoeff–Van Gieson stain.)

frequently also in the retina and within the walls of arteries, particularly the gastric mucosal arteries, coronary arteries, and large peripheral arteries. The inheritance is autosomal recessive. Pseudoxanthoma elasticum is caused by mutations in the ABCC6 gene, which encodes a putative transmembrane efflux transporter that is primarily expressed in the liver (110). The cutaneous lesions usually appear first in the second or third decade of life and are generally progressive in extent and severity. They consist of soft, yellowish, coalescing papules, and the affected skin appears loose and wrinkled. The sides of the neck, the axillae, and the groin are the most common sites of

lesions. In the eyes, so-called angioid streaks of the fundi may cause progressive impairment of vision. Involvement of the arteries of the gastric mucosa may lead to gastric hemorrhage; coronary artery involvement may result in attacks of angina pectoris; involvement of the large peripheral arteries may cause intermittent claudication. Radiologic examination in such cases reveals extensive calcification of the affected arteries.

HISTOPATHOLOGY. Histologic examination of the involved skin reveals in the middle and lower thirds of the dermis considerable accumulations of swollen and irregularly clumped fibers staining like elastic fibers with orcein or Verhoeff stain. With routine hematoxylin-eosin, the altered elastic fibers stain faintly basophilic because of their calcium imbibition, and staining for calcium with the von Kossa method shows them well. In the vicinity of the altered elastic fibers, there may be accumulations of a slightly basophilic mucoid material, which stains strongly positive with the colloidal iron reaction or with alcian blue. In some cases with pronounced elastic tissue calcification, a macrophage and giant cell reaction may be present.

The angioid streaks occur in Bruch membrane, which is located between the retina and the choroid and possesses numerous elastic fibers in its outer portion, the lamina elastica. Calcification of these fibers causes fissures to form in the lamina elastica. These fissures result in repeated hemorrhages and exudates, which in turn cause scarring and pigment shifting in the retina. Gastric bleeding is the result of calcification of elastic fibers in the thin-walled arteries located immediately beneath the gastric mucosa. The internal elastic lamina is particularly affected. In muscular arteries, such as the coronary arteries and the large peripheral arteries, calcification begins in the internal and external elastic laminae, leading to their fragmentation, and subsequently extends to the media and intima.

Conditions to consider in the differential diagnosis:

> pseudoxanthoma elasticum
> penicillamine-induced elastosis perforans
> solar elastosis
> erythema ab igne
> annular elastolytic giant cell granuloma (actinic granuloma)

VF4 Fiber Disorders, Elastin Reduced

Elastin may be reduced focally or diffusely as part of an inborn error of its metabolism, or as an acquired phenomenon. These disorders are uncommon. Anetoderma is prototypic (111).

Anetoderma (Macular Atrophy)

CLINICAL SUMMARY. Macular atrophy, or anetoderma, is characterized by atrophic patches located mainly on the upper trunk. The skin of the patches is thin and blue-white and bulges slightly. The lesions may give the palpating finger the same sensation as a hernial orifice. In many patients, new lesions continue to appear over a period of several years. Primary anetoderma occurs on previously healthy skin, and has been associated with the presence of antiphospholipid antibodies and autoimmune conditions including LE and the antiphospholipid syndrome. Secondary anetoderma results because of abnormal healing of a prior skin lesion such as acne vulgaris (112). Anetoderma of prematurity occurs in ill premature

neonates and commonly occurs at the site of monitoring leads (113).

HISTOPATHOLOGY. Early, erythematous lesions usually show a moderate perivascular infiltrate of mononuclear cells. Occasionally, neutrophils and eosinophils predominate and nuclear dust is present, resulting in a histologic picture of LCV. The elastic tissue may still appear normal in an early lesion, but usually, it is already decreased or even absent. Mononuclear cells may be seen adhering to elastic fibers. Longstanding, lesions generally show a more or less complete loss of elastic tissue, either in the papillary and upper reticular dermis or in the upper reticular dermis only.

Conditions to consider in the differential diagnosis:

> cutis laxa
> anetoderma
> middermal elastolysis

VF5 Fiber Disorders, Perforating

Abnormal elastin or collagen fibers may be extruded through the epidermis, which may form channels that extend down into the dermis. Elastosis perforans serpiginosa (EPS) is prototypic (123).

Elastosis Perforans Serpiginosa

CLINICAL SUMMARY. In EPS, increased numbers of thickened elastic fibers are present in the upper dermis and altered elastic fibers are extruded through the epidermis. It is a rare disorder that affects young individuals, men more often than women, with a peak incidence in the second decade. EPS is primarily a papular eruption localized to one anatomic site and most commonly affecting the nape of the neck, the face, or the upper extremities. The papules are typically 2 to 5 mm in diameter and are arranged in arcuate or serpiginous groups and may coalesce.

Important associations of EPS with systemic diseases include Down syndrome, Ehlers–Danlos syndrome, osteogenesis imperfecta, pseudoxanthoma elasticum, and Marfan syndrome. In addition, on rare occasions EPS is observed in association with Rothmund–Thompson syndrome or other connective tissue disorders, and it also may occur as a complication of penicillamine administration.

HISTOPATHOLOGY. The essential findings include a narrow transepidermal channel of acantholytic epidermis that may be straight, wavy, or of corkscrew shape, containing thick, coarse elastic fibers admixed with granular basophilic staining debris. A mixed inflammatory cell infiltrate accompanies the fibers in the channel. Abnormal elastic fibers are present in the upper dermis in the vicinity of the channel. In this zone the elastic fibers are increased in size

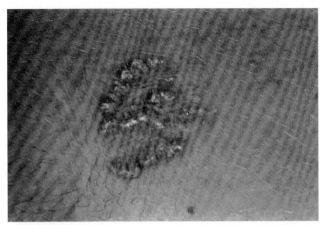

Clin. Fig. VF5.a

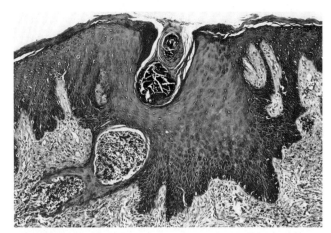

Fig. VF5.a

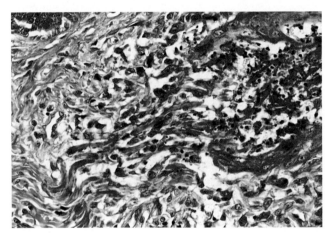

Fig. VF5.b

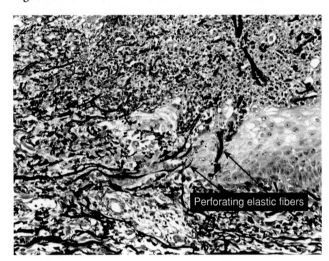

Fig. VF5.c

Clin. Fig. VF5.a. *Elastosis perforans serpiginosa.* Papules in an annular and serpiginous configuration appeared on the volar forearms in a healthy adult female.

Fig. VF5.a. *Elastosis perforans serpiginosa, low power.* There is a narrow, curved channel extending through an acanthotic epidermis. The upper portion of the channel contains basophilic degenerate material. The lower portion of the channel contains elastic fibers, in addition to the degenerate material. (E. Heilman and R. Friedman.)

Fig. VF5.b. *Elastosis perforans serpiginosa, high power.* There are thickened degenerated elastic fibers at the origin of the epidermal channel. (E. Heilman and R. Friedman.)

Fig. VF5.c. *Elastosis perforans serpiginosa, high power, Verhoeff–Van Gieson stain.* Black elastic fibers are seen perforating through the epidermis.

and number. As these fibers enter the lower portion of the channel, they maintain their normal staining characteristics, but as they approach the epidermal surface they may not stain as expected with elastic stains.

Reactive Perforating Collagenosis

Reactive perforating collagenosis (RPC) is a rare disease in the spectrum of primary perforating dermatoses. It clinically presents with brown erythematous papules with a central plug that develops after minor skin trauma. Histologically there is epidermal perforation and transepidermal elimination of altered dermal collagen. Familial and acquired forms have been described. The acquired forms are usually associated with systemic diseases, most commonly diabetes mellitus and renal failure (114).

Perforating Folliculitis

See Fig. VF5.g.

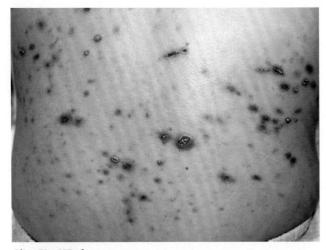

Clin. Fig. VF5.b

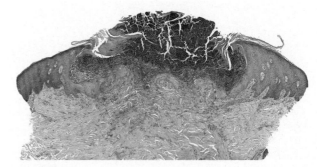

Fig. VF5.d

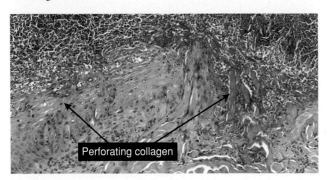

Fig. VF5.e

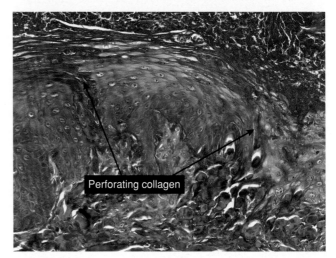

Fig. VF5.f

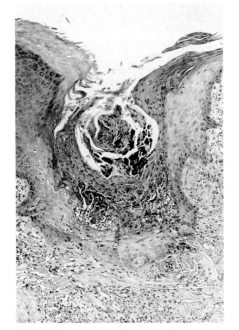

Fig. VF5.g

Clin. Fig. VF5.b. *Reactive perforating collagenosis.* A 48-year-old woman with diabetes and renal failure developed brown papules and plaques, some of which developed a central plug.

Fig. VF5.d. *Reactive perforating collagenosis, low power.* A cup-shaped channel containing degenerated collagen bundles and basophilic material.

Fig. VF5.e. *Reactive perforating collagenosis, medium power.* Pink collagen fibers are seen perforating vertically through the epidermis.

Fig. VF5.f. *Reactive perforating collagenosis, trichrome stain, medium power.* Blue stained collagen fibers perforating the channel and extending to the surface.

Fig. VF5.g. *Perforating folliculitis, medium power.* A dilated follicular unit contains a keratotic plug with an admixture of basophilic debris. The follicular epithelium is perforated, and there are degenerated collagen fibers in the adjacent dermis. (E. Heilman and R. Friedman.)

Conditions to consider in the differential diagnosis:

elastosis perforans serpiginosa
Kyrle disease
perforating folliculitis
reactive perforating collagenosis
perforating disorder of renal failure and diabetes
perforating calcific elastosis
perforating granuloma annulare

VG DEPOSITION OF MATERIAL IN THE DERMIS

The dermis serves as a reaction site for a variety of inflammatory, infiltrative, and desmoplastic processes, which may include accumulations of matrix molecules that may either be indigenous to the normal dermis, or foreign to it.

1. Increased Normal Nonfibrous Matrix Constituents
2. Increased Material Not Normally Present in the Dermis
3. Parasitic Infestations of the Dermis and/or Subcutis

VG1 Increased Normal Nonfibrous Matrix Constituents

Ground substance (hyaluronic acid) is increased, associated with a varying inflammatory infiltrate that can include lymphocytes, plasma cells, and eosinophils. Digital mucous cysts and cutaneous focal mucinosis (CFM) (115) are common examples.

Digital Mucous Cysts and Cutaneous Focal Mucinosis

CLINICAL SUMMARY. Two types of digital mucous cysts exist. One type presents as a pale papule, analogous to focal mucinosis. It differs from CFM only by its location near the proximal nail fold and by its greater tendency to fluctuate (116). The other type is located on the dorsum of a finger near the distal interphalangeal joint and is due to a herniation of the joint lining, thus representing a ganglion (117). Digital mucous cysts commonly cause a longitudinal indentation in the nail plate.

HISTOPATHOLOGY. The *myxomatous* type of digital mucous cyst in its early stage has the same histologic appearance as that seen in focal mucinosis, namely, an ill-defined area of mucinous material. Subsequently, multiple clefts form and then coalesce into one large cystic space containing mucin composed largely of hyaluronic acid, which stains with alcian blue and colloidal iron. The cystic space in early lesions is separated from the epidermis by mucinous stroma but in older lesions is found in a subepidermal location with thinning of the overlying epidermis. The collagen at the periphery of the cyst appears compressed. No lining of the cyst wall is apparent. In the *ganglion type* of digital mucous cyst, on surgical exploration the cyst shows a flattened lining and evidence of a pedicle leading to the joint spaces.

It has been suggested to use the term "solitary CFM" for isolated lesions, to distinguish them from multiple CFM associated with mucinosis-associated systemic diseases.

Mucinosis in Lupus Erythematosus

See Fig. VG1.d.

Mucinoses

Six types of primary cutaneous mucinosis include: (1) generalized myxedema; (2) pretibial myxedema; (3) lichen myxedematosus or papular mucinosis; (4) reticular

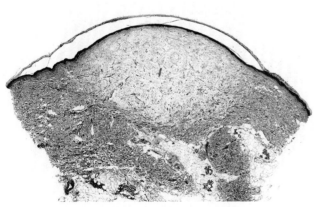

Fig. VG1.a

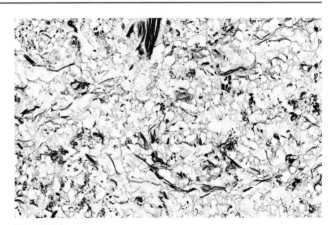

Fig. VG1.b

Fig. VG1.a. *Cutaneous focal mucinosis, low power.* There is a zone of pallor in the superficial dermis, extending up to the epidermis.

Fig. VG1.b. *Cutaneous focal mucinosis, medium power.* The collagen bundles are separated by ground substance (mucin) which can be shown by a colloidal iron stain to contain abundant hyaluronic acid. (*continues*)

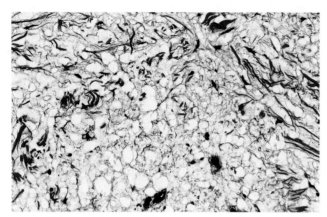

Fig. VG1.c

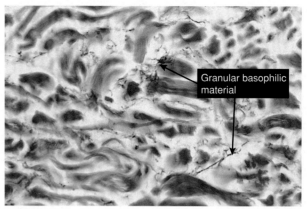

Fig. VG1.d

Fig. VG1.c. *Cutaneous focal mucinosis, high power.* There is an increase in interstitial mucin, and an apparent diminution in collagen, but vessels are not increased.

Fig. VG1.d. *Lupus erythematosus, high power.* Basophilic mucinous material is present diffusely between otherwise unaltered collagen bundles in a lesion from a patient with lupus.

erythematous mucinosis or plaque-like mucinosis; (5) self-healing juvenile cutaneous mucinosis; and (6) scleredema. Regular demonstration of the presence of mucin in the dermis is possible only in pretibial myxedema, self-healing juvenile cutaneous mucinosis, and lichen myxedematosus. In reticular erythematous mucinosis, it is possible in most cases. In generalized myxedema, the amount of mucin usually is too small to be demonstrable, and in scleredema, mucin may be present only in the early stage.

Pretibial Myxedema

CLINICAL SUMMARY. In pretibial myxedema, the lesions are limited to the anterior aspects of the legs, but they may extend to the dorsa of the feet and rarely the forearms. They consist of raised, nodular, yellow, waxy plaques with prominent follicular openings that give a peau d'orange appearance (118).

Pretibial myxedema usually occurs in association with thyrotoxicosis and not infrequently becomes more pronounced after treatment of the thyrotoxicosis. Rarely, it occurs in nonthyrotoxic thyroid disease such as chronic lymphocytic thyroiditis.

HISTOPATHOLOGY. The epidermis and papillary dermis are usually normal. Mucin in large amounts is present in the dermis, particularly in the upper half. As a result, the dermis is greatly thickened. The mucin occurs not only as individual threads and granules but also as extensive deposits resulting in the splitting up of collagen bundles into fibers and wide separation of the fibers. As a result of shrinkage of the mucin during the process of fixation and dehydration, there are empty spaces within

the mucin deposits. The number of fibroblasts is not increased as a rule, but in areas in which there is much mucin, some fibroblasts have a stellate shape and are then referred to as mucoblasts. A perivascular infiltrate of lymphocytes may be seen in some cases and mast cells are moderately increased in number.

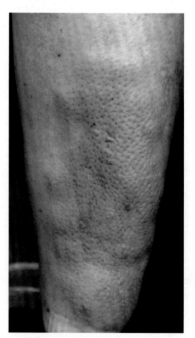

Clin. Fig. VG1.a

Clin. Fig. VG1.a. *Pretibial myxedema.* Raised, nodular, yellow, waxy plaque with a peau d'orange appearance related to follicular orifices.

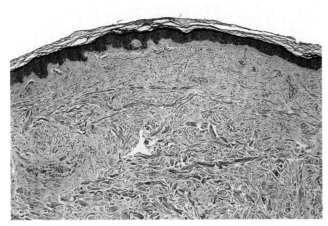

Fig. VG1.e

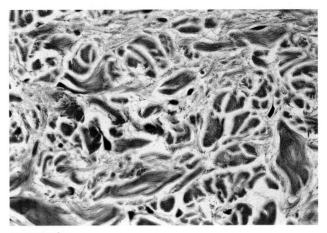

Fig. VG1.f

Fig. VG1.e. *Myxedema, low power.* Increased mucin is present in the dermis, particularly in the upper half. As a result, the dermis is greatly thickened.

Fig. VG1.f. *Myxedema, high power.* The mucin appears as threads and granules resulting in the splitting up of collagen bundles into fibers and wide separation of the fibers. As a result of shrinkage of the mucin during the process of fixation and dehydration, there are empty spaces within the mucin deposits. The number of fibroblasts is not increased.

Scleredema

CLINICAL SUMMARY. Scleredema is a rare scleromucinous connective tissue disease of unknown etiology. Despite continuing use by some of the term "scleredema adultorum," scleredema occurs in individuals of all ages. Three types of scleredema have been distinguished. Type 1, the classic "Buschke" type, 55% of cases usually follows a febrile infection (especially streptococcal or viral respiratory tract infection) and affects mainly children. Type 2 (25%) is associated with paraproteinemia. Type 3 (20%) has been named scleredema diabeticorum because of its association with diabetes mellitus. Other associated diseases are numerous, and uncommon. In the early stages, scleredema presents as woody, nonpitting, indurated plaques of the skin of the neck, which later spread to shoulders and upper trunk, sparing hands and feet. The skin wrinkles or takes on a "peau d'orange" appearance when pinched (117).

HISTOPATHOLOGY. The skin is greatly thickened, with thickened collagen bundles separated by clear spaces, causing "fenestration" of the collagen, and containing colloidal iron–positive interstitial mucin. There is no significant inflammation.

Lichen Myxedematosus and Scleromyxedema

According to a modern classification two main clinicopathologic subsets of lichen myxedematosus (papular mucinosis) should be distinguished: a generalized papular and sclerodermoid form, also called scleromyxedema, and a localized papular form (119). Diagnosis of scleromyxedema should fulfill the following criteria: (1) generalized papular and sclerodermoid eruption; (2) mucin deposition, fibroblast proliferation, and fibrosis; (3) monoclonal gammopathy; and (4) the absence of thyroid disease. The criteria for localized lichen myxedematosus are as follows:

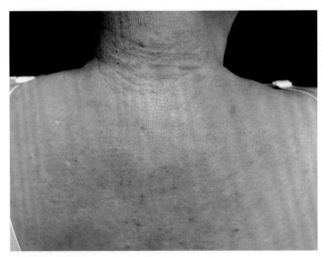

Clin. Fig. VG1.b

Clin. Fig. VG1.b. *Scleredema.* A 53-year-old woman with a 10-year-history of diabetes developed woody, nonpitting, indurated patches of the skin of the neck, which later spread to the shoulders and upper back. (*continues*)

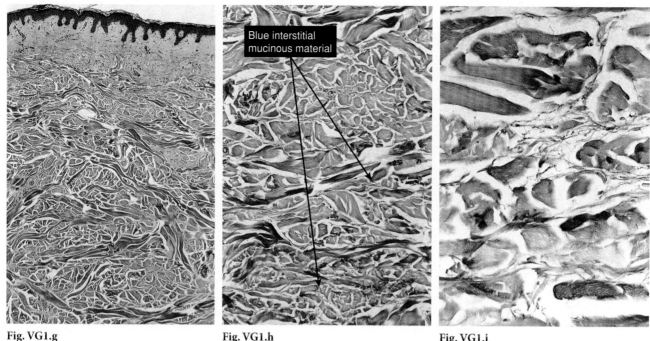

Blue interstitial mucinous material

Fig. VG1.g   Fig. VG1.h   Fig. VG1.i

Fig. VG1.g. *Scleredema, low power.* The dermis is greatly thickened. The collagen bundles are thickened and separated by clear spaces, causing "fenestration" of the collagen.

Fig. VG1.h. *Scleredema, medium power, colloidal iron.* The separation of collagen bundles is not accompanied by an increase in cellularity.

Fig. VG1.i. *Scleredema, high power, colloidal iron.* In this and the previous figure, the separation is seen to be due to interstitial mucin, which is highlighted by the colloidal iron reaction.

---

(1) papular or nodular/plaque eruption; (2) mucin deposition with variable fibroblast proliferation; and (3) the absence of both monoclonal gammopathy and thyroid disease.

Histologically, in the diffusely thickened skin of scleromyxedema, there is extensive proliferation of fibroblasts throughout the dermis, associated with irregularly arranged bundles of collagen. In many areas, the collagen bundles are split into individual fibers by mucin. As a rule, the amount of mucin is greater in the upper half than in the lower half of the dermis. A paraprotein, usually IgG, is present in the sera of most patients with scleromyxedema, and is often associated with hyperplasia of bone marrow plasma cells, which synthesize the monoclonal IgG. In some cases, these cells may be atypical, however frank multiple myeloma is uncommon.

In localized lichen myxedematosus (papular mucinosis), clinically the patients exhibit small, firm, waxy papules, which may become confluent, but confined to only a few sites, usually upper and lower limbs and trunk. Histopathologic examination reveals mucin deposition with variable fibroblast proliferation without sclerotic features, paraproteinemia, systemic involvement, or thyroid disease. Clinicopathologic correlation may be required to establish a definitive diagnosis.

Conditions to consider in the differential diagnosis:

granuloma annulare
pretibial myxedema
generalized myxedema
juvenile cutaneous mucinosis
papular mucinosis (lichen myxedematosus)
scleromyxedema
reticulated erythematous mucinosis (REM)
scleredema
focal dermal mucinosis
digital mucous cyst/myxoid cyst
cutaneous myxoma
mucocoele, mucinous mucosal cyst
lupus erythematosus
hereditary progressive mucinous histiocytosis

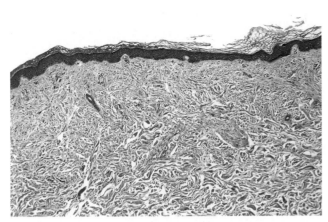

Fig. VG1.j

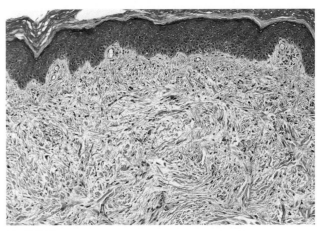

Fig. VG1.k

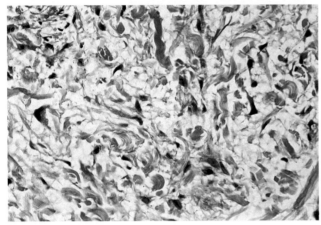

Fig. VG1.l

Fig. VG1.j. *Scleromyxedema, low power.* The skin is diffusely thickened, and there is an appearance of increased cellularity.

Fig. VG1.k. *Scleromyxedema, medium power.* The increased cellularity is due to extensive proliferation of fibroblasts throughout the dermis, associated with irregularly arranged bundles of collagen.

Fig. VG1.l. *Scleromyxedema, high power.* The collagen bundles tend to be split into individual fibers by mucin. As a rule, the amount of mucin is greater in the upper half than in the lower half of the dermis.

VG2 | Increased Material Not Normally Present in the Dermis

Materials not present in substantial amounts in the normal dermis are deposited, as crystals (gout), amorphous deposits (calcinosis), hyaline material (colloid milium, amyloidosis, porphyria), or as pigments. Gout is prototypic (120).

Gout

CLINICAL SUMMARY. In the early stage of gout, there usually are irregularly recurring attacks of acute arthritis. In the late stage, deposits of monosodium urate form within and around various joints, leading to chronic arthritis with destruction in the joints and the adjoining bone. During this late stage, urate deposits, called tophi, may occur in the subcutaneous tissue and occasionally the dermis. Tophi are observed most commonly on the helix of the ears, over the bursae of the elbows, and on the fingers and toes. They may attain a diameter of several centimeters and when large may discharge a chalky material. In rare instances, gout may present as tophi on the fingertips or as panniculitis on the legs without the coexistence of a gouty arthritis.

HISTOPATHOLOGY. For the histologic examination of tophi, fixation in absolute ethanol or an ethanol-based fixative, such as Carnoy fluid, is preferable to fixation in formalin; aqueous fixatives such as formalin dissolve the characteristic urate crystals, leaving only amorphous material which however can usually be recognized as the residue of a tophus because of the characteristic rim of foreign-body giant cells and macrophages which surrounds the aggregates of amorphous material. Anhydrous tissue processing is also important to preserve the urate crystals. On fixation in alcohol, tophi can be seen to consist of variously sized, sharply demarcated aggregates of needle-shaped urate crystals lying closely packed in the form of bundles or sheaves. The crystals often have a brownish color and are doubly refractile on polariscopic examination.

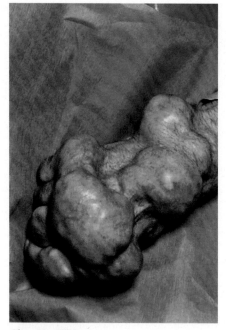

Clin. Fig. VG2.a

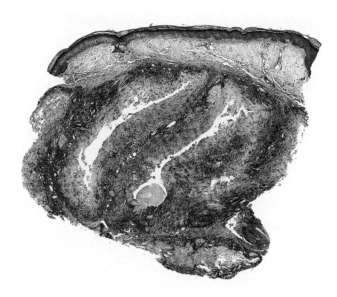

Fig. VG2.a

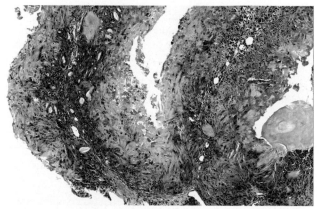

Fig. VG2.b

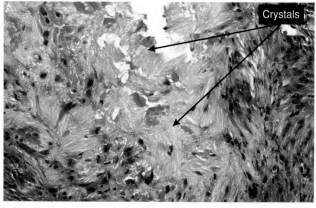

Crystals

Fig. VG2.c

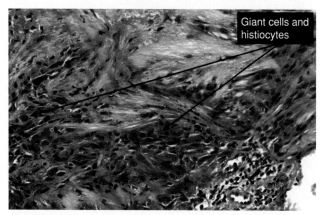

Giant cells and histiocytes

Fig. VG2.d

Clin. Fig. VG2.a. *Gout.* This elderly female had a 17-year history of large, globular tophi which become tender and required drainage.

Fig. VG2.a. *Gout, low power.* Irregular masses of pale material are present in the dermis and subcutis.

Fig. VG2.b. *Gout, medium power.* Granulomatous inflammation surrounds the amorphous material.

Fig. VG2.c,d. *Gout, high power.* The material consists of narrow elongated crystals, best seen post fixation in alcohol. After aqueous fixation, as here, a negative impression of the dissolved crystals can usually be discerned. There is a surrounding foreign-body giant cell reaction.

Oxalosis

CLINICAL SUMMARY. Deposition of oxalate crystals within the skin is seen with hyperoxaluria (121). Hyperoxaluria may be primary (familial) or secondary (acquired from exogenous sources or underlying disease). There are three types of primary hyperoxaluria: Type I is a deficiency in the enzyme alanine glyoxalate aminotransferase; type II is a deficiency in D-glycerate dehydrogenase; type III is secondary to increased oxalate absorption without any known intestinal pathology. Secondary hyperoxaluria can be secondary to increased absorption of oxalates, and to small bowel resection or inflammatory bowel disease, end-stage renal disease, pyridoxine deficiency and excess intake of oxalate or oxalate precursors. This latter category includes ethylene glycol poisoning, methoxyflurane anesthesia, or large doses of ascorbic acid.

With hyperoxaluria, oxalate will precipitate as calcium oxalate in virtually all tissues of the body. There are some preferential sites including the bones which have metabolic activity, and tissues where calcium modulates electric current, such as myocardium and smooth muscle of blood vessels. Patients with primary hyperoxaluria generally develop renal failure, cardiac disease, severe peripheral vascular ischemia, retinal deposits, and liver failure. Without a liver–kidney transplant, many patients die in the third to fourth decades.

Skin manifestations generally are secondary to calcium oxalate deposition in blood vessels resulting in livedo reticularis, ulcerations, skin infarctions, acrocyanosis, or gangrene (122,123). Calcified nodules may also be seen.

HISTOPATHOLOGY. Yellow-brown calcium oxalate deposits are most commonly seen within the walls of both small and large blood vessels. Crystals may also been seen deposited as nodular aggregates in the subcutaneous tissue. The crystals characteristically show a radial array or rosette-like appearance. The birefringent crystalline material is highlighted with polaroscopy. Frequently there is an associated sparse mononuclear cell infiltrate as well as multinucleated giant cells. The overlying epidermis and superficial dermis may show secondary necrosis and/or ulceration (124).

Colloid Milium

Adult colloid milium (ACM) is a rare cutaneous deposition disorder that presents with multiple nodules on the sun-exposed areas of the face, neck, and dorsum of the hands. A full-thickness skin biopsy may be required to diagnose ACM and to distinguish it from amyloid (125).

Idiopathic Calcinosis Cutis

CLINICAL SUMMARY. Calcinosis cutis is often associated with a connective tissue disease such as scleroderma.

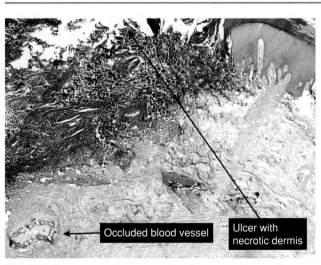

Occluded blood vessel

Ulcer with necrotic dermis

Fig. VG2.e

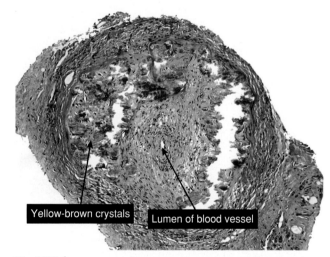

Yellow-brown crystals

Lumen of blood vessel

Fig. VG2.f

Fig. VG2.e. *Oxalosis, low power.* The epidermis is ulcerated and there is superficial dermal necrosis. Beneath the ulceration, there is a medium-sized blood vessel with a thickened wall.

Fig. VG2.f. *Oxalosis, medium power.* At the base of the tissue of the same specimen, there is a detached piece of connective tissue which contains a medium-sized vessel which shows marked thickening of the vascular wall with a very small lumen. Within the wall of the vessel are large aggregates of crystalline material. (*continues*)

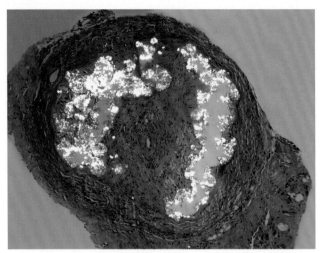

Fig. VG2.g

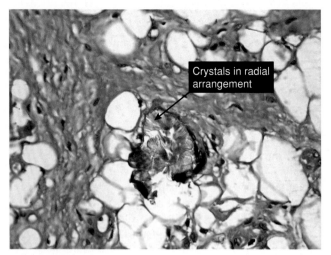

Fig. VG2.h

Fig. VG2.g. *Oxalosis, medium power.* The blood vessel visualized with polarized lights reveals refractile crystalline material in the vessel wall.

Fig. VG2.h. *Oxalosis, high power.* Upon close inspection, some of the crystals show a radial arrangement.

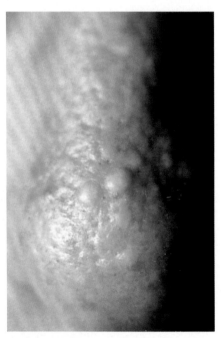

Clin. Fig. VG2.b

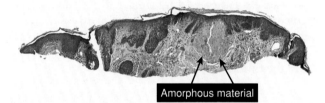

Fig. VG2.i

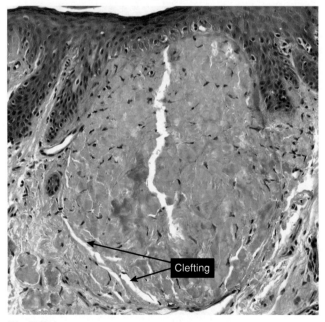

Fig. VG2.j

Clin. Fig. VG2.b. *Colloid milium.* These asymptomatic, whitish, soft papules on the nose were an incidental finding on examination.

Fig. VG2.i. *Colloid milium, low power.* A nodule of pink amorphous material is present in the papillary dermis.

Fig. VG2.j. *Colloid milium, medium power.* The amorphous material may show this characteristic clefting artifact.

In some instances of this *dystrophic calcinosis cutis* the underlying disease may be mild and can be overlooked unless specifically searched for. There remain cases of idiopathic calcinosis cutis that resemble dystrophic calcinosis cutis but there is no underlying disease. Tumoral calcinosis is regarded as a special manifestation of idiopathic calcinosis cutis (126). It consists of numerous large, subcutaneous, calcified masses that may be associated with papular and nodular skin lesions of calcinosis. The disease usually is familial and is associated with hyperphosphatemia. Otherwise, the resemblance of tumoral calcinosis to the dystrophic calcinosis universalis observed with dermatomyositis is great.

HISTOPATHOLOGY. Tumoral calcinosis shows in the subcutaneous tissue large masses of calcium surrounded by a foreign-body reaction. Intradermal aggregates are present in some cases. Discharge of calcium may take place through areas of ulceration or by means of transepidermal elimination.

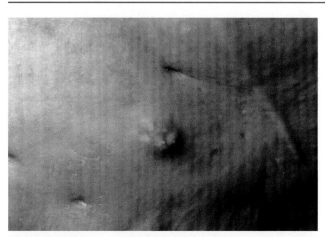

Clin. Fig. VG2.c

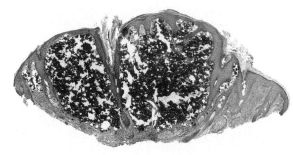

Fig. VG2.k

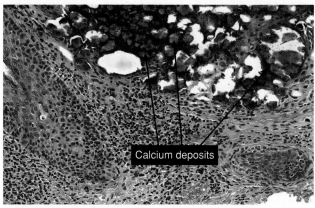

Calcium deposits

Fig. VG2.l

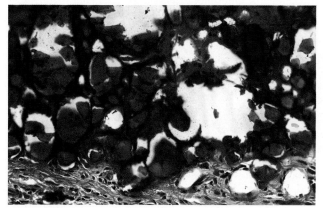

Fig. VG2.m

Clin. Fig. VG2.c. *Calcinosis cutis.* Firm, grouped whitish papules on the trunk of an individual without obvious predisposing factors for calcification.

Fig. VG2.k. *Idiopathic calcinosis cutis, low power.* A tumoral mass of calcium is present in the dermis. There are no obvious changes of associated connective tissue disease, or other predisposing condition for dystrophic calcification.

Fig. VG2.l. *Idiopathic calcinosis cutis, medium power.* An amorphous mass of calcium in the dermis, with an adjacent inflammatory reaction.

Fig. VG2.m. *Idiopathic calcinosis cutis, high power.* There are irregular aggregates of purple material without nuclei.

Cryoglobulinemia

See Fig. VG2.n.

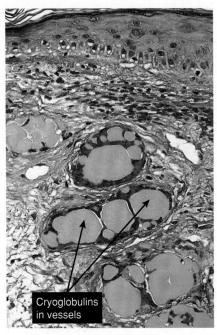

Fig. VG2.n

Fig. VG2.n. *Cryoglobulinemia, medium power.* In type I cryoglobulinemia, amorphous material (precipitated monoclonal cryoglobulins in this case of Waldenstrom macroglobulinemia) is deposited subjacent to endothelium and throughout the vessel wall as well as within the vessel lumen, resulting in a noninflammatory thrombus-like appearance.

Fig. VG2.o. *Keratin granuloma, low power.* There is a collection of keratin in the dermis, representing the site of rupture of an epidermal cyst. There is a foreign-body giant cell reaction at the periphery.

Fig. VG2.p. *Keratin granuloma, medium power.* Gray-pink keratin flakes are present in the center of the lesion and in giant cells at its periphery.

Fig. VG2.q. *Keratin granuloma, high power.* In some lesions, the flakes of keratin may be difficult to appreciate, but may be found within the cytoplasm of giant cells. Their color is often gray, rather than the expected pink.

Keratin Granuloma

A keratin granuloma is a common finding at the site of a ruptured epidermal cyst (which may not be evident in any given biopsy).

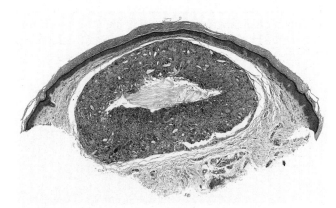

Fig. VG2.o

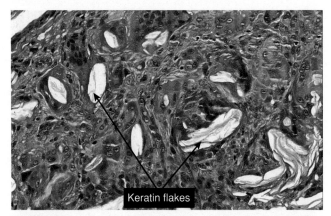

Fig. VG2.p

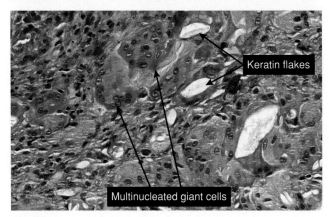

Fig. VG2.q

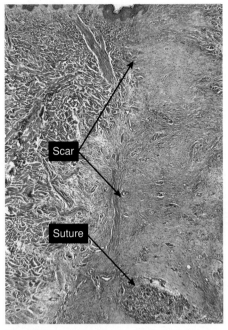

Fig. VG2.r

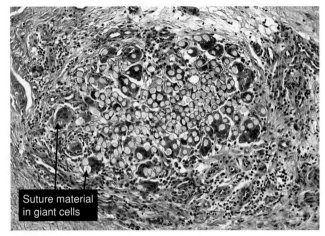

Fig. VG2.s

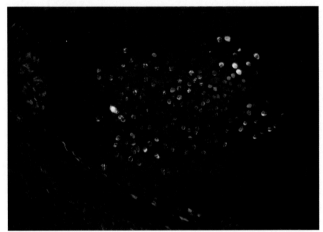

Fig. VG2.t

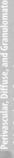

Fig. VG2.r. *Suture granuloma, low power.* At the base of a scar to the right, there is a cluster of pink cells and gray fibers.

Fig. VG2.s. *Suture granuloma, medium power.* The cells are foreign-body giant cells and the fibers are those of a suture cut in cross-section.

Fig. VG2.t. *Suture granuloma, high power.* Many man-made fibers are birefringent as viewed here between crossed polarizing filters.

Suture Granuloma

Suture and other foreign medical materials may give rise to a foreign-body reaction with prominent histiocytes and giant cells.

Minocycline Pigmentation

CLINICAL SUMMARY. Presenting as macular blue-black pigmentation of the skin, the pigmentation is often seen in a perifollicular location or at the sites of prior inflammation such as old acne scars. The pigmentation is most prominent in sun-exposed sites, such as the face. Diffuse pigmentation is another clinical variation exhibiting a "slate-gray" hue most commonly on the extremities, with the legs exhibiting the most striking change, or the pigmentation may be generalized over the body. This latter presentation also occurs with medications other than minocycline (127). Other parts of the body affected by minocycline pigmentation include the nail beds, sclera, teeth, thyroid, and bone (128).

HISTOPATHOLOGY. There may be an increase in basilar pigment in the epidermis; this can be seen in all clinical types but is most striking in the diffuse type. In the dermis there are aggregates of brown-black granules, in macrophages and in perivascular and perieccrine locations. Pigment granules may be found only in the subcutis. The granules stain with silver (Fontana-Masson) and iron (Perls) stains. The differential diagnosis includes postinflammatory hyperpigmentation and other drug causes of dermal pigmentation include amiodarone, antimalarials, cyclophosphamide, phenytoin, chlorpromazine, gold, silver, and clofazimine (129).

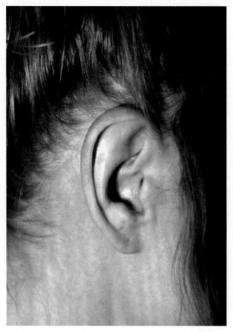

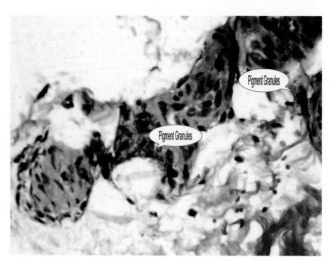

Clin. Fig. VG2.d   **Fig. VG2.u**

Clin. Fig. VG2.d. *Minocycline pigmentation.* Note grayish-blue discoloration resulting from pigmentation of ear cartilage.

Fig. VG2.u. *Minocycline pigmentation.* Pigment granules in a perivascular location in the dermis.

Conditions to consider in the differential diagnosis:

gout
oxalosis
colloid milium
calcinosis cutis
    calcinosis universalis, circumscripta (scleroderma)
    tumoral calcinosis
    idiopathic calcification of the scrotum
    subepidermal calcified nodule
    calciphylaxis
    Monckeberg calcification
polyarteritis nodosa
amyloidosis
dermal pigments
    minocycline
    argyria
    chrysiasis
    mercury pigmentation
    hemochromatosis
    alkaptonuric ochronosis
    calcaneal petechiae (hemoglobin)
lipoid proteinosis (hyalinosis cutis et mucosae, Urbach–Wiethe)
cryoglobulinemia
porphyria cutanea tarda
foreign material—dirt, glass, paraffin, grease, etc.
    tattoo reactions
    silicone, talc, starch

cactus, sea urchin, hair granulomas
intralesional steroids
vaccines
Hunter syndrome (lysosomal storage granules)

VG3 Parasitic Infestations of the Dermis and/or Subcutis

Macroscopically visible parasitic agents may infest the epidermis, dermis, and subcutis. Creeping eruption (larva migrans) is a good example (130).

Cutaneous Larva Migrans

Cutaneous larva migrans presents with the clinical sign known as creeping eruption. It is caused by filariform larvae of the dog and cat hookworms *Ancylostoma braziliensis*, *A. caninum*, and *Uncinaria stenocephala*. Migration is manifested by an irregularly linear, thin, raised burrow, 2 to 3 mm wide. The first sign is an erythematous papule which later develops the characteristic serpiginous erythematosus elevated track. The larva moves a few millimeters per day. The eruption is self-limited because humans are abnormal hosts. The feet and buttocks are the areas most commonly involved. Most cases in developed countries are seen in travelers. The organism is transmitted when bare skin comes in contact with contaminated soil (131).

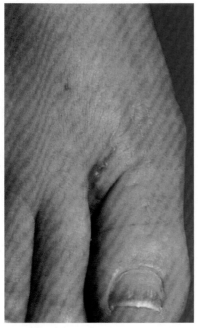

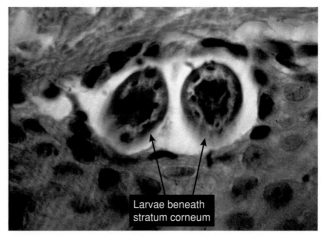

Larvae beneath
stratum corneum

Clin. Fig. VG3   **Fig. VG3.a**

Clin. Fig. VG3. *Larva migrans.* Shortly after vacationing in Jamaica, a patient noticed a pruritic creeping movement which manifested as a serpiginous plaque. Aggressive cryotherapy resulted in resolution.

Fig. VG3.a. *Larva migrans, high power.* Cross-section of larva of Ancylostoma in the stratum corneum (PAS stain). (From Johnson BJ Jr, Honig P, Jaworsky C, eds. *Pediatric Dermatopathology.* Newton, MA: Butterworth-Heineman; 1994. Reprinted with permission.)

HISTOPATHOLOGY. The larva is found in a specimen taken from just beyond the leading edge of the track. It is located in a burrow in the superficial epidermis. The lesion, aside from the larva which is often not observed in the biopsies, shows spongiosis and intraepidermal vesicles containing necrotic keratinocytes. The epidermis and the upper dermis contain a chronic inflammatory infiltrate with many eosinophils.

Conditions to consider in the differential diagnosis:

larva migrans (Ancylostoma)
subcutaneous dirofilariasis
onchocerciasis
strongyloidiasis
schistosomiasis
subcutaneous cysticercosis
myiasis

References

1. Kim KJ, Chang SE, Choi JH, et al. Clinicopathologic analysis of 66 cases of erythema annulare centrifugum. *J Dermatol* 2002; 29(2):61–67.
2. Kim DH, Lee JH, Lee JY, et al. Erythema annulare centrifugum: analysis of associated diseases and clinical outcomes according to histopathologic classification. *Ann Dermatol* 2016;28(2): 257–259.
3. Ruiz H, Sanchez JL. Tumid lupus erythematosus. *Am J Dermatopathol* 1999;12(4):356–360.
4. Wick MR. Disorders characterized by predominant or exclusive dermal inflammation. *Semin Diagn Pathol* 2017;34(3): 273–284.
5. Shaffer B, Jacobsen C, Beerman H. Histopathologic correlation of lesions of papular urticaria and positive skin test reactions to insect antigens. *AMA Arch Derm Syphilol* 1954;70(4): 437–442.
6. Jordaan HF, Schneider JW. Papular urticaria: a histopathologic study of 30 patients. *Am J Dermatopathol* 1997;19(2):119–126.
7. Barzilai A, Sagi L, Baum S, et al. The histopathology of urticaria revisited-clinical pathological study. *Am J Dermatopathol* 2017;39(10):753–759.
8. Cohen LM, Capeless EL, Krusinski PA, et al. Pruritic urticarial papules and plaques of pregnancy and its relationship to maternal-fetal weight gain and twin pregnancy. *Arch Dermatol* 1989;125(11):1534–1536.
9. Ambros-Rudolph CM. Dermatoses of pregnancy—clues to diagnosis, fetal risk and therapy. *Ann Dermatol* 2011;23(3): 265–275.
10. Jeerapaet P, Ackerman AS. Histologic patterns of secondary syphilis. *Arch Dermatol* 1973;107(3):373–377.
11. Flamm A, Parikh K, Xie Q, et al. Histologic features of secondary syphilis: a multicenter retrospective review. *J Am Acad Dermatol* 2015;73(6):1025–1030.
12. Hoang MP, High WA, Molberg KH. Secondary syphilis: a histologic and immunohistochemical evaluation. *J Cutan Pathol* 2004;31(9):595–599.

13. Phelps RG, Knispel J, Tu ES, et al. Immunoperoxidase technique for detecting spirochetes in tissue sections: comparison with other methods. *Int J Dermatol* 2000;39(8):609–613.

14. Buffet M, Grange PA, Gerhardt P, et al. Diagnosing Treponema pallidum in secondary syphilis by PCR and immunohistochemistry. *J Invest Dermatol* 2007;127(10):2345–2350.

15. Berger BW. Erythema chronicum migrans of Lyme disease. *Arch Dermatol* 1984;120(8):1017–1021.

16. Miraflor AP, Seidel GD, Perry AE, et al. The many masks of cutaneous Lyme disease. *J Cutan Pathol* 2016;43(1):32–40.

17. Miloslavsky EM, Stone JH, Unizony SH. Challenging mimickers of primary systemic vasculitis. *Rheum Dis Clin North Am* 2015;41(1):141–160.

18. Wobser M, Burger M, Trautmann A. Images in dermatology. The red flag. *Am J Med* 2010;123(1):31–33.

19. Ferrara G, Cerroni L. Cold-associated perniosis of the thighs ("Equestrian-Type" Chilblain): a reappraisal based on a clinicopathologic and immunohistochemical study of 6 cases. *Am J Dermatopathol* 2016;38(10):726–731.

20. Boada A, Bielsa I, Fernández-Figueras MT, et al. Perniosis: clinical and histopathological analysis. *Am J Dermatopathol* 2010;32(1):19–23.

21. Zang JB, Coates SJ, Huang J, et al. Pityriasis lichenoides: long-term follow-up study. *Pediatr Dermatol* 2018;35(2):213–219.

22. D'Alessandro M, Buoncompagni A, Minoia F, et al. Cytomegalovirus-related necrotising vasculitis mimicking Henoch-Schönlein syndrome. *Clin Exp Rheumatol* 2014;32(3 Suppl 82):S73–S75.

23. Diaz-Perez JL, Winkelmann RK. Cutaneous polyarteritis nodosa. *Arch Dermatol* 1974;110(3):407–414.

24. Morgan AJ, Schwartz RA. Cutaneous polyarteritis nodosa: a comprehensive review. *Int J Dermatol* 2010;49(7):750–756.

25. Villiger PM, Guillevin L. Microscopic polyangiitis: clinical presentation. *Autoimmun Rev* 2010;9(12):812–819.

26. Carlson JA. The histological assessment of cutaneous vasculitis. *Histopathology* 2010;56(1):3–23.

27. Sunderkötter CH, Zelger B, Chen KR, et al. Nomenclature of cutaneous vasculitis: dermatologic addendum to the 2012 Revised International Chapel Hill Consensus Conference Nomenclature of Vasculitides. *Arthritis Rheumatol* 2018;70(2):171–184.

28. Tirumalae R, Yeliur IK, Antony M, et al. Papulonecrotic tuberculid-clinicopathologic and molecular features of 12 Indian patients. *Dermatol Pract Concept* 2014;4(2):17–22.

29. Jordaan HF, Van Niekerk DJ, Louw M. Papulonecrotic tuberculid. A clinical, histopathological, and immunohistochemical study of 15 patients. *Am J Dermatopathol* 1994;16(5):474–485.

30. Fischer AH, Morris DJ. Pathogenesis of calciphylaxis: study of three cases with literature review. *Hum Pathol* 1995;26(10):1055–1064.

31. Chen TY, Lehman JS, Gibson LE, et al. Histopathology of calciphylaxis: cohort study with clinical correlations. *Am J Dermatopathol* 2017;39(11):795–802.

32. Ng AT, Peng DH. Calciphylaxis. *Dermatol Ther* 2011;24(2):256–262.

33. Akasu R, Kahn HJ, From L. Lymphocyte markers on formalin-fixed tissue in Jessner's lymphocytic infiltrate and lupus erythematosus. *J Cutan Pathol* 1992;19(1):59–65.

34. Rémy-Leroux V, Léonard F, Lambert D, et al. Comparison of histopathologic-clinical characteristics of Jessner's lymphocytic infiltration of the skin and lupus erythematosus tumidus:

35. Von Den Driesch P. Sweet's syndrome: acute febrile neutrophilic dermatosis. *J Am Acad Dermatol* 1994;31(4):535–556; quiz 557–560.

36. Bisno AL, Stevens DL. Streptococcal infections of skin and soft tissues. *N Engl J Med* 1996;334(4):240–245.

37. Nofal A, Abdelmaksoud A, Amer H, et al. Sweet's syndrome: diagnostic criteria revisited. *J Dtsch Dermatol Ges* 2017;15(11):1081–1088.

38. DiCaudo DJ, Connolly SM. Neutrophilic dermatosis (pustular vasculitis) of the dorsal hands. *Arch Dermatol* 2002;138(3):361–365.

39. Weenig RH, Bruce AJ, McEvoy MT, et al. Neutrophilic dermatosis of the hands: four new cases and review of the literature. *Int J Dermatol* 2004;43(2):95–102.

40. Gilaberte Y, Coscojuela C, Garcia-Prats MD. Neutrophilic dermatosis of the dorsal hands versus pustular vasculitis. *J Am Acad Dermatol* 2002;46(6):962–963.

41. Krasagakis K, Samonis G, Valachis A, et al. Local complications of erysipelas: a study of associated risk factors. *Clin Exp Dermatol* 2011;36(4):351–354.

42. Ridley DS. Histological classification and the immunological spectrum of leprosy. *Bull World Health Organ* 1974;51(5):451–465.

43. Massone C, Belachew WA, Schettini A. Histopathology of the lepromatous skin biopsy. *Clin Dermatol* 2015;33(1):38–45.

44. Risdall RJ, Dehner LP, Duray P, et al. Histiocytosis X (Langerhans' cell histiocytosis): prognostic role of histopathology. *Arch Pathol Lab Med* 1983;107(2):59–63.

45. Crickx E, Bouaziz JD, Lorillon G, et al. Clinical spectrum, quality of life, BRAF mutation status and treatment of skin involvement in adult langerhans cell histiocytosis. *Acta Derm Venereol* 2017;97(7):838–842.

46. Marchand-Senécal X, Barkati S, Bouffard D, et al. A secondary syphilis rash with scaly target lesions. *Oxf Med Case Reports* 2018;2018(2):omx089.

47. Matito A, Azaña JM, Torrelo A, et al. Cutaneous mastocytosis in adults and children: new classification and prognostic factors. *Immunol Allergy Clin North Am* 2018;38(3):351–363.

48. Fisher GB, Greer KE, Copper PH. Eosinophilic cellulitis (Wells' syndrome). *Int J Dermatol* 1985;24(2):101–107.

49. Räßler F, Lukács J, Elsner P. Treatment of eosinophilic cellulitis (Wells syndrome)—a systematic review. *J Eur Acad Dermatol Venereol* 2016;30(9):1465–1479.

50. Gandhi RK, Coloe J, Peters S, et al. Wells syndrome (eosinophilic cellulitis): a clinical imitator of bacterial cellulitis. *J Clin Aesthet Dermatol* 2011;4(7):55–57.

51. Gleim ER, Garrison LE, Vello MS, et al. Factors associated with tick bites and pathogen prevalence in ticks parasitizing humans in Georgia, USA. *Parasit Vectors* 2016;9:125.

52. Handler MZ, Patel PA, Kapila R, et al. Cutaneous and mucocutaneous leishmaniasis: differential diagnosis, diagnosis, histopathology, and management. *J Am Acad Dermatol* 2015;73(6):911–926; 927–928.

53. Kopf AW, Weidman AI. Nevus of Ota. *Arch Dermatol* 1962;85:195–208.

54. Goldman-Lévy G, Rigau V, Bléchet C, et al. Primary melanoma of the leptomeninges with BAP1 expression-loss in the setting of a nevus of Ota: a clinical, morphological and genetic study of 2 cases. *Brain Pathol* 2016;26(4):547–550.

multicenter study of 46 cases. *J Am Acad Dermatol* 2008;58(2):217–223.

55. Al Wahbi A. Autoamputation of diabetic toe with dry gangrene: a myth or a fact? *Diabetes Metab Syndr Obes* 2018;11:255–264.

56. O'Brien TJ. Iodic eruptions. *Australas J Dermatol* 1987;28(3): 119–122.

57. Castillo CG, Kauffman CA, Miceli MH. Blastomycosis. *Infect Dis Clin North Am* 2016;30(1):247–264.

58. Mercurio MG, Elewski BE. Cutaneous blastomycosis. *Cutis* 1992;50(6):422–424.

59. Noe MH, Rosenbach M. Cutaneous sarcoidosis. *Curr Opin Pulm Med* 2017;23(5):482–486.

60. Dalle Vedove C, Colato C, Girolomoni G. Subcutaneous sarcoidosis: report of two cases and review of the literature. *Clin Rheumatol* 2011;30(8):1123–1128.

61. Farina MC, Gegundez MI, Pique E, et al. Cutaneous tuberculosis: a clinical, histopathologic, and bacteriologic study. *J Am Acad Dermatol* 1995;33(3):433–440.

62. Amiruddin D, Mii S, Fujimura T, et al. Clinical evaluation of 35 cases of lupus miliaris disseminatus faciei. *J Dermatol* 2011; 38(6):618–620.

63. Piette EW, Rosenbach M. Granuloma annulare: clinical and histologic variants, epidemiology, and genetics. *J Am Acad Dermatol* 2016;75(3):457–465.

64. Lowitt MH, Dover JS. Necrobiosis lipoidica. *J Am Acad Dermatol* 1991;25(5 Pt 1):735–748.

65. Sibbald C, Reid S, Alavi A. Necrobiosis lipoidica. *Dermatol Clin* 2015;33(3):343–360.

66. Mehregan DA, Winkelmann RK. Necrobiotic xanthogranuloma. *Arch Dermatol* 1992;128(1):94–100.

67. Wood AJ, Wagner MV, Abbott JJ, et al. Necrobiotic xanthogranuloma: a review of 17 cases with emphasis on clinical and pathologic correlation. *Arch Dermatol* 2009;145(3):279–284.

68. Higgins LS, Go RS, Dingli D, et al. Clinical features and treatment outcomes of patients with necrobiotic xanthogranuloma associated with monoclonal gammopathies. *Clin Lymphoma Myeloma Leuk* 2016;16(8):447–452.

69. Veys EM, De Keyser F. Rheumatoid nodules: differential diagnosis and immunohistological findings. *Ann Rheum Dis* 1993;52(9):625–626.

70. Ziemer M, Müller AK, Hein G, et al. Incidence and classification of cutaneous manifestations in rheumatoid arthritis. *J Dtsch Dermatol Ges* 2016;14(12):1237–1246.

71. Chu P, Connolly MK, LeBoit PE. The histopathologic spectrum of palisaded neutrophilic and granulomatous dermatitis in patients with collagen vascular disease. *Arch Dermatol* 1994; 130(10):1278–1283.

72. Sangueza OP, Caudell MD, Mengesha YM, et al. Palisaded neutrophilic granulomatous dermatitis in rheumatoid arthritis. *J Am Acad Dermatol* 2002;47(2):251–257.

73. Mahmoodi M, Ahmad A, Bansal C, et al. Palisaded neutrophilic and granulomatous dermatitis in association with sarcoidosis. *J Cutan Pathol* 2011;38(4):365–368.

74. Gordon K, Miteva M, Torchia D, et al. Allopurinol-induced palisaded neutrophilic and granulomatous dermatitis. *Cutan Ocul Toxicol* 2012;31(4):338–340.

75. Rosenbach M, English JC 3rd. Reactive granulomatous dermatitis: a review of palisaded neutrophilic and granulomatous dermatitis, interstitial granulomatous dermatitis, interstitial granulomatous drug reaction, and a proposed reclassification. *Dermatol Clin* 2015;33(3):373–387.

76. Molina-Ruiz AM, Requena L. Foreign body granulomas. *Dermatol Clin* 2015;33(3):497–523.

77. Adler BL, Krausz AE, Minuti A, et al. Epidemiology and treatment of angiolymphoid hyperplasia with eosinophilia (ALHE): a systematic review. *J Am Acad Dermatol* 2016;74(3):506–512.

78. Ko JS, Billings SD. Diagnostically challenging epithelioid vascular tumors. *Surg Pathol Clin* 2015;8(3):331–351.

79. Thompson MJ, Engelman D, Gholam K, et al. Systematic review of the diagnosis of scabies in therapeutic trials. *Clin Exp Dermatol* 2017;42(5):481–487.

80. Hashimoto K, Fujiwara K, Punwaney J, et al. Post-scabetic nodules: a lymphohistiocytic reaction rich in indeterminate cells. *J Dermatol* 2000;27(3):181–194.

81. Quintella LP, Passos SR, do Vale AC, et al. Histopathology of cutaneous sporotrichosis in Rio de Janeiro: a series of 119 consecutive cases. *J Cutan Pathol* 2011;38(1):25–32.

82. Gonzalez-Santiago TM, Drage LA. Nontuberculous mycobacteria: skin and soft tissue infections. *Dermatol Clin* 2015; 33(3):563–577.

83. Travis WD, Travis LB, Roberts GD, et al. The histopathologic spectrum in Mycobacterium marinum infection. *Arch Pathol Lab Med* 1985;109(12):1109–1113.

84. Sirka CS, Dash G, Pradhan S, et al. Cutaneous botryomycosis in immunocompetent patients: a case series. *Indian Dermatol Online J* 2019;10(3):311–315.

85. Yang CS, Chen CB, Lee YY, et al. Chromoblastomycosis in Taiwan: a report of 30 cases and a review of the literature. *Med Mycol* 2018;56(4):395–405.

86. Correia RT, Valente NY, Criado PR, et al. Chromoblastomycosis: study of 27 cases and review of medical literature. *An Bras Dermatol* 2010;85(4):448–454.

87. Chavan SS, Kulkarni MH, Makannavar JH. 'Unstained' and 'de stained' sectionsin the diagnosis of chromoblastomycosis: a clinico-pathological study. *Indian J Pathol Microbiol* 2010; 53(4):666–671.

88. Bernardeschi C, Foulet F, Ingen-Housz-Oro S, et al; French Mycosis Study Group. Cutaneous invasive aspergillosis: retrospective multicenter study of the French invasive-aspergillosis registry and literature review. *Medicine (Baltimore)* 2015; 94(26):e1018.

89. Copeland NK, Decker CF. Other sexually transmitted diseases chancroid and donovanosis. *Dis Mon* 2016;62(8):306–313.

90. Hadi A, Lebwohl M. Clinical features of pyoderma gangrenosum and current diagnostic trends. *J Am Acad Dermatol* 2011; 64(5):950–954.

91. Braswell SF, Kostopoulos TC, Ortega-Loayza AG. Pathophysiology of pyoderma gangrenosum (PG): an updated review. *J Am Acad Dermatol* 2015;73(4):691–698.

92. Upile T, Patel NN, Jerjes W, et al. Advances in the understanding of chondrodermatitis nodularis chronica helicis: the perichondrial vasculitis theory. *Clin Otolaryngol* 2009;34(2):147–150.

93. Ferreli C, Gasparini G, Parodi A, et al. Cutaneous manifestations of scleroderma and scleroderma-like disorders: a comprehensive review. *Clin Rev Allergy Immunol* 2017;53(3):306–336.

94. Fett N, Werth VP. Update on morphea: part I. Epidemiology, clinical presentation, and pathogenesis. *J Am Acad Dermatol* 2011;64(2):217–228; quiz 229–230.

95. Senecal JL, Henault J, Raymond Y. The pathogenic role of autoantibodies to nuclear autoantigens in systemic sclerosis (scleroderma). *J Rheumatol* 2005;32(9):1643–1649.

96. Graf SW, Hakendorf P, Lester S, et al. South Australian scleroderma register: autoantibodies as predictive biomarkers of phenotype and outcome. *Int J Rheum Dis* 2012;15(1):102–109.

Perivascular, Diffuse, and Granulomatous Infiltrates of the Reticular Dermis

97. Kreuter A, Wischnewski J, Terras S, et al. Coexistence of lichen sclerosus and morphea: a retrospective analysis of 472 patients with localized scleroderma from a German tertiary referral center. *J Am Acad Dermatol* 2012;67(6):1157–1162.

98. Boncher J, Bergfeld WF. Fluoroscopy-induced chronic radiation dermatitis: a report of two additional cases and a brief review of the literature. *J Cutan Pathol* 2012;39(1):63–67.

99. LeBoit PE. Subacute radiation dermatitis: a histologic imitator of acute cutaneous graft-versus-host disease. *J Am Acad Dermatol* 1989;20(2 Pt 1):236–241.

100. Girardi M, Kay J, Elston DM, et al. Nephrogenic systemic fibrosis: clinicopathological definition and workup recommendations. *J Am Acad Dermatol* 2011;65(6):1095–1106.

101. Haemel AK, Sadowski EA, Shafer MM, et al. Update on nephrogenic systemic fibrosis: are we making progress? *Int J Dermatol* 2011;50(6):659–666.

102. Knobler R, Moinzadeh P, Hunzelmann N, et al. European dermatology forum S1-guideline on the diagnosis and treatment of sclerosing diseases of the skin, Part 2: scleromyxedema, scleredema and nephrogenic systemic fibrosis. *J Eur Acad Dermatol Venereol* 2017;31(10):1581–1594.

103. Kucher C, Xu X, Pasha T, et al. Histopathologic comparison of nephrogenic fibrosing dermopathy and scleromyxedema. *J Cutan Pathol* 2005;32(7):484–490.

104. Chen AY, Zirwas MJ, Heffernan MP. Nephrogenic systemic fibrosis: a review. *J Drugs Dermatol* 2010;9(7):829–834.

105. Braverman IM, Cowper S. Nephrogenic systemic fibrosis. *F1000 Med Rep* 2010;2:84.

106. Elder DE. Melanoma progression. *Pathology* 2016;48(2):147–154.

107. Goltz RW, Henderson RR, Hitch JM, et al. Focal dermal hypoplasia syndrome. *Arch Dermatol* 1970;101(1):1–11.

108. Maalouf D, Mégarbané H, Chouery E, et al. A novel mutation in the PORCN gene underlying a case of almost unilateral focal dermal hypoplasia. *Arch Dermatol* 2012;148(1):85–88.

109. Danielsen L, Kohayasi T, Larsen HW, et al. Pseudoxanthoma elasticum. *Acta Derm Venereol (Stockh)* 1970;50(5):355–373.

110. Uitto J, Bercovitch L, Terry SF, et al. Pseudoxanthoma elasticum: progress in diagnostics and research towards treatment: summary of the 2010 PXE International Research Meeting. *Am J Med Genet A* 2011;155A(7):1517–1526.

111. Andrés-Ramos I, Alegría-Landa V, Gimeno I, et al. Cutaneous elastic tissue anomalies. *Am J Dermatopathol* 2019;41(2):85–117.

112. Staiger H, Saposnik M, Spiner RE, et al. Primary anetoderma: a cutaneous marker of antiphospholipid antibodies. *Skinmed* 2011;9(3):168–171.

113. Goujon E, Beer F, Gay S, et al. Anetoderma of prematurity: an iatrogenic consequence of neonatal intensive care. *Arch Dermatol* 2010;146(5):565–567.

114. Kanitakis J. Reactive perforating collagenosis. *Skinmed* 2018;16(6):390–396.

115. Kuo KL, Lee LY, Kuo TT. Solitary cutaneous focal mucinosis: a clinicopathological study of 11 cases of soft fibroma-like cutaneous mucinous lesions. *J Dermatol* 2017;44(3):335–338.

116. Salasche SJ. Myxoid cysts of the proximal nail fold. *J Dermatol Surg Oncol* 1984;10(1):35–39.

117. Armijo M. Mucoid cysts of the fingers. Differential diagnosis, ultrastructure, and surgical treatment. *J Dermatol Surg Oncol* 1981;7(4):317–322.

118. Lan C, Wang Y, Zeng X, et al. Morphological diversity of pretibial myxedema and its mechanism of evolving process and outcome: a retrospective study of 216 cases. *J Thyroid Res* 2016;2016:2652174.

119. Rongioletti F, Rebora A. Updated classification of papular mucinosis, lichen myxedematosus, and scleromyxedema. *J Am Acad Dermatol* 2001;44(2):273–281.

120. Molina-Ruiz AM, Cerroni L, Kutzner H, et al. Cutaneous deposits. *Am J Dermatopathol* 2014;36(1):1–48.

121. Maldonado I, Prasad V, Reginato AJ. Oxalate crystal deposition disease. *Curr Rheumatol Rep* 2002;4(3):257–264.

122. Blackmon JA, Jeffy BG, Malone JC, et al. Oxalosis involving the skin: case report and literature review. *Arch Dermatol* 2011;147(11):1302–1305.

123. Shih HA, Kao DM, Elenitsas R, et al. Livedo reticularis, ulcers, and peripheral gangrene: cutaneous manifestations of primary hyperoxaluria. *Arch Dermatol* 2000;136(10):1272–1274.

124. Trent JT, Kirsner RS. Ulcerations in primary hyperoxaluria. *Adv Skin Wound Care* 2005;18(5 Pt 1):244–247.

125. Mehregan D, Hooten J. Adult colloid milium: a case report and literature review. *Int J Dermatol* 2011;50(12):1531–1534.

126. Pursley TV, Prince MJ, Chausmer AB, et al. Cutaneous manifestations of tumoral calcinosis. *Arch Dermatol* 1979;115(9):1100–1102.

127. Dereure O. Drug induced skin pigmentation. Epidemiology, diagnosis and treatment. *Am J Clin Dermatol* 2001;2(4):253–262.

128. Tavares J, Leung WW. Discoloration of nail beds and skin from minocycline. *CMAJ* 2011;183(2):224.

129. Argenyi ZB, FInell L, Bergfeld WF, et al. Minocycline related cutaneous hyperpigmentation as demonstrated by light microscopy, electron microscopy and x-ray energy spectroscopy. *J Cutan Pathol* 1987;14(3):176–180.

130. Sulica VJ, Berberian B, Kao GF. Histopathologic findings in cutaneous larva migrans (abstr). *J Cutan Pathol* 1988;15:346.

131. Feldmeier H, Schuster A. Mini review: hookworm-related cutaneous larva migrans. *Eur J Clin Microbiol Infect Dis* 2012;31(6):915–918.

Tumors and Cysts of the Dermis and Subcutis

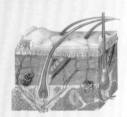

Neoplasms in the reticular dermis may arise from any of the tissues included in the dermis—lymphoreticular tissue, connective tissue, and epithelial tissue of the skin appendages. In addition, metastases commonly present in the dermis and subcutis. A neoplastic nodule is a circumscribed collection of neoplastic cells in the dermis. Abscesses, granulomas and cysts may also present as nodules. Cysts are considered separately. In general, neoplastic nodules can be differentiated from reactive and inflammatory nodules by the presence of a monotonous population of cells consistent with a clonal proliferation, while inflammatory nodules are composed of inflammatory cell types (lymphocytes, neutrophils, histiocytes etc.), generally in a heterogeneous mixture.

VIA SMALL AND INTERMEDIATE CELL TUMORS

The cells of this group of tumors range in size from that of a small lymphocyte to approximately that of a histiocyte. These tumors in general are characterized by having very scant cytoplasm, so that the nuclei are closely apposed to one another and may even mold on one another as is characteristic in small cell carcinomas of the lung. The nuclei, while larger than those of lymphocytes (except in the case of a well-differentiated small cell lymphoma) are relatively small by virtue of having compact hyperchromatic chromatin and, usually, absent or inconspicuous nucleoli.

1. Tumors of Lymphocytes or Hemopoietic Cells
2. Tumors of Lymphocytes and Mixed Cell Types
3. Tumors of Plasma Cells
4. Small Round Cell Tumors

VIA1 Tumors of Lymphocytes or Hemopoietic Cells

Nodular infiltrates or extensive diffuse infiltrates of normal and/or atypical lymphocytes are found in the dermis. In a single center follow-up study of 299 patients with primary cutaneous lymphomas, 63% expressed a T-cell phenotype and 37% a B-cell phenotype (1). The most common primary cutaneous T-cell entities were mycosis fungoides (31%, with an overall disease-specific 5-year survival of 80%), lymphomatoid papulosis (16% with a 100% survival), and anaplastic large cell lymphoma (9%, 92% survival). The most common primary cutaneous B-cell entities were follicular center cell lymphoma (17% with a 98% survival), marginal zone B-cell lymphoma (BCL) (10%, 100% survival), and diffuse large B-cell lymphoma (DLBCL), leg type (9%, 63% survival). Primary cutaneous mantle cell lymphoma, with a very poor prognosis, is very rare (2). Primary cutaneous follicular center lymphoma (PCFCL) is prototypic (3,4). The final diagnosis of most of these conditions should be made by experts with specialization in cutaneous lymphoma pathology; however, it is necessary to recognize the conditions as they present in routine practice so as to allow for appropriate disposition of them.

Cutaneous B-Cell Follicle Center Lymphoma

CLINICAL SUMMARY. The clinical presentation of PCFCL stereotypically comprises one or several nodules situated in a single area, most often the skin of the scalp or forehead. The lesions are red to purple and can have intact or ulcerated surfaces. In general, the prognosis of cutaneous BCLs is favorable if the disease is primary and unfavorable if the skin is secondarily involved from a nodal or systemic lymphoma. Spread to the skin is observed in about 4% of the cases of nodal FCL.

Tumors and Cysts of the Dermis and Subcutis

VI

HISTOPATHOLOGY. The infiltrates of cutaneous BCLs are most easily diagnosed when they are "bottom-heavy" (the larger proportion of the tumor is in the lower dermis or subcutaneous fat), but top-heavy patterns also occur. In primary cutaneous FCL, the neoplastic follicles can be of uniform size, with mantles that are thin or absent, resulting in coalescence of follicles. Tingible body macrophages, which represent cells engulfing the remnants of apoptotic lymphocytes, are rare. In contrast, a heterogeneous composition of follicles, with many tingible body macrophages and well-formed mantles of small lymphocytes around them, would favor a benign interpretation. The mitotic rate is low in cases in which small cleaved cells (centrocytes) predominate, and higher as the proportion of large non-cleaved cells or centroblasts increases. Most of the many variations of follicular lymphoma (FL) that occur in lymph nodes, such as irregularly shaped follicles, follicles with serrated outlines, follicles with thick mantles, conspicuous follicular dendritic cells, many tingible body macrophages, and follicles with extracellular amorphous material, can also occur in cutaneous lesions. In lesions with an immunophenotype-resembling MALToma (marginal zone lymphoma), the cells can resemble centrocytes, which are small lymphocytes with indented nuclei and varying amounts of pale cytoplasm, and/or may be plasmacytoid.

By immunohistochemistry, the B cells of primary cutaneous FL may express monotypic cell surface immunoglobulin (more commonly in frozen sections or by flow cytometry), or may fail to express immunoglobulin at all (so-called "immunoglobulin-negative" FL). Light chain restriction can be used to demonstrate clonality. Genotypic studies can detect clonal rearrangement of the immunoglobulin heavy or light chain genes, or both. PCFCL express the B-cell markers CD19+, CD20+, CD22+, and are bcl-2−, bcl-6+, and CD10+/−. Large cell lymphomas that occur most commonly on the leg of women, but also on other sites, and are therefore classified as DLBCL, leg type, have the immunophenotype CD20+ CD70a+, CD10−, CD138−, bcl-6 +/−, bcl2+, MUM-1/RF-4+. Mantle cell lymphomas are typically CD20+, CD10−, CD23−, cyclin D+, BCL-6−, and characteristically but not always CD5+. The vast majority of mantle cell lymphomas have a translocation involving the cyclin D locus with subsequent overexpression of this gene (5–8). See Table VI.1 for a summary of immunohistochemical profiles of the major B-cell proliferations.

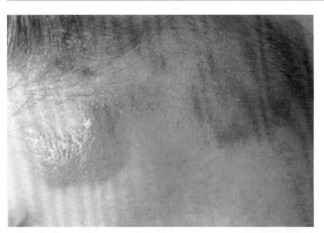

Clin. Fig. VIA1.a

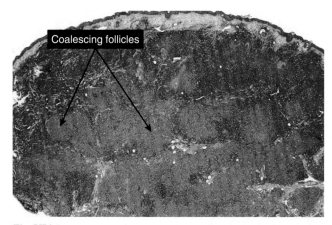

Fig. VIA1.a

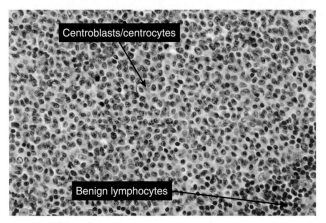

Fig. VIA1.b

Clin. Fig. VIA1.a. *Cutaneous lymphoma (secondary)*. A 57-year-old woman with B-cell lymphoma developed asymptomatic erythematous-lavender plaques and tumors on the face and scalp.

Fig. VIA1.a. *Primary cutaneous follicular center cell lymphoma, low power*. A multinodular pattern is clearly evident in this lymphomatous infiltrate situated at the dermal-subcutaneous junction, composed of small, cleaved follicular center cells arranged as coalescing follicles. (G Murphy.)

Fig. VIA1.b. *Primary cutaneous follicular center cell lymphoma, medium power*. Higher magnification of follicular centrocytes and centroblasts. Note the absence of tingible-body macrophages. Although mostly "small," the cells are larger than benign lymphocytes. (G Murphy.)

TABLE VI.1. Immunophenotype of B-Cell Cutaneous Lymphoid Proliferations

	CD20 & CD79a	BCL6	BCL2	CD10	CD5	CCND
CLH	+	+	−	+	−	−
PCMZL	+	−	−	−	−	−
PCFCL	+	+	+/−	−	−	−
2° FCL in skin	+	+	+	+	−	−
MCL	+	−	+	−	+	+
CLL/SLL	+	−	+	−	+	

CLH: cutaneous lymphoid hyperplasia; PCMZL: primary cutaneous (PC) mantle cell lymphoma; PCFCL: PC follicular cell lymphoma; 2° FCL: secondary cutaneous FCL; MCL: mantle cell lymphoma; CLL/SLL: chronic lymphocytic leukemia/small lymphocytic lymphoma.

Data from Jaffe ES, Arber DA, Campo E, et al. Hematopathology. 2nd ed. Elsevier; 2016.

Cutaneous Diffuse B-Cell Lymphoma

PCFCL can have follicular (nodular), follicular and diffuse, or diffuse patterns. The diffuse patterns are typically comprised of larger cells than the follicular patterns. The differential diagnosis for this appearance (when the cells are smaller) could include a chronic lymphocytic leukemia/small lymphocytic lymphoma (CLL/SLL) of systemic origin. See Table VI.1.

Primary Cutaneous Marginal Zone (MALT) Lymphoma

Primary cutaneous marginal zone lymphoma (PCMZL) is an indolent lymphoma comprised of neoplastic small B cells, plasma cells, and a variable number of T cells. It presents histologically as a dense dermal multinodular infiltrate of small lymphocytes, plasma cells and includes follicles with reactive germinal centers (9). See Table VI.1.

The immunophenotype of marginal zone lymphoma is positive for the B-cell markers CD19+, CD20+, CD22+, CD79a+, and is bcl-2+, CD5−, CD10−, bcl6−, CD23−. In contrast, reactive germinal centers are bcl-6+, bcl-2−.

Cutaneous T-Cell Lymphoma, Tumor Stage

Mycosis fungoides is the prototype of cutaneous T-cell lymphomas (CTCLs). From an initial patch and plaque stages (illustrated in IIID1, IIIF1, and IIIF5), the lesions may progress to a tumor stage in which the dermal

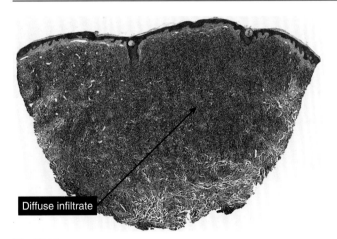

Diffuse infiltrate

Fig. VIA1.c

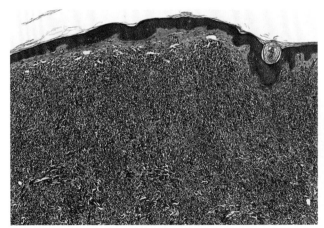

Fig. VIA1.d

Fig. VIA1.c. *Cutaneous diffuse B-cell lymphoma, low power.* There is a dense dermal infiltrate of basophilic cells which does not involve the overlying epidermis. Typically, in cutaneous B-cell lymphoma, the infiltrate is "bottom-heavy," meaning that a significant portion of the infiltrate involves the lower dermis.

Fig. VIA1.d. *Cutaneous diffuse B-cell lymphoma, medium power.* The dermal infiltrate may be nodular in appearance, however, as seen here the cells frequently permeate between bundles of reticular dermal collagen. (*continues*)

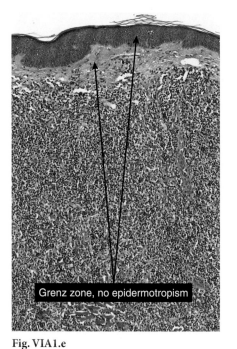

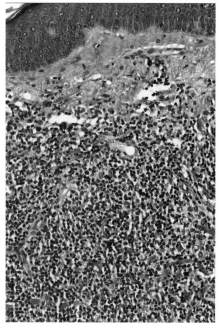

Fig. VIA1.e. *Cutaneous diffuse B-cell lymphoma, high power.* High power reveals cytologically atypical lymphoid cells admixed with nuclear fragments. With little pressure from a punch biopsy, these cells frequently show crush artifact.

Fig. VIA1.f. *Cutaneous diffuse B-cell lymphoma, high power.* Not all cells in cutaneous B-cell lymphoma are large and atypical. In this example, the cells are small, hyperchromatic, and monotonous in appearance.

Fig. VIA1.e

Fig. VIA1.f

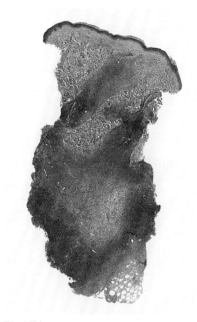

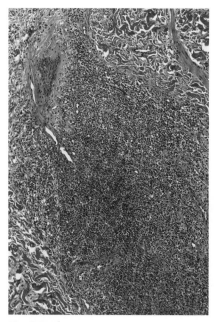

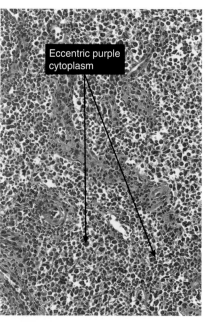

Fig. VIA1.g

Fig. VIA1.h

Fig. VIA1.i

Fig. VIA1.g. *Primary cutaneous marginal zone lymphoma, low power.* A dense tumor with a "bottom heavy" configuration in the dermis and subcutis and a multinodular appearance.

Fig. VIA1.h. *Primary cutaneous marginal zone lymphoma, medium power.* The tumor is comprised of sheets of monotonous small cells.

Fig. VIA1.i. *Primary cutaneous marginal zone lymphoma, high power.* The cells have a plasmacytoid configuration, with eccentric purple cytoplasm.

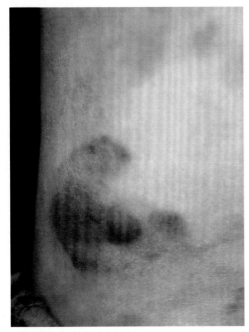

Clin. Fig. VIA1.b

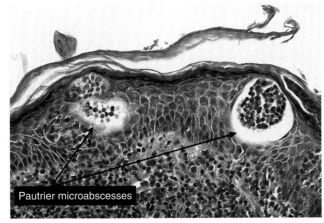

Fig. VIA1.j

Grenz zone, no epidermotropism

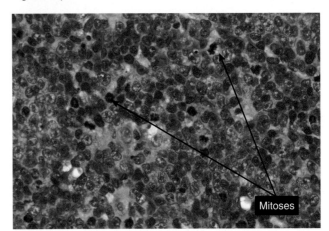

Fig. VIA1.k

Pautrier microabscesses

Fig. VIA1.l

Mitoses

Clin. Fig. VIA1.b. *Cutaneous T-cell lymphoma, tumor stage.* A tumor nodule has arisen in a pre-existing plaque stage of mycosis fungoides in a 41-year-old woman.

Fig. VIA1.j. *Cutaneous T-cell lymphoma, tumor stage, low power.* In tumor stage mycosis fungoides, there are dense aggregates of lymphoid cells filling the papillary and reticular dermis. The overlying epidermis may or may not be involved by these atypical cells.

Fig. VIA1.k. *Cutaneous T-cell lymphoma, tumor stage, medium power.* Focally, one may identify collections of epidermotropic T cells ("Pautrier microabscesses"), a feature which helps differentiate this lesion from cutaneous B-cell lymphoma.

Fig. VIA1.l. *Cutaneous T-cell lymphoma, tumor stage, high power.* Upon close inspection the lymphoid cells have enlarged nuclei and there are numerous mitotic figures.

VI Tumors and Cysts of the Dermis and Subcutis

infiltrates become diffuse, epidermotropism may be lost, and the cells are larger. The immunophenotype is typically CD2+, CD3+, CD4+, CD5+, CD45RO+, CD8−, CD30−. During progression of the disease, loss of CD2, CD5 and CD7 can occur, and CD30 expression may be acquired. The CD4+ cells may have a cytotoxic phenotype of TIA-1+, granzyme +. Occasionally the phenotype is CD8+ CD4− (10).

Conditions to consider in the differential diagnosis:

> cutaneous T-cell lymphoma
> > lymphoblastic lymphoma, T-cell type
> > tumor-stage mycosis fungoides
> > adult T-cell /lymphoma
>
> cutaneous B-cell lymphoma
> > lymphoblastic lymphoma, B-cell type
> > small lymphocytic lymphoma
> > immunocytoma (lymphoplasmacytoid lymphoma)
> > primary cutaneous follicular lymphoma
> > diffuse large B-cell lymphoma (centroblastic/immunoblastic)
>
> drug-induced pseudolymphoma
> aluminum granuloma
> pseudolymphomatous tattoo reaction
> leukemia cutis

VIA2 | Tumors of Lymphocytes and Mixed Cell Types

Nodular infiltrates or extensive diffuse infiltrates of normal lymphocytes are found in the dermis. Other reactive cell types (plasma cells, histiocytes) are admixed. B-cell cutaneous lymphoid hyperplasia is prototypic (11).

B-Cell Cutaneous Lymphoid Hyperplasia (B-CLH, Pseudolymphoma, Lymphocytoma Cutis)

CLINICAL SUMMARY. The term "pseudolymphoma" loosely refers to a group of conditions in which the microscopic appearance of lymphocytic infiltrates in the skin resembles that of one of the cutaneous lymphomas. There are many cutaneous pseudolymphomas, including lymphoid proliferations of B-cell or T-cell composition. B-CLH is often referred simply to as pseudolymphoma, because it was the first simulant of cutaneous lymphoma to be studied comprehensively. In B-CLH, nodules or plaques result from the recapitulation in the skin of the elements found in the cortices of reactive lymph nodes. Clinically, B-CLH generally presents with red to purple nodules or plaques, usually on the face or scalp. Lesions are usually solitary but may be multiple. Patients with multiple lesions often have only a few lesions affecting a circumscribed area (most often the skin of the head or neck), but rare patients have generalized lesions. Most lesions persist for months or years, sometimes to resolve spontaneously.

HISTOPATHOLOGY. The infiltrates of B-CLH are nodular or diffuse, and involve the dermis and/or the subcutis. A "top-heavy" pattern is often observed at scanning magnification—that is, the infiltrate is denser in the dermis than in the subcutis. Follicles may be distinct or inconspicuous. In the follicular pattern, distinct germinal centers are present, identical in composition to secondary follicles in reactive lymph nodes. These consist of follicular center cells which include small cleaved and large lymphocytes, and tingible body macrophages surrounded by a mantle of small lymphocytes. Mitotic figures are commonly found in these reactive follicles. The polarization seen in reactive lymph nodes is usually not evident. The mantle zone is composed of small lymphocytes. Peripheral to the follicles and their mantles is an admixture of cells that consist of T cells with small but irregularly shaped nuclei, immunoblasts (large cells with large vesicular nuclei and prominent, central nucleoli), histiocytes and rarely histiocytic giant cells, eosinophils, polyclonal plasma cells, and plasmacytoid monocytes. The venules found in these interfollicular areas resemble the "high endothelial venules" of lymph nodes in that their endothelial cells have protuberant nuclei.

The nonfollicular pattern of B-CLH can present as a nodular or diffuse infiltrate with a mixture of cell types. A *sine qua non* is the presence of follicular center cells, but there are often eosinophils, macrophages, and plasma cells. Hints of follicles are sometimes apparent at scanning magnification as zones of pale-staining cells; the presence of follicular elements in such areas can be confirmed by immunostaining for antigens such as CD21 and CD23 that recognize follicular dendritic cells, whose processes form a meshwork in lymphoid follicles. See Table VI.1 for immunohistochemical profiles.

In a study of 24 cases, the lesions were classified according to characteristic histologic features and immunophenotypic staining patterns as follows: 10 cases with presence of germinal center (GC) cell clusters forming well-defined lymphoid follicles; 6 with clusters of GC cells not forming well-defined lymphoid follicles; 1 case of persistent arthropod assault type CLH; 4 cases of CLH with a prominent histiocytic component; and 3 of CLH without specific histologic and immunophenotypic features, that is, nonspecific mixed T-cell and B-cell CLH. Most of the CLH cases did not demonstrate clonal T-cell receptor and/or immunoglobulin heavy chain gene rearrangements except for 3 cases in which long-term follow-up was uneventful (12).

Conditions to consider in the differential diagnosis:

> cutaneous lymphoid hyperplasia/lymphocytoma cutis
> angioimmunoblastic lymphadenopathy
> Borrelial lymphocytoma cutis
> chronic myelogenous leukemia

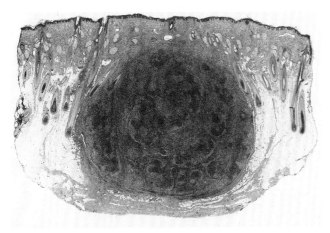

Fig. VIA2.a

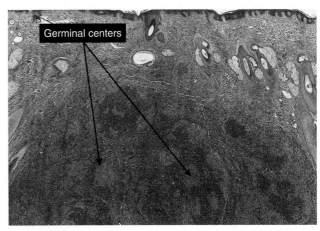

Fig. VIA2.b

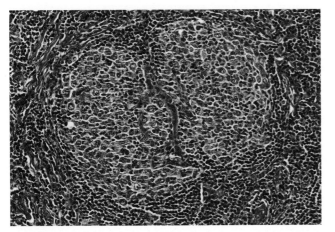

Fig. VIA2.c

Fig. VIA2.a. *Cutaneous lymphoid hyperplasia, low power.* In cutaneous lymphoid hyperplasia there are nodular aggregates of mononuclear cells within the dermis which may extend into the subcutaneous fat. The infiltrate may be diffuse, or as seen here, nodular in architecture.

Fig. VIA2.b. *Cutaneous lymphoid hyperplasia, medium power.* The lymphoid infiltrate mimics the pattern seen in lymph nodes with formation of germinal centers.

Fig. VIA2.c. *Cutaneous lymphoid hyperplasia, high power.* The germinal center consists of central large mononuclear cells with vesicular nuclei. These are surrounded by a mantle of small lymphocytes. Confirming immunostains and perhaps gene rearrangement studies should be considered in cases like this; there should be evidence of polyclonality, and the reactive germinal centers should be bcl-6+, bcl-2−.

VIA3 Tumors of Plasma Cells

Nodular plasma cell infiltrates, with scattered lymphocytes. Cutaneous plasmacytoma (13) and multiple myeloma (14) exemplify this reaction pattern.

Cutaneous Plasmacytoma and Multiple Myeloma (MM)

CLINICAL SUMMARY. Cutaneous lesions of MM or plasmacytoma are usually circumscribed, violaceous papules or nodules. Diffusely infiltrated plaques are occasionally observed. Cutaneous deposits of myeloma are rare, occurring in only about 2% of myeloma patients. Patients with myeloma can also develop a variety of nonspecific cutaneous complications (15), including deposits of light-chain derived amyloid (primary systemic amyloidosis), purpuric lesions resulting from monoclonal cryoglobulinemia, diffuse normolipemic plane xanthoma, pyoderma gangrenosum, Sweet syndrome, leukocytoclastic vasculitis, and erythema elevatum diutinum.

Monoclonal gammopathies can complicate a variety of other cutaneous diseases, such as scleromyxedema, necrobiotic xanthogranuloma with paraproteinemia, POEMS syndrome (polyneuropathy, organomegaly, endocrinopathy, M protein, and skin lesions), and scleredema. Myeloma supervenes in a small minority of patients with any of these disorders.

HISTOPATHOLOGY. In cutaneous lesions of MM and in plasmacytomas, there are monomorphous infiltrates of plasma cells, arrayed as densely cellular nodules or interstitially between collagen bundles. In the nodular pattern, clusters of macrophages are sometimes present. Multinucleate plasma cells, plasmacytes with large atypical nuclei, and mitotic figures can be observed. Plasma cell bodies, round eosinophilic fragments of plasma cell cytoplasm, can be present in the background between intact cells, but are not specific for MM. Intranuclear inclusions of immunoglobulin, known as Dutcher bodies, are rare in MM. Infiltrates that are composed of nuclei with a "clock-face" clumping of chromatin typical of mature, or Marshalko-type, plasma cells have been referred to as the plasmacytic variant. Infiltrates that are composed of cells with nuclei that resemble those of immunoblasts are sometimes

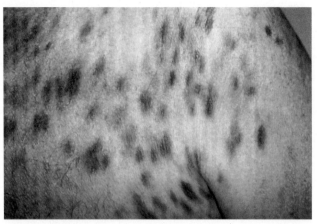

Clin. Fig. VIA.3

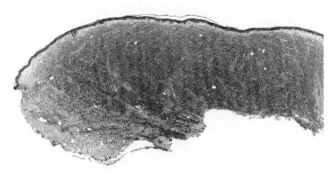

Fig. VIA3.a

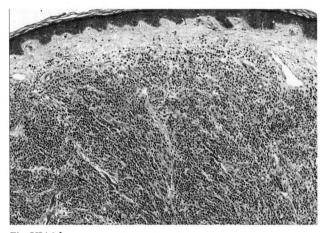

Fig. VIA3.b

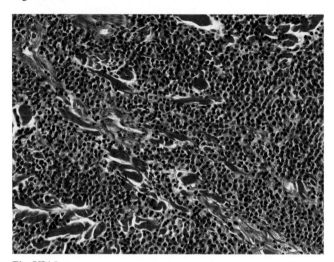

Fig. VIA3.c

Clin. Fig. VIA.3. *Systemic plasmacytosis, low power.* A middle-aged woman suddenly developed multiple nodules and papules.

Fig. VIA3.a. *Plasmacytoma, low power.* Biopsy of a papule shows a dense interstitial infiltrates.

Fig. VIA3.b. *Plasmacytoma, low power.* The tumor cells do not involve the epidermis.

Fig. VIA3.c. *Plasmacytoma, high power.* The infiltrate consists of a monotonous population of histologically typical plasma cells. These appearances, taken in isolation, are suspicious but not diagnostic of an evolving myeloma. Demonstration of clonality would confirm the impression of a neoplastic rather than reactive infiltrate. Myeloma would need to be ruled out clinically.

referred to as plasmablastic plasmacytoma, whereas an even greater degree of nuclear atypia is observed in the anaplastic variant. The lesions are typically light chain restricted, although this does not necessarily correlate with prognosis, which may be good for a localized lesion.

Conditions to consider in the differential diagnosis:

cutaneous plasmacytoma
multiple myeloma

VIA4 **Small Round Cell Tumors**

Tumors of small cells with scant cytoplasm, and with small dark nuclei, constitute a group of tumors that can usually be distinguished from one another with appropriate immunohistochemical investigations, in conjunction with light microscopic and clinical information. Some of these tumors arise in the deep soft tissue, but they may rarely present in a deep skin biopsy. Merkel cell tumors are prototypic (16).

Cutaneous Small Cell Undifferentiated Carcinoma (Merkel Cell Tumor)

CLINICAL SUMMARY. Cutaneous small-cell undifferentiated carcinoma (CSCUC) (Merkel cell, neuroendocrine, or trabecular carcinoma), an uncommon tumor, mostly occurs as a solitary nodule, usually on the head or on the extremities, often in an immunosuppressed or elderly patient. The tumors are usually few in number but occasionally are multiple. The lesions of Merkel cell tumors are firm, nodular, and red-pink. They usually are nonulcerated and range in size from 0.8 to 4.0 cm. The prognosis is quite poor with an overall disease-specific survival of 64%; however, when lymph nodes are pathologically negative, the prognosis improves dramatically to 97% (17). A subset of the tumors is associated with Merkel cell polyomavirus (18).

HISTOPATHOLOGY. Tumor cells with scanty cytoplasm and plump, round or irregular nuclei are closely spaced in sheets and trabecular patterns, and less commonly in ribbons and festoons. Pseudorosettes are an occasional feature. The nuclear chromatin often is dense and uniformly distributed. In some examples, nuclei focally or uniformly show margination of chromatin. Nucleoli generally are inconspicuous or absent. Nuclear molding may be a feature. Mitoses and nuclear fragments are regular features. In some tumors, the nests of cells are supported by scant, delicate, and paucicellular stroma. Lymphoid infiltrates are common at the margin and focally in the stroma. Contact with the epidermis is rare, but if a lesion invades the epidermis, the patterns may include rounded "pagetoid" defects in which tumor cells are collected.

Keratinocytic dysplasia or carcinoma *in situ* in the overlying epidermis is not uncommon, and islands of squamous cell differentiation in the dermal nests occur uncommonly. Lymphatic invasion is commonly present.

The immunohistochemical profile is positive for NSE, chromogranin, Ber-EP4, and CD57. A single punctate zone of cytoplasmic immunoreactivity for cytokeratins, especially CK20, or neurofilaments is most characteristic. EMA is expressed in 75% to 80% of CSCUC. A reaction for CK20 is evidence against the diagnosis of metastatic small cell carcinoma of the lung. Ultrastructurally, cytoplasmic, membrane-bound, round, dense-core granules of neuroendocrine type measure 100 to 200 nm in diameter. Perinuclear bundles or whorls of intermediate filaments 7- to 10-nm wide and small desmosomes are regularly present. Tonofilaments attached to the desmosomes have been found in only a few cases.

Metastatic Small Cell Carcinoma

Metastatic carcinoma of any kind tends to present as an initially small papule that grows rapidly and may over time become multiple. The lesions initially at least are relatively symmetrical and well circumscribed, and can simulate a benign lesion.

Conditions to consider in the differential diagnosis:

primitive neuroepithelial tumors (PNET)
peripheral neuroblastoma/neuroepithelioma
Ewing sarcoma
cutaneous small cell undifferentiated carcinoma (CSCUC/Merkel cell tumor)

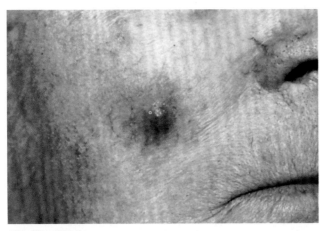

Clin. Fig. VIA4.a

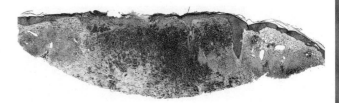

Fig. VIA4.a

Clin. Fig. VIA4.a. *Merkel cell tumor.* A smooth-topped erythematous nodule appeared suddenly and grew on the cheek of an elderly woman.

Fig. VIA4.a. *Merkel cell carcinoma, low power.* Scanning magnification reveals a dense dermal infiltrate of small basophilic cells. At this magnification the differential diagnosis includes cutaneous lymphoma and metastatic small cell carcinoma. (*continues*)

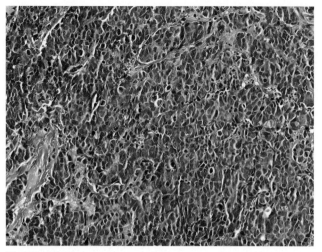

Fig. VIA4.b

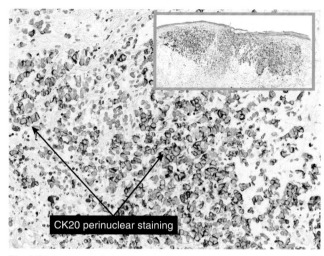

Fig. VIA4.c

Fig. VIA4.b. *Merkel cell carcinoma, high power.* The individual cells are small, compared to most carcinoma cells, although larger than small lymphocytes. They are round and have scant cytoplasm. The nuclei show a characteristic stippled appearance. Mitoses and apoptotic cells are frequently seen.

Fig. VIA4.c. *Merkel cell carcinoma, high power, CK20 immunoperoxidase stain.* Stains for cytokeratin 20 reveal a characteristic perinuclear dot staining pattern, helping to differentiate the lesion from a metastatic small cell carcinoma of the lung.

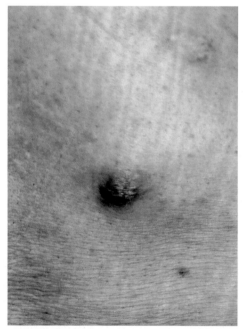

Clin. Fig. VIA4.b

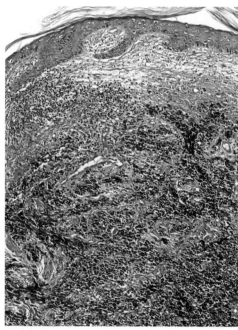

Fig. VIA4.d

Clin. Fig. VIA4.b. *Metastatic small cell carcinoma.* A tumor nodule located on the back, in a 62-year-old man with a history of small cell lung cancer. He also had brain metastases. The differential diagnosis would be broad in the absence of history.

Fig. VIA4.d. *Metastatic small cell carcinoma.* There is an asymmetrical nodular and diffuse collection of cells in the reticular dermis.

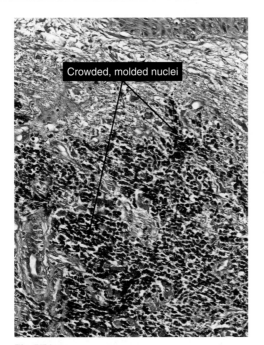

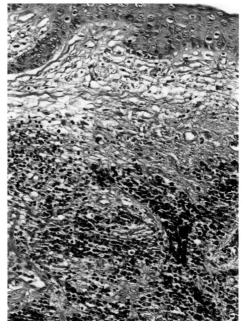

Fig. VIA4.e   **Fig. VIA4.f**

Fig. VIA4.e. *Metastatic small cell carcinoma.* The tumor consists of a monotonous population of small blue cells, infiltrating and disrupting the dermal architecture.

Fig. VIA4.f. *Metastatic small cell carcinoma.* The small cells have scant cytoplasm, resulting in molding of nuclei against one another. The nuclei are small, but larger than those of a lymphocyte. They have homogeneous chromatin and lack nucleoli. Crush artifact is common. Immunohistochemistry may be needed to rule out a lymphoma in a case like this. CK20 staining is typically negative.

melanotic neuroepithelial tumor of infancy
lymphoma/leukemia
rhabdomyosarcoma
metastatic neuroendocrine carcinoma
small cell melanoma
small cell carcinoma (squamous or adenocarcinoma)
eccrine spiradenoma

VIB   LARGE POLYGONAL AND ROUND CELL TUMORS

Large polygonal and round cell tumors have large round to oval nuclei that often exhibit relatively open chromatin. Especially in adenocarcinomas and in melanomas, there may be prominent nucleoli. The cytoplasm is abundant, and often amphophilic because of an abundant content of ribosomes.

1. Squamous Cell Tumors
2. Adenocarcinomas
3. Melanocytic Tumors
4. Eccrine Tumors
5. Apocrine Tumors
6. Pilar Tumors
7. Sebaceous Tumors
8. "Histiocytoid" and Miscellaneous Clear Cell Tumors
9. Tumors of Large Hematolymphoid Cells
10. Mast Cell Tumors
11. Tumors With Prominent Necrosis
12. Miscellaneous and Undifferentiated Epithelial Tumors

VIB1   Squamous Cell Tumors

Proliferations of large cells with more or less abundant cytoplasm, and with evidence of desmosome formation and/or keratin production occupy the dermis as nodular masses. Primary tumors may show evidence of origin from the epidermis in the form of a contiguous precursor (actinic keratosis) or, less specifically, of blending between the tumor cells and the epidermal cells. The possibility of metastatic squamous cell carcinoma must be considered and differentiated from the possibility of a primary cutaneous squamous cell carcinoma.

Squamous Cell Carcinoma

CLINICAL SUMMARY. Squamous cell carcinoma may occur anywhere on the skin and on mucous membranes with squamous epithelium. Clinically, squamous cell

VI   Tumors and Cysts of the Dermis and Subcutis

carcinoma of the skin most commonly consists of a shallow ulcer surrounded by a wide, elevated, indurated border and often covered by a crust that conceals a red, granular base. Occasionally, raised, fungoid, verrucous lesions without ulceration occur. Most commonly, it arises in sun-damaged skin, either as such or from an actinic keratosis. Next to sun-damaged skin, squamous cell carcinomas arise most commonly in scars from burns and in stasis ulcers, termed *Marjolin ulcers*. Carcinomas arising in sun-damaged skin in general have a very low propensity to metastasize, except for carcinomas of the lower lip, even though in most cases these are also induced by exposure to the sun (19).

HISTOPATHOLOGY. The tumors consist of irregular masses of epidermal cells that proliferate downward into the dermis. The invading tumor masses are composed in varying proportions of more or less mature squamous cells and of atypical (anaplastic) squamous cells. The latter are characterized by such changes as great variation in the size and shape of the cells, hyperplasia and hyperchromasia of the nuclei, absence of intercellular bridges, keratinization of individual cells, and the presence of atypical mitotic figures. Differentiation in squamous cell carcinoma is in the direction of keratinization, which often takes place in the form of horn pearls. These are very characteristic structures composed of concentric layers of squamous cells showing gradually increasing usually incomplete keratinization toward the center. Keratohyaline granules within the horn pearls

are sparse or absent. High-risk prognostic features for squamous cell carcinoma include primary site on the ear or lip, poor differentiation, tumor thickness greater than 2 mm, Clark's level IV or V invasion, and perineural invasion of nerves greater than 0.1 mm in diameter (20).

Keratoacanthoma

Solitary keratoacanthoma, a common lesion, occurs in elderly persons usually as a single lesion, and consists of a firm, dome-shaped nodule 1.0 to 2.5 cm in diameter with a horn-filled crater in its center. The lesions may occur on any hairy cutaneous site, with a predilection for exposed areas. They usually reach their full size within 6 to 8 weeks and involute spontaneously leaving a slightly depressed scar, generally in less than 6 months. Healing takes place. An increased incidence of keratoacanthoma is observed in immunosuppressed patients, and in the Muir–Torre syndrome of sebaceous neoplasms and keratoacanthomas associated with visceral carcinomas. "Giant" and locally destructive forms of keratoacanthoma exist. In the 2018 WHO classification of tumors of the skin, keratoacanthoma is listed as a form of squamous cell carcinoma, "with distinct clinical behavior" (21).

HISTOPATHOLOGY. The architecture of the lesion is as important to the diagnosis as the cellular characteristics. Therefore, if the lesion cannot be excised in its entirety, it is advisable that a fusiform specimen be excised for biopsy

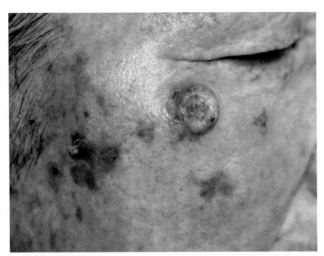

Clin. Fig. VIB1.a

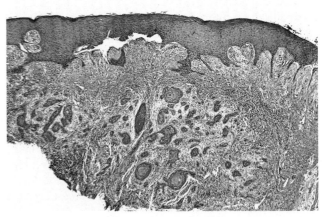

Fig. VIB1.a

Clin. Fig. VIB1.a. *Squamous cell carcinoma.* A 78-year-old woman had an asymmetrical ulcerated nodule, on the malar face with severe solar damage. She also had a cutaneous horn and multiple actinic keratosis.

Fig. VIB1.a. *Squamous cell carcinoma, invasive, low power.* Arising from the base of the epidermis there are endophytic proliferative lobules of atypical epithelium which are associated with a patchy lymphocytic infiltrate.

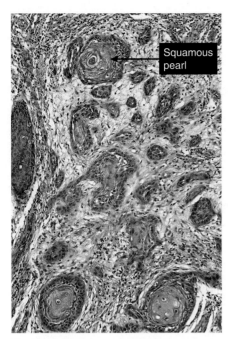

Fig. VIB1.b

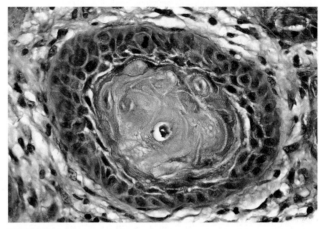

Fig. VIB1.c

Fig. VIB1.b. *Squamous cell carcinoma, invasive, medium power.* Haphazardly oriented lobules are of varying shapes and sizes and show an infiltrative growth pattern within the dermis. The lobule at the top of this photomicrograph shows formation of a squamous pearl, a whorled aggregate of parakeratin within the epithelial island.

Fig. VIB1.c. *Squamous cell carcinoma, high power.* The atypical keratinocytes may show a spectrum of cytologic atypia from mild to severe.

from the center of the lesion and that this specimen includes the edge at least of one side and preferably of both sides of the lesion. A shave biopsy is inadvisable, since the histologic changes at the base of the lesion are often of great importance in the differentiation from squamous cell carcinoma.

In the early proliferative stage, there is a horn-filled cup-shaped invagination of the epidermis from which strands of epidermis protrude into the dermis. These strands are poorly demarcated from the surrounding stroma in many areas and may contain cells showing nuclear atypia as well as many mitotic figures including occasionally atypical mitoses. Perineural invasion is occasionally seen. A fully developed lesion shows in its center a large, irregularly shaped crater filled with keratin. The nondysplastic adjacent epidermis extends like a lip or a buttress over the sides of the crater. At the base of the crater, irregular epidermal proliferations extend downward. There are only one or two layers of basophilic, nonkeratinized cells at the periphery of the proliferations, whereas the cells within this shell appear eosinophilic and glassy as a result of keratinization. There are many horn pearls, most of which show complete keratinization in their center. The base appears regular and well demarcated and

usually does not extend below the level of the sweat glands. In the involuting stage, proliferation has ceased, and most cells at the base of the crater have undergone keratinization. The distinction between keratoacanthoma and well-differentiated squamous cell carcinoma is often difficult, however most such lesions can now be interpreted as "squamous cell carcinoma, well-differentiated, keratoacanthoma type" (21). Keratoacanthomas and keratoacanthoma-like squamous cell carcinomas occur with some frequency in patients on targeted therapy for melanoma and perhaps other cancers (22).

Inverted Follicular Keratosis

Inverted follicular keratosis (IFK) may be regarded as an endophytic form of the irritated, or activated, type of seborrheic keratosis, in which the characteristic feature is the presence of numerous whorls or eddies composed of eosinophilic flattened squamous cells arranged in an onion-peel fashion, somewhat resembling poorly differentiated keratin pearls (23). These "squamous eddies" can be differentiated from the horn pearls of squamous cell carcinoma by their large number, small size, and circumscribed configuration. Frequently, some of these proliferations are

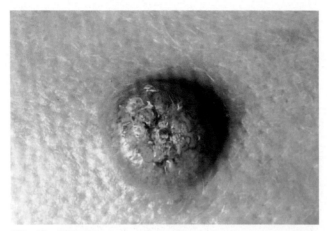

Clin. Fig. VIB1.b

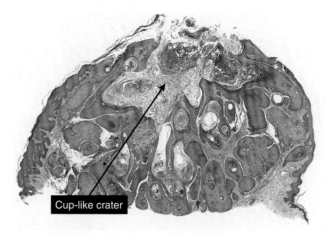

Fig. VIB1.d

Cup-like crater

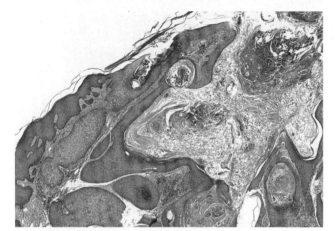

Fig. VIB1.e

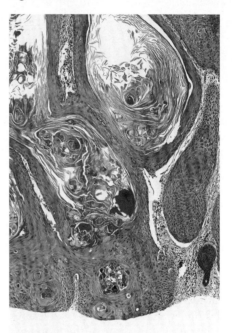

Fig. VIB1.f

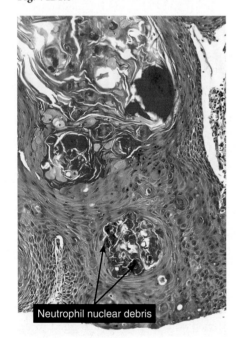

Neutrophil nuclear debris

Fig. VIB1.g

Clin. Fig. VIB1.b. *Keratoacanthoma.* A symmetrical tumor with a keratin-filled cup-shaped center developed suddenly in chronically sun-damaged skin of an elderly man.

Fig. VIB1.d. *Keratoacanthoma, low power.* The epidermis is invaginated forming a cup-like crater, which is filled with masses of keratin. At the dermal–epidermal junction there is an infiltrate of mononuclear cells.

Fig. VIB1.e. *Keratoacanthoma, medium power.* The epidermis shows an abrupt transition from relatively normal to a proliferation of eosinophilic hyalinized ground-glass–appearing atypical keratinocytes. At the dermal-epidermal junction there is a brisk infiltrate of lymphocytes that are exocytotic to this proliferative atypical epithelium.

Fig. VIB1.f. *Keratoacanthoma, high power.* The dermal–tumor junction shows a dense infiltrate of mononuclear cells that are exocytotic to this proliferative, eosinophilic, hyalinized ground-glass–appearing tumor.

Fig. VIB1.g. *Keratoacanthoma, medium power.* Within the proliferative epithelium of a cup-shaped tumor, there are intraepidermal collections of polymorphonuclear leukocytes (which may be considerable more numerous than in this example).

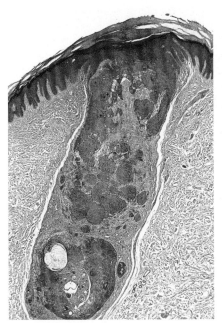

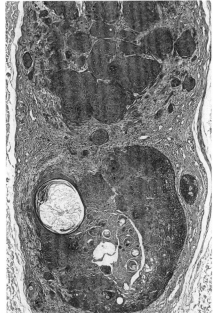

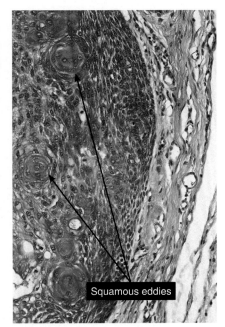

Fig. VIB1.h   Fig. VIB1.i   Fig. VIB1.j

Fig. VIB1.h. *Inverted follicular keratosis, low power.* This epithelial neoplasm arises from the epidermis and shows an endophytic architecture which vaguely resembles that of a hair follicle.

Fig. VIB1.i. *Inverted follicular keratosis, medium power.* This epithelial proliferation is embedded in a fibrotic stroma and it is sharply separated from the adjacent reticular dermal collagen. Keratin-filled cystic structures are seen within it.

Fig. VIB1.j. *Inverted follicular keratosis, high power.* Numerous squamous eddies as depicted here are a characteristic feature of an inverted follicular keratosis.

seen to originate from the walls of keratin-filled invaginations. The combination of an inverted or invaginated architectural pattern and the squamous eddies can falsely suggest the possibility of squamous cell carcinoma. IFK can be seen in association with trichoblastoma, supporting its follicular derivation (24).

Pseudoepitheliomatous Hyperplasia (PEH)

PEH is a reaction pattern of squamous epithelium that usually occurs in association with certain neoplasms or over a chronic inflammatory process and may be regarded as reparative in nature (25). Conditions that may be associated with PEH are listed below in the differential diagnosis section. The reactive epithelium may extend into the superficial reticular dermis, simulating a carcinoma. However, the epithelium is typically very bland, with a single layer of basal cells maturing continuously to the surface. Although mitoses may be present, they are not abnormal. There may be evidence of the underlying stimulus in the dermis. Without such a finding, the distinction between PEH and well-differentiated invasive squamous cell carcinoma may be almost impossible to make on histologic grounds alone.

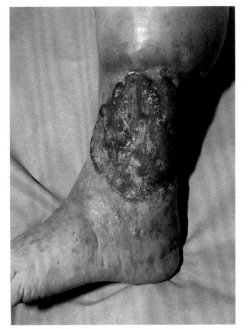

Clin. Fig. VIB1.c

Clin. Fig. VIB1.c. *Pseudoepitheliomatous hyperplasia.* An elderly woman had an ulcer of 10 years' duration characterized by granulation tissue and a hypertrophic, irregular border. Multiple biopsies ruled out squamous cell carcinoma. (*continues*)

VI | Tumors and Cysts of the Dermis and Subcutis

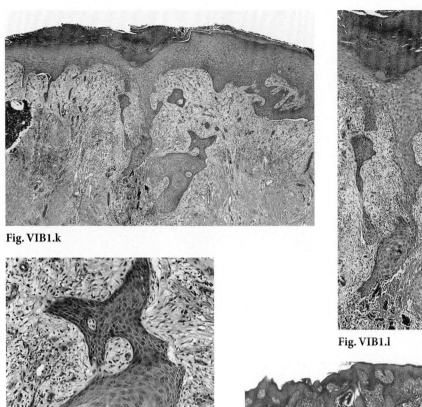

Fig. VIB1.k

Fig. VIB1.l

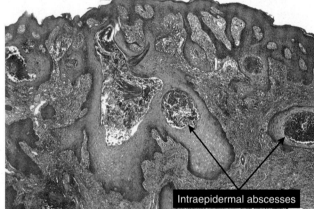

Intraepidermal abscesses

Fig. VIB1.m

Fig. VIB1.n

Fig. VIB1.k. *Pseudoepitheliomatous hyperplasia, low power.* This reactive epithelial hyperplasia is present adjacent to a healing biopsy site. Squamous cell carcinoma should always be considered in the differential diagnosis of this process and a careful search for cytologic atypia and/or adjacent actinic keratosis or carcinoma *in situ* should be undertaken. The epidermis reveals marked irregular acanthosis with endophytic tongues extending into the superficial dermis. There is associated hyperkeratosis.

Fig. VIB1.l. *Pseudoepitheliomatous hyperplasia, medium power.* PEH can be difficult to differentiate from invasive squamous cell carcinoma. The presence of dermal fibrosis as seen in this example suggests a reactive process such as previous procedure at this site, or a healing ulceration.

Fig. VIB1.m. *Pseudoepitheliomatous hyperplasia, high power.* Despite the irregular architecture and infiltrative pattern of the epithelial tongues, there is no high-grade atypia and the lesional cells appear to mature smoothly from a basal layer.

Fig. VIB1.n. *Pseudoepitheliomatous hyperplasia in North American blastomycosis, low power.* There is florid irregular epidermal hyperplasia extending deeply into the reticular dermis, associated with a mixed-cell inflammatory infiltrate and with multiple intraepithelial abscesses, a clue to the diagnosis of a deep fungal infection. This should be demonstrated with special stains and if possible with culture.

Proliferating Trichilemmal Cyst (Pilar Tumor)

CLINICAL SUMMARY. The proliferating trichilemmal cyst (26) is nearly always a single lesion, usually located on the scalp or on the back, most commonly in an elderly woman. Starting as a subcutaneous nodule suggestive of a wen, the tumor may grow into a large, elevated, lobulated mass that may undergo ulceration and thus greatly resemble a squamous cell carcinoma. The lesions may recur after simple local excision, and malignant transformation may occur (27).

HISTOPATHOLOGY. The lesion usually is well demarcated from the surrounding tissue, and is composed of variably sized lobules of squamous epithelium. Some of the lobules are surrounded by a vitreous layer and show palisading of their peripheral cell layer. Characteristically, the epithelium in the center of the lobules abruptly changes into eosinophilic amorphous keratin of the same type as that seen in the cavity of ordinary trichilemmal cysts. In addition to this trichilemmal pattern of keratinization, some proliferating trichilemmal cysts exhibit epidermoid changes resembling that of the follicular infundibulum. This may result in horn pearls, some of which resemble "squamous eddies." The tumor cells in many areas show some degree of nuclear atypia, as well as individual cell keratinization, which at first glance may suggest a squamous cell carcinoma. The tumor differs from a squamous cell carcinoma by its rather sharp demarcation from the surrounding stroma as well as by its abrupt mode of keratinization. Malignant proliferating trichilemmal tumors may arise focally within a benign lesion and are characterized by increased cytologic atypia and an infiltrative growth pattern (22). Mutations of tp53 and loss of heterozygosity at 17p have been found in malignant proliferating trichilemmal tumor (28).

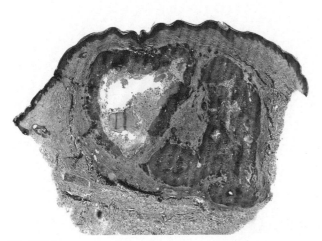

Fig. VIB1.o

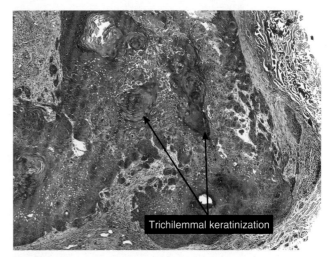

Trichilemmal keratinization

Fig. VIB1.p

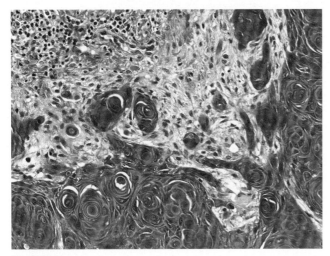

Fig. VIB1.q

Fig. VIB1.o. *Proliferating trichilemmal cyst, low power.* There is a neoplasm in the dermis comprised of multiple lobules of interconnecting epithelium with multiple associated cystic spaces.

Fig. VIB1.p. *Proliferating trichilemmal cyst, medium power.* There are large bands of connected epithelial tissue with zones of trichilemmal keratinization, that is keratinization without formation of a granular cell layer.

Fig. VIB1.q. *Proliferating trichilemmal cyst, high power.* The epithelial cells may be large with an abundance of cytoplasm and may appear infiltrative into the tumor stroma at the periphery of the nodule, but they fail to reveal high-grade cytologic atypia, and the tumor does not infiltrate into the surrounding native tissue.

Tumors and Cysts of the Dermis and Subcutis

VI

Prurigo Nodularis

CLINICAL SUMMARY. This is a chronic dermatitis characterized by discrete, raised, firm hyperkeratotic papulonodules, usually from 5 to 12 mm in diameter but occasionally larger (29). They occur chiefly on the extensor surfaces of the extremities and are intensely pruritic. The disease usually begins in middle age and women are more frequently affected than men. The condition may coexist with lesions of lichen simplex chronicus and there may be transitional lesions. The cause remains unknown but local trauma, insect bites, atopic background, and metabolic or systemic diseases have been implicated as predisposing factors in some cases.

HISTOPATHOLOGY. There is pronounced hyperkeratosis and irregular acanthosis. In addition, there may be papillomatosis and irregular downward proliferation of the epidermis and adnexal epithelium approaching pseudoepitheliomatous hyperplasia. The papillary dermis shows a predominantly lymphocytic inflammatory infiltrate and vertically oriented collagen bundles. Occasionally, prominent neural hyperplasia may be observed; however, this is an uncommon finding and is not considered to be an essential feature for the diagnosis of prurigo nodularis. In some cases, silver stains or cholinesterase stains demonstrate the increased number of cutaneous nerves.

Eosinophils and marked eosinophil degranulation may be seen more frequently in patients with an atopic background. Dermal Langerhans cells are increased, and there may be enlarged dendritic mast cells in the dermis.

PATHOGENESIS. It is generally assumed that the neural proliferation in prurigo nodularis is a secondary

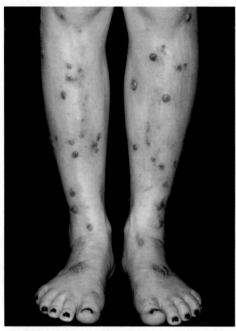

Clin. Fig. VIB1.d

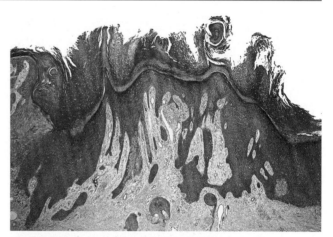

Fig. VIB1.r

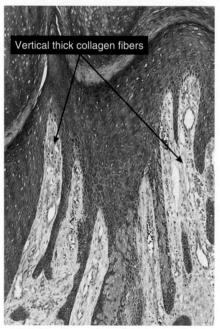

Fig. VIB1.s

Clin. Fig. VIB1.d. *Prurigo nodularis.* Multiple "picker's nodules" on accessible regions of the anterior legs.

Fig. VIB1.r. *Prurigo nodularis, low power.* There is hyperkeratosis and the epidermis is hyperplastic and highly irregular, with protrusion of tongues of cells well into the reticular dermis. The appearances, caused by chronic irritation, are reminiscent of pseudoepitheliomatous hyperplasia.

Fig. VIB1.s. *Prurigo nodularis, medium power.* The hyperplastic epithelium is well differentiated, without substantial cytologic atypia. As in lichen simplex chronicus, there may be vertically oriented thick collagen fibers in the elongated dermal papillae.

phenomenon due to chronic trauma by scratching. Still, it may be that the extreme pruritus is related to the increased number of dermal nerves. It has been shown that nerve growth factor (NGF) and its receptors are overexpressed in lesional skin of prurigo nodularis, compared to normal controls, with the inflammatory cell infiltrate being the source of NGF with resulting neural hyperplasia (30).

Conditions to consider in the differential diagnosis:

   primary squamous cell carcinoma
   metastatic squamous cell carcinoma
   proliferating trichilemmal cyst
   inverted follicular keratosis
   keratoacanthoma
   prurigo nodularis

VIB2 Adenocarcinomas

Proliferations of atypical cells with more or less abundant cytoplasm, and with evidence of gland formation and/or mucin production occupy the dermis as nodular masses. The possibility of metastatic adenocarcinoma must be considered and differentiated from the possibility of a primary cutaneous adenocarcinoma of skin appendages (refer to eccrine, apocrine, pilar, sebaceous tumor sections below).

Metastatic Adenocarcinoma

CLINICAL SUMMARY. In women, the majority of all cutaneous metastases are mammary or pulmonary adenocarcinomas. The latter are the most common in men.

Colon in both sexes and ovaries in women account for most of the rest. Cutaneous metastatic disease as the first sign of internal cancer is most commonly seen with adenocarcinomas of the lung, kidney, and ovary. Inflammatory mammary carcinoma is a distinctive disorder that is characterized by an erythematous patch or plaque with an active spreading border that resembles erysipelas and usually affects the breast and nearby skin. The inflammatory appearance and warmth are attributed to capillary congestion. En cuirasse or scirrhous metastatic mammary carcinoma is characterized by a diffuse morphea-like induration of the skin and rarely involves skin from other primary carcinomas. It usually begins as scattered papular lesions coalescing into a sclerodermoid plaque without inflammatory changes.

HISTOPATHOLOGY. In scirrhous mammary carcinoma, the indurated areas are fibrotic and may contain only a few tumor cells. The tumor cells may be confused with fibroblasts. They have elongated nuclei similar to those of fibroblasts, but larger, more angular, and more deeply basophilic. The tumor cells often lie singly, but in some areas they may form small groups or single rows between fibrotic and thickened collagen bundles. This latter feature of "single filing" is of diagnostic importance. In inflammatory carcinoma there is extensive invasion of the dermal and often the subcutaneous lymphatics by groups and cords of tumor cells. These cells are similar to those in the primary growth and atypical in character with large, pleomorphic, hyperchromatic nuclei. Adenocarcinomas metastatic to skin from lung are often moderately differentiated, but some show well-formed, mucin-secreting,

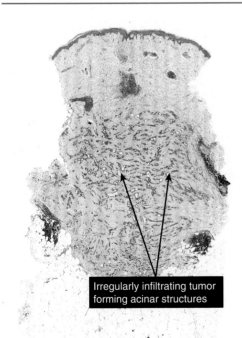

Irregularly infiltrating tumor forming acinar structures

Fig. VIB2.a

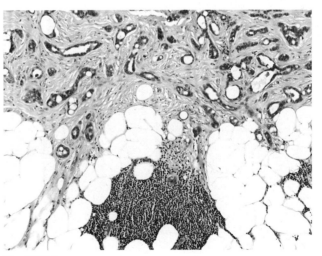

Fig. VIB2.b

Fig. VIB2.a. *Metastatic adenocarcinoma, low power.* There is a tumor forming glands in the dermis and extending into the subcutis.

Fig. VIB2.b. *Metastatic adenocarcinoma, medium power.* There is a patchy lymphocytic infiltrate. (*continues*)

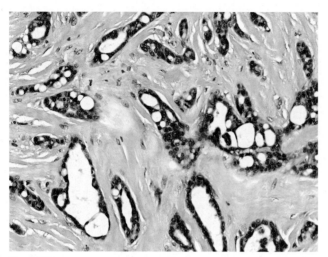

Fig. VIB2.c

Fig. VIB2.c. *Metastatic adenocarcinoma, medium power.* The cribriform architecture of this lesion would be fairly characteristic but not diagnostic of a metastasis from a mammary carcinoma.

glandular structures. Individual tumor cells sometimes contain abundant cytoplasmic mucin, but usually lack large pools of mucin, which is more characteristically seen from gastrointestinal metastatic adenocarcinomas.

Metastatic Mammary Ductal Carcinoma

Metastatic mammary carcinoma can be difficult to distinguish from primary sweat gland tumors in some cases. In a comparative study, immunoreactivity for p63, CK5/6, D2-40, GATA3, and mammaglobin was respectively observed in 81%, 71%, 52%, 71%, and 5% of sweat gland carcinomas compared with 6%, 6%, 6%, 91%, and 45% of metastatic breast carcinomas. For the diagnosis of metastatic breast carcinoma, GATA3 and mammaglobin were >90% specific for breast carcinoma but had limited sensitivity (45%) in this context. These data suggested that p63 and CK5/6 are specific determinants for sweat gland carcinoma in this context (31).

Mammary Carcinoma, "Inflammatory" Type

See Figs. VIB2.g,h.

Conditions to consider in the differential diagnosis:

primary adenocarcinoma of skin adnexal origin (see below)
mucin-producing squamous cell carcinoma (mucoepidermoid, adenosquamous carcinoma)
metastatic adenocarcinoma

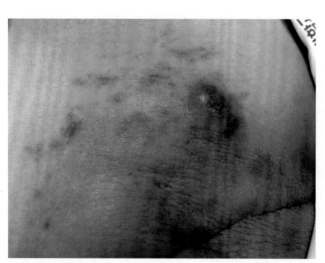

Clin. Fig. VIB.2

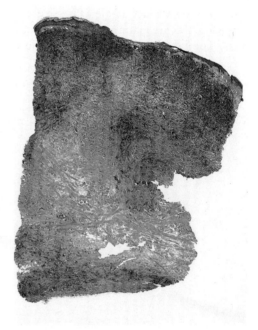

Fig. VIB2.d

Clin. Fig. VIB.2. *Metastatic mammary carcinoma.* En cuirasse pattern of scirrhous metastatic mammary carcinoma creates diffuse morphea-like induration of the skin and begins as scattered papular lesions coalescing into a sclerodermoid plaque.

Fig. VIB2.d. *Metastatic mammary carcinoma, infiltrating ductal type, low power.* The entire dermis is expanded and replaced by an infiltrative tumor. The tumor has replaced the adnexal structures.

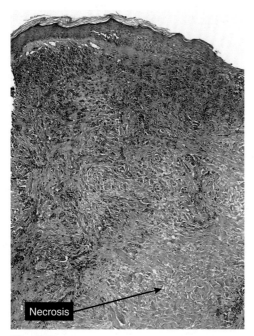

Fig. VIB2.e

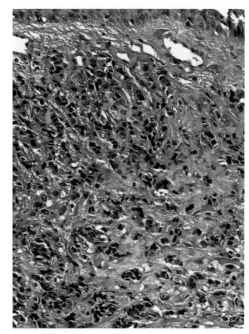

Fig. VIB2.f

Fig. VIB2.e. *Metastatic mammary carcinoma, infiltrating ductal type, medium power.* Throughout the dermis there are multiple small tumor aggregates permeating between bundles of reticular dermal collagen. Many of the tumor aggregates form small ducts. There is an area of confluent necrosis, characterized by eosinophilia with loss of nuclear and cytoplasmic cellular detail.

Fig. VIB2.f. *Metastatic mammary carcinoma, infiltrating ductal type, high power.* Infiltrating cords of cells are characteristic of this subtype, which is also known as "scirrhous carcinoma" because of its tendency to have a dense collagenous stroma. The tumor cells show enlarged hyperchromatic nuclei and eosinophilic cytoplasm. The cytoplasm may show small clear vacuoles.

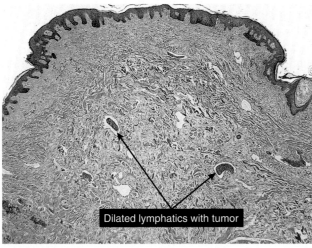

Fig. VIB2.g

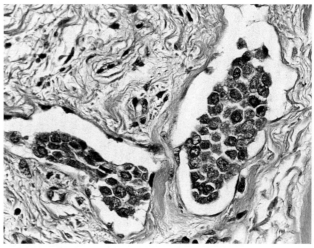

Fig. VIB2.h

Fig. VIB2.g. *Inflammatory carcinoma, low power.* In this example of breast carcinoma there are dilated lymphatics containing clusters of tumor cells. The appearances are consistent with "inflammatory carcinoma," a condition in which there is extensive lymphatic involvement with slight if any inflammation.

Fig. VIB2.h. *Inflammatory carcinoma, high power.* Solid collections of malignant cells are seen within dilated lymphatics. They have irregular, hyperchromatic nuclei and high nuclear to cytoplasmic ratios.

Tumors and Cysts of the Dermis and Subcutis

VI

VIB3 Melanocytic Tumors

The proliferations in the dermis are melanocyte derived, pigmented or amelanotic, benign, atypical, or malignant. Superficial lesions may involve the epidermis (junctional component). There may be a fibrous and inflammatory host response. S100, Sox10, Melan-A, HMB45, tyrosinase and MITF stains may be of value in recognizing melanocytic differentiation in amelanotic tumors (32). Intradermal melanocytic nevi, halo nevi, cellular blue nevi, Spitz nevi, and primary melanomas of the "nodular" type, and metastatic melanomas will be discussed here as examples of dermal melanocytic tumors (33,34), even though many of these have an epidermal as well as a dermal component. Nontumorigenic primary melanomas have been discussed elsewhere (IIB1, IID2).

VIB3a Melanocytic Lesions With Little or No Cytologic Atypia

With rare exceptions, such as perhaps a few nevoid melanomas (at least at first glance), malignant melanocytic tumors are characterized by cytologic atypia and usually also by mitotic activity in the dermis. Benign melanocytic nevi, in contrast, tend to lack these features. If atypia is present at all, it tends to be "random" (confined to a minority of the lesional cells) rather than "diffuse" as in most melanomas.

Melanocytic Nevi, Acquired and Congenital Types

CLINICAL SUMMARY. At least 5 types of melanocytic nevi can be distinguished as viewed histologically, namely (1) flat lesions which are for the most part are histologically junctional nevi, and compound nevi which include (2) slightly elevated lesions often with raised centers and flat peripheries many of which are histologically dysplastic nevi (see Section IIC), (3) papillomatous lesions, (4) dome-shaped lesions, and (5) pedunculated lesions (see IIA.2). Most nonpigmented papillomatous, dome-shaped, and pedunculated nevi are intradermal nevi. Strictly defined congenital melanocytic nevi are by definition present at birth. They may be "small" (<1.5 cm and especially when <1 cm generally indistinguishable from acquired nevi), "intermediate" (amenable to excision with primary closure) or "large" (not amenable to excision except with extraordinary measures). Pigment is variable in nevi, and often absent in dermal nevi.

In the 2018 WHO classification of skin tumors, nevi are classified according to their relationships to the various categories of melanomas which in turn are classified on the basis of clinical features, histologic features, and also on epidemiology and genomic characteristics. The superficial spreading melanomas and lentigo maligna

TABLE VI.2. Melanocytic Skin Tumors in Intermittently Sun-Exposed Skin (WHO 2018)

Low-CSD melanoma (superficial spreading melanoma)
Simple lentigo and lentiginous nevus
Junctional, compound and dermal nevi
Dysplastic nevus
Nevus spilus
Special site nevi (e.g., breast, axilla, scalp, ear)
Halo nevus
Meyerson nevus
Recurrent nevus
Deep penetrating nevus
Pigmented epithelioid melanocytoma
Combined nevus including combined BAP-1 inactivated nevus

melanomas, which predominate in Western populations, and also the less common desmoplastic melanomas, are in the general category of lesions related to cumulative solar damage (CSD). Superficial spreading melanoma is categorized as "low CSD," and nevi in its lineage include common acquired nevi, dysplastic nevi, deep penetrating nevi, and BRAF deficiency nevi, and some examples of pigmented epithelioid melanocytoma. These lesions tend to have activating mutations of the oncogene BRAFV600E. Lentigo maligna melanoma is classified as "high CSD" melanoma, in which NRAS and Kit mutations predominate. Well-defined nevi are not a feature of this lineage (Table VI.2) (35).

HISTOPATHOLOGY. The lesional cells of nevi ("nevus cells") tend to be arranged in more-or-less well-defined nests and to contain variable pigment, especially superficially within the lesion. In nonpigmented lesions, the tendency to nesting is often the key feature in recognizing that a lesion is melanocytic. The most important architectural features that distinguish a dermal nevus from a melanoma are their overall smaller size and greater symmetry, and the decrease in size of lesional cells from superficial to deep within the dermis which is often referred to as "maturation." If dermal nevus cells are confined to the papillary dermis, they often retain a discrete, or "pushing" border with the stroma. However, nevus cells that enter the reticular dermis tend to disperse among collagen fiber bundles as single cells or attenuated single files of cells, differing from melanomas, where groups rather than single cells tend to dissect and displace the collagen. Nevus cells entering the reticular dermis are seen in many congenital nevi, but also in acquired nevi, which may be termed "congenital pattern nevi." Relatively more specific indicators of congenital nevus include size greater than 1.5 cm, and nevus cells within skin appendages, especially sebaceous units. Cytologically, nevus cells differ from melanoma cells by lacking high-grade and uniform cytologic atypia, and mitoses are totally absent in the vast majority of benign nevi.

Lesions where nevus cells extend into the lower reticular dermis and the subcutaneous fat, or are located within nerves, hair follicles, sweat ducts, and sebaceous glands, are termed "congenital pattern nevi" because these

patterns may be seen, though not exclusively, in nevi that have been present since birth.

Acquired Nevi, Compound and Dermal

Most acquired compound in dermal nevi have the BRAFV600E mutation which is also seen in the common melanomas of the superficial spreading type ("low-CSD melanoma") (36).

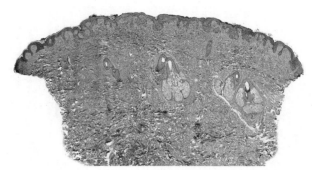

Fig. VIB3a.a

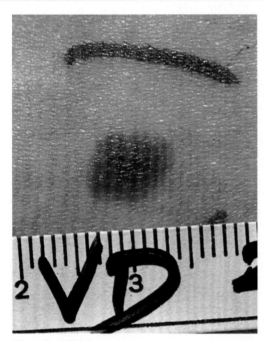

Clin. Fig. VIB3a.a

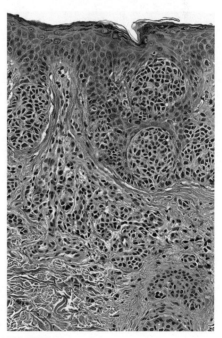

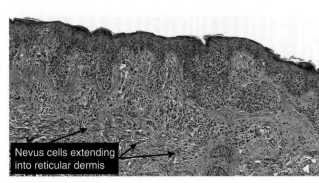

Fig. VIB3a.b

Nevus cells extending into reticular dermis

Fig. VIB3a.c

Clin. Fig. VIB3a.a. *Compound nevus.* An 8 mm well circumscribed, symmetrical and uniformly colored papule. A lesion of this size could be an acquired nevus or a small congenital pattern nevus.

Fig. VIB3a.a. *Compound melanocytic nevus, low power.* There is a superficial symmetrical moderately cellular proliferation of cells in the epidermis and the dermis.

Fig. VIB3a.b. *Compound nevus, medium power.* As in the junctional component of a nevus, the dermal nevus cells are recognized at this power chiefly by their tendency to be arranged in nests.

Fig. VIB3a.c. *Compound nevus, high power.* The nests of nevus cells in the epidermis overly a dermal component of orderly nevus cells, which extend into the reticular dermis in a "congenital pattern." (*continues*)

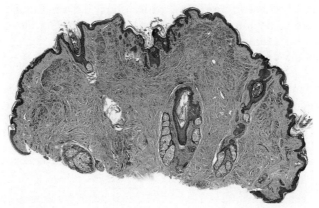

Fig. VIB3a.d

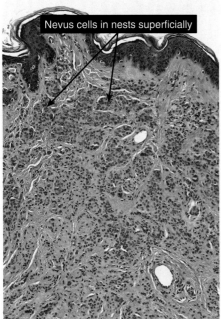

Nevus cells in nests superficially

Fig. VIB3a.e

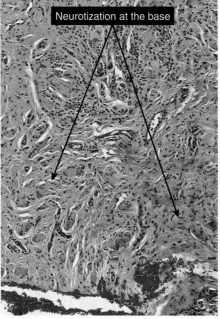

Neurotization at the base

Fig. VIB3a.f

Fig. VIB3a.d. *Predominantly dermal nevus with neurotization ("neurotized nevus" or "neurone-vus"), low power.* A symmetrical, moderately symmetrical proliferation of cells with an ill-defined nested arrangement.

Fig. VIB3a.e. *Predominantly dermal nevus, medium power.* Cells at the top of the dermal component are arranged in a nevoid nested pattern and they blend with a different patter at the base of the image.

Fig. VIB3a.f. *Predominantly dermal nevus, high power.* The cells at the base tend to be more spindled and they are arranged in leaf-like structures that recapitulate sensory nerve appendages such as Wagner–Meissner corpuscles.

Balloon Cell Nevus

Although not separately classified in the WHO classification, balloon cell nevi are distinctive and likely represent an usual cytologic variant of "nevi of intermittently sun-exposed skin."

Halo Nevus

CLINICAL SUMMARY. A halo nevus, also known as Sutton nevus, nevus depigmentosa centrifugum, or leukoderma acquisitum centrifugum (36), represents a pigmented nevus surrounded by a depigmented zone. A similar halo reaction may be seen in relation to a primary or metastatic melanoma. In the common type of halo nevus, the central nevus gradually involutes over a period of several months. The area of depigmentation shows no clinical signs of inflammation and ultimately

disappears in most cases often after many months or even years. Most persons with halo nevi are children or young adults, and the back is the most common site. Not infrequently, halo nevi are multiple, occurring either simultaneously or successively. Halo nevi may arise from a variety of nevi, mostly in intermittently sun-exposed skin, and most of which are not dysplastic nevi (37).

HISTOPATHOLOGY. In the early stage there are nests of nevus cells embedded in a dense inflammatory infiltrate, in the upper dermis and at the epidermal–dermal junction. Later, more scattered nevus cells than nests are observed. Even when melanin is still present in the nevus cells, these cells often show evidence of damage to their nuclei and cytoplasm, and some frankly apoptotic nevus cells are commonly observed. Some cells, especially

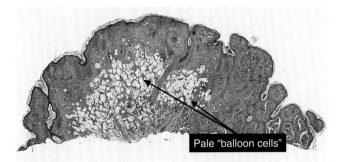

Fig. VIB3a.g

Pale "balloon cells"

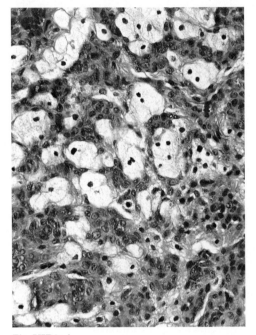

Fig. VIB3a.i

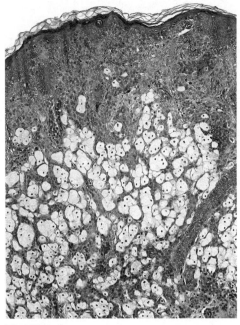

Fig. VIB3a.h

Fig. VIB3a.g. *Balloon cell nevus, low power.* This shave biopsy shows a compound nevus with a slightly papillomatous architecture. In the upper/mid dermis there is a collection of clear cells.

Fig. VIB3a.h. *Balloon cell nevus, medium power.* At the dermal–epidermal junction and within the superficial dermis there are nests of orderly pigmented melanocytic cells. These cells blend with larger melanocytic cells which show an abundance of clear cytoplasm.

Fig. VIB3a.i. *Balloon cell nevus, high power.* Upon close inspection the clear cells all show small, uniform centrally placed nuclei. The lack of cytologic atypia and mitotic activity help differentiate this lesion from a balloon cell melanoma.

superficially, may have enlarged ovoid nucleoli, changes that may be regarded as a form of "reactive atypia," but high-grade and uniform nuclear atypia is not observed, and lesional cell mitoses are usually absent. Importantly, the lesional cells tend to show evidence of "maturation," becoming smaller with descent from superficial to deep within the lesion. Most of the cells in the dense inflammatory infiltrate are lymphocytes. However, some of them are macrophages containing various amounts of melanin. As the infiltrate invades the nevus cell nests, it often is difficult to distinguish between the lymphoid cells of the infiltrate and the type B nevus cells in the mid-dermis, because they, too, have the appearance of lymphoid cells. At a later stage, only a few and finally no distinct nevus cells can be identified. Gradually, after all nevus cells have disappeared, the inflammatory infiltrate subsides. The epidermis of the halo, lateral to the dermal nevus cells, may show subtle lymphocytic inflammation with damage

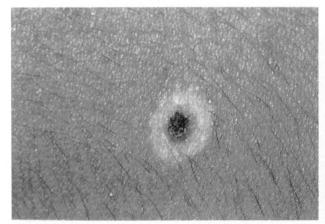

Clin. Fig. VIB3a.b

Clin. Fig. VIB3a.b. *Halo nevus.* A small compound nevus in a teenager was found to have a clear halo after the development of a tan in late spring. (*continues*)

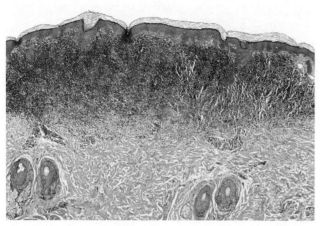

Fig. VIB3a.j   Fig. VIB3a.k

Fig. VIB3a.j. *Halo nevus.* The nevus architecture is obscured by a dense lymphocytic infiltrate.

Fig. VIB3a.k. *Halo nevus.* Lymphocytes infiltrate among the dermal nevus cells, which eventually degenerate and disappear.

to melanocytes followed by their disappearance, and a progressive absence of melanin.

Acral Nevus

Some acral nevi have BRAFV600E mutations and likely represent examples of acquired nevi. Others share genomic features with acral melanomas (38), and likely represent lesions that are not primarily related to sun exposure, as is also believed to be the case for acral melanomas (36) (Table VI.3).

TABLE VI.3.	Melanocytic Tumors in Skin That Is Generally Not Sun-Exposed (or sun exposure is considered to be incidental)

Spitz tumors
Malignant Spitz tumor (Spitz melanoma)
Spitz nevus
Pigmented spindle cell nevus

Melanocytic tumors in acral skin
Acral melanoma
Acral nevus

Genital and mucosal melanocytic tumors
Mucosal melanomas
Genital nevi

Melanocytic tumors arising in blue nevus
Melanoma arising in blue nevus
Blue nevus NOS
Cellular blue nevus
Mongolian spot, nevus of Ito and nevus of Ota

Melanocytic tumors arising in congenital nevi
Melanoma arising in giant congenital nevus
Congenital melanocytic nevus
Proliferative nodules in congenital melanocytic nevus

Congenital Nevus

See Clin. Fig. VIB3a.c and Figs. VIB3a.n,o.

Blue Nevus

Blue nevi differ from most acquired nevi in that they are present in the reticular dermis, yet contain abundant pigment, and are comprised of spindle cells. They also have a different genomic architecture, having activation mutations of GNAQ or GNA11 rather than BRAF or NRAS, which characterize most acquired and congenital nevi respectively (36).

Cellular Blue Nevus

CLINICAL SUMMARY. A cellular blue nevus (39) presents as a blue nodule that is usually larger than the common blue nevus. It generally measures 1 to 3 cm in diameter, but it may be larger. It shows either a smooth or an irregular surface. About half of all cellular blue nevi have been located over the buttocks or in the sacrococcygeal region. Although rare, malignant degeneration of cellular blue nevi can occur (malignant blue nevus).

HISTOPATHOLOGY. In the most common "mixed-biphasic" pattern, areas of deeply pigmented dendritic melanocytes, as observed also in common blue nevi, are admixed with cellular islands composed of closely aggregated, rather large spindle-shaped cells with ovoid nuclei and abundant pale cytoplasm often containing little or no melanin. Not infrequently, the cellular islands penetrate into the subcutaneous fat, often forming a bulbous expansion there that is highly characteristic of cellular blue nevi. In some of the intersecting bundles, the cells appear rounded, perhaps as a result of cross sectioning. Melanophages with abundant melanin may be present between

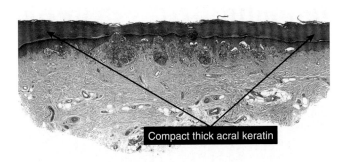

Fig. VIB3a.l

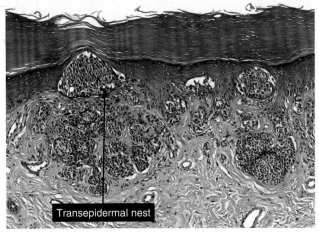

Fig. VIB3a.m

Fig. VIB3a.l. *Compound nevus, acral type, low power.* One can identify that this biopsy is from an acral site because of the thick, compact stratum corneum. The nevus is small and symmetrical and shows both a junctional and superficial dermal component.

Fig. VIB3a.m. *Compound nevus, acral type, medium power.* The nests in the papillary dermis are small, orderly, and lack atypia. Slight or even marked upward pagetoid scatter of cells as seen here is acceptable in the absence of other indicators of melanoma. The nest at the top left is an example of "transepidermal elimination," a phenomenon often seen in benign acral nevi (and also Spitz nevi).

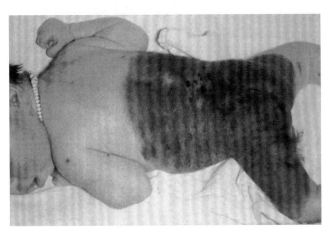

Clin. Fig. VIB3a.c

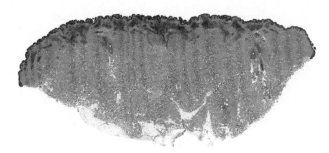

Fig. IVB3a.n

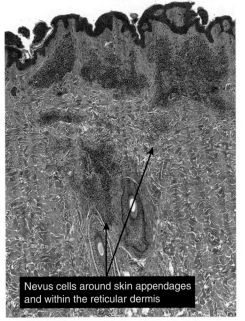

Fig. IVB3a.o

Clin. Fig. VIB3a.c. *Congenital nevus.* This giant, hairy nevus was present at birth and covers a "garment"-like or "bathing-trunk" distribution.

Fig. IVB3a.n. *Congenital pattern nevus, low power.* This relatively large nevus is compound but is predominantly in the dermis. The lesion extends to the mid and deep reticular dermis.

Fig. IVB3a.o. *Congenital pattern nevus, medium power.* The dermal component is composed of bland, uniform ovoid melanocytic cells. These cells extend into the reticular dermis and also around eccrine ducts and a hair follicle. This pattern may be seen in truly congenital nevi but may also be seen in some acquired nevi.

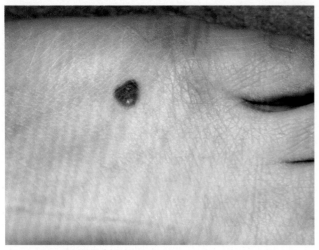

Clin. Fig. VIB3a.d

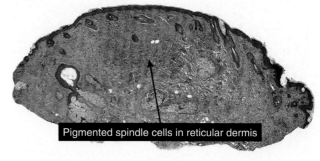

Pigmented spindle cells in reticular dermis

Fig. VIB3a.p

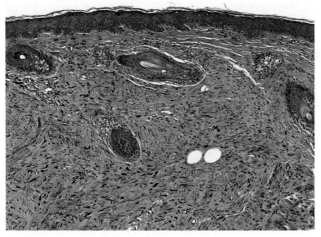

Fig. VIB3a.q

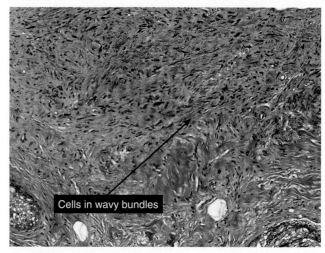

Cells in wavy bundles

Fig. VIB3a.r

Clin. Fig. VIB3a.d. *Blue nevus.* A 28-year-old woman had a 3-year history of a bluish papule on the left foot dorsum.

Fig. VIB3a.p. *Blue nevus, low power.* Within the dermis there is a poorly defined but symmetrical spindle cell proliferation which is dark brown in color. There is no significant change in the overlying epidermis.

Fig. VIB3a.q. *Blue nevus, medium power.* The spindled, heavily pigmented cells encircle collagen bundles in the reticular dermis, a pattern which is also seen in dermatofibromas.

Fig. VIB3a.r. *Blue nevus, high power.* The lesion is composed of elongate cells which are heavily pigmented and show prominent pigmented dendrites. The nuclei are small. The cells may be arranged in wavy fiber bundles consistent with schwannian differentiation.

---

the islands. The diagnosis of cellular blue nevus is generally easy in these "biphasic" lesions with both dendritic and spindle-shaped cells and with areas that resemble common blue nevi, but it can be difficult in occasional lesions without dendritic cells and in a few lesions that lack readily appreciable melanin. Larger islands composed of spindle-shaped cells may consist of many intersecting bundles of cells extending in various directions and resembling the storiform pattern observed in a neurofibroma. Some

lesions consist entirely of pigmented spindle cells extending into the dermis. These lesions, referred to as the "monophasic spindle cell type" of cellular blue nevus, overlap histologically with Spitz nevi, deep penetrating nevi, and spindle cell melanomas. They tend to differ from the latter by overall architectural symmetry, by their monotony of cell type, and by lacking necrosis or frequent mitoses. Although frank anaplastic high-grade nuclear atypia is generally absent in cellular blue nevi, the nuclei may be

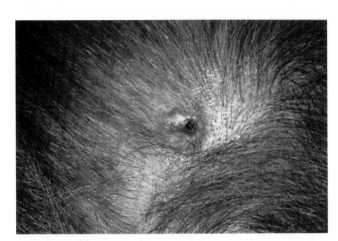

Clin. Fig. VIB3a.e

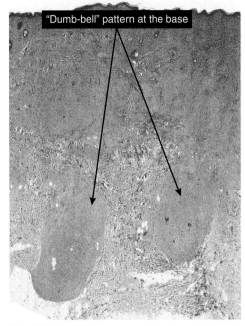

"Dumb-bell" pattern at the base

Fig. VIB3a.s

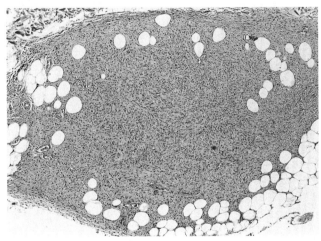

Fig. VIB3a.t

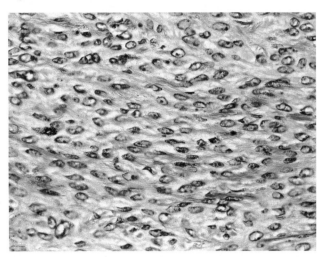

Fig. VIB3a.u

Clin. Fig. VIB3a.e. *Blue nodule in the scalp.* This blue nodule on clinical grounds could represent a cellular blue nevus, a malignant blue nevus, or malignant melanoma (primary or metastatic). Despite the symmetry of the lesion and its relatively small size, a malignant diagnosis is favored clinically by the presence of focal ulceration.

Fig. VIB3a.s. *Cellular blue nevus, low power.* Cellular blue nevi are frequently relatively large, involving a good portion of the reticular dermis and extending deeply as tongue-like aggregates of tumor cells at the base of the lesion. The dendritic melanocytic component that resembles a common blue nevus can be seen at the periphery of the lesion.

Fig. VIB3a.t. *Cellular blue nevus, medium power.* Involvement of the subcutaneous fat is common and does not imply a malignant diagnosis.

Fig. VIB3a.u. *Cellular blue nevus, high power.* The cellular areas are composed of uniform spindled melano-cytic cells with more cytoplasm and larger nuclei than what is seen in common blue nevus. There are irregularly distributed collections of coarse melanin pigment within the cells.

large with prominent nucleoli. Although most of these lesions have a benign course, a few have been locally aggressive or have metastasized at least to regional lymph nodes, and a guarded prognosis is appropriate in the presence of more than a few mitoses (melanocytic tumor of uncertain malignant potential). The absence or scarcity of mitotic figures and the absence of areas of necrosis are evidence against a diagnosis of malignant blue nevus, and the presence of areas of dendritic cells elsewhere in the tumor, as well as the lack of a characteristic intraepidermal component, argue against a diagnosis of melanoma.

VIB3b Melanocytic Lesions With Cytologic Atypia

Although some benign lesions may exhibit "significant" cytologic atypia, in most such cases, such as deep penetrating nevi, the atypia is "random," or confined to a minority population of scattered lesional cells. Spitz nevi are an exception; in these lesions there is a characteristic nuclear morphology of large nuclei with open chromatin, regular nuclear membranes, and large nucleoli. This nuclear morphology is uniform across the lesion, and needs to be distinguished from the more hyperchromatic nuclei with irregular nuclear membranes and clumped chromatin seen in most melanomas.

Deep Penetrating Nevus

CLINICAL SUMMARY. This is a distinctive entity that has some features of combined nevus, blue nevus, and Spitz nevus (40). In the first report of 70 cases from a referral center, many cases had previously been misdiagnosed histologically as melanomas. Similar lesions have also been described as plexiform spindle cell nevi. The lesions occur in children as well as adults, and the head, neck, and shoulder are the most frequent sites of involvement. The lesions range in size up to about 10 mm, and are darkly pigmented papules and nodules, often diagnosed clinically as blue nevi or cellular blue nevi. Occasional recurrences have been described, and there are anecdotal examples of metastasis from lesions with many if not all features of deep penetrating nevi (41,42). On cross section, the lesions extended at least halfway into the dermis, with a smooth, dome-shaped elevation of the epidermis. Lesions termed "nevi with focal atypical epithelioid component" or "clonal" or "combined" nevi may represent a superficial variant. These distinctions are of little or no importance; the key distinction is from melanoma.

HISTOPATHOLOGY. At scanning magnification, the lesions are circumscribed and pyramidal in shape, with a broad base abutting the epidermis, and an apex extending into or toward the fat. Nests of nevus cells at the dermal–epidermal junction are usually present. The dermal component is composed of loosely-arranged nests or plexiform fascicles of large pigmented spindle and

epithelioid cells interspersed with melanophages. There is a tendency of formation of narrow spindle cells at the periphery of the nests, reminiscent of sustentacular cell differentiation. In many cases there is an admixture of smaller, more conventional nevus cells. The lesional cell nests tend to surround skin appendages, and to infiltrate the collagen at the periphery of the lesion. The cells do not tend to "mature" with descent into the dermis. Some lesions have a patchy mild lymphocytic infiltrate.

At higher magnification, nuclear pleomorphism may be striking in some lesions, with variation in size and shape, hyperchromasia, and nuclear pseudoinclusions. The atypia tends to be confined to randomly scattered cells rather than being "uniform," or present in a majority of the cells. Nucleoli are usually inconspicuous but a few large eosinophilic nucleoli may be observed. Importantly, mitoses are absent or very rare, with no more than one or two in multiple sections of any given lesion. The cytoplasm is abundant, and contains finely-divided brown melanin pigment. The lesional cells react positively for S-100 protein and HMB-45 antigen, and other melanocytic markers.

Spitz Tumor/Nevus

CLINICAL SUMMARY. The importance of recognizing Spitz tumors is that the histology often resembles a nodular melanoma because of the large size of the lesional cells, often with considerable nuclear and cytoplasmic pleomorphism and an inflammatory infiltrate (43). This lesion, described by Sophie Spitz in 1948 as "juvenile melanoma," is known also as spindle and epithelioid cell nevus or as "nevus of large spindle and/or epithelioid cells." It occurs in children, and in young to early middle-aged (and occasionally older) adults. Typically, it consists of a dome-shaped, hairless pink nodule, usually smaller than 6 mm to 1 cm, and encountered most commonly on the lower extremities and face. The color is usually pink, and the lesion is then often diagnosed clinically as granuloma pyogenicum, angioma, or dermal nevus. However, it may be tan, brown, or even black. After an initial period of growth, most Spitz nevi are stable. In rare instances, there are multiple tumors, either agminated (grouped) in one area or widely disseminated. Some lesions exhibit atypical features histologically and there is overlap with nevoid or "Spitzoid" melanomas, so that the term "tumor" (or "melanocytoma") is currently preferred to that of a "nevus" with its implication of an invariably benign neoplasm (44). Nevertheless, the vast majority of Spitz tumors, especially in children, will have a benign course. Even after the discovery of lymph node metastases in a Spitzoid lesion, long survivals have been reported (45). Spitz nevi/tumors lack the BRAF mutations that characterize most common nevi. Most of them have activated fusion genes including ALK, ROS1, NTRK and others. Some atypical lesions have an activating mutation of H-RAS, which is rare in other nevi and in melanomas (46). These genetic findings may have some utility in diagnosis (47).

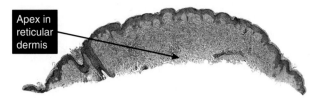

Fig. VIB3b.a

Apex in reticular dermis

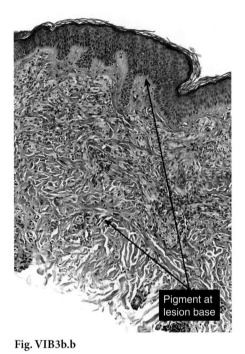

Fig. VIB3b.b

Pigment at lesion base

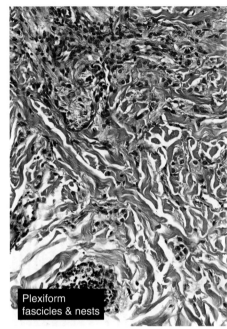

Fig. VIB3b.c

Plexiform fascicles & nests

Fig. VIB3b.a. *Deep penetrating nevus, low power.* There is a relatively small and symmetrical melanocytic lesion which in this instance is entirely in the dermis although other such lesions may have a junctional component. Although more superficial and plaque like than some such lesions, it has a wedge-shaped architecture with an apex in the reticular dermis.

Fig. VIB3b.b. *Deep penetrating nevus, medium power.* The lesion is composed of nests and fascicles of heavily pigmented melanocytic cells which extend deeply into the reticular dermis.

Fig. VIB3b.c. *Deep penetrating nevus, high power.* The tumor cells are epithelioid with an abundance of cytoplasm containing fine melanin pigment. Heavily pigmented melanophages are frequent. The majority of the nuclei are small and uniform, however, mild random nuclear atypia may be seen in these lesions. Mitotic figures are absent or exceedingly rare.

HISTOPATHOLOGY. In their overall architectural pattern, Spitz nevi resemble junctional or compound nevi. They are small, symmetrical, and well circumscribed. The epidermis is often hyperplastic with elongated rete ridges. The epidermal component is arranged in nests that tend to be oriented vertically and, although large, do not vary a great deal in size and shape or tend to become confluent. In Spitz nevi with junctional activity, there are often artifactual clefts between the nests of nevus cells and the surrounding keratinocytes, a feature that is less often seen in melanoma. Pagetoid permeation of the epidermis by tumor cells is usually slight, except occasionally and especially in young children.

Important cytologic features of Spitz nevi include especially the "large spindle and/or epithelioid cells," which define the lesion histologically. Apart from the shape of their cell bodies, the spindle cells and epithelioid cells in any given Spitz nevus resemble one another in nuclear and cytoplasmic consistency, suggesting that they may represent dimorphic expression of a single cell type. They have abundant amphophilic cytoplasm and prominent eosinophilic nucleoli. A useful although not pathognomonic cytologic criterion for Spitz nevi is the presence within the epidermis of coalescent red globular "Kamino

bodies." Of special importance is maturation of the cells with increasing depth, so that they become smaller and look more like the cells of a common nevus. Also important is the uniformity of the lesional cells from one side of the lesion to the other: at any given level of the lesion from the epidermis to its base, the lesional cells look the same. The small lesional cells at the base of most Spitz nevi tend to disperse as single cells or files of single cells among reticular dermis collagen bundles. Mitoses are found in about half of the cases, usually in small numbers (<2/sq.mm). Atypical mitoses are rare or absent. The complete absence of mitoses in 50% of Spitz nevi is very helpful in ruling out melanoma in these cases.

Bulky tumors with spitzoid cytology occur and cause difficulty in diagnosis. A series of such cases was recently reported as "epithelioid melanocytomas of uncertain malignant potential" (48). Features in these lesions that were associated with more aggressive behavior (which was usually but not always limited to bulky regional nodal metastases) included mitoses in the lower third of the lesion, and the presence of a lymphocytic infiltrate. These authors concluded that "The major outcome of this study of a series of 'MELTUMPs' suggests as a preliminary observation that these lesions as a group exist and that

TABLE VI.4. Spitz Tumor Versus Atypical Spitz Tumor Versus Nodular Melanoma

Feature	Spitz Tumor	Atypical Spitz Tumor/ MELTUMP	Nodular Melanoma
Size	Smaller	Larger	Larger
Symmetry	Good	Fair	May be good but often imperfect
Cytology	Uniform large spindle and/or epithelioid cells	May be somewhat variable from side to side	More variable—large and small, pigmented and nonpigmented etc.
Ulceration and necrosis	Rare	Occasionally	Often
Consumption of Epidermis	Epidermis thickened	Usually thickened	Often thinned
Mitoses	Very few if any	More readily detectable	Often frequent
Kamino bodies	Usually	Usually	Hardly ever
Maturation	Good	Fair	Poor
Dispersion into reticular dermis	Single cells at base	May be clusters/nests	Clusters at base
Lymphocytic infiltrate	Often absent	Often present	Often present

they may be biologically different from conventional melanoma and benign melanocytic nevi. The terminology remains highly controversial, reflecting the uncertainty in classification and interpretation of these atypical melanocytic tumors." Genomic studies including comparative genomic hybridization (CGH) and fluorescence *in situ* hybridization (FISH) may be helpful in decision making in these difficult cases, but are not at present likely to be independently diagnostic (49). See Table VI.4.

Nodular Melanoma

CLINICAL SUMMARY. Nodular melanoma, by definition, contains only tumorigenic vertical growth (29). The lesion starts as an elevated, variably pigmented papule that increases in size quite rapidly to become a nodule and often ulcerates. The ABCD criteria reviewed earlier do not apply to nodular melanomas, which are often quite small, symmetrical, and well-circumscribed. They may be conspicuously pigmented,

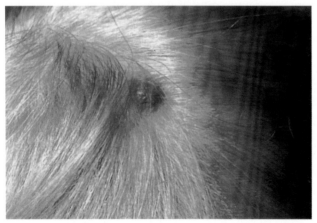

Clin. Fig. VIB3b.a

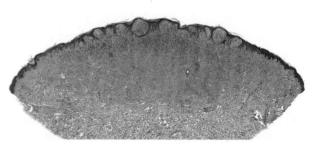

Fig. VIB3b.d

Clin. Fig. VIB3b.a. *Spitz nevus.* A symmetrical pink nodule which appeared suddenly in a child but then remained stable for several weeks before excision was arranged.

Fig. VIB3b.d. *Spitz nevus/tumor, low power.* At scanning magnification there is a symmetrical zone of epithelial hyperplasia. Because Spitz nevi are frequently amelanotic, the melanocytic component may be difficult to appreciate at low magnification.

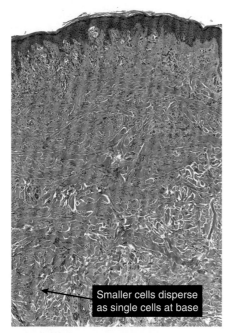

Smaller cells disperse as single cells at base

Fig. VIB3b.e

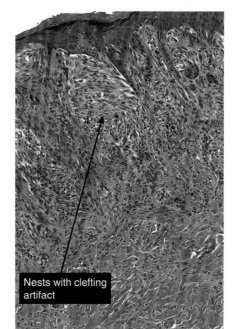

Nests with clefting artifact

Fig. VIB3b.f

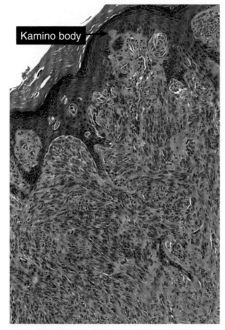

Kamino body

Fig. VIB3b.g

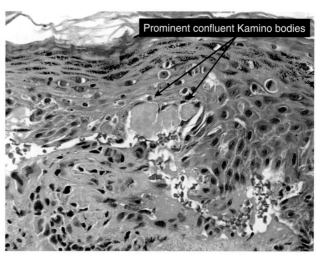

Prominent confluent Kamino bodies

Fig. VIB3b.h

Fig. VIB3b.e. *Spitz nevus/tumor, medium power.* Lesional cells show a characteristic pattern of maturation and dispersion as single cells into the reticular dermis at the base of the tumor.

Fig. VIB3b.f. *Spitz nevus/tumor, medium power.* Nests of spindled melanocytes in the epidermis demonstrate clefting artifact, a common finding in Spitz tumors.

Fig. VIB3b.g. *Spitz nevus/tumor, medium power.* Higher magnification reveals the cytology of the cells to be predominantly spindled in form. There may also be epithelioid cells with an abundance of cytoplasm. Eosinophilic nucleoli are frequently prominent. A small eosinophilic globule (Kamino body) is seen in the epidermal component.

Fig. VIB3b.h. *Spitz nevus, high power.* Prominent globoid Kamino bodies in another case from a 7-year-old child.

oligomelanotic, or amelanotic. When other risk factors such as thickness are controlled, the prognosis of nodular melanoma is not worse than that of other forms of melanoma. In terms of the WHO 2018 classification of melanomas, nodular melanomas can occur probably in all of the different pathways to melanoma (low CSD, high CSD, no CSD).

HISTOPATHOLOGY. There is contiguous growth of uniformly atypical melanocytes in the dermis, forming an often asymmetrical tumor mass. Asymmetry is often apparent at the cytologic level as variation in cell size, shape, and pigmentation, and in the distribution of the host response, such that one half of the lesion is not a mirror image of the other half. However, the silhouette of the entire lesion may be quite symmetrical in a nodular melanoma because of the lack of an adjacent component. There is a variable lymphocytic infiltrate around the base or within the tumor. The epidermis is frequently ulcerated, or there is an adherent scale-crust. In a nodular melanoma, "pagetoid" permeation of the epidermis with tumor cells is limited to that portion overlying the dermal tumor, and in some cases, the epidermal involvement may be quite limited in degree. For this reason, nodular melanoma may be difficult or impossible to distinguish from a metastatic melanoma in the skin, and when the tumor is amelanotic, the distinction from other malignancies may require immunohistochemistry.

Cytologically, the tumor cells in the dermis tend to vary greatly in size and shape. Nevertheless, two major types of cells—epithelioid and spindle-shaped—can be recognized. Usually one type predominates. The epithelioid cells tend to lie in nested or alveolar formations surrounded by delicate collagen fibers, and the spindle-shaped cells in irregularly branching formations. Tumors in which spindle cells predominate may resemble sarcomas but in most cases differ from them by the presence of junctional melanocytic activity. The uniformly atypical nuclei of the melanoma cells are larger than those of melanocytes or nevus cells, with irregular nuclear membranes, hyperchromatic chromatin, and often prominent nucleoli that tend to be irregular in size, shape, and number. There is also a diagnostically important failure of the melanocytes in the deeper layers of the dermis to decrease in size (absence of "maturation"). Mitotic figures are usually present and often numerous in the lesional cells of the dermal and epidermal compartments of tumorigenic melanomas.

Superficial Spreading Melanoma (Tumorigenic)

CLINICAL SUMMARY. Unlike nodular melanoma, most melanomas evolve through a clinically evident stage of tumor progression termed the radial growth phase (RGP) in which they enlarge as it were along the radii of an imperfect circle in the skin. Subsequently a tumorigenic phase may ensue, in which a vertical growth phase (VGP) nodule appears within the pre-existing RGP plaque. The ABCD criteria reviewed earlier apply mostly to the RGP component. Histologic criteria, reviewed below, also apply mainly to the RGP. The tumorigenic VGP differs not at all from that in most "nodular melanomas" (which by definition lack an RGP), and prognosis is the same when all of the microstaging attributes are taken into consideration.

HISTOPATHOLOGY. Key features that define a superficial spreading melanoma, compared to the other most common RGP subtype, lentigo maligna melanoma, include the following: the lesions tend to be characterized by a

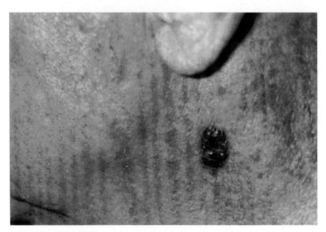

Clin. Fig. VIB3b.b

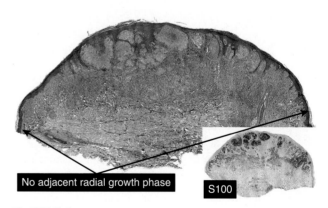

No adjacent radial growth phase

S100

Fig. VIB3b.i

Clin. Fig. VIB3b.b. *Malignant melanoma, tumorigenic.* An elderly man presented with an asymmetrical black tumor and cervical adenopathy.

Fig. VIB3b.i. *Nodular melanoma, low power.* This subtype of malignant melanoma frequently shows a dome-shaped or polypoid architecture, which may seem deceptively symmetrical at scanning magnification. S100 staining (inset) demonstrates asymmetrical arrangements of the cells in the dermis. There is no radial growth phase to this lesion, the feature which distinguishes it from other forms of melanoma.

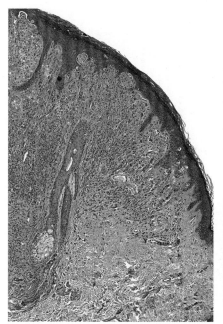

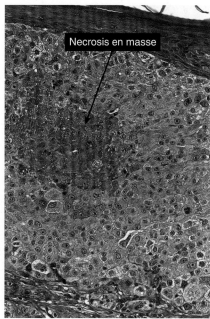

Necrosis en masse

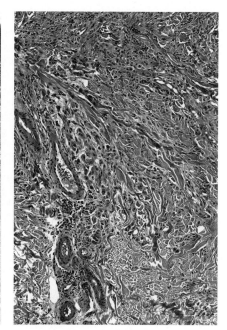

Fig. VIB3b.j

Fig. VIB3b.k

Fig. VIB3b.l

Fig. VIB3b.j. *Nodular melanoma, medium power.* The tumor shows its origination from the overlying epidermis which shows single and nested atypical melanocytes at the dermal–epidermal interface. In nodular melanoma, pagetoid spread may not be prominent.

Fig. VIB3b.k. *Nodular melanoma, high power.* Mitotic figures are generally identified and occasional cells show brown pigment within the cytoplasm. Necrosis "en masse" and/or ulceration are commonly seen in bulky vertical growth phase tumors.

Fig. VIB3b.l. *Nodular melanoma, high power.* The tumor cells infiltrate the reticular dermis as pushing fascicles rather than as single cells as is the rule in Spitz and congenital pattern nevi, benign lesions that also involve the reticular dermis.

hyperplastic epidermal contour rather than the atrophic pattern seen in lentigo maligna melanoma. Pagetoid scatter of lesional cells into the epidermis is a striking feature even at scanning magnification. Lesional cells tend to be arranged in a prominent nested pattern, with nests varying in size, shape, orientation, and distribution within the epidermis. The cells tend to be large epithelioid cells, and pigment is more abundant in superficial spreading than in lentigo maligna melanoma. Superficial spreading melanoma is also more likely than lentigo maligna melanoma to be associated with a nevus, and less likely to be associated with severe chronic solar damage. In recently published genotype–phenotype correlation studies which have helped to refine the criteria for the subtypes of melanoma, these features of superficial spreading melanoma correlate generally with mutations of the oncogene BRAF (50,51).

Nevoid Melanoma

Nevoid melanomas are defined as lesions that, to a considerable extent, mimic a benign nevus histologically, especially in terms of lesional architecture (52,53). Usually, the resemblance is most apparent at scanning magnification,

where lesions may appear symmetrical, nested, and devoid of radial growth. These features can lead to a missed diagnosis if sufficient attention is not paid to cytologic and subtle architectural features including the presence of multiple mitoses. In a seminal study by Schmoeckel, useful discriminating attributes included cellular atypia, mitoses, infiltration of adnexa, infiltrative growth in the deeper dermis, and absence of maturation. Tumor thickness was the most important prognostic criterion (26). Nevoid melanomas are generally considered to have the same biologic potential as other melanomas with similar microstaging attributes. Key to the recognition of a nevoid melanoma is a high index of suspicion, and the identification of high cellularity, mitotic activity and cytologic atypia in the dermal component of the lesion.

Metastatic Malignant Melanoma

CLINICAL SUMMARY. Metastatic malignant melanoma most commonly presents as a firm, red-purple to blue-black subcutaneous mass. Epidermotropic metastatic melanoma presents as small symmetrical papules that may simulate a benign nevus (54).

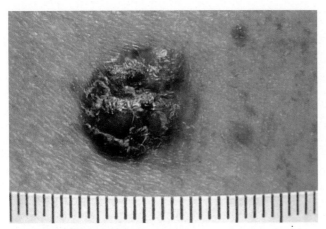

Clin. Fig. VIB3b.c

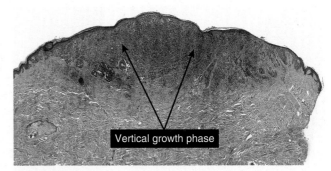

Fig. VIB3b.m

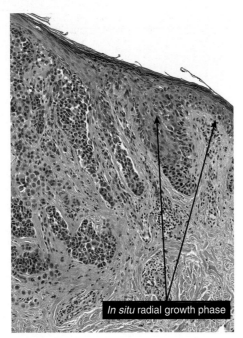

Fig. VIB3b.n

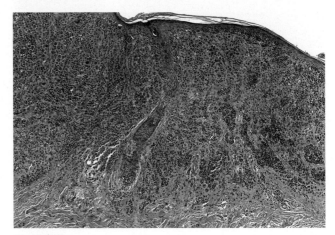

Fig. VIB3b.o

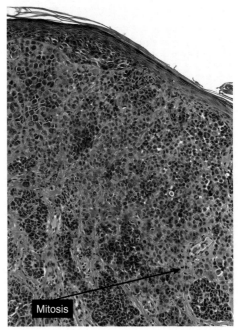

Fig. VIB3b.p

Clin. Fig. VIB3b.c. *Malignant melanoma, superficial spreading type, tumorigenic.* This lesion has a prominent blue-black tumorigenic vertical growth phase nodule, and an adjacent tan plaque component which represents an associated radial growth phase.

Fig. VIB3b.m. *Superficial spreading melanoma, with bulky tumorigenic vertical growth phase, low power.* An asymmetric tumor nodule is the prominent feature at scanning magnification.

Fig. VIB3b.n. *Superficial spreading melanoma, with bulky tumorigenic vertical growth phase, medium power.* Adjacent to the nodule there is pagetoid scatter of uniformly atypical epithelioid cells arranged singly and in illdefined nests. The presence and pagetoid/nested morphology of this adjacent radial growth phase component define this lesion as a superficial spreading melanoma.

Fig. VIB3b.o. *Superficial spreading melanoma, with bulky tumorigenic vertical growth phase, medium power.* The nodule is very cellular and there is little or no evidence of maturation from superficial to deep.

Fig. VIB3b.p. *Superficial spreading melanoma, with bulky tumorigenic vertical growth phase.* The cells in the nodule are large epithelioid melanoma cells which have abundant cytoplasm and large, irregular nuclei with prominent nucleoli. Mitoses are readily detected.

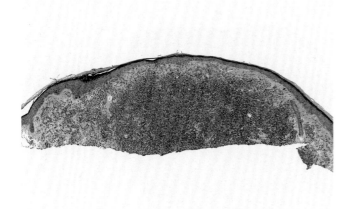

Fig. VIB3b.q

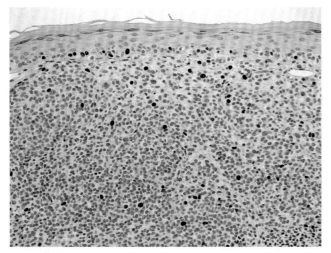

Fig. VIB3b.s

Fig. VIB3b.r

Fig. VIB3b.q. *Nevoid melanoma, low power.* Although there is an impression of a nevoid configuration at first glance, the cellularity of this lesion is high, with extensive confluent sheetlike growth of the small nevoid lesional cells in the dermis.

Fig. VIB3b.r. *Nevoid melanoma, high power.* At high magnification, the cells demonstrate uniform albeit mild to moderate atypia, and dermal mitotic figures are present although not frequent.

Fig. VIB3b.s. *Nevoid melanoma, medium power.* A Ki-67 study demonstrates more than a sprinkling of cycling cells. Although not diagnostic in and of itself, this finding supports the diagnosis of nevoid melanoma when taken in conjunction with the high cellularity, confluent growth, failure of maturation and mitotic activity seen in this lesion.

HISTOPATHOLOGY. The histologic appearance usually differs from that of a primary melanoma by the absence of an inflammatory infiltrate and of junctional activity. However, primary melanomas may occasionally fail to involve the epidermis, and may also not show an inflammatory infiltrate, particularly when they are deeply invasive. Furthermore, some metastases exhibit a prominent lymphocytic infiltrate, and can contact the overlying epidermis in a way that is suggestive of junctional activity. *Epidermotropic metastatic melanoma* refers to a metastatic deposit that is initially localized in the papillary dermis and involves the overlying epidermis. Most of these lesions occur in an extremity regional to a distal primary melanoma. Epidermotropic metastasis is characterized by (1) thinning of the epidermis by aggregates of atypical melanocytes within the dermis, (2) inward turning of the rete ridges at the periphery of the lesion, and (3) usually no lateral extension of atypical melanocytes within the epidermis beyond the concentration of the metastasis in the dermis. However, this distinction can be very difficult in a few lesions where extension beyond the dermal component

occurs. In some of these cases, the metastatic cells are small and nevoid, with few if any mitoses, and in these instances of *differentiated epidermotropic metastatic melanoma* the lesions can be mistaken for compound nevi.

Metastatic Malignant Melanoma, Satellite Lesion

See Figs. VIB3b.v,w.

Epidermotropic Metastatic Melanoma

This term refers to a metastatic deposit that is initially localized to the papillary dermis and involves the overlying epidermis. Most of these lesions occur in an extremity regional to a distal primary melanoma. Epidermotropic metastasis is characterized by thinning of the epidermis by aggregates of atypical melanocytes within the dermis, inward turning of the rete ridges at the periphery of the lesion, and usually no lateral extension of atypical melanocytes within the epidermis beyond the concentration of the metastasis in the dermis. However, this distinction can be very difficult at times, and cases have been reported

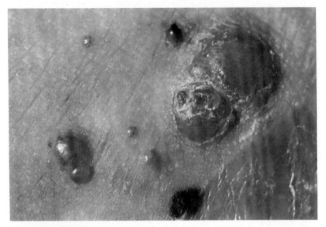

Clin. Fig. VIB3b.d

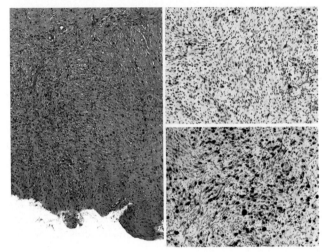

Fig. VIB3b.u

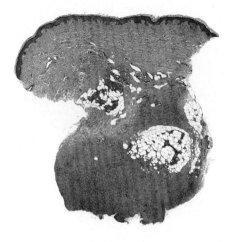

Fig. VIB3b.t

Clin. Fig. VIB3b.d. *Metastatic malignant melanoma.* A 69-year-old man presented with translucent erythematous and black nodules and papules surrounding the skin graft at the site of a previous melanoma of the foot.

Fig. VIB3b.t. *Metastatic malignant melanoma, low power.* In this example of metastatic melanoma there is a nodular tumor within the subcutaneous fat and lower dermis. There is no overlying tumor in the dermis or epidermis.

Fig. VIB3b.u. *Metastatic malignant melanoma, high power.* The tumor is composed of large atypical cells with an abundance of cytoplasm, large nuclei and prominent nucleoli. Brown melanin pigment is seen within the cytoplasm of these cells. Mitotic figures, which may be few or numerous, can generally be identified in metastatic lesions. This tumor has a brisk lymphocytic infiltrate and appears to be undergoing partial regression. Melan A (upper panel) and S100 stains are positive in scattered residual melanoma cells.

in which there was such lateral extension. In some other cases, the metastatic cells are small and nevoid, with few if any mitoses, and in these instances of *differentiated or nevoid epidermotropic metastatic melanoma* or "epidermotropic metastatic melanomas with maturation" the lesions can be mistaken for compound nevi. A molecular study of 21 lesions suggested that epidermotropic metastatic melanomas are clonally related to their primary lesion in many cases. Interestingly, the data also indicated that some cases so diagnosed might be divergent clones or even new primaries rather than metastases (55).

Pigmented Epithelioid Melanocytoma (PEM)/Epithelioid Blue Nevus

CLINICAL SUMMARY. This heavily pigmented melanocytic tumor closely resembles epithelioid blue nevi as seen in Carney complex, and also some cellular blue nevi (56,57). This lesion appears to represent a distinctive

tumor that affects males and females equally with a median age of occurrence of 27 years (range 0.6–78 years). Multiple body sites may be affected, with extremities being the most common. Loss of expression due to a loss of function mutation of a presumptive suppressor gene (protein kinase A regulatory subunit 1alpha, PRKAR1a) has been described in these lesions (58). Another subset has fusions of PRKCA, a possibly related gene, while others have loss of expression of PRKAR1a but no detectable mutations. PEM-like lesions with GNAQ or GNA11 mutations should be classified as blue nevi (59).

HISTOPATHOLOGY. Histologically there is a deep dermal nodule of heavily-pigmented epithelioid and/or spindled melanocytes. Some lesions occur as a component of a combined nevus. Ulceration may be present in occasional lesions; a finding generally not present in epithelioid blue nevi. Although tumor cells may be bland and mitoses and

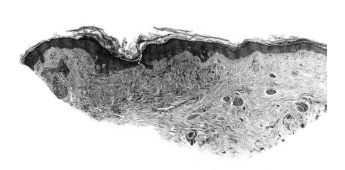

Fig. VIB3b.v

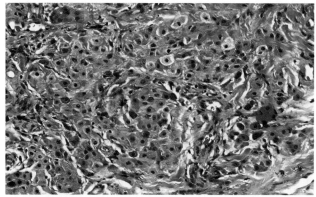

Fig. VIB3b.w

Fig. VIB3b.v. *Metastatic malignant melanoma, satellite lesion, low power.* This small black papule was present adjacent to a malignant melanoma. Within the upper dermis there are collections of heavily pigmented melanocytic cells without an overlying epidermal component.

Fig. VIB3b.w. *Malignant melanoma, satellite lesion, high power.* Small satellite lesions histologically may look nevic. However, the aggregates are of various sizes and the individual cells are large with hyperchromatic nuclei. Atypia is not always severe in these lesions, as in this example. The presence of mitotic figures, although not always numerous, is helpful in differentiating these lesions from nevi.

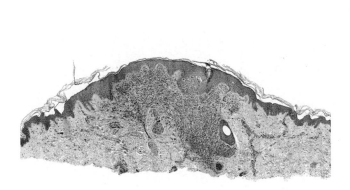

Fig. VIB3b.x

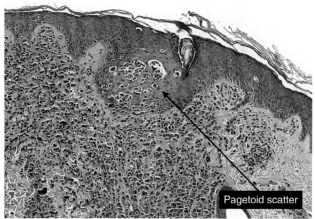

Fig. VIB3b.y

Fig. VIB3b.x. *Epidermotropic metastatic malignant melanoma, medium power.* In this example of epidermotropic metastatic melanoma, the cells lack melanin pigment and they show pagetoid scatter of atypical cells into the epidermis, a pattern which mimics a primary malignant melanoma.

Fig. VIB3b.y. *Epidermotropic metastatic malignant melanoma, medium power.* Pagetoid scatter is typically confined to the epidermis above the dermal component in these lesions. Readily detectable lymphatic invasion (not shown) may be a clue to the diagnosis but is often absent.

necrosis inconspicuous or absent, regional lymph node involvement has been seen in 46% of cases studied. Nonetheless, extranodal spread is rare, and even with involvement of draining lymph nodes, the clinical course may be remarkably indolent. Similar or identical lesions associated with the Carney complex appear to be benign.

Melanocytic Tumor of Uncertain Malignant Potential

Some lesions present conflicting histologic criteria, making it impossible to clearly distinguish between a benign nevus (or tumor) and a tumorigenic melanoma which could have metastasizing as well as locally recurring potential. A recent study described the difficulties and lack of agreement in the histopathologic diagnosis of particular melanocytic tumors, such as atypical Spitz tumors (AST), atypical blue nevi, and deep penetrating nevi (38). These lesions are often referred to as "melanocytic tumors of uncertain malignant potential" (MELTUMP). This of course is a descriptive term and not a definitive diagnosis or a homogeneous category. Principles of

VI Tumors and Cysts of the Dermis and Subcutis

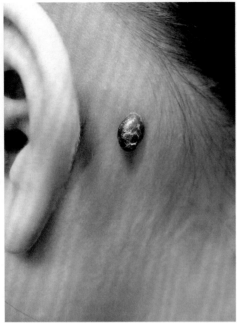

Clin. Fig. VIB3b.e

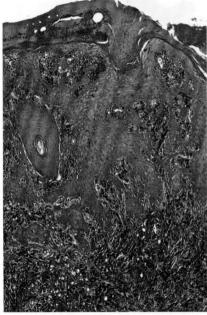

Fig. VIB3b.z

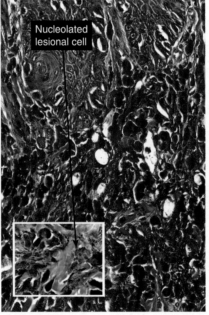

Fig. VIB3b.za

Nucleolated
lesional cell

Fig. VIB3b.zb

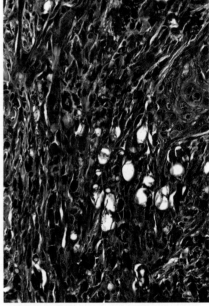

Fig. VIB3b.zc

Clin. Fig. VIB3b.e. *A large heavily pigmented exophytic blue-black nodule in a 3-year-old girl.* In contrast to many melanomas of this size, the lesion is not ulcerated and there is no adjacent RGP component.

Fig. VIB3b.z. *Pigmented Epithelioid Melanocytoma (PEM), low power.* A heavily pigmented nodule spanning the dermis. There is a bulbous expansion into the subcutis similar to what is often seen in cellular blue nevi.

Fig. VIB3b.za. *PEM.* The lesion is comprised of heavily pigmented cells which are melanophages and more lightly pigmented cells which are the lesional cells. There is often as here a prominent junctional component with marked keratinocytic hyperplasia.

Fig. VIB3b.zb. *PEM, high power.* The lesional cells (inset) are epithelioid or sometimes spindled in configuration, and have prominent nucleoli with open chromatin and regular nuclear membranes. Mitoses are usually present but not numerous.

Fig. VIB3b.zc. *PEM, medium power.* A melanin bleach stain reveals the nuclear detail of the characteristic lesional cells (smooth contour, pale chromatin, prominent nucleolus, see also inset in previous image), and the infiltrating melanophages.

classification of these lesions have been discussed above. The term "melanocytoma" has been proposed as a designation that is noncommittal as to the predicted behavior of some of these difficult and controversial lesions (38). Even when these lesions are found to have metastasized to regional nodes in a sentinel node staging procedure, the subsequent course is usually benign, based on multiple follow-up studies reviewed in a recent report (60).

Conditions to consider in the differential diagnosis:

Superficial Melanocytic Nevi
    compound melanocytic nevus
    dermal melanocytic nevus, acquired type
    dermal recurrent melanocytic nevus
    dysplastic nevi, compound
    nevus of genital skin
    nevus of acral skin
    halo nevus
    combined nevus
    pigmented spindle cell nevus of Reed
    balloon cell nevus

Superficial and Deep Melanocytic Nevi
    small congenital nevus
    intermediate and giant congenital nevi
    deep penetrating nevus
    spindle and epithelioid cell nevus (Spitz nevus)

Pigment-Synthesizing Dermal Neoplasms
    metastatic melanoma

    common blue nevus
    cellular blue nevus
    combined nevus
    deep penetrating nevus
    malignant blue nevus
    proliferative nodules in congenital melanocytic nevi
    malignant melanomas in congenital melanocytic nevi
    malignant melanocytic schwannoma
    dermal melanocytic tumors of uncertain malignant potential (MELTUMP)
    nevus of Ota
    melanotic neuroepithelial tumor of infancy

Tumorigenic Primary Melanomas
    nodular melanomas
    tumorigenic melanomas with radial and vertical growth phase
    superficial spreading type
    lentigo maligna type
    acral lentiginous type
    mucosal-lentiginous type
    desmoplastic melanoma
    neurotropic melanoma
    minimal deviation melanoma

Metastatic Malignant Melanoma
    epidermotropic metastatic melanoma
    satellites and in-transit metastatic melanoma
    dermal and subcutaneous metastatic melanoma

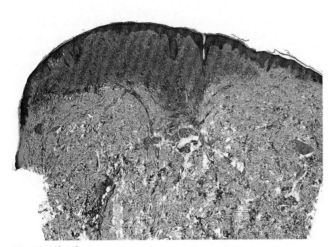

Fig. VIB3b.zd

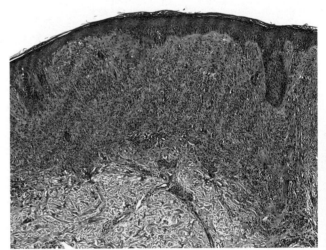

Fig. VIB3b.ze

Fig. VIB3b.zd. *Melanocytic Tumor of Uncertain Malignant Potential (MELTUMP).* At scanning magnification this lesion from the back of a teenager is quite large and very cellular, but relatively symmetrical.

Fig. VIB3b.ze. *MELTUMP/AST/Spitzoid melanoma.* Large epithelioid cells are uniform from side to side. Mitoses were present. There is only slight evidence of maturation to the base. (*continues*)

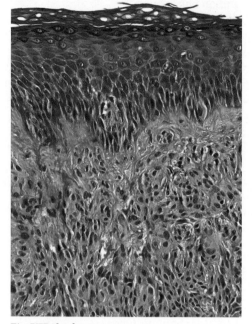

Fig. VIB3b.zf

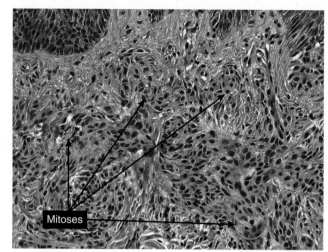

Mitoses

Fig. VIB3b.zg

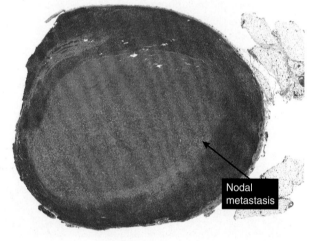

Nodal
metastasis

Fig. VIB3b.zh

Fig. VIB3b.zf. *MELTUMP/AST/Spitzoid melanoma.* The cells near the surface are large, with generally moderate atypia.

Fig. VIB3b.zg. *MELTUMP/AST/Spitzoid melanoma.* Although generally rare, focally several mitoses are present (green circles).

Fig. VIB3b.zh. *Metastatic MELTUMP/AST/Spitzoid melanoma.* There is a lymph node metastasis, found in a sentinel node procedure. Especially in a young individual, there is a growing body of literature to indicate that systemic metastasis is very uncommon in these "metastatic nodal spitzoid melanocytomas" which may be best regarded as of "uncertain malignant potential."

VIB4 | Eccrine Tumors

Proliferations of eccrine ductal (small dark cells usually forming tubules at least focally) or glandular tissue or both in a hyalinized or sclerotic dermis. The inflammatory infiltrate is mainly lymphocytic. Malignant examples of most of the tumor categories exist. These are rare, and are characterized in general by infiltration of the native dermis and other adjacent structures beyond the stroma of the tumor itself, by severe uniform cytologic atypia, increased mitotic activity, and necrosis or ulceration. Immunohistochemical studies have been proposed to help distinguish between primary adnexal carcinomas and metastatic adenocarcinomas;

p63 and D2-40 expression appear to be especially useful as markers of adnexal origin (61). Eccrine spiradenoma and nodular hidradenoma are the prototypic examples of the benign tumors.

VIB4a | Circumscribed, Symmetrical Eccrine Tumors

Eccrine Spiradenoma

CLINICAL SUMMARY. As a rule, eccrine spiradenoma (62) occurs as a solitary intradermal nodule measuring 1 to 2 cm in diameter. Occasionally, there are several nodules, and rarely, there are numerous small nodules in a

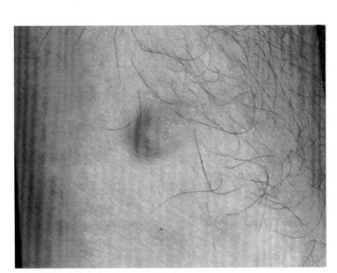

Clin. Fig. VIB4a.a

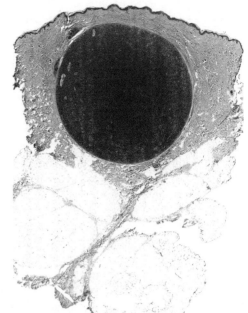

Fig. VIB4a.a

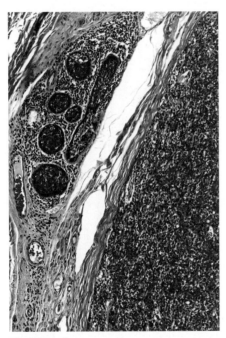

Fig. VIB4a.b

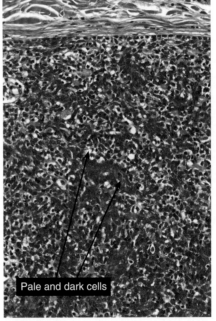

Pale and dark cells

Fig. VIB4a.c

Clin. Fig. VIB4a.a. *Eccrine spiradenoma.* A 55-year-old man had a 30-year history of a bluish nodulocystic lesion of the wrist, with a history of recent enlargement and tenderness.

Fig. VIB4a.a. *Eccrine spiradenoma, low power.* This adnexal neoplasm is a basaloid nodular tumor within the dermis. The lesion is sharply circumscribed and separated from the adjacent dermal collagen.

Fig. VIB4a.b. *Eccrine spiradenoma, medium power.* This tumor may be separated from the surrounding dermis by a thin fibrous capsule. At this power, the tumor cells form an interlocking pattern. "Satellite" tumors are common as seen here and are not indicators of malignancy.

Fig. VIB4a.c. *Eccrine spiradenoma, high power.* The tumor is composed of small basaloid cells with small nuclei and scant cytoplasm. A second population of cells is also present with slightly larger, vesicular nuclei, and more cytoplasm.

zosteriform pattern or large nodules in a linear arrangement. The nodules are often tender and occasionally painful.

HISTOPATHOLOGY. The tumor may consist of one large, sharply demarcated lobule, or of several such lobules located in the dermis without connections to the epidermis. There may be a fibrous capsule. The tumor lobules often appear deeply basophilic because of the close aggregation of the nuclei. The epithelial cells within the tumor lobules are arranged in intertwining cords, which may enclose small, irregularly shaped islands of edematous connective tissue. Two types of epithelial cells are present in the cords, both with only scant cytoplasm. The cells of the first type have small, dark nuclei; they are generally located at the periphery of the cellular aggregates. The cells of the second type have large, pale nuclei; they are located in the center of the aggregates and may be arranged partially around small lumina observed in about half of the tumors, or in a rosette arrangement. The lumina frequently contain small amounts of a PAS-positive granular, eosinophilic material. In some cases, hyaline material is focally present in the stroma that surrounds the cords of tumor cells. A heavy diffuse lymphocytic infiltrate may be present.

Cylindroma

CLINICAL SUMMARY. Cylindromas present as slow-growing, soft or firm dermal pink to reddish nodules, usually as solitary lesions on the head, neck and scalp. They arise predominantly in elderly and middle-aged females, with a female-to-male ratio of reportedly 9:1. Cylindroma can undergo malignant transformation, with potential for metastatic disease. These usually benign tumors may occur in the Brooke–Spiegler syndrome, an autosomal dominantly inherited disease in which multiple cylindromas develop. Mutations in the CYLD tumor suppressor gene have been associated with this syndrome. Cutaneous cylindromas are benign and should not be confused with adenoid cystic carcinomas which may occur in the skin as in other sites such as salivary glands.

HISTOPATHOLOGY. Cylindromas most frequently occur in the dermis of scalp and facial skin, and are comprised of irregularly shaped islands of basaloid cells surrounded by an eosinophilic hyaline sheath. The tumor islands typically consist of two types of cells: a peripheral palisade of cells with small dark nuclei, representing relatively undifferentiated

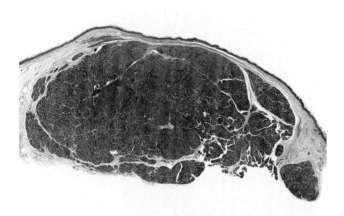

Fig. VIB4a.d

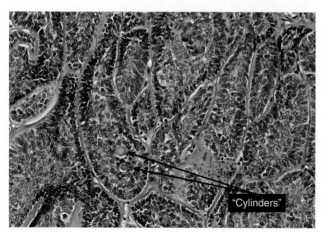

Fig. VIB4a.f

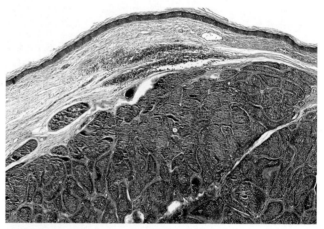

Fig. VIB4a.e

Fig. VIB4a.d. *Cylindroma, low power.* There is a relatively well-circumscribed basophilic tumor within the dermis. There is no association with the overlying epidermis which shows an effaced rete ridge pattern.

Fig. VIB4a.e. *Cylindroma, medium power.* The tumor is composed of multiple islands of basaloid cells which fit neatly together, adjacent to one another; the close proximity and interdigitating nature resemble the pieces of a jigsaw puzzle.

Fig. VIB4a.f. *Cylindroma, high power.* These tumors are composed of two populations of cells similar to what is seen in spiradenomas. The basaloid islands are surrounded by a homogenous eosinophilic basement membrane–like material. Also present within the islands are round aggregates of similar eosinophilic material.

basaloid tumor cells; and more centrally located, more differentiated cells with large, pale nuclei that resemble ductal or secretory cells. The thickened basement membrane zone of cylindromas is abnormal in terms of laminin, integrin and collagen expression, and in lack of hemidesmosomes (63).

Poroma

Poromas are benign neoplasms with differentiation toward the intraepidermal portion of the sweat apparatus. They are comprised of poroid and cuticular cells. Poroid cells have a rounded oval nucleus and scant cytoplasm while cuticular cells have more abundant cytoplasm and a central nucleus. Ductal differentiation may take the form of small intracytoplasmic vacuoles or formation of authentic ductal structures, which classically have an eosinophilic cuticular lining (64).

Syringoma

Syringoma is a small benign sweat gland tumor which commonly affects older women although the eruptive variant is most common in young women. Most arise in the lower eyelids and periorbital area. Eruptive lesions tend to occur on the neck, chest, axilla, pubic area, umbilicus, and genital regions. The lesions present as skin colored or slightly yellow smooth papules. Histologically they are well-circumscribed lesions typically located in the upper half of the dermis, occasionally deeper. There are epithelial cells forming ducts, cords, tubules and cysts, in a homogeneous and sclerotic stroma. The lumens are lined by a double layer of cuboidal cells. The ducts often have characteristic extensions resembling a tadpole tail. Small cysts are often present (65).

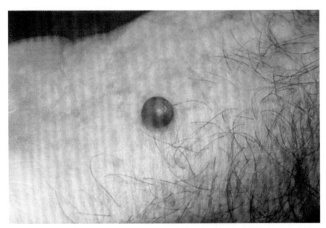

Clin. Fig. VIB4a.b

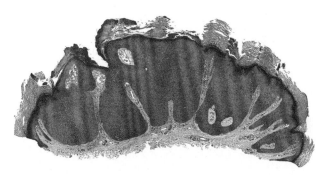

Fig. VIB4a.g

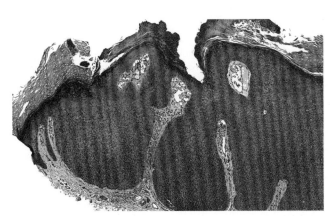

Fig. VIB4a.h

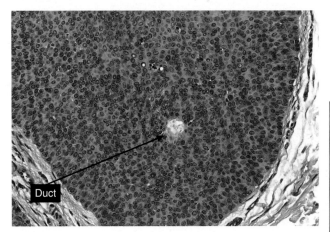

Fig. VIB4a.i

Clin. Fig. VIB4a.b. *Eccrine poroma.* A firm slightly erythematous papule on the volar aspect of the wrist.

Fig. VIB4a.g. *Eccrine poroma, low power.* A circumscribed proliferation of cells extending from the epidermis into the dermis.

Fig. VIB4a.h. *Eccrine poroma, medium power.* The epithelial cells form monotonous sheets.

Fig. VIB4a.i. *Eccrine poroma, high power.* A structure within the tumor is consistent with an abortive duct. In other examples, ducts may be lined by an eosinophilic cuticle similar to that of an eccrine duct.

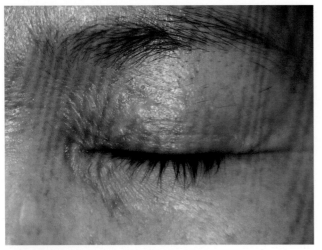

Clin. Fig. VIB4a.c

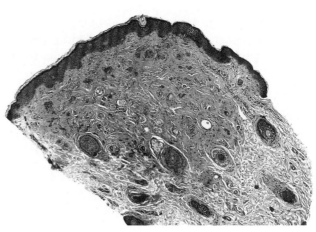

Fig. VIB4a.j

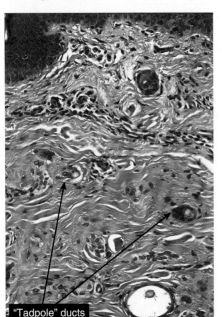

"Tadpole" ducts

Fig. VIB4a.k

Clin. Fig. VIB4a.c. *Multiple syringomas.* A 55-year-old woman with an 8-year history of multiple smooth-topped slightly yellow papules around the eye and eyelid.

Fig. VIB4a.j. *Syringoma, low power.* Within the upper half of the dermis there is a well-circumscribed adnexal tumor which is embedded in an eosinophilic stroma. Although this lesion has no capsule, the edge of the lesion is defined by the edge of the stroma.

Fig. VIB4a.k. *Syringoma, medium power.* The tumor is composed of multiple small islands of bland-appearing epithelial cells. Many of the islands form small ducts lined by an eosinophilic cuticle. The islands may show a "tad-pole" or "comma-like" appearance.

Nodular Hidradenoma

CLINICAL SUMMARY. Nodular hidradenoma (66) is presently also called *clear cell hidradenoma* and *eccrine acrospiroma*, although apocrine features are seen in many of these neoplasms (67). It is a fairly common tumor without a preferred site. The tumors present as intradermal nodules in most instances between 0.5 and 2.0 cm in diameter, although they may be larger. They are usually covered by intact skin, but some tumors show superficial ulceration and discharge serous material. Although clinically the tumor only rarely gives the impression of being cystic, gross examination of the specimen often reveals cysts.

HISTOPATHOLOGY. The tumor is well circumscribed and may appear encapsulated. It is composed of lobulated masses located in the dermis and often extending into the subcutaneous fat, usually with no connection to the surface epidermis. The tumor nodules are frequently separated by a characteristic eosinophilic hyalinized stroma. Within the lobulated masses, tubular lumina of various sizes are often present. However, these may be absent or few in number. The tubular lumina may be branched or straight, and are lined by cuboidal ductal cells or by columnar secretory cells, which may show evidence of decapitation secretion (i.e., apocrine differentiation). There are often cystic spaces, which may be of considerable size and contain a faintly eosinophilic, homogeneous

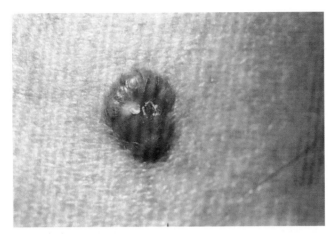

Clin. Fig. VIB4a.d

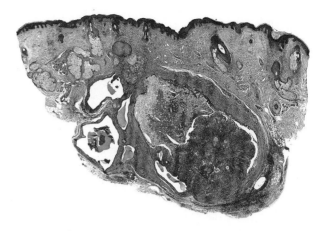

Fig. VIB4a.l

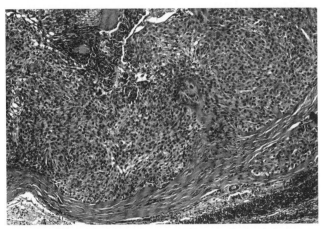

Fig. VIB4a.m

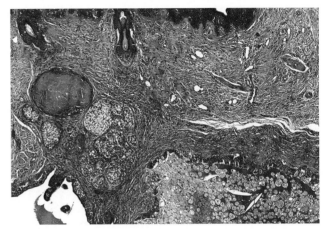

Fig. VIB4a.n

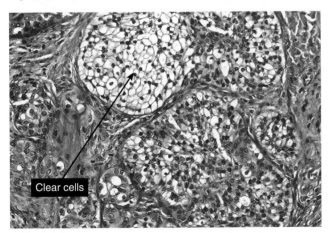

Clear cells

Fig. VIB4a.o

Clin. Fig. VIB4a.d. *Nodular hidradenoma.* A 55-year-old man presented with an asymptomatic 1 cm pink, telangiectatic slightly scaly nodule on the lateral forearm. The lower pole was pigmented.

Fig. VIB4a.l. *Nodular hidradenoma, low power.* Within the dermis, this neoplasm is composed of several well-circumscribed tumor lobules.

Fig. VIB4a.m. *Nodular hidradenoma, medium power.* These tumor aggregates are well circumscribed from the surrounding normal dermis and subcutaneous fat. The tumor islands may be surrounded by a thin fibrous capsule.

Fig. VIB4a.n. *Nodular hidradenoma, medium power.* Within the tumor islands there may be small or large, cystic spaces containing amorphous fluid. The spaces are lined by two rows of flattened epithelial cells.

Fig. VIB4a.o. *Nodular hidradenoma, high power.* The epithelial cells frequently show clear cell change with the small basophilic nucleus pushed to the side of the cell. The clear cell change is secondary to glycogen deposition and stains positively with PAS.

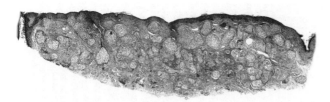

Fig. VIB4a.p

Fig. VIB4a.p. *Clear cell syringoma, low power.* Within the superficial dermis there are multiple small lobules of clear cells embedded in an eosinophilic sclerotic stroma.

Fig. VIB4a.q. *Clear cell syringoma, high power.* Similar to the nodular (clear cell) hidradenoma, these epithelial cells are clear because of the presence of glycogen. In the center of these islands one can identify small eccrine-type ducts lined by an eosinophilic cuticle.

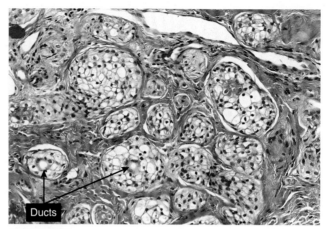

Fig. VIB4a.q

---

material. In solid portions of the tumor, two types of cells can be recognized in varying proportions, and with transitional forms. One type of cell is usually polyhedral or fusiform with a rounded nucleus and slightly basophilic cytoplasm. The second type of cell is usually round with very clear cytoplasm, so that the cell membrane is distinctly visible. Its nucleus appears small and dark. In some tumors, epidermoid differentiation is seen, with the cells appearing large and polyhedral and showing eosinophilic cytoplasm. There even may be keratinizing cells with formation of horn pearls or structures reminiscent of the follicular infundibulum, and there may also be sebaceous differentiation. In other tumors, groups of squamous cells

are arranged around small lumina that are lined with a well-defined eosinophilic cuticle and thus resemble the intraepidermal portion of the eccrine duct.

Clear Cell Syringoma

Clear cell change is occasionally seen in syringomas.

Mixed Tumor (Chondroid Syringoma)

Mixed tumor is a benign sweat gland tumor comprised of three components, namely epithelial, myoepithelial and chondroid elements, and is the cutaneous analog of pleomorphic adenoma of the salivary gland. This tumor

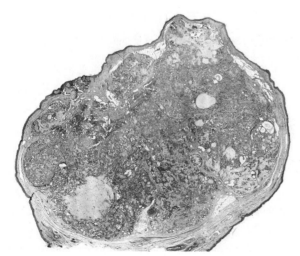

Fig. VIB4a.r

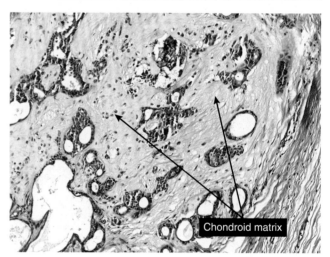

Fig. VIB4a.s

Fig. VIB4a.r. *Chondroid syringoma/hidradenoma, low power.* This nodular tumor shows multiple tiny epithelial islands embedded in a bluish, myxoid matrix.

Fig. VIB4a.s. *Chondroid syringoma/hidradenoma, medium power.* The small epithelial islands form small ductal lumina typical of eccrine differentiation. The bluish chondroid matrix resembles cartilage. In other areas, this lesion has features overlapping with nodular hidradenoma.

is most common in middle-aged men. The scalp and face are commonly involved and also external ear canal, eyelids, hands and arms, but rarely the trunk and genital regions. There are apocrine and less common eccrine variants (68).

Conditions to consider in the differential diagnosis:

> eccrine nevus
> papillary eccrine adenoma
> clear cell (nodular) hidradenoma (eccrine acrospiroma)
> syringoma
> chondroid syringoma
> eccrine spiradenoma

> cylindroma (some consider apocrine)
> eccrine syringofibroadenoma
> mucinous syringometaplasia

VIB4b Infiltrative, Asymmetrical Eccrine Tumors

Microcystic Adnexal Carcinoma

CLINICAL SUMMARY. Microcystic adnexal carcinoma (69), or sclerosing sweat duct carcinoma, may best be considered as a sclerosing variant of ductal eccrine carcinoma.

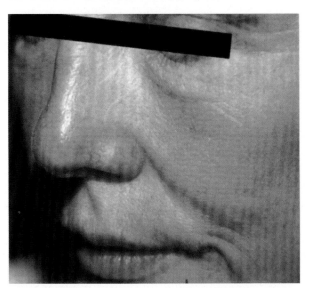

Clin. Fig. VIB4b.a

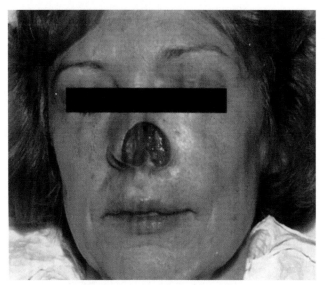

Clin. Fig. VIB4b.b

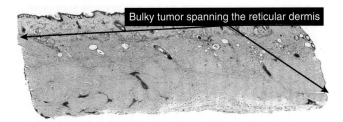

Bulky tumor spanning the reticular dermis

Fig. VIB4b.a

Clin. Fig. VIB4b.a. *Microcystic adnexal carcinoma.* A middle-aged woman developed a visually inconspicuous indurated swelling on the ala of the nose.

Clin. Fig. VIB4b.b. *Microcystic adnexal carcinoma.* Mohs micrographic surgery was used to delineate the extent and to excise the tumor, resulting in the large defect seen here.

Fig. VIB4b.a. *Microcystic adnexal carcinoma, low power.* In another case treated by surgical excision, a poorly circumscribed dermal tumor extends through the dermis to the base of the biopsy.

Fig. VIB4b.b. *Microcystic adnexal carcinoma, medium power.* Ducts and solid cords of cells are present in a desmoplastic stroma. (*continues*)

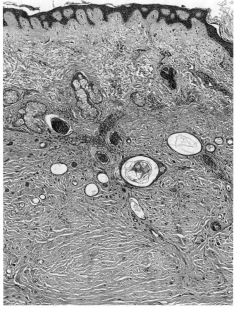

Fig. VIB4b.b

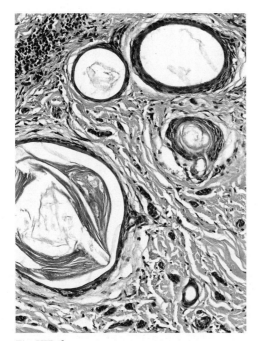

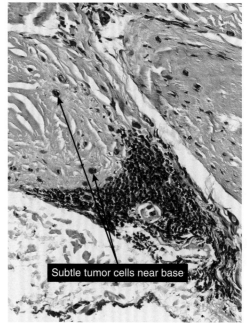

Subtle tumor cells near base

Fig. VIB4b.c

Fig. VIB4b.d

Fig. VIB4b.c. *Microcystic adnexal carcinoma, medium power.* Some of the ducts are lined by a single layer of cells; others may appear to have two layers.

Fig. VIB4b.d. *Microcystic adnexal carcinoma, high power.* Subtle lesional cells infiltrating to near the base of the tumor. Perineural invasion was not seen in this example.

This tumor, which is most commonly seen on the skin of the upper lip, but occasionally also on the chin, nasolabial fold, or cheek, is an aggressive neoplasm that invades deeply. Local recurrence is common; however, metastases have not been reported.

HISTOPATHOLOGY. Microcystic adnexal carcinoma is a poorly circumscribed dermal tumor that may extend into the subcutis and skeletal muscle. Continuity with the epidermis or follicular epithelium may be seen. Two components within a desmoplastic stroma may be evident. In some areas, basaloid keratinocytes are seen, some of which contain horn cysts and abortive hair follicles; in other areas, ducts and gland-like structures lined by a two-cell layer predominate. The tumor islands typically reduce in size as the tumor extends deeper into the dermis. Cells with clear cytoplasm may be present, and sebaceous differentiation has been reported. Cytologically, the cells are bland without significant atypia; mitoses are rare or absent. Perineural invasion may be seen, a feature that may account for the high recurrence rate. Lack of circumscription, deep dermal involvement, and perineural involvement all aid in diagnosis, since the cytology mimics benign adnexal neoplasms.

Mucinous Carcinoma (Mucinous Eccrine Carcinoma)

Mucinous carcinoma of the skin is a rare adnexal carcinoma identical to homologous lesions in the breast.

There are some tumors that are solid, with a minimal mucus component and express neuroendocrine markers that are considered by some to be a precursor entity and are diagnosed as endocrine mucin-producing sweat gland carcinoma. The lesions present as a solitary, slow-growing nodule or cyst-like lesion that is flesh colored, blue or erythematous. The prototypic presentation is of neoplastic cells arranged in nests, strands or as individual cells floating in lakes of extracellular mucin sometimes with thin fibrous septa. Mitoses are generally infrequent. The epithelial cells express low–molecular-weight cytokeratins, EMA, CEA, E-cadherin, and GCSDP15. Estrogen and progesterone receptors are expressed in most cases. The CK7+/CK20− phenotype is characteristic. Neuroendocrine differentiation can be encountered (70).

Digital Papillary Adenocarcinoma

CLINICAL SUMMARY. This is an uncommon tumor that arises from the sweat glands, and presents as cutaneous nodules, usually on the hands (85%) and feet (15%) (71,72). These tumors are more common in men in the fifth decade with an age range of 17 to 85 years. The clinical differential diagnosis includes glomus tumor, pyogenic granuloma, foreign-body granuloma and other tumors or tumor-like lesions. The diagnosis is based on the histologic findings.

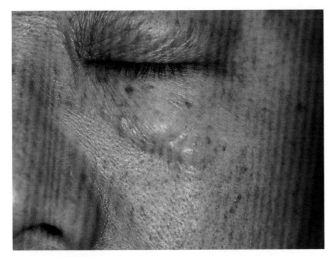

Clin. Fig. VIB4b.c

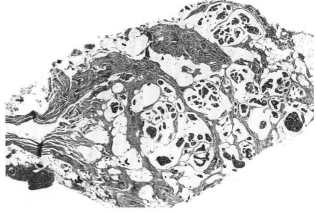

Fig. VIB4b.e

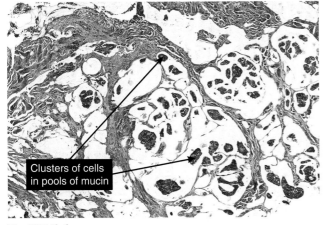

Clusters of cells in pools of mucin

Fig. VIB4b.f

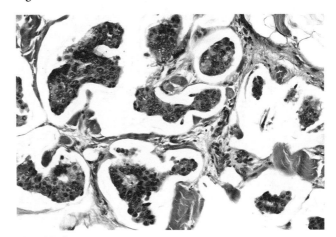

Fig. VIB4b.g

Clin. Fig. VIB4b.c. *Mucinous carcinoma.* A 60-year-old man had a multinodular, bluish tumor located on the cheek, which recurred 5 years after the first excision.

Fig. VIB4b.e. *Mucinous eccrine carcinoma, low power.* Within the deep dermis and subcutaneous fat there are basophilic islands of tumor cells embedded in a mucinous matrix. The islands are of various sizes. The overlying epidermis and superficial dermis are generally uninvolved.

Fig. VIB4b.f. *Mucinous eccrine carcinoma, medium power.* These basaloid islands appear to be floating in the abundant hypocellular mucinous matrix.

Fig. VIB4b.g. *Mucinous eccrine carcinoma, high power.* The epithelial islands are composed of crowded basaloid cells which focally show formation of small ducts. Cytologic atypia may be minimal.

HISTOPATHOLOGY. The epidermis may have tumor connections but is usually effaced and unaffected. In the dermis is a multilobular tumor composed of tubuloalveolar and ductal structures, cystic areas are also seen. Papillary projections can be seen in the cystic portions of the tumors. Cysts are thought to be formed secondary to tumor necrosis. The tumors may be poorly circumscribed and have a cribriform pattern. p63 may be a useful marker for distinguishing primary from metastatic adenocarcinomas, and in addition, the proliferation marker Ki67 may be an indicator of aggressive behavior and thus be helpful in therapeutic decision making (73).

The tumors are thought to be of eccrine origin although they may exhibit apocrine characteristics. Cytologic atypia is variable. Mitoses are present in almost all tumors with an average range of 0 to 50 per high-power field. The tumors stain positively with Cytokeratin, S100, CEA and EMA. The differential diagnosis includes digital papillary adenoma, metastatic carcinoma, and apocrine carcinoma.

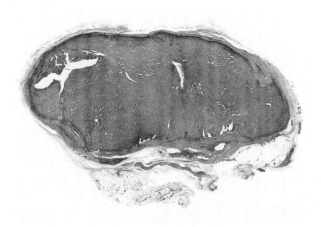

Fig. VIB4b.h

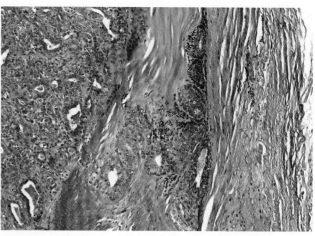

Fig. VIB4.i

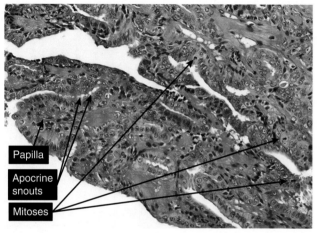

Papilla

Apocrine snouts

Mitoses

Fig. VIB4.j

Fig. VIB4b.h. *Digital papillary adenocarcinoma.* Multilobular tumor in dermis and subcutis.

Fig. VIB4.i. *Digital papillary adenocarcinoma.* Tubular structures and a focus of invasion of the tumor capsule but not the surrounding native tissue.

Fig. VIB4.j. *Digital papillary adenocarcinoma.* Papillary projections within the tumor; apocrine snouts and mitoses in the tumor cells.

Conditions to consider in the differential diagnosis:

   sclerosing sweat duct carcinoma
   microcystic adnexal carcinoma
   malignant chondroid syringoma
   malignant clear cell (nodular) hidradenoma
   malignant eccrine spiradenoma
   malignant eccrine poroma (porocarcinoma)
   eccrine adenocarcinoma
   mucinous eccrine carcinoma
   adenoid cystic eccrine carcinoma
   aggressive digital papillary adenoma/adenocarcinoma
   syringoid eccrine carcinoma

VIB5 Apocrine Tumors

Tumors in the dermis are composed of proliferations of apocrine ductal and glandular epithelium (large pink cells with decapitation secretion). The stroma is sclerotic, well vascularized and the inflammatory cells are mainly lymphocytes.

Tubular Apocrine Adenoma

CLINICAL SUMMARY. This tumor (74) consists of a well-defined nodule that is commonly located on the scalp. Most tumors have a smooth surface and are under 2 cm in diameter.

HISTOPATHOLOGY. The characteristic feature of this tumor is the presence of numerous irregularly shaped tubular structures that are usually lined by two layers of epithelial cells. The peripheral layer consists of cuboidal or flattened cells, and the luminal layer is composed of columnar cells. Some of the tubules have a dilated lumen with papillary projections extending into it. Decapitation secretion of the luminal cells is seen in many areas, and cellular fragments are seen in some lumina.

Syringocystadenoma Papilliferum

CLINICAL SUMMARY. Syringocystadenoma papilliferum (75) occurs most commonly on the scalp or the

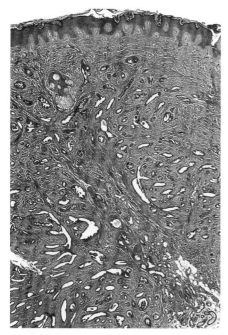

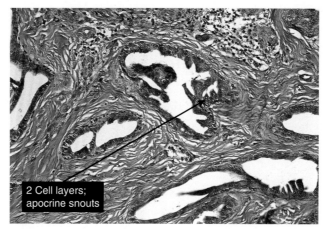

Fig. VIB5.a   **Fig. VIB5.b**

Fig. VIB5.a. *Tubular apocrine adenoma, low power.* Irregularly shaped tubules lined by two layers of cells extend through the reticular dermis.

Fig. VIB5.b. *Tubular apocrine adenoma, medium power.* The double layer of cells and the presence of decapitation secretion differentiate this lesion from a microcystic adnexal carcinoma. The absence of high-grade atypia helps to eliminate a metastatic adenocarcinoma.

face. It is usually first noted at birth or in early childhood and consists of either one papule or several papules in a linear arrangement, or of a solitary plaque. The lesion increases in size at puberty, becoming papillomatous and often crusted. On the scalp, syringocystadenoma papilliferum frequently arises around puberty within a nevus sebaceous that has been present since birth.

HISTOPATHOLOGY. The epidermis shows varying degrees of papillomatosis. One or several cystic invaginations extend downward from the epidermis, lined in their upper portions by squamous, keratinizing cells similar to those of the surface epidermis. In the lower portion of the cystic invaginations, numerous papillary projections extend into the lumina, lined by glandular epithelium often with two rows of cells. The luminal row of cells consists of high columnar cells with oval nuclei, faintly eosinophilic cytoplasm and, occasionally, active decapitation secretion. The outer row consists of small cuboidal cells with round nuclei and scanty cytoplasm. Beneath the cystic invaginations, deep in the dermis, one can often find groups of tubular glands with large lumina, lined by apocrine cells with evidence of active decapitation secretion. A helpful diagnostic feature is the almost invariable presence of a fairly dense cellular infiltrate composed nearly entirely of plasma cells in the stroma of this tumor,

especially in the papillary projections. In about one-third of the cases, syringocystadenoma papilliferum is associated with a nevus sebaceous.

Syringocystadenocarcinoma papilliferum is extremely rare and may present within a pre-existing lesion as *in situ* and/or invasive adenocarcinoma, or rarely squamous cell carcinoma. Ductal changes analogous to those in mammary carcinoma are often present and have suggested a transformation that may involve a pathway from usual ductal hyperplasia to atypical ductal hyperplasia to *in situ* to invasive adenocarcinoma (76).

Conditions to consider in the differential diagnosis:

Circumscribed, Symmetrical Apocrine Tumors
apocrine nevus
tubular apocrine adenoma ("tubulopapillary hidradenoma")
cylindroma (some consider eccrine)
hidradenoma papilliferum
syringocystadenoma papilliferum
apocrine hidrocystoma
Infiltrative, Asymmetrical Apocrine Tumors
apocrine adenocarcinoma
malignant cylindroma
erosive adenomatosis (florid papillomatosis of the nipple)

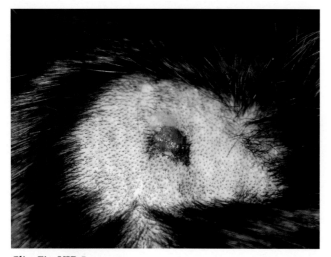

Clin. Fig. VIB.5

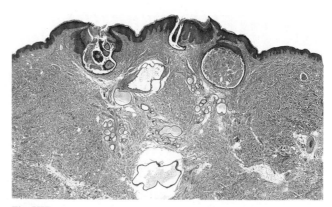

Fig. VIB5.c

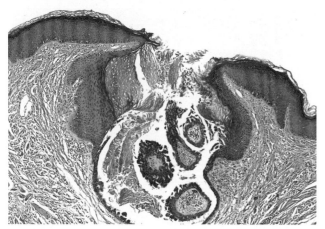

Fig. VIB5.d

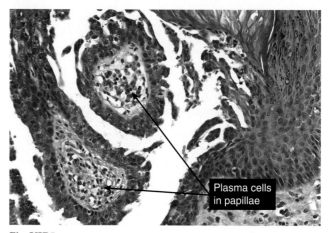

Plasma cells in papillae

Fig. VIB5.e

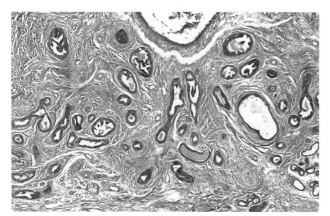

Fig. VIB5.f

Clin. Fig. VIB.5. *Syringocystadenoma papilliferum.* A 40-year-old woman had a long-standing nevus sebaceous lesion of the scalp since birth, which came to attention because of ulceration and bleeding that had started 5 years ago.

Fig. VIB5.c. *Syringocystadenoma papilliferum, low power.* There is an endophytic epithelial neoplasm which arises from the surface epidermis. There are numerous papillary projections into the cystic lumen.

Fig. VIB5.d. *Syringocystadenoma papilliferum, high power.* The papillary projections are lined by two layers of cells: luminal columnar cells which show decapitation secretion, and basilar cuboidal cells.

Fig. VIB5.e. *Syringocystadenoma papilliferum, high power.* The stroma contains numerous plasma cells.

Fig. VIB5.f. *Syringocystadenoma papilliferum, high power.* Glands at the base resemble apocrine adenoma.

VIB6 Pilar Tumors

The dermal infiltrating tumor is composed of epithelium that differentiates toward hair, or is a proliferation of portions of the follicular structure and its stroma. The inflammatory cell infiltrate is mainly lymphocytic, and the dermis is fibrocellular. Trichoepithelioma is prototypic (77).

Trichoepithelioma

CLINICAL SUMMARY. The differentiation in this tumor is directed toward hair structures. It occurs either in multiple lesions or as a solitary lesion. Multiple trichoepithelioma is transmitted as an autosomal dominant and may occur in association with the Brooke–Spiegler syndrome

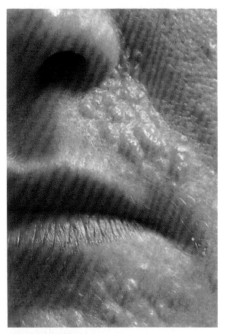

Clin. Fig. VIB.6

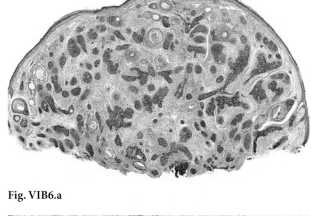

Fig. VIB6.a

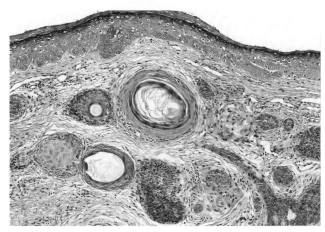

Fig. VIB6.b

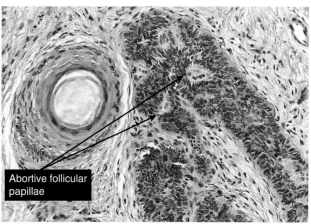

Abortive follicular papillae

Fig. VIB6.c

Clin. Fig. VIB.6. *Trichoepithelioma.* Since early childhood, a 22-year-old woman had developed firm flesh-colored discrete papules and nodules over the face around the nose and mouth.

Fig. VIB6.a. *Trichoepithelioma, low power.* At scanning magnification there is a dome-shaped epithelial neoplasm within the dermis. The epithelial islands do not connect to the overlying epidermis.

Fig. VIB6.b. *Trichoepithelioma, medium power.* These basaloid epithelial islands are associated with small cystic structures filled with laminated keratin.

Fig. VIB6.c. *Trichoepithelioma, medium power.* The epithelial islands show follicular differentiation mimicking the follicular bulb. The stroma is fibrotic and closely associated with these epithelial islands. Retraction artifact as one sees in basal cell carcinoma is absent in these lesions.

VI   Tumors and Cysts of the Dermis and Subcutis

and a CYLD mutation (49). Typically, the first lesions appear in childhood and gradually increase in number. There are numerous rounded, skin-colored, firm papules and nodules located mainly in the nasolabial folds but also elsewhere on the face, and occasionally also the scalp, neck, and upper trunk. Solitary trichoepithelioma is not inherited and consists of a firm, elevated, flesh-colored nodule usually less than 2 cm in diameter. Its onset usually is in childhood or early adult life, and it is commonly located in the anterior facial triangle.

HISTOPATHOLOGY. As a rule, the lesions of multiple trichoepithelioma are superficial, well circumscribed, small, and symmetrical. Horn cysts are the most characteristic histologic feature, present in most lesions. They consist of a fully keratinized center surrounded by basophilic cells that lack high-grade atypia and mitoses. The keratinization is abrupt and complete, in the manner of so-called "trichilemmal" keratinization, not gradual and incomplete as in the horn pearls of squamous cell carcinoma. As a second major component, tumor islands composed of basophilic cells are arranged in a lacelike or adenoid network and occasionally also as solid aggregates. These tumor islands show peripheral palisading of their cells and are surrounded by a fibroblastic stroma. This stroma lacks the retraction artifact typical of basal cell carcinoma, and frequently contains foci of granulomatous inflammation about fragments of keratin. The epithelial aggregates form invaginations, which contain numerous fibroblasts and thus resemble follicular papillae. *Solitary*

trichoepithelioma is used as a histologic designation only for highly differentiated lesions. Solitary lesions with relatively little differentiation toward hair structures are best classified as keratotic basal cell carcinoma. If a lesion is to qualify for the diagnosis of solitary trichoepithelioma, it should contain numerous horn cysts and abortive hair papillae. Mitotic figures should be very rare or absent, and the lesion should not be unduly large, asymmetrical, or infiltrative.

Desmoplastic Trichoepithelioma

CLINICAL SUMMARY. This tumor occurs most commonly as a morpheaform plaque, having slightly raised borders and a central depression (78). The tumors are typically located on the face, mainly on the cheeks, and rarely occur on other areas of the head and neck. It is seen most frequently in the second decade usually in women. The history is of slow progressive growth of many years duration.

HISTOPATHOLOGY. A dermal tumor composed of streams and cords of basaloid cells immersed in a dense fibrocellular stroma that compresses the tumor islands into thin delicate strands (79). Calcification and cystic keratinization occur on or within the basaloid tumor. Mitoses and cytologic atypia are uncommon. An inflammatory response is variable and is usually lymphatic. Tumors do not usually extend into the subcutis. Differential diagnoses include sclerosing basal cell carcinoma, microcystic adnexal carcinoma, trichoepithelioma, poroma, tumor of the follicular infundibulum, and syringomas (80).

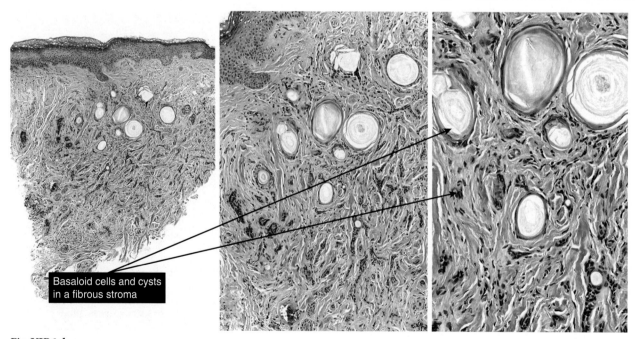

Basaloid cells and cysts in a fibrous stroma

Fig. VIB6.d

Fig. VIB6.d. *Desmoplastic trichoepithelioma.* Low, medium and high powers. Basaloid cells in a dense fibrocellular stroma, with cystic structures.

Dilated Pore of Winer

See Figs. VIB6.e,f.

Pilar Sheath Acanthoma

See Figs. VIB6.g,h.

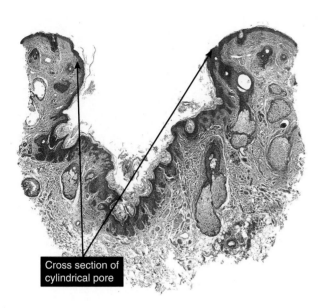

Fig. VIB6.e

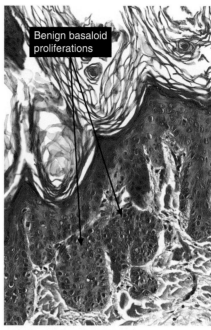

Fig. VIB6.f

Fig. VIB6.e. *Dilated pore of Winer, low power.* There is a sinus-like structure which originates from the surface epidermis. The center of the lesion may contain laminated keratin and there is a proliferative epithelial wall.

Fig. VIB6.f. *Dilated pore of Winer, medium power.* The epithelial wall shows a verrucous inner surface with elongation of rete ridges. There is infundibular keratinization with formation of a granular cell layer.

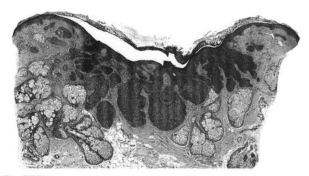

Fig. VIB6.g

Fig. VIB6.g. *Pilar sheath acanthoma, low power.* This lesion shows the architecture of an epithelial cyst as well as that of a dilated pore of Winer. There is an invagination of epithelium filled with keratin opening to the skin surface. The wall of the cystic structure is, however, quite proliferative.

Fig. VIB6.h. *Pilar sheath acanthoma, medium power.* The wall of the cystic structure is composed of a proliferation of basaloid and squamous cells which focally show follicular differentiation mimicking the outer root sheath portion of the hair follicle in this image.

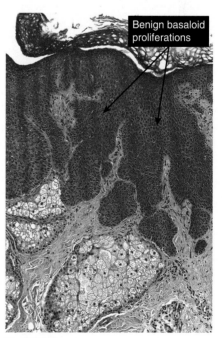

Fig. VIB6.h

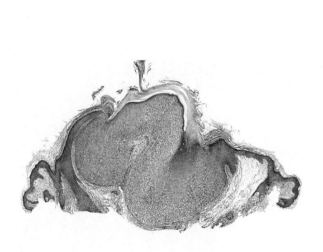

Fig. VIB6.i

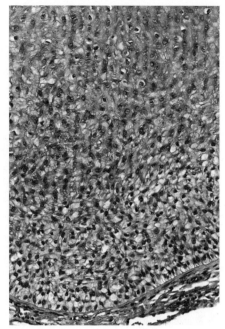

Fig. VIB6.j

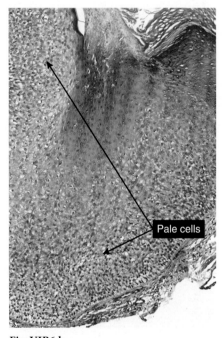

Pale cells

Fig. VIB6.k

Fig. VIB6.i. *Trichilemmoma, low power.* This epithelial neoplasm is well circumscribed and shows both an endophytic architecture as well as a verrucous and hyperkeratotic surface.

Fig. VIB6.j. *Trichilemmoma, medium power.* The endophytic lobule is composed of bland-appearing epithelial cells which may show clear cell change. At the periphery the basal cells show a palisaded architecture and there may be a thickened basement membrane. These lesions do not have a mucinous stroma, a feature which helps differentiate them from basal cell carcinomas.

Fig. VIB6.k. *Trichilemmoma, high power.* At the edge of this lesion the verrucous surface may show hypergranulosis.

Trichilemmoma

See Figs. VIB6.i–k.

Trichofolliculoma

See Figs. VIB6.l–n.

Fibrofolliculoma/Trichodiscoma

Fibrofolliculoma, and also trichodiscoma and possibly acrochordon may occur in association with the Birt–Hogg–Dubé syndrome which is a rare autosomal dominant genodermatosis that is caused by germline mutations in the folliculin (FLCN) gene, encoding the folliculin tumor-suppressor protein. Phenotypic manifestations related to this disease include lung cysts, leading to pneumothorax, and a markedly increased risk for renal neoplasia. Other neoplastic manifestations have been described including correlations between FLCN mutations and risk of colon or breast cancer (81).

Trichoadenoma

See Figs. VIB6.r,s.

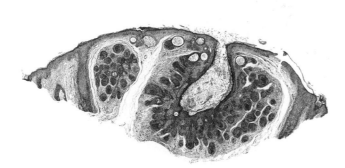

Fig. VIB6.l

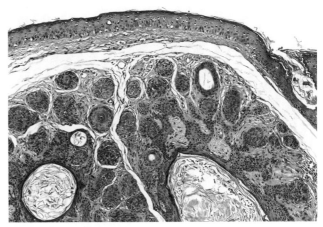

Fig. VIB6.m

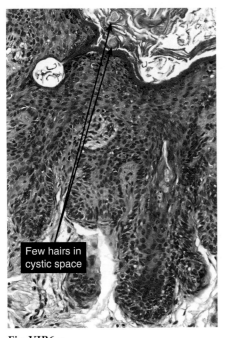

Few hairs in cystic space

Fig. VIB6.n

Fig. VIB6.l. *Trichofolliculoma, low power.* A central cystic structure is filled with keratin and is associated with a hyperplastic wall, from which secondary hairs extend into the stroma.

Fig. VIB6.m. *Trichofolliculoma, medium power.* The secondary hair follicles arise from the central cystic structure. Tertiary follicles may also be present, branching from the secondary follicles.

Fig. VIB6.n. *Trichofolliculoma, medium power.* The secondary follicles produce hair shafts seen within the cystic canal.

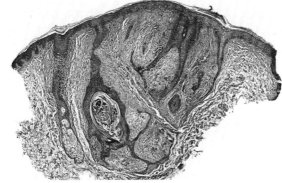

Fig. VIB6.o

Fig. VIB6.o. *Fibrofolliculoma/trichodiscoma, low power.* Note the fibrous stroma enveloping the epithelial proliferation which may include a cystic space and/or epithelial strands as here. (*continues*)

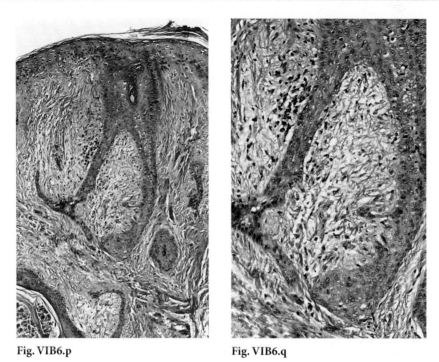

Fig. VIB6.p

Fig. VIB6.q

Fig. VIB6.p. *Fibrofolliculoma/trichodiscoma, medium power.* The thin, delicate strands of epithelium show follicular differentiation, which may in some cases include formation of sebaceous lobules.

Fig. VIB6.q. *Fibrofolliculoma/trichodiscoma, medium power.* The characteristic thin strands of epithelium ramifying in a fibrous stroma.

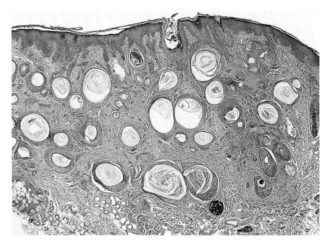

Fig. VIB6.r

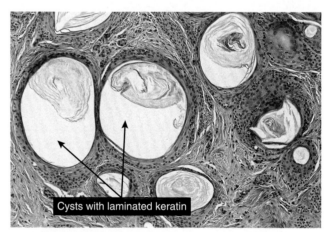

Cysts with laminated keratin

Fig. VIB6.s

Fig. VIB6.r. *Trichoadenoma, low power.* Within the upper two-thirds of the dermis is a well-circumscribed lesion composed of multiple cystic structures embedded in a fibrotic stroma.

Fig. VIB6.s. *Trichoadenoma, medium power.* The cystic structures are formed by mature squamous epithelium which shows infundibular differentiation. They contain laminated keratin. Although not shown here, they may be associated with a granulomatous infiltrate secondary to rupture of these cysts.

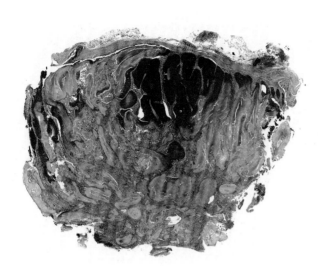

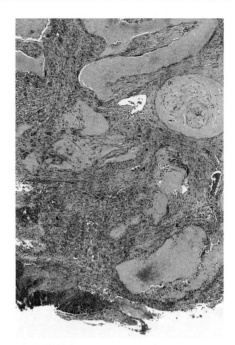

Fig. VIB6.t

Fig. VIB6.u

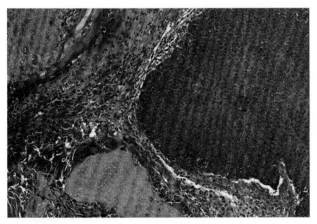

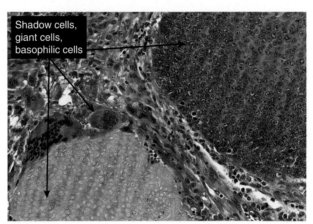

Shadow cells, giant cells, basophilic cells

Fig. VIB6.v

Fig. VIB6.w

Fig. VIB6.t. *Pilomatricoma, low power.* This well-circumscribed tumor shows both basophilic and eosinophilic elements.

Fig. VIB6.u. *Pilomatricoma, medium power.* The basophilic areas are composed of crowded areas of small basaloid cells which are in contiguity with the eosinophilic areas.

Fig. VIB6.v. *Pilomatricoma, high power.* The basaloid cells are small and crowded however they lack significant atypia. These cells blend with the eosinophilic shadow cells which show the ghost of an epithelial cell without viable basophilic staining.

Fig. VIB6.w. *Pilomatricoma, high power.* Adjacent to the shadow cells seen here are foreign body–type giant cells, a frequent finding in these lesions.

Pilomatricoma

See Figs. VIB6.t–w.

Trichoblastoma

CLINICAL SUMMARY. Trichoblastoma presents as a solitary nodule, rarely multiple, most commonly on the scalp and is often associated with nevus sebaceous of Jadassohn (82). The tumor does not have a distinctive enough clinical appearance that would allow for diagnosis without biopsy. Trichoblastomas occur on most body surfaces but not on non–hair-bearing sites such as the mucosa, palms and soles.

HISTOPATHOLOGY. A dermal tumor without epidermal connection composed of collections of basaloid cells

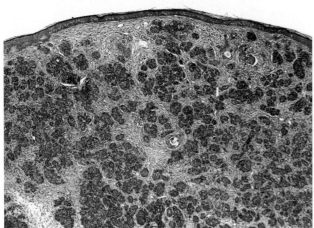

Fig. VIB6.x

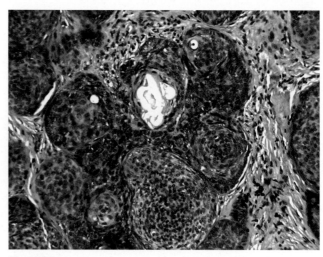

Fig. VIB6.y

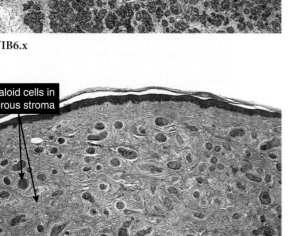

Basaloid cells in a fibrous stroma

Fig. VIB6.z

Fig. VIB6.x. *Trichoblastoma, medium power.* These lesions typically present as a vertically oriented tumor in the dermis, typically well circumscribed and often "shelling out" from the surrounding dermis.

Fig. VIB6.y. *Trichoblastoma, medium power.* This tumor is comprised of basaloid cells, but without the atypia, clefting artifact or specialized stroma of a basal cell carcinoma. Nevertheless, the distinction can sometimes be difficult.

Fig. VIB6.z. *Trichoblastic fibroma, medium power.* The tumor is embedded in a dense, typically well circumscribed, fibrous stroma.

that may nest (83). The tumor may extend into the subcutaneous tissue. When there is a mixture of fibrocellular stroma and epithelial islands the tumors have been designated "trichoblastic fibromas." When the epithelial component predominates, tumors are designated "trichoblastomas." This is an arbitrary distinction and probably not warranted in practice. In some tumors immature follicular structures are seen and these have been called the trichogenic trichoblastoma variety. There is no significant inflammatory response unless ulceration occurs.

Histologic variants include the so-called "rippled" pattern, in which there are basaloid cells in linear rows parallel to each other giving a rippled appearance, and the adamantoid, pigmented and clear cell patterns. Immunohistochemically, the tumors express cytokeratins 5/6, 14,7 and focally CK17 and CK19. The stromal cells are positive for vimentin and CD34. The differential diagnosis includes basal cell carcinoma, trichoepithelioma, poroma, acrospiroma, spiradenoma, and melanoacanthoma (84).

Conditions to consider in the differential diagnosis:

Follicular infundibular neoplasms
dilated pore of Winer
pilar sheath acanthoma
trichilemmoma
tumor of the follicular infundibulum
Branching and lobular pilosebaceous neoplasms
trichofolliculoma
trichoepithelioma
tumor of follicular infundibulum
top of nevus sebaceus
Nodular pilosebaceous neoplasms
hair follicle nevus
keratoacanthoma
trichoepithelioma
desmoplastic trichoepithelioma
immature trichoepithelioma
hair follicle hamartoma
pilomatricoma
trichoblastoma

trichoblastic fibroma
trichoadenoma
proliferating trichilemmal cyst (pilar tumor)
inverted follicular keratosis
Tumors of pilosebaceous mesenchyme
trichodiscoma
fibrofolliculoma
tumors of the erector pilae muscle
Infiltrative, asymmetrical tumors
pilomatrix carcinoma (malignant pilomatricoma)
trichilemmal carcinoma
basal cell carcinoma with follicular differentiation

VIB7 | Sebaceous Tumors

The dermal masses are proliferations of the germinative epithelium and of mature sebocytes. The admixture of these cells varies from one tumor to the other. The dermis is fibrocellular. Sebaceous adenomas, epitheliomas and carcinomas are the prototypes (85). These tumors are often seen in association with the Muir–Torre syndrome, which is a subset of the hereditary nonpolyposis colorectal carcinoma (HNPCC) syndrome, that is, an autosomal dominant cancer predisposition syndrome due to inheritance of a defective gene encoding a DNA mismatch repair protein. These proteins function to detect and repair errors in base pairing occurring during DNA replication, leading to genomic instability (86).

Sebaceous Adenoma and Sebaceous Epithelioma (Sebaceoma)

CLINICAL SUMMARY. Sebaceous adenoma presents as a yellow, circumscribed nodule located on either the face or

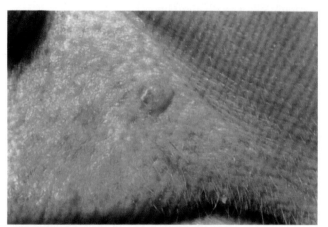

Clin. Fig. VIB7.a

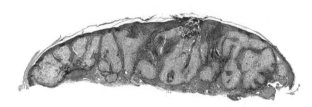

Fig. VIB7.a

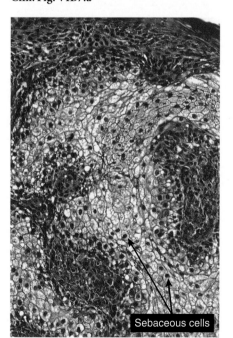
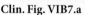

Fig. VIB7.b

Clin. Fig. VIB7.a. *Sebaceous adenoma.* A 67-year-old woman with bladder cancer and colon cancer and a history of keratoacanthoma and sebaceous adenoma (Muir–Torre syndrome) presented with an illdefined flesh-colored yellowish papule on the upper lip.

Fig. VIB7.a. *Sebaceous adenoma, low power.* Arising from the surface epidermis is a multilobated epithelial neoplasm with clear cell change.

Fig. VIB7.b. *Sebaceous adenoma, medium power.* The clear cell change represents sebaceous differentiation manifested by vacuolated cytoplasm which indents the central nucleus. These cells compose at least 50% of the lesion. The second population of cells is composed of an increased number of basaloid cells at the periphery of the lobules.

scalp. Sebaceous epithelioma, or sebaceoma, varies from a circumscribed nodule to that of an ill-defined plaque. Some of the lesions are yellow. Sebaceous epithelioma occasionally arises within a nevus sebaceus. Sebaceous epitheliomas and adenomas may also be found among the multiple sebaceous neoplasms that occur in association with multiple visceral carcinomas in the Muir–Torre syndrome.

HISTOPATHOLOGY. On histologic examination, sebaceous adenoma is sharply demarcated from the surrounding tissue. It is composed of incompletely differentiated sebaceous lobules that are irregular in size and shape. Two types of cells are present in the lobules. The first are undifferentiated basaloid cells identical to the cells at the periphery of normal sebaceous glands. The second are mature sebaceous cells. In most lobules, the two types of cells occur in approximately equal proportions, often arranged in such a way that groups of sebaceous cells are surrounded by basaloid cells. There may be foci of squamous epithelium with keratinization.

The histologic spectrum of sebaceous epithelioma (sebaceoma) extends from that in sebaceous adenoma to lesions that may be difficult to distinguish from sebaceous carcinoma. Generally, a sebaceoma shows irregularly shaped cell masses in which more than half of the cells are undifferentiated basaloid cells but in which there are significant aggregates of sebaceous cells and of transitional cells. Lesions verging on a sebaceous carcinoma show some degree of irregularity in the arrangement of the cell masses, and, although the majority of cells are basaloid cells, many cells show differentiation toward sebaceous cells. Sebaceous adenoma and sebaceous epithelioma lack nuclear atypia and invasive, asymmetric growth patterns, which are hallmarks of sebaceous carcinoma. Considerable mitotic activity in the basaloid regions may be present in either, however.

Sebaceous Hyperplasia

See Clin. Fig. VIB7.b and Figs. VIB7.c,d.

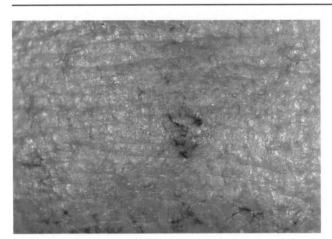

Clin. Fig. VIB7.b

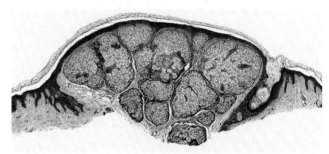

Fig. VIB7.c

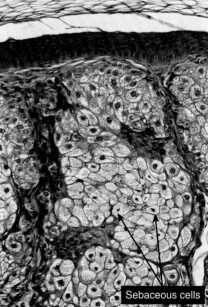

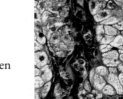

Clin. Fig. VIB7.b. *Sebaceous hyperplasia.* This yellowish, umbilicated papule is often mistaken for basal cell carcinoma.

Fig. VIB7.c. *Sebaceous hyperplasia, low power.* At scanning magnification there is an increased number of mature sebaceous lobules which are located superficially in the dermis, closer than normal to the overlying epidermis.

Fig. VIB7.d. *Sebaceous hyperplasia, medium power.* The sebaceous lobules are composed almost entirely of mature sebocytes with only a single row of undifferentiated basaloid cells at the periphery.

Fig. VIB7.d

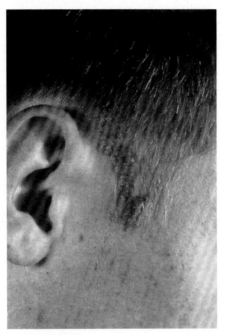

Clin. Fig. VIB7.c

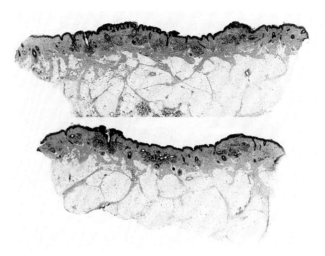

Fig. VIB7.e

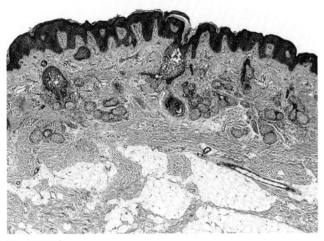

Fig. VIB7.f

Clin. Fig. VIB7.c. *Nevus sebaceus of Jadassohn.* A well-defined, yellow-brown verrucous plaque on the scalp that was present at birth.

Fig. VIB7.e. *Nevus sebaceus of Jadassohn, prepubertal, low power.* At scanning magnification there is an area in the center of this specimen which shows a decreased number of terminal hairs in the subcutaneous fat. This corresponds with the alopecia noted clinically.

Fig. VIB7.f. *Nevus sebaceus of Jadassohn, prepubertal, medium power.* In this area there are several abortive follicular structures in the superficial dermis which fail to produce a hair shaft. This nevus sebaceus is from a one-year-old child. In this age group, the lesions do not show the characteristic verrucous epidermal hyperplasia and large mature sebaceous lobules which show direct association with the overlying epidermis.

Nevus Sebaceus of Jadassohn

See Clin. Fig. VIB7.c and Figs. VIB7.e,f.

Sebaceous Epithelioma

See Figs. VIB7.g,h.

Sebaceous Carcinoma

CLINICAL SUMMARY. Carcinomas of the sebaceous glands occur most frequently on the eyelids, but they may occur elsewhere on the skin. The tumors usually manifest as a nodule that may or may not be ulcerated. Sebaceous carcinomas of the eyelids quite frequently cause death resulting from visceral metastases. Sebaceous carcinomas arising on the skin away from the eyelids may cause regional metastases, but visceral metastasis resulting in death is very rare. The histopathology of sebaceous tumors and their association with the Muir–Torre syndrome have been recently reviewed (68).

HISTOPATHOLOGY. The tumors are characterized at scanning magnification by asymmetry and an infiltrative border formed by irregular lobular formations that vary greatly in size and shape. Although many cells are undifferentiated, distinct sebaceous cells showing a foamy cytoplasm are present in the center of most lobules. Many cells are atypical, showing considerable variation in the shape and size of their nuclei. Some of the large lobules contain areas composed of atypical keratinizing cells, as seen in

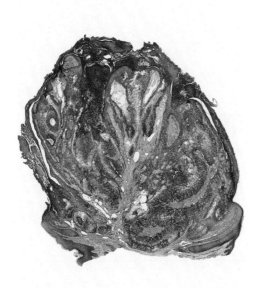

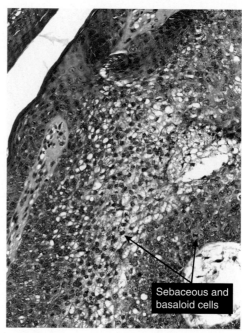

Fig. VIB7.g   **Fig. VIB7.h**

Fig. VIB7.g. *Sebaceous epithelioma/sebaceoma, low power.* There is a well-circumscribed neoplasm with a surface crust. At scanning magnification, it resembles a basal cell carcinoma but lacks the typical mucinous stroma with retraction artifact.

Fig. VIB7.h. *Sebaceous epithelioma/sebaceoma, medium power.* This lesion is composed of greater than 50% basaloid cells with a smaller population of mature sebaceous cells.

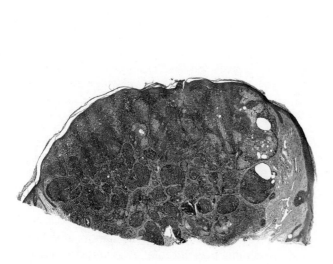

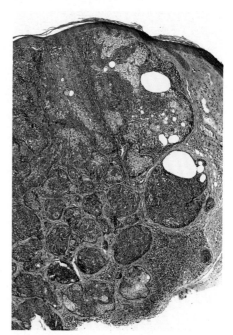

Fig. VIB7.i   **Fig. VIB7.j**

Fig. VIB7.i. *Sebaceous carcinoma, low power.* This lesion shows focal ulceration, an infiltrative growth pattern, and an associated inflammatory reaction. At this magnification it has many features which resemble an invasive squamous cell carcinoma.

Fig. VIB7.j. *Sebaceous carcinoma, medium power.* Although in some areas the lesion may resemble squamous cell carcinoma, the characteristic feature is focal sebaceous differentiation characterized by vacuolated cytoplasm which indents the central nucleus.

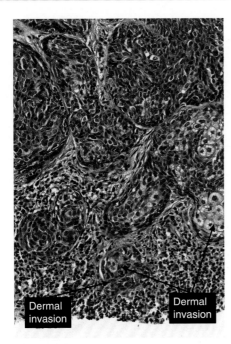

Fig. VIB7.k

Fig. VIB7.k. *Sebaceous carcinoma.* Stromal invasion by a cluster of basaloid cells with focal minimal sebaceous differentiation is seen at the base of this image. Other clusters are better differentiated.

squamous cell carcinoma. Sebaceous carcinomas of the eyelids often show pagetoid spread of malignant cells in the conjunctival or adjacent epithelium, a change that is seen very rarely in extraocular sebaceous carcinoma.

Conditions to consider in the differential diagnosis:

> **Symmetrical, Circumscribed Sebaceous Neoplasms**
> sebaceous hyperplasia
> Fordyce condition (ectopic sebaceous glands in mucosae)
> rhinophyma
> nevus sebaceus
> sebaceous adenoma
> sebaceous epithelioma
> sebaceous trichofolliculoma
> **Infiltrative, Asymmetrical Sebaceous Neoplasms**
> sebaceous carcinoma
> basal cell carcinoma with sebaceous differentiation

VIB8 | "Histiocytoid" and Miscellaneous Clear Cell Tumors

"Histiocytes" may have foamy cytoplasm reflecting the accumulation of lipids, or may have eosinophilic or amphophilic cytoplasm surrounding an ovoid nucleus with open chromatin. Some nonhistiocytic lesions whose cells may simulate histiocytes are also included here. There

is a great diversity of primary histiocytic dermatoses (87). The conditions may be divided into Langerhans histiocytosis, and non-Langerhans histiocytosis. The latter have been recently reviewed and include juvenile xanthogranuloma, multicentric reticulohistiocytosis (MRH), sea-blue histiocyte syndrome, sinus histiocytosis with massive lymphadenopathy, also known as Rosai–Dorfman syndrome, necrobiotic xanthogranuloma, xanthoma disseminatum (XD), and hemophagocytic lymphohistiocytosis, which although not formally malignant can all show aggressive behavior to a greater or lesser extent (88). Xanthelasma and juvenile xanthogranuloma are prototypic. Reticulohistiocytoma is an important differential (89).

Xanthomas and Xanthelasma

CLINICAL SUMMARY. Tuberous and tuberoeruptive xanthomas are found predominantly in patients with an increase in chylomicron and VLDL remnants. They are large nodes or plaques located most commonly on the elbows, knees, fingers, and buttocks. Most of the lipid in these xanthomas is in the form of cholesterol. Xanthelasmata consist of slightly raised, yellow, soft plaques on the eyelids. Although xanthelasmata are the commonest of the cutaneous xanthomas, they are also the least specific because they occur frequently in persons with normal lipoprotein levels. Plane xanthomas typically develop in skin folds and especially in the palmar creases. Diffuse plane xanthomas are typically seen as multiple grouped papules and poorly defined yellowish plaques in normolipemic patients, often with paraproteinemia, lymphoma, or leukemia.

HISTOPATHOLOGY. The histologic appearance of xanthomas of the skin and the tendons is characterized by foam cells, which are macrophages that have engulfed lipid droplets. There may be varying degrees of fibrosis, giant cells, and clefts, depending on the type and site of xanthoma sampled, but most are surprisingly similar. Most of these foam cells or "xanthoma cells" are mononuclear, but giant cells, especially of the Touton type with a wreath of nuclei, may be found. Larger extracellular deposits of cholesterol and other sterols leave behind clefts. Xanthelasmata located on the eyelids are characterized by the fairly superficial location of foam cells and the nearly complete absence of fibrosis. Superficial striated muscles, vellus hairs, small vessels, and a thinned epidermis all suggest location on the eyelid and serve as clues to the histologic diagnosis of xanthelasma.

Xanthelasma

See Clin. Fig. VIB8.a and Figs. VIB8.a,b.

Eruptive Xanthoma

See Clin. Fig. VIB8.b and Figs. VIB8.c–e.

Verruciform Xanthoma

See Figs. VIB8.f,g.

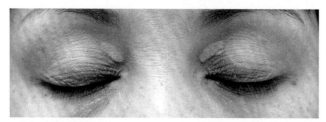

Clin. Fig. VIB8.a

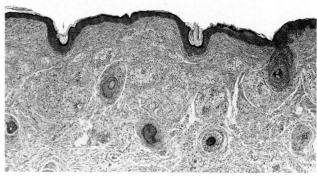

Fig. VIB8.a

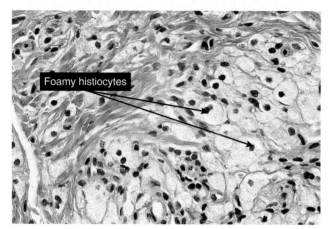

Fig. VIB8.b

Clin. Fig. VIB8.a. *Xanthelasma.* Strikingly yellow papular lesions of the eyelids in a 37-year-old woman with hyperlipidemia.

Fig. VIB8.a. *Xanthelasma, low power.* Throughout the dermis there are poorly defined aggregates of pale-staining cells.

Fig. VIB8.b. *Xanthelasma, high power.* These foam cells are seen throughout the dermis without an organized pattern. They have small nuclei and prominent vacuolated cytoplasm.

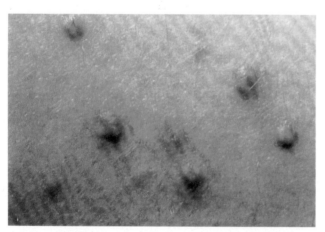

Clin. Fig. VIB8.b

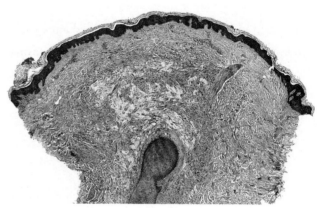

Fig. VIB8.c

Clin. Fig. VIB8.b. *Eruptive xanthomas.* Multiple yellow-red papules-nodules developed suddenly on the buttock skin of a 35-year-old woman. Testing revealed markedly elevated triglycerides.

Fig. VIB8.c. *Eruptive xanthoma, low power.* Within the mid dermis there is an inflammatory infiltrate associated with clear spaces forming clefts.

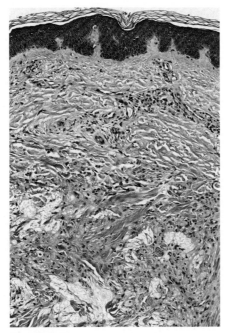

Fig. VIB8.d

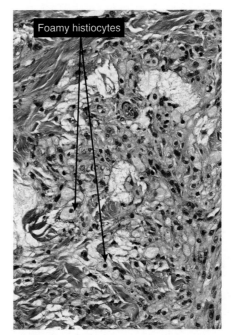

Foamy histiocytes

Fig. VIB8.e

Fig. VIB8.d. *Eruptive xanthoma, medium power.* These variably-sized clefts represent the lipid deposition. In the lower half of this photomicrograph is foam cells (macrophages).

Fig. VIB8.e. *Eruptive xanthoma, high power.* Multiple foamy histiocytes are found throughout the dermis. In eruptive xanthomas, neutrophils are often admixed with these histiocytes.

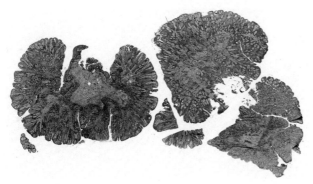

Fig. VIB8.f

Fig. VIB8.f. *Verruciform xanthoma, low power.* The epidermis shows prominent hyperplasia as well as hyperkeratosis. There is a mixed infiltrate in the papillary and superficial reticular dermis.

Fig. VIB8.g. *Verruciform xanthoma, high power.* Within the tips of the dermal papillae there are large histiocytes with an abundance of foamy cytoplasm.

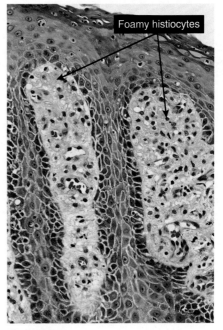

Foamy histiocytes

Fig. VIB8.g

Juvenile Xanthogranuloma (JXG)

CLINICAL SUMMARY. JXG (90) is a benign disorder in which one, several, or occasionally numerous red to yellow nodules are present. Despite the name, the lesions are also seen in adults but are most common in young children. In children the lesions may grow rapidly but almost always regress within a year. Lesions in adults are not uncommon but are usually solitary and persistent. JXG has also been identified in many other organ systems,

usually in association with macronodular lesions. A number of systemic complications are associated with JXG. Ocular involvement including glaucoma and bleeding into the anterior chamber is the most common, and bone involvement may occur.

HISTOPATHOLOGY. The typical JXG contains histiocytes with a variety of cellular features. Early lesions may show large accumulations of histiocytes without any lipid infiltration intermingled with only a few lymphoid cells

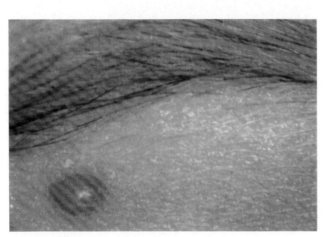

Clin. Fig. VIB8.c

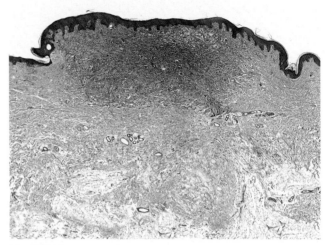

Fig. VIB8.h

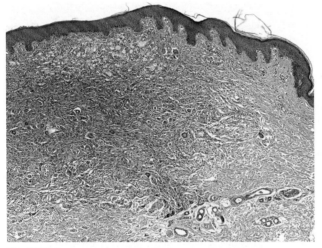

Fig. VIB8.i

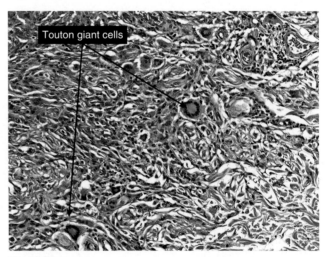

Fig. VIB8.j

Clin. Fig. VIB8.c. *Juvenile xanthogranuloma.* A 10-year-old girl developed several discrete red to yellow nodules and papules on the face and trunk, which later resolved spontaneously.

Fig. VIB8.h. *Juvenile xanthogranuloma, low power.* In a xanthogranuloma there is a dense infiltrate forming a solid mass occupying nearly the entire thickness of the dermis.

Fig. VIB8.i. *Juvenile xanthogranuloma, medium power.* There is a dense mixed infiltrate composed predominantly of histiocytes. There may be few or multiple multinucleated giant cells. Eosinophils and neutrophils are frequently seen, especially in early lesions.

Fig. VIB8.j. *Juvenile xanthogranuloma, high power.* Characteristic Touton giant cells show a wreath of nuclei surrounded by a peripheral rim of cytoplasm which is often vacuolated.

and eosinophils. When no foam cells or giant cells are seen, the possibility of JXG is often overlooked. Usually some degree of lipidization is present, even in very early lesions, manifested by pale-staining histiocytes. In mature lesions, a granulomatous infiltrate is usually present containing foam cells, foreign-body giant cells, and Touton giant cells as well as histiocytes, lymphocytes, and eosinophils. Older, regressing lesions show proliferation of fibroblasts and fibrosis replacing part of the infiltrate. The oncocytic or reticulohistiocytic type of histiocyte with an eosinophilic cytoplasm is uncommon in childhood lesions but may be seen in adult lesions. The spindle cell variant is also more common in adults. Here one sees predominantly a spindle cell proliferation, similar to blue nevus or dermatofibroma, with few foamy or giant cells.

Reticulohistiocytosis

CLINICAL SUMMARY. Two types of reticulohistiocytosis (91) are recognized: giant cell reticulohistiocytoma (GCRH) and multicentric reticulohistiocytosis (MRH). Both types occur almost exclusively in adults. The histologic picture is very similar in the two types. In GCRH there is usually a single nodule "solitary reticulohistiocytoma," but occasionally multiple lesions are seen, most commonly on the head and neck. The nodules are smooth and 0.5 to 2.0 cm in diameter. They may involute spontaneously. Even patients with multiple lesions show no sign of systemic involvement.

In MRH, the patients tend to be middle-aged females, with widespread cutaneous involvement and a destructive arthritis. Nodules ranging in size from a few millimeters to several centimeters are most common on the extremities. The polyarthritis may be mild or severe, and may be mutilating, especially on the hands, through destruction of articular cartilage and subarticular bone. The disease tends to wax and wane over many years, with mutilating arthritis and disfigurement being real possibilities.

HISTOPATHOLOGY. The characteristic histologic feature in both GCRH and MRH is the presence of numerous multinucleate giant cells and oncocytic histiocytes showing abundant eosinophilic, finely granular cytoplasm, often with a "ground glass" appearance. In older lesions giant cells and fibrosis are more common. There may be subtle differences between the two lesions. For example, in MRH the giant cells are smaller (50–100 mm), have fewer nuclei (perhaps 10), and are almost always strikingly PAS-positive. However, the two conditions often cannot be separated microscopically. The polyarthritis present in nearly all instances of MRH is caused by the same type of infiltrate as found in the cutaneous lesions, and similar infiltrates of uncertain clinical significance have been described in other organs.

Metastatic Renal Cell Carcinoma

Metastatic renal cell carcinoma, which can mimic a histiocytic infiltrate or a sweat gland tumor, should always be considered when there is a proliferation of clear cells in the skin. Cytologic atypia and mitotic activity may be deceptively minimal.

Conditions to consider in the differential diagnosis:

Foamy Histiocytes
Xanthomas—eruptive, plane, tuberous, tendon verruciform xanthoma

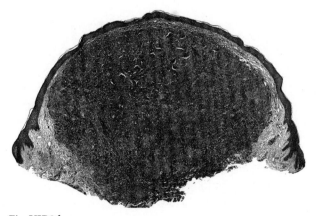

Fig. VIB8.k

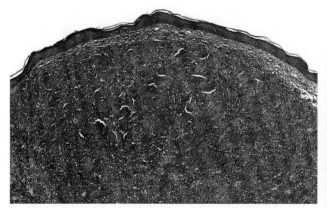

Fig. VIB8.l

Fig. VIB8.k. *Reticulohistiocytoma, low power.* At this magnification the lesion resembles a xanthogranuloma with a dense nodular infiltrate in the dermis; the overlying epidermis shows an effaced architecture.

Fig. VIB8.l. *Reticulohistiocytoma, medium power.* This dense infiltrate is mixed but there are scattered giant cells whose cytoplasm show an eosinophilic "ground glass" appearance. They may show a ring of nuclei but they lack the foamy cytoplasm typical of a Touton giant cell. (*continues*)

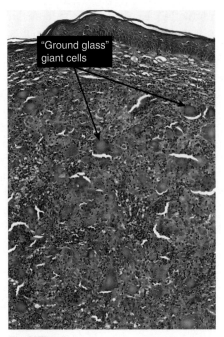

Fig. VIB8.m

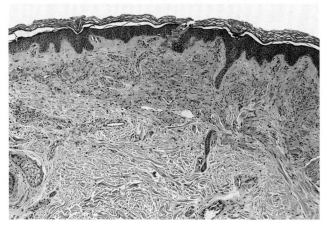

Fig. VIB8.n

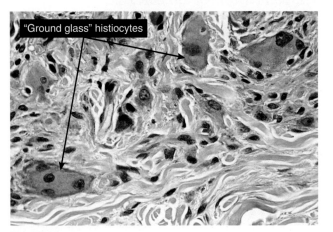

Fig. VIB8.o

Fig. VIB8.m. *Reticulohistiocytoma, high power.* The infiltrate is mixed with numerous histiocytes as well as lymphocytes and eosinophils. One giant cell seen here shows an eosinophilic cytoplasm without a vacuolated periphery.

Fig. VIB8.n. *Multicentric reticulohistiocytosis, low power.* In the upper third of the reticular dermis there are poorly defined cellular aggregates.

Fig. VIB8.o. *Multicentric reticulohistiocytosis, high power.* This infiltrate is mixed but contains large giant cells with one or more nuclei and eosinophilic "ground glass" cytoplasm.

xanthelasma
cholestanolemia, phytosterolemia
xanthoma disseminatum
diffuse normolipemic plane xanthoma
papular xanthoma
eruptive normolipemic xanthoma
progressive nodular histiocytoma (superficial)
Langerhans cell histiocytosis (rare xanthomatous
    type)
histoid leprosy
Non-Foamy Histiocytes
dermatofibroma/histiocytoma
Langerhans cell histiocytosis
congenital self-healing reticulohistiocytosis
indeterminate cell histiocytosis
granuloma annulare

eruptive histiocytomas
benign cephalic histiocytosis
sinus histiocytosis with massive lymphadenopathy
juvenile xanthogranuloma
Giant Cells Prominent
juvenile xanthogranuloma
multicentric reticulohistiocytosis
solitary reticulohistiocytoma
giant cell reticulohistiocytoma
necrobiotic xanthogranuloma with paraproteinemia
xanthoma disseminatum
Histiocytic Simulants
pleomorphic large cell lymphoma (Ki-1, usually T-cells)
epithelioid sarcoma
leukemia cutis
metastatic renal cell carcinoma

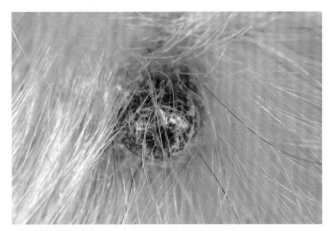

Clin. Fig. VIB8.d

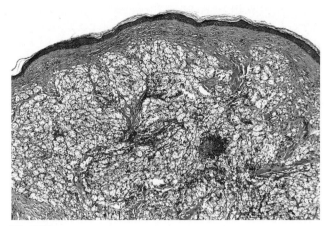

Fig. VIB8.p

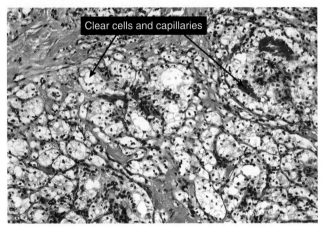

Clear cells and capillaries

Fig. VIB8.q

Clin. Fig. VIB8.d. *Metastatic renal cell carcinoma to the scalp.* Because of prominent blood supply, nodules have a characteristic hemorrhagic component, mimicking a pyogenic granuloma.

Fig. VIB8.p. *Metastatic renal cell carcinoma, low power.* In the dermis is a nonencapsulated tumor composed of clear cells with an increased number of small vascular channels. The clear cell type may suggest an adnexal tumor such as a nodular ("clear cell") hidradenoma.

Fig. VIB8.q. *Metastatic renal cell carcinoma, high power.* The individual cells contain an abundance of clear cytoplasm. The nuclei are small and bland in appearance. There is an increased number of small blood vessels with associated hemorrhage.

VIB9 Tumors of Large Hematolymphoid Cells

Large lymphoid cells may be mistaken for carcinoma or melanoma cells, but may be distinguished morphologically by their tendency to less cohesive growth in large sheets, by the absence of epithelial or melanocytic differentiation, and by immunopathology. Anaplastic large cell lymphoma is prototypic (92). Lymphomatoid papulosis (93) and leukemia cutis are important differentials.

Cutaneous CD30+ (Ki-1+) Anaplastic Large Cell Lymphoma (ALCL)

CLINICAL SUMMARY. The entity historically described as "Ki-1+ lymphoma" was first recognized as a neoplasm manifested as cutaneous nodules composed of lymphocytes with large, strikingly atypical nuclei. The neoplastic cells, usually of T-cell lineage, by definition expressed the Ki-1 (now known as CD30) antigen. The CD30 antigen is an inducible marker of lymphocyte activation that can be identified on either B or T cells. CD30 expression can also be observed in tumor stage MF, some pleomorphic T-cell

lymphomas, and some nonneoplastic eruptions including lymphomatoid papulosis (see below). CD30+ ALCL lesions typically present as a single or a few large nodules or tumors located on the extremities, and ulceration and crusting are common. The lymphoma can present at any age. Patients with cutaneous ALCL do not usually develop systemic symptoms, in contrast to patients with nodal involvement at presentation. CD30+ ALCL appears to be the most common cutaneous lymphoma in patients with HIV. In contrast to immunocompetent individuals, HIV-seropositive patients with CD30+ ALCL have a dismal prognosis (94).

HISTOPATHOLOGY. It is now established that CD30+ lymphoproliferative disorders do not constitute a single entity but comprise a spectrum of disorders linked by the presence of a common neoplastic cell type. The spectrum includes CD30+ ALCL and lymphomatoid papulosis (LyP). CD30+ ALCL is characterized by a nodular dermal and subcutaneous infiltrate of large lymphocytes with abundant, faintly basophilic cytoplasm; large, irregularly shaped vesicular nuclei with coarsely clumped chromatin along nuclear membranes; and large, irregularly shaped nucleoli. Wreath-shaped multinucleated cells are often present, as are "embryo"-shaped nuclei. Sarcomatoid (spindled) cellular morphology is encountered in rare cases. Epidermal hyperplasia or ulceration and an inflammatory infiltrate rich in neutrophils are commonly observed. The neoplastic cells have an activated CD4+ T-cell phenotype (occasionally CD8 +), with variable loss of CD2, CD5, CD7 and CD3, and frequent expression of cytotoxic molecules including granzyme B, TIA1, and perforin. CD30 is by definition expressed by greater than 75% of the neoplastic cells. Most cutaneous ALCL do not express EMA or ALK, in contrast to systemic ALCL. CD15 is expressed in about 40% of cases and staining for IRF (MUM1) is almost always positive (94). Because of the abundant cytoplasm and the compact arrangement of the lesional cells, some examples may simulate a carcinoma

or a sarcoma. Conversely, CD30 can be expressed by a variety of carcinomas, including embryonal carcinoma. Lesions of LyP are usually separable histologically in that atypical lymphocytes are arrayed in small numbers or in small clusters rather than sheets, within a heterogeneous infiltrate in which neutrophils and/or eosinophils are usually conspicuous.

Lymphomatoid Papulosis

CLINICAL SUMMARY. The atypical cells of lymphomatoid papulosis (49) (LyP) and ALCL share similar cellular morphology, CD30 expression, and clonal rearrangement of the T-cell receptor gene. Thus, a strong case can be made that these conditions comprise a disease spectrum. Within this spectrum, the overall number of clinical

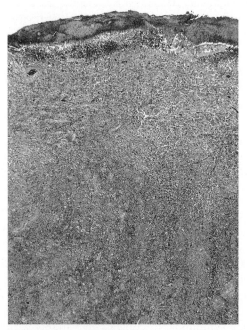

Fig. VIB9.a

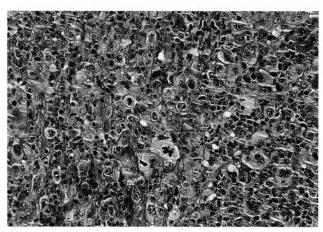

Fig. VIB9.b

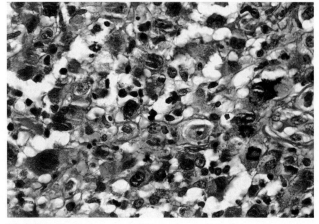

Fig. VIB9.c

Fig. VIB9.a. *Cutaneous anaplastic large cell lymphoma, low power.* This relatively large tumor is composed of a dense infiltrate occupying the entire dermis. There is associated ulceration of the overlying epidermis.

Fig. VIB9.b. *Large cell anaplastic lymphoma, medium power.* There are dense sheets of atypical cells admixed with inflammatory cells, frequently eosinophils. A number of the atypical cells show more than one nucleus.

Fig. VIB9.c. *Large cell anaplastic lymphoma, high power.* Many of the cells are large with large hyperchromatic nuclei; bizarre forms and mitotic figures are frequently seen.

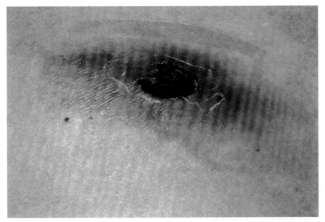

Clin. Fig. VIB9.a

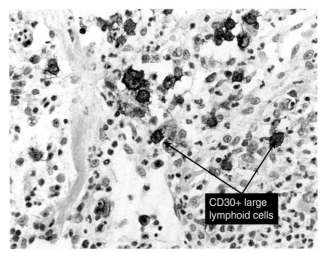

Fig. VIB9.d

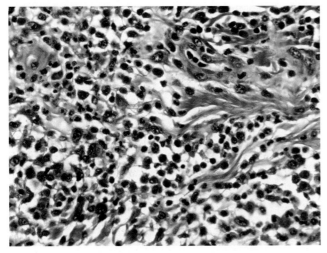

Fig. VIB9.e

CD30+ large
lymphoid cells

Fig. VIB9.f

Clin. Fig. VIB9.a. *Lymphomatoid papulosis.* Indurated erythematous nodules, some with ulcerated centers, developed on a recurrent basis in this elderly man.

Fig. VIB9.d. *Lymphomatoid papulosis, low power.* Scanning magnification reveals a dense cellular infiltrate extending well into the reticular dermis.

Fig. VIB9.e. *Lymphomatoid papulosis, medium power.* There is a mixture of large and small lymphoid cells, and neutrophils.

Fig. VIB9.f. *Lymphomatoid papulosis, high power, CD30 immunoperoxidase stain.* The scattered large atypical cells in lymphomatoid papulosis stain positive with an antibody to CD30. In contrast to anaplastic large cell lymphoma these cells do not form large sheets or nodular clusters.

lesions is roughly inversely proportional to the durability of the lesions. Thus, lesions of LyP tend to be numerous, short-lived, and recurrent in most instances, whereas ALCL lesions tend to be few in number and persistent.

HISTOPATHOLOGY. Lesions of LyP are usually separable histologically from cutaneous anaplastic large cell lymphoma in that atypical lymphocytes are arrayed in small numbers or in small clusters rather than sheets, within a heterogeneous infiltrate in which neutrophils and/or eosinophils are usually conspicuous. The epidermis can

show a variety of patterns in LyP biopsies, including infiltration by small- to medium-sized convoluted lymphocytes, an interface reaction with necrotic keratinocytes, or necrosis and ulceration.

Leukemia Cutis

CLINICAL SUMMARY. Leukemias are neoplasms of hematolymphoid cells that usually present with prominent involvement of the peripheral blood. They can be broadly grouped into acute and chronic forms of either lymphoid or myeloid lineage. Cutaneous leukemic infiltrates present as macules, papules, plaques, nodules, and ulcers. Lesions can be erythematous or purpuric. Extramedullary deposits of acute myelogenous leukemia (AML) are commonly referred to as granulocytic or myeloid sarcomas or chloromas. In addition to these specific infiltrates of leukemia, there are various inflammatory skin diseases that occur in conjunction with leukemia, sometimes referred to as leukemids. These disorders include leukocytoclastic vasculitis, pyoderma gangrenosum, Sweet syndrome, urticaria, erythroderma, erythema nodosum, and erythema multiforme.

HISTOPATHOLOGY. The most common pattern of skin involvement consists of an interstitial (reticular) infiltrate marked by diffuse permeation of the reticular dermis by leukemic cells in horizontal strands between collagen bundles. Nodular infiltrates of leukemic cells can also occur. Dense, bandlike infiltrates in the superficial dermis and sparse superficial and deep perivascular infiltrates are occasionally observed.

AML can assume either an interstitial or a nodular pattern. The epidermis is spared, but the subcutis is often involved. The diagnosis hinges in large part on the recognition of myeloblasts, which have scant cytoplasm, large vesicular nuclei, and nucleoli of variable size. Eosinophilic myelocytes or metamyelocytes are not pathognomonic of AML, but strongly favor that diagnosis in the proper context. These immature cells have the granules of mature eosinophils with monolobed nuclei. Cutaneous infiltrates of chronic myeloid leukemia (CML) are less common than those of AML. Similar diffuse or nodular patterns occur. The infiltrates contain a range of myelocytic differentiation from myeloblasts to segmented neutrophils. Acute lymphocytic (lymphoblastic) leukemia (ALL) shares features with lymphoblastic lymphoma, presenting typically as diffuse or nodular monomorphous infiltrates of lymphoblasts, cells with scant cytoplasm and round nuclei that are slightly to moderately convoluted with thin but well-defined nuclear membranes and finely dispersed chromatin. Histochemical and immunophenotypic studies can help in the identification of leukemic infiltrates. As recently summarized, a minimal panel of immunohistochemical markers should include anti-CD43 or antilysozyme as sensitive markers of myeloid sarcoma. Use of more specific markers of myeloid disease, such as CD33, myeloperoxidase, CD34 and CD117 is necessary to establish the diagnosis. Other antibodies may be added depending on the differential diagnosis; the choice of these can be guided by flow cytometry if this has been done. Identification of acute myeloid leukemia-associated genetic lesions may also be helpful in arriving at the correct diagnosis (95).

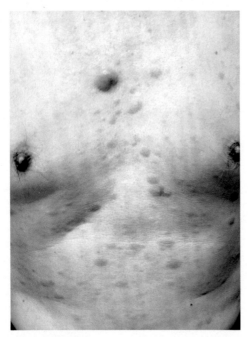

Clin. Fig. VIB9.b

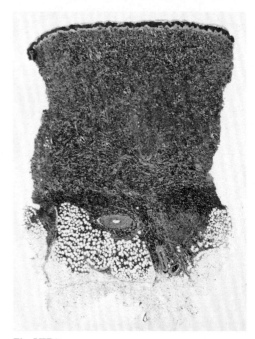

Fig. VIB9.g

Clin. Fig. VIB9.b. *Leukemia cutis.* A 66-year-old man first presented with multiple nodules in the skin, and bone marrow biopsy revealed acute myeloid leukemia.

Fig. VIB9.g. *Leukemia cutis, acute myelogenous leukemia, low power.* There is a dense infiltrate occupying the entire dermis extending into the subcutaneous fat. At this magnification, the predominant differential diagnosis is lymphoma cutis.

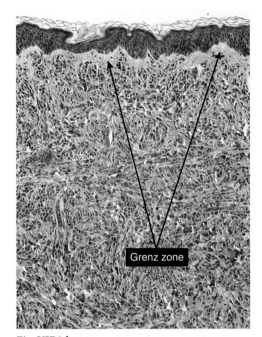

Fig. VIB9.h

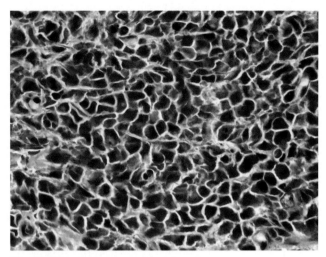

Fig. VIB9.i

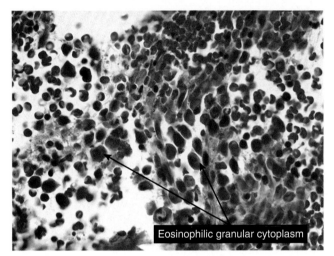

Fig. VIB9.j

Fig. VIB9.h. *Leukemia cutis, acute myelogenous leukemia, medium power.* This dense infiltrate is separated from the overlying normal-appearing epidermis forming a "grenz zone." The cells show an infiltrative pattern in between collagen bundles without organization.

Fig. VIB9.i. *Leukemia cutis, acute myelogenous leukemia, high power.* The infiltrate is composed entirely of atypical cells with hyperchromatic nuclei and eosinophilic cytoplasm; the cells are monotonous indicating a clonal process.

Fig. VIB9.j. *Acute myelogenous leukemia, high power.* Eosinophilic cytoplasm and indented nuclei can be seen in this image.

Conditions to consider in the differential diagnosis:

pleomorphic peripheral T-cell lymphoma
cutaneous anaplastic large cell lymphoma (CD30 (Ki-1) lymphoma (regressing atypical histiocytosis)
leukemia cutis
cutaneous Hodgkin disease

Primary Cutaneous Diffuse Large B-Cell Lymphoma, Leg Type

CLINICAL SUMMARY. Primary cutaneous diffuse large B-cell lymphoma leg type (PCLBCL-LT) is a large B-cell lymphoma comprised exclusively of centroblasts and immunoblasts, most commonly arising in leg. This tumor account for 4% of all primary cutaneous lymphomas, and most frequently occurs in elderly women. The lesions present as often rapidly growing tumors on one or both legs; 10% to 15% of cases occur at other sites. Extracutaneous spread is common. The historical 5-year survival of approximately 50% has been improved by combination of rituximab and multiagent chemotherapy regimens.

HISTOPATHOLOGY. PCLBCL-LT presents as a monotonous diffuse nonepidermotropic infiltrate of confluent sheets of centroblasts and immunoblasts. There are frequent mitoses. The neoplastic B cells express monotypic immunoglobulin, CD20 and CD79a. Unlike primary cutaneous follicle center lymphomas, these tumors strongly express Bcl2, IRF4, (MUM1), FOXP1, MYC, and

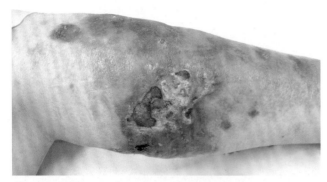

Clin. Fig. VIB9.c

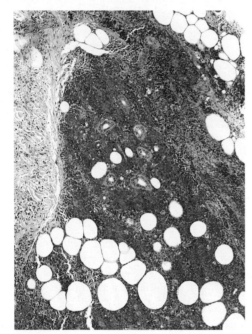

Fig. VIB9.l

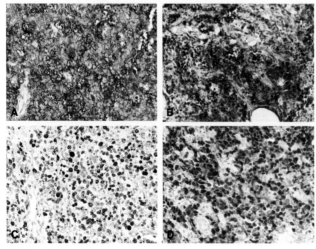

Fig. VIB9.n

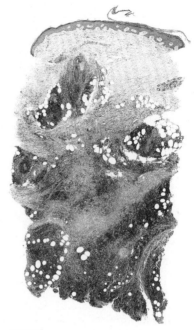

Fig. VIB9.k

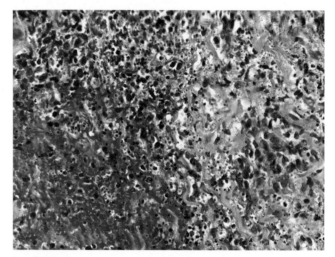

Fig. VIB9.m

Clin. Fig. VIB9.c. *Primary cutaneous diffuse large B-cell Lymphoma, leg type.* A 74-year-old woman had a large complex ulcerated tumor which was comprised of large B cells that were MUM-1 positive.

Fig. VIB9.k. *Primary cutaneous diffuse large B-cell lymphoma, leg type, low power.* A highly cellular tumor located in the dermis and subcutis. (D. Frank.)

Fig. VIB9.l. *Primary cutaneous diffuse large B-cell lymphoma, leg type, medium power.* The tumor cells infiltrate and subcutaneous fat, and around skin appendages. (D. Frank.)

Fig. VIB9.m. *Primary cutaneous diffuse large B-cell lymphoma, leg type, high power.* The cells have large moderately irregular nuclei, and prominent nucleoli. There is necrosis and hemorrhage. (D. Frank.)

Fig. VIB9.n. *Primary cutaneous diffuse large B-cell lymphoma, leg type.* Strong cytoplasmic staining for CD20 (A) and BCL2 (B), and strong nuclear staining for Ki-67 (C), and IRF4 (MUM1, D). (D. Frank.)

cytoplasmic IgM. The Ki-67 proliferation rate is high. BCL6 is expressed by most cases and CD10 is negative. PCLBCL-LT should be differentiated from PCFCL with a diffuse growth pattern, and also other rare types of cutaneous DLBCL, iatrogenic immunodeficiency–associated lymphoproliferative disorders, and secondary cutaneous diffuse large B-cell lymphoma. Cases that cannot otherwise be classified can be diagnosed as primary cutaneous DLBCL-NOS (96).

VIB10 | Mast Cell Tumors

Mast cells predominate in a nodular dermal infiltrate, with scattered eosinophils.

Urticaria Pigmentosa, Nodular Lesions (See also IIIA.2)

CLINICAL SUMMARY. Children or adults with urticaria pigmentosa (20) may present with multiple brown nodules

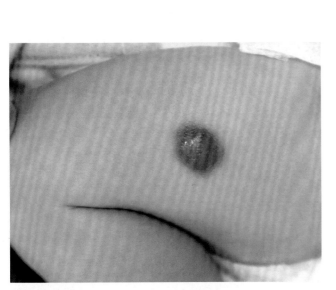

Clin. Fig. VIB10

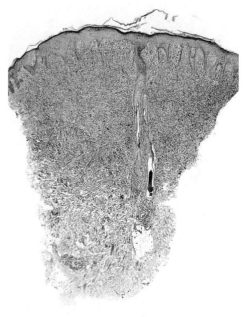

Fig. VIB10.a

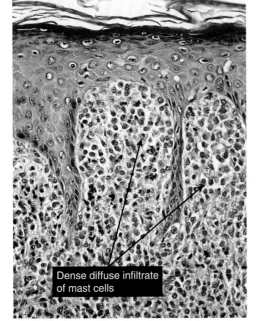

Dense diffuse infiltrate of mast cells

Fig. VIB10.b

Clin. Fig. VIB10. *Mastocytoma.* A nodular tumor developed in a 2-month-old boy.

Fig. VIB10.a. *Mastocytoma, low power.* There is a dense nodular infiltrate involving the upper half of the dermis. The overlying epidermis shows mild hyperplasia.

Fig. VIB10.b. *Mastocytoma, medium power.* The infiltrate is composed of uniform ovoid cells which are present densely in the reticular dermis but also fill the papillary dermis. The cells do not involve the overlying epidermis. (*continues*)

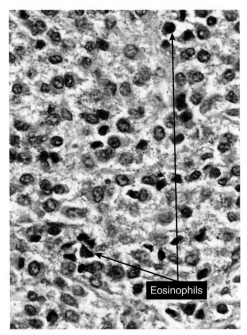

Fig. VIB10.c

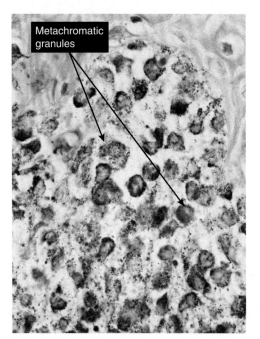

Metachromatic granules

Fig. VIB10.d

Fig. VIB10.c. *Mastocytoma, high power.* The individual cells have small uniform ovoid nuclei and an abundance of granular cytoplasm. Scattered eosinophils are frequently seen in all forms of mastocytosis, a clue to the diagnosis.

Fig. VIB10.d. *Mastocytoma, Giemsa stain.* The mast cell granules metachromatically stain purple with Giemsa stain.

or plaques which, on stroking, show urtication and occasionally blister formation. Infants, almost exclusively, may present with a usually solitary, large cutaneous nodule, which on stroking often shows not only urtication but also large bullae. Adults with urticaria pigmentosa have macular lesions with telangiectasia; urtication on stroking is variable. Mast cells are of myeloid lineage and the disease may be associated with mutation of the c-kit oncogene (97). Mast cell tumors (mastocytomas) may occur in a background of urticaria pigmentosa, or de novo.

HISTOPATHOLOGY. In these nodular or plaque lesions, the mast cells lie closely packed in tumorlike aggregates. The infiltrate may extend through the entire dermis and even into the subcutaneous fat. The mast cells nuclei in these tumors are cuboidal rather than spindle shaped, and the cells have ample eosinophilic cytoplasm and a well-defined cell border. In adults, the diagnosis can be difficult. An increase in interstitial mast cells is helpful in establishing the diagnosis. Giemsa, toluidine blue and tryptase stains, and also c-kit immunostaining, may be helpful in supporting the diagnosis. In a mastocytoma, the tumor cells present as a dense nodular infiltrate.

Conditions to consider in the differential diagnosis:

mastocytosis (urticaria pigmentosa, nodular lesions)

VIB11 Tumors With Prominent Necrosis

Necrosis is a striking feature in epithelioid sarcoma, which may be in consequence be mistaken for a granulomatous process. In addition, many advanced malignancies, often metastatic, have prominent necrosis.

Epithelioid Sarcoma

CLINICAL SUMMARY. This is a distinctive rare malignant soft tissue neoplasm of uncertain origin, occurring most commonly in the distal extremities of young adult males as a slowly growing dermal or subcutaneous nodule. However, the tumor has been reported in a wide range of anatomic sites. This aggressive neoplasm is characterized by multiple recurrences, often producing ulcerated nodules and plaques in the dermis and subcutis, and by regional and systemic metastases resulting in a poor prognosis (98). An aggressive subtype has been identified, known as the proximal axial type. Clinically, this differs from the classic type by its multinodular growth pattern, more frequent occurrence in older patients, more proximal/axial distribution (mainly, but not exclusively, involving the pelvic, perineal, and genital areas), more deep-seated location, and more aggressive clinical behavior from the outset. Angiomatoid or angiosarcoma-like and fibrous histiocytoma-like or fibroma-like subtypes have also been described (99).

HISTOPATHOLOGY. The tumors are composed of irregular nodules of atypical epithelioid cells with abundant eosinophilic cytoplasm and pleomorphic nuclei, merging with spindle cells. These aggregates are embedded in collagenous fibrous tissue in which there may be focal hemorrhage, hemosiderin, and mucin deposition with a patchy lymphocytic infiltrate. Mitoses are present in varied frequency, vascular invasion is a common feature, and foci of necrosis are present in the centers of tumor nodules. Ulceration follows epidermal involvement by the larger tumor nodules, and invasion extends diffusely into the subcutis and deeper soft tissues. A fibromalike variant of epithelioid sarcoma has also been reported, in which the spindle cell pattern predominates without the characteristic epithelioid cells and nodularity. At low power, the neoplasm may suggest a granulomatous process such as granuloma annulare, necrobiosis lipoidica, or rheumatoid nodule. The cellular atypia, diffuse stromal invasion, and foci of necrosis involving tumor cells and not only stroma, as in the necrobiotic granulomatous processes, identify the process as malignant. The diagnosis is supported by positive immunostaining for cytokeratin, epithelial membrane antigen and vimentin, and negativity for leucocyte common antigen. Histologically, the proximal subtype differs from the classic type by its larger size and deeper invasion often into muscle, and by larger epithelioid cells, with

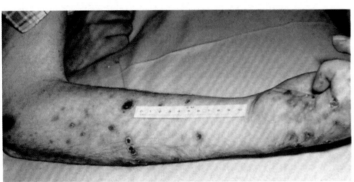

Clin. Fig. VIB11

Fig. VIB11.a

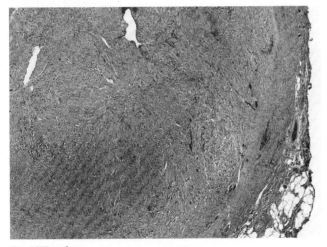

Fig. VIB11.b

Fig. VIB11.c

Clin. Fig. VIB11. *Epithelioid sarcoma.* Flexion contractures of the fingers, with multiple ulcerating nodules of the hand and forearm. (Image from P. Heenan MD.)

Fig. VIB11.a. *Epithelioid sarcoma, low power.* Poorly fragmented specimen of a multinodular lesion involving the dermis and subcutis defined nodules in the dermis with central foci of necrosis. (Case from PJ Zhang MD.)

Fig. VIB11.b. *Epithelioid sarcoma, medium power.* Multinodular patterns of epithelioid and spindle cells.

Fig. VIB11.c. *Epithelioid sarcoma, high power.* Atypical epithelioid predominate in some areas, with cellular degeneration and hemorrhage. (*continues*)

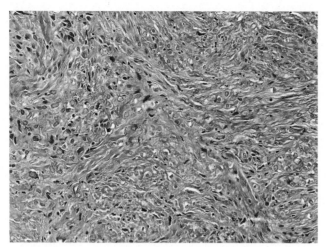

Fig. VIB11.d

Fig. VIB11.d. *Epithelioid sarcoma, low power.* Other areas present a more paucicellular spindle cell pattern. Immunostaining (not shown) supported the diagnosis.

vesicular nuclei, and prominent nucleoli; copious, eccentric cytoplasm; marked cytologic atypia; and frequent rhabdoid features. Tumoral necrosis is also a common finding in the proximal subtype, but usually without the granuloma-like appearance of the classic type.

Conditions to consider in the differential diagnosis:

    epithelioid sarcoma
    metastatic carcinomas, sarcomas, melanomas
    occasional advanced primary malignant tumors

VIB12 | Miscellaneous and Undifferentiated Epithelial Tumors

Proliferations of atypical cells with more or less abundant cytoplasm and contiguous cell borders occupy the dermis as nodular masses.

Granular Cell Tumor

Granular cell tumor is a benign neuroectodermal tumor comprised of large, round to oval cells with abundant and distinctly granular cytoplasm. The age range is broad but most arise in the fourth to sixth decades. Common sites include head and neck (particularly the tongue), breast, proximal extremities, gastrointestinal tract and respiratory tract. Skin, subcutis and submucosa are commonly involved but visceral involvement can occur. The tumors have poorly defined borders and are comprised of packets and trabeculae of large round to oval cells with granular and abundant cytoplasm. The nuclei range from small and uniform to enlarged with prominent nucleoli. The granular cytoplasm results from massive numbers of lysosomes, along with larger granules surrounded by a clear halo called pustular ovoid bodies of Milian. Perineural involvement is frequent. Malignant granular cell tumor is exceedingly rare. The lesions stain positively for S100, CD68, CD63, and NSE. HMB45 is negative and Melan-A is rare and focal (100).

Cellular Neurothekeoma

Cellular neurothekeoma may mimic melanoma, and may express some "melanoma markers" such as MITF

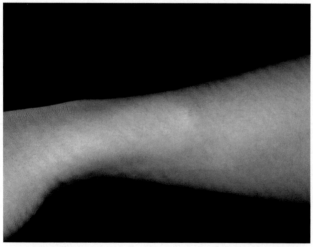

Clin. Fig. VIB12

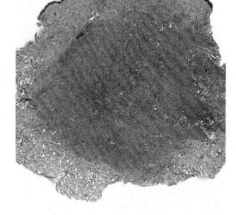

Fig. VIB12.a

Clin. Fig. VIB12. *Granular cell tumor.* A 19-year-old man with a 10-year history of a subcutaneous nodule in the forearm.

Fig. VIB12.a. *Granular cell tumor, medium power.* There is a cellular tumor in the dermis. Epidermal hyperplasia overlying a granular cell tumor may be absent or minimal as seen here or there may be striking pseudoepitheliomatous hyperplasia resembling a squamous cell carcinoma.

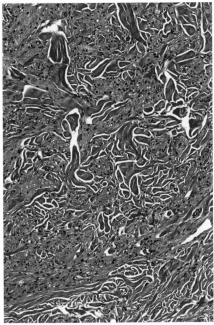

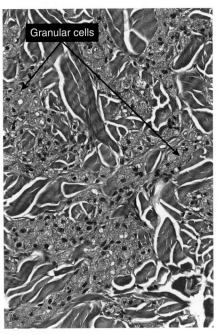

Granular cells

Fig. VIB12.b

Fig. VIB12.c

Fig. VIB12.b. *Granular cell tumor, high power.* The individual cells are large with an abundance of eosinophilic granular cytoplasm. There are small nuclei granules can be highlighted using the PAS stain.

Fig. VIB12.c. *Granular cell tumor with pseudoepitheliomatous hyperplasia, high power.* These granules can be highlighted with a PAS stain, and the tumors are typically S100 positive (not shown).

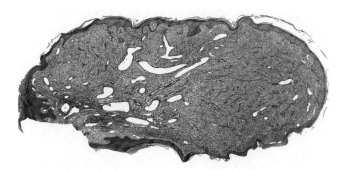

Fig. VIB12.d

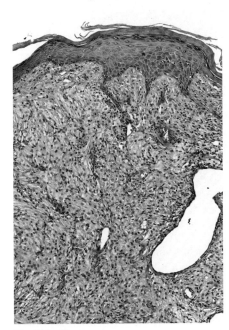

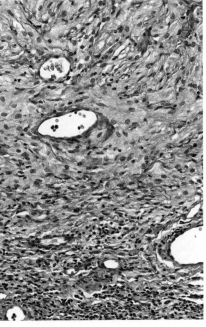

Fig. VIB12.e

Fig. VIB12.f

Fig. VIB12.d. *Cellular neurothekeoma, low power.* There is a relatively well-circumscribed nodule within the dermis.

Fig. VIB12.e. *Cellular neurothekeoma, medium power.* The neoplasm is composed of multiple interlacing clusters of cells which may be reminiscent of a neuroma at this magnification.

Fig. VIB12.f. *Cellular neurothekeoma, high power.* The cells are spindle and epithelioid in form, some with an abundance of eosinophilic cytoplasm. The nuclei are relatively small and uniform with minimal atypia and minimal mitotic activity. (*continues*)

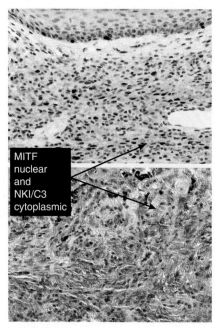

Fig. VIB12.g

Fig. VIB12.g. *Cellular neurothekeoma, high power.* Positive staining for MITF (top) and NKI/C3, while not specific, are characteristic for this tumor. S100 and other melanoma markers were negative.

and NKI/C3. However, it is negative for S100, Melan A, HMB45 and tyrosinase.

Metastatic Malignant Melanoma

See Figs. VIB12.h,i.

Conditions to consider in the differential diagnosis:

Epithelial Tumors
    undifferentiated carcinoma (large cell, small cell)
    neuroendocrine tumor
Epithelial Simulants
    anaplastic large cell lymphoma (CD30/Ki-1, usually T-cells)
    epithelioid sarcoma
    granular cell nerve sheath tumor (granular cell tumor/schwannoma)
    plexiform granular cell nerve sheath tumor
    malignant granular cell tumor
    epithelioid angiosarcoma
    cellular neurothekeoma (immature nerve sheath myxoma)
    ganglioneuroma
    cephalic brain–like hamartoma (nasal glioma)
    encephalocele
    cutaneous meningiomas

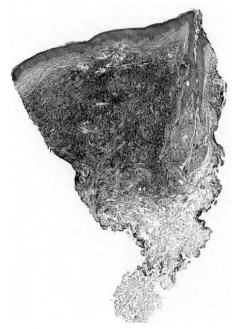

Fig. VIB12.h   **Fig. VIB12.i**

Fig. VIB12.h. *Metastatic malignant melanoma, low power.* A pale staining, poorly defined tumor has replaced the reticular dermis.

Fig. VIB12.i. *Metastatic malignant melanoma, high power.* The tumor is composed of pleomorphic anaplastic cells. Many cells show multiple nuclei as well as atypical nuclei and prominent nucleoli. If melanin pigment were absent, immunoperoxidase stains would be necessary to definitively identify this as metastatic melanoma and not some other tumor.

SPINDLE CELL, PLEOMORPHIC, AND CONNECTIVE TISSUE TUMORS

In the dermis there is a proliferation of elongated tapered "spindle cells"; these may be of fibrohistiocytic, muscle, neural (Schwannian), melanocytic or unknown origin. Immunohistochemistry may be essential in making these distinctions.

1. Fibrohistiocytic Spindle Cell Tumors
2. Schwannian/Neural Spindle Cell Tumors
3. Spindle Cell Tumors of Muscle
4. Melanocytic Spindle Cell Tumors
5. Tumors and Proliferations of Angiogenic Cells
6. Tumors of Adipose Tissue
7. Tumors of Cartilaginous Tissue
8. Tumors of Osseous Tissue

VIC1 Fibrohistiocytic Spindle Cell Tumors

There is a proliferation of spindle to pleomorphic cells that may synthesize collagen, or be essentially undifferentiated. Because there are no useful specific markers for fibroblasts, immunohistochemistry is of little diagnostic utility except to rule out nonfibrous spindle cell tumors. Morphology is critical for accurate diagnosis.

VIC1a Fibrohistiocytic Tumors With Minimal or No Atypia

In most benign lesions there is no atypia. Random atypia that may be seen in some dermatofibromas is an exception. Low-grade malignancies such as dermatofibrosarcoma protruberans may show little or no atypia.

Dermatofibroma

CLINICAL SUMMARY. Dermatofibromas (101) occur in the skin as firm, indolent red to red-brown or occasionally blue-black single or multiple nodules, usually only a few millimeters in diameter. The cut surface of the lesions varies in color from white to yellowish brown, depending on the proportions of fibrous tissue, lipid, and hemosiderin present. The lesions usually persist indefinitely.

HISTOPATHOLOGY. The epidermis is usually hyperplastic, with hyperpigmentation of the basal layer and elongation of the rete ridges, separated by a clear (Grenz) zone from a spindle cell tumor in the dermis. The highly characteristic hyperplasia of the overlying epidermis in the center of the lesion may mimic basal cell carcinoma and has considerable value in establishing the diagnosis of dermatofibroma. The dermal tumor is composed of fibroblast-like spindle cells, histiocytes, and blood vessels in varying proportions. Foamy histiocytes and multinucleated giant cells containing lipid or hemosiderin may be present, sometimes in large numbers, forming xanthomatous aggregates. Capillaries may be plentiful in the stroma, giving the lesion an angiomatous component; when associated with a sclerotic stroma, such lesions have been referred to as "sclerosing hemangioma." In some small lesions the spindle cells are distributed singly between the collagen bundles, forming a zone of subtly increased cellularity, whereas in larger tumors there is much denser cellularity and the spindle cells are arranged in sheets or interlocking strands in storiform pattern. The dermal

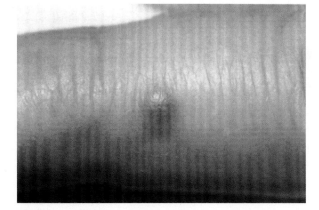

Clin. Fig. VIC1a.a

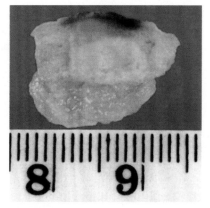

Clin. Fig. VIC1a.b

Clin. Fig. VIC1a.a. *Dermatofibroma.* A 47-year-old man presented with a 4-mm deep firm smooth red nodule on the extensor finger.

Clin. Fig. VIC1a.b. *Dermatofibroma.* A sectioned gross specimen demonstrating a circumscribed yellowish nodule in the reticular dermis. The epidermis is hyperplastic and hyperpigmented, and is separated from the epidermis by a clear zone. (P. Heenan.) (*continues*)

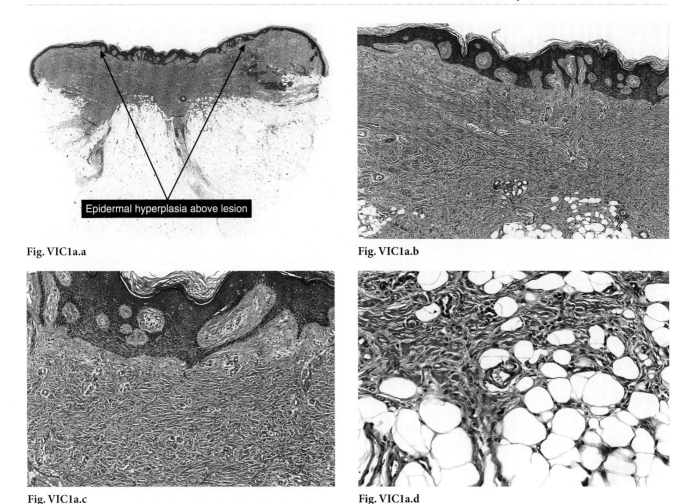

Fig. VIC1a.a

Epidermal hyperplasia above lesion

Fig. VIC1a.b

Fig. VIC1a.c

Fig. VIC1a.d

Fig. VIC1a.a. *Dermatofibroma, low power.* There is a symmetrical but noncircumscribed area of hypercellularity in the mid dermis. This proliferation is associated with retraction of the overlying epidermis which produces the "dimple" sign which is seen clinically.

Fig. VIC1a.b. *Dermatofibroma, medium power.* Within the mid dermis there is a proliferation of bland-appearing spindled cells. These cells encircle bundles of reticular dermal collagen.

Fig. VIC1a.c. *Dermatofibroma, medium power.* The overlying epidermis becomes hyperplastic as well as hyperpigmented.

Fig. VIC1a.d. *Dermatofibroma, high power.* There is only slight (or usually no) "honeycombing" of fat at the base.

tumor is poorly demarcated on both sides, so that the fibroblasts and the young basophilic collagen extend between the mature, eosinophilic collagen bundles of the dermis and surround them, trapping normal collagen bundles at the periphery of the tumor nodule.

Cellular dermatofibroma is a very densely cellular tumor with fascicular and storiform growth patterns and frequent extension into the subcutis. The neoplasm shares some features, therefore, with dermatofibrosarcoma protuberans (DFSP), from which it is distinguished by the overlying epidermal hyperplasia, polymorphism of the tumor cell population, extension of tumor cells at the edge of the lesion to surround individual hyalinized collagen bundles, and the absence of immunostaining for CD34. The cellular dermatofibroma also extends into the subcutis along the septa or in a bulging, expansile pattern, rather than in the more diffusely infiltrative pattern of DFSP, which produces a typical honeycomb-like pattern and extends far along interlobular septa of the panniculus. Cellular dermatofibromas may recur and rare cases have even been reported to have metastasized to the lung (102). These lesions should therefore be completely excised.

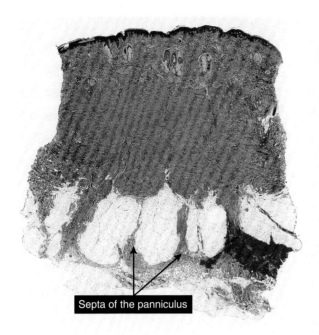

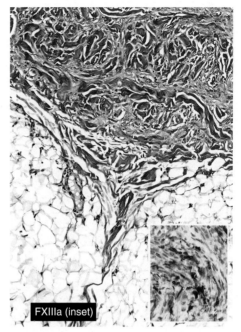

FXIIIa (inset)

Fig. VIC1a.e

Fig. VIC1a.f

Fig. VIC1a.e. *Cellular dermatofibroma, medium power.* The tumor consists of spindle cells arranged in densely cellular fascicular and storiform patterns.

Fig. VIC1a.f. *Cellular dermatofibroma, high power.* There is little or no honeycombing of the fat or extension down septa. Factor XIIIa is positive in the lesional cells. A negative immunohistochemical stain for CD34 (not shown) assists in differentiating a cellular dermatofibroma from a dermatofibrosarcoma protuberans.

Cellular Dermatofibroma

See Figs. VIC1a.e,f.

Sclerosing/Angiomatoid Spitz Nevus (Desmoplastic Spitz Nevus)

In a few examples of this condition the Spitz nevus cells may be so inconspicuous that a regressing or desmoplastic melanoma, or a fibrosing disorder or an angiomatous lesion may be simulated (103).

Dermatofibrosarcoma Protuberans

CLINICAL SUMMARY. Dermatofibrosarcoma protuberans (104) (DFSP) is a slowly growing dermal spindle cell neoplasm of intermediate malignancy that usually forms an indurated plaque on which multiple reddish purple, firm nodules subsequently arise, sometimes with ulceration. A characteristic COL1-PDGF fusion gene is present (see below). The tumors occur most frequently on the trunk or the proximal extremities of young adults and only rarely in the head and neck. A small proportion of cases have been reported in childhood and, rarely, as congenital lesions. Local recurrence is common but metastasis is rare.

HISTOPATHOLOGY. DFSP is composed of densely packed, monomorphous, plump spindle cells arranged in a storiform (mat-like) pattern in the central areas of tumor nodules, whereas at the periphery there is diffuse infiltration of the dermal stroma, frequently extending into the subcutis and producing a characteristic honeycomb pattern. Infiltration into the underlying fascia and muscle is a late event. The peripheral elements of the tumor may have a deceptively bland appearance, and may extend far along septa of the panniculus, which can cause difficulties in determining the true extent of the tumor. Myxoid areas, sometimes resembling liposarcoma, include a characteristic vascular component of slitlike anastomosing thin-walled blood vessels presenting a crow's foot or chicken wire appearance. Melanin-containing cells may be present in a small proportion of tumors, so-called Bednar tumor (pigmented DFSP, storiform neurofibroma). Giant cells are seen in a small proportion of otherwise typical DFSP; it has been suggested that giant cell fibroblastoma is a juvenile variant of DFSP. Fibrosarcomatous areas are seen in a small proportion of DFSP, characterized by a fascicular or herringbone growth pattern of the spindle cells, usually presenting with larger size, more expansile patterns of invasion of the subcutis and with muscle invasion, p53 expression, and increased proliferative activity. This

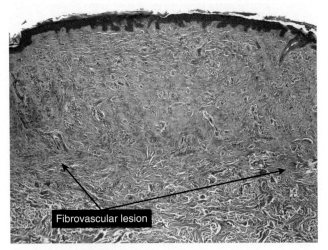

Fig. VIC1a.g

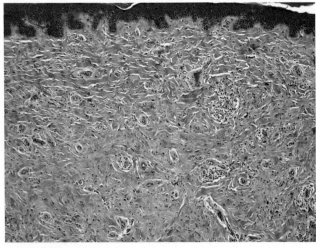

Fig. VIC1a.h

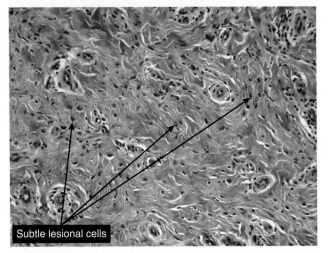

Fig. VIC1a.i

Fig. VIC1a.g. *Sclerosing/angiomatoid Spitz nevus.* There is an illdefined area of altered collagen in the dermis.

Fig. VIC1a.h. *Sclerosing/angiomatoid Spitz nevus.* At intermediate magnification prominent vessels are the major feature.

Fig. VIC1a.i. *Sclerosing/angiomatoid Spitz nevus.* At high power, with searching, one can appreciate the large spindle and/ or epithelioid lesional cells among the altered collagen bundles. In case of doubt, an S100 stain will reliably highlight these cells.

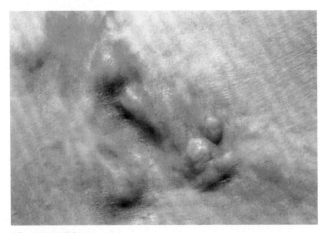

Clin. Fig. VIC1a.c

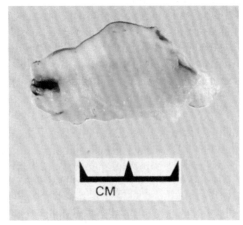

Clin. Fig. VIC1a.d

Clin. Fig. VIC1a.c. *Dermatofibrosarcoma protuberans, recurrent.* An elderly woman presented with multiple variably shaped flesh-colored nodules and papules in a chest wall excision scar.

Clin. Fig. VIC1a.d. *Dermatofibrosarcoma protuberans.* A sectioned gross specimen reveals an asymmetric tumor spanning the dermis and infiltrating the subcutis. (P. Heenan.)

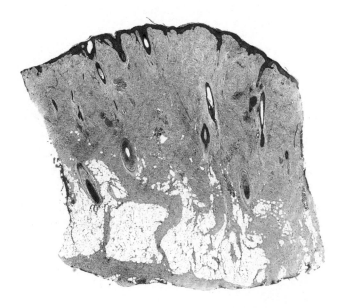

Fig. VIC1a.j

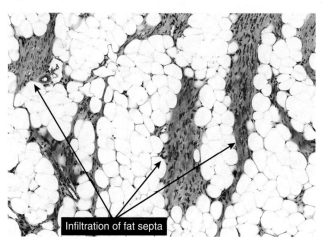

Fig. VIC1a.k

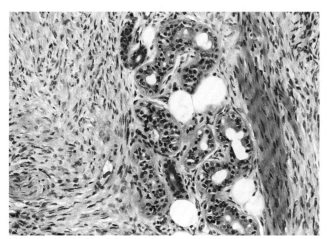

Fig. VIC1a.l

Infiltration of fat septa

Fig. VIC1a.m

Fig. VIC1a.j. *Dermatofibrosarcoma protuberans, low power.* There is a tumor which occupies nearly the entire dermis and extends into the underlying subcutaneous fat.

Fig. VIC1a.k. *Dermatofibrosarcoma protuberans, medium power.* The spindle cell proliferation shows a storiform or cartwheel pattern.

Fig. VIC1a.l. *Dermatofibrosarcoma protuberans, high power.* The neoplasm is composed of relatively uniform spindled cells whose nuclei are elongate with tapered ends. Mitoses may be identified but are usually few in numbers.

Fig. VIC1a.m. *Dermatofibrosarcoma protuberans, medium power.* This spindle cell proliferation characteristically infiltrates the subcutaneous fat, producing a "honey-comb" pattern.

VI Tumors and Cysts of the Dermis and Subcutis

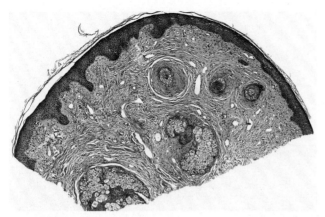

Fig. VIC1a.n. *Fibrous papule (angiofibroma), low power.* This dome-shaped neoplasm shows a normal overlying epidermis and a fibrovascular core.

Fig. VIC1a.o. *Fibrous papule (angiofibroma), medium power.* The dermis is fibrotic and one cannot identify a distinction between papillary and reticular dermis. There is an increased number of small, mature vascular channels which contain erythrocytes.

Fig. VIC1a.p. *Fibrous papule (angiofibroma), high power.* The stroma is composed of collagen and stellate fibroblasts around the small vascular channels.

Fig. VIC1a.n

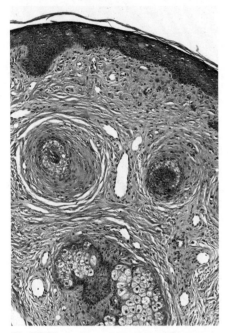

Fig. VIC1a.o

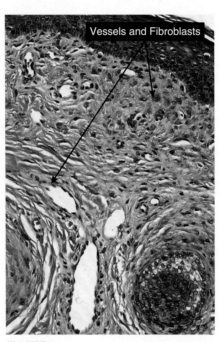

Vessels and Fibroblasts

Fig. VIC1a.p

may have increased propensity for local recurrence and rarely for metastasis. Demonstration of the presence of a COL1A1-PDGFB fusion gene may be a useful tool for diagnosis of DFSP and particularly for the fibrosarcomatous variant (105).

Fibrous Papule (Angiofibroma)

See Figs. VIC1a.n–p.

Recurrent Infantile Digital Fibromatosis

See Figs. VIC1a.q–s.

Keloid

CLINICAL SUMMARY. Keloids and hypertrophic scars are caused by a variety of injuries to the skin. Superficial injuries that do not reach the reticular dermis do not cause these phenomena. Aberrant word healing in these conditions is thought to be due to continuous inflammation, suggesting that proinflammatory genes in the skin are more sensitive to trauma in these situations (106).

HISTOPATHOLOGY. Keloids differ from hyperplastic scars in having characteristic thickened hyalinized eosinophilic collagen bundles. There is often a background of hyperplastic scar and there is usually associated inflammation. Clinically, keloids tend to persist more or less indefinitely, while hyperplastic scars tend to regress, especially after treatment, for example with corticosteroids.

Acquired Digital Fibrokeratoma

See Clin. Fig. VIC1a.f and Figs. VIC1a.v,w.

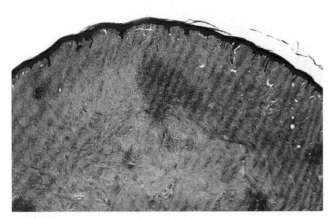

Fig. VIC1a.q

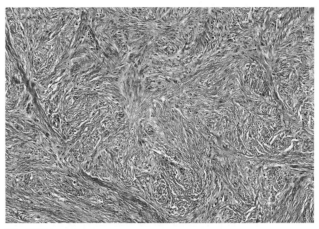

Fig. VIC1a.r

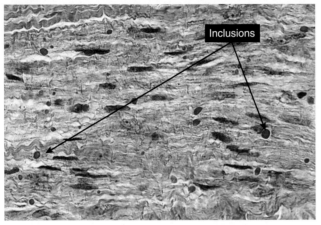

Inclusions

Fig. VIC1a.s

Fig. VIC1a.q. *Recurrent infantile digital fibromatosis, low power.* The dermis is replaced by a tumor which is relatively uniform and symmetrical.

Fig. VIC1a.r. *Recurrent infantile digital fibromatosis, medium power.* The tumor is composed of uniform spindled cells embedded in a collagenous stroma. There is no atypia.

Fig. VIC1a.s. *Recurrent infantile digital fibromatosis, high power.* High magnification reveals elongate nuclei with tapered ends. The collagenous stroma is wavy in appearance. The characteristic finding in these lesions is the eosinophilic cytoplasmic inclusions. These inclusions stain red using the Masson-Trichrome stain.

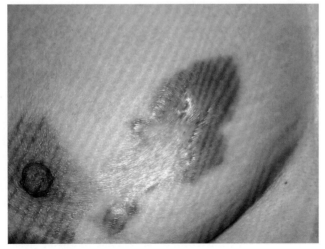

Clin. Fig. VIC1a.e

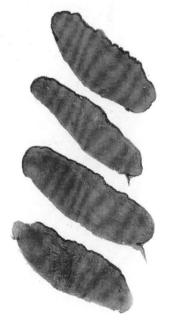

Clin. Fig. VIC1a.e. *Keloid.* This scar at the site of a prior injury became large, raised, rubbery firm, and red, and persisted for many years in a 27-year-old woman.

Fig. VIC1a.t. *Keloid, low power.* This lesion can be diagnosed at scanning magnification. No adnexal structures are seen within the dermis. Within the dermis, there are multiple bundles of thick eosinophilic collagen. (*continues*)

Fig. VIC1a.t

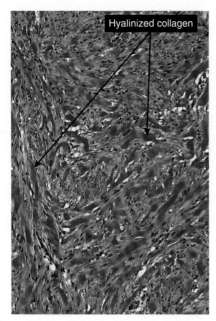

Fig. VIC1a.u

Fig. VIC1a.u. *Keloid, high power.* The collagen bundles are markedly thickened and eosinophilic. Scattered small fibroblasts are seen between these hyalinized collagen bundles.

Tenosynovial Giant Cell Tumor (Giant Cell Tumor of Tendon Sheath)

CLINICAL SUMMARY. Tenosynovial giant cell tumor (TGCT) was formerly known as pigmented villonodular synovitis and is a benign proliferative condition arising from synovium of joints, bursae or tendon sheaths. TGCT can present either as a single nodule, as localized TGCT or as multiple nodules (diffuse TGCT). Although large joints are usually affected, other joints including fingers may be involved, and also soft tissue not necessarily related to a joint. The etiology is thought to have inflammatory and neoplastic components, resulting from activation of CSF1 expression by a translocation in a minority of tumor cells, or by other unknown mechanisms (107). The lifetime recurrence risk is said to be up to 15% for localized and 55% for diffuse TGCT (108).

HISTOPATHOLOGY. Localized TGCT presents as a lobulated lesion usually arising from the tendon sheath of the digit (109). These lesions generally have a fibrous capsule and are less cellular than the diffuse type, with

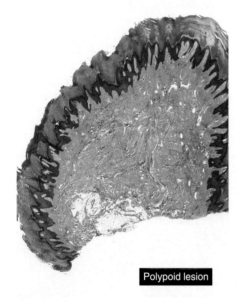

Fig. VIC1a.v

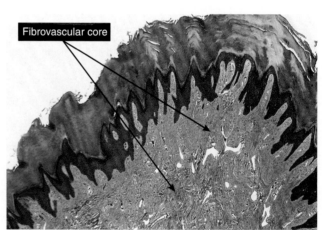

Fig. VIC1a.w

Fig. VIC1a.v. *Acquired digital fibrokeratoma, low power.* This biopsy of acral skin shows a dome-shaped lesion which is hyperkeratotic. There is a fibrovascular core.

Fig. VIC1a.w. *Acquired digital fibrokeratoma, medium power.* The epidermis shows mild, uniform, verrucous hyperplasia. There are no viral cytopathic changes. The core shows fibrosis and a few small vascular channels.

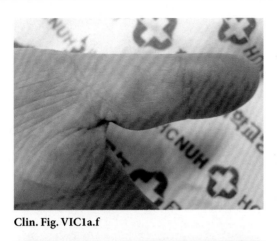

Clin. Fig. VIC1a.f

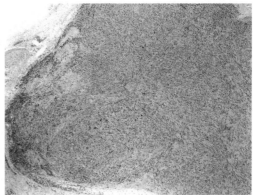

Fig. VIC1a.x

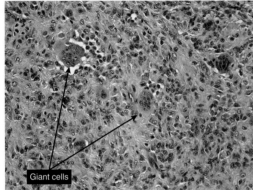

Fig. VIC1a.y

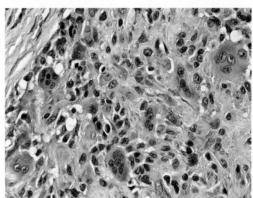

Fig. VIC1a.z

Clin. Fig. VIC1a.f. *Tenosynovial giant cell tumor.* A 45-year-old woman had a dome-shaped movable nodule on the left volar thumb.

Fig. VIC1a.x. *Tenosynovial giant cell tumor, low power.* Within the deep tissue there is a large, irregularly shaped nodular fibrohistiocytic proliferation.

Fig. VIC1a.y. *Tenosynovial giant cell tumor, medium power.* The tumor is composed of plump histiocytes and numerous multinucleated giant cells.

Fig. VIC1a.z. *Tenosynovial giant cell tumor, high power.* These osteoclast-like giant cells have multiple nuclei. There are also scattered lymphocytes throughout the lesion.

prominent hyalinization of the stroma. Giant cells are usually more prominent than in the diffuse type. The background cells have characteristics of histiocytes and there may also be dendritic cells with possible myofibroblastic differentiation that may stain with desmin. Malignancy is rare even in the diffuse type. Atypical histologic features may include a very high mitotic rate, necrosis, monomorphism and spindling of mononuclear cells, unusually abundant eosinophilic cytoplasm in histiocyte-like cells, and large nuclei with nucleoli and stromal myxoid change. Giant cell tumor of bone should be excluded by clinical and radiographic information (108).

Nodular Fasciitis

See Figs. VIC1a.za–zc.

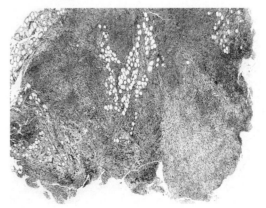

Fig. VIC1a.za

Fig. VIC1a.za. *Nodular fasciitis, low power.* There is a poorly defined hypercellular lesion which infiltrates the subcutaneous fat. (*continues*)

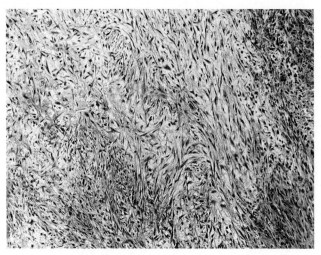

Fig. VIC1a.zb

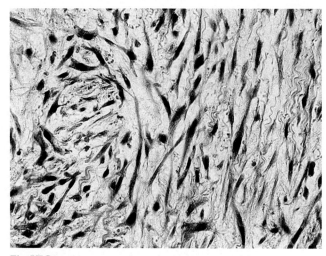

Fig. VIC1a.zc

Fig. VIC1a.zb. *Nodular fasciitis, medium power.* There are numerous haphazardly arranged spindled cells, some of which are embedded in a mucinous stroma.

Fig. VIC1a.zc. *Nodular fasciitis, high power.* In the mucinous area there is a proliferation of plump, but cytologically bland-appearing fibroblasts in a haphazard arrangement and a pale-staining stroma. Mitotic figures may be frequent (not shown).

VIC1b Fibrohistiocytic Tumors With High-Grade Atypia

High-grade cytologic atypia is often a sign of malignancy. However, atypical fibroxanthoma is a lesion that demonstrates often startling atypia yet usually follows a benign course.

Atypical Fibroxanthoma

CLINICAL SUMMARY. Atypical fibroxanthoma (110) is a fairly common pleomorphic spindle cell neoplasm of the dermis that, despite apparently malignant histologic features, usually follows an indolent or locally aggressive course. Because a small number of metastases have been reported, atypical fibroxanthoma is regarded as a neoplasm of low-grade malignancy related to malignant fibrous histiocytoma (pleomorphic dermal sarcoma). According to this view, the more favorable prognosis of atypical fibroxanthoma is related to its small size and superficial location. The disease usually presents as a solitary nodule less than 2 cm in diameter on the exposed skin of the head and neck or dorsum of the hand of elderly patients, often with a short history of rapid growth. The

---

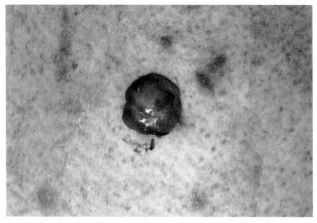

Clin. Fig. VIC1b.a

Fig. VIC1b.a

Clin. Fig. VIC1b.a. *Atypical fibroxanthoma.* A symmetrical nodule appeared suddenly and grew rapidly in sun-damaged skin of an elderly man.

Fig. VIC1b.a. *Atypical fibroxanthoma, high power.* The ulcerated tumor is composed of elongate spindle cells with a somewhat haphazard arrangement.

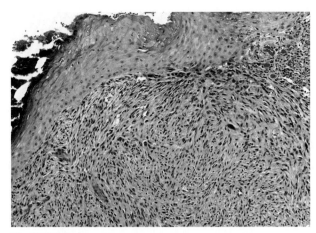

Fig. VIC1b.b

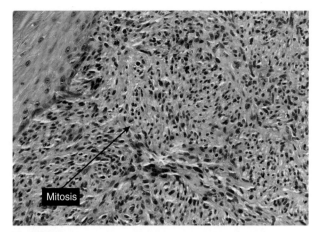

Mitosis

Fig. VIC1b.c

Fig. VIC1b.b. *Atypical fibroxanthoma, medium power.* There is prominent nuclear pleomorphism, often much more pronounced than in this example.

Fig. VIC1b.c. *Atypical fibroxanthoma, high power.* Other spindle cell tumors (melanoma, squamous cell carcinoma, soft tissue tumors) must be excluded with immunostains.

lesions are usually associated with severe actinic damage, and a few have arisen in areas treated by radiation.

HISTOPATHOLOGY. Atypical fibroxanthoma is an exophytic, densely cellular neoplasm, unencapsulated but with only limited infiltration of the stroma, frequently with an epidermal collaret. The tumor may extend to the dermoepidermal junction, but there is no direct continuity with the squamous epithelium, although ulceration is often present. Severe solar elastosis is present in the adjacent dermis. The classical tumor is composed of pleomorphic histiocytelike cells and atypical giant cells, often with bizarre nuclei, prominent nucleoli, and numerous mitotic figures, including abnormal forms. The cells are arranged in a compact, disorderly pattern, surrounding but not destroying adnexal structures. Fibroblast-like spindle cells are present in variable numbers; cells of morphology intermediate between these spindle cells and histiocytelike cells are also present. Scattered inflammatory cells and numerous small blood vessels are present, commonly with focal hemorrhage.

Malignant Fibrous Histiocytoma (Pleomorphic Dermal Sarcoma)

See Figs. VIC1b.d–g.

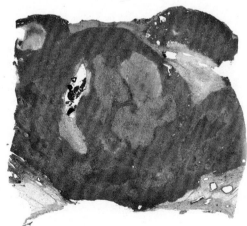

Fig. VIC1b.d

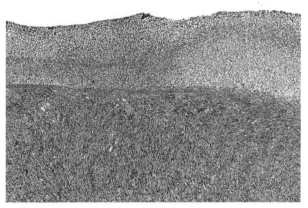

Fig. VIC1b.e

Fig. VIC1b.d. *Malignant fibrous histiocytoma (pleomorphic dermal sarcoma), low power.* Scanning magnification of a large spindle cell tumor shows extensive involvement of the subcutaneous fat and dermis.

Fig. VIC1b.e. *Malignant fibrous histiocytoma, low power.* The size, location, and depth of involvement distinguish this lesion from an atypical fibroxanthoma, a smaller, more superficial lesion. *(continues)*

Tumors and Cysts of the Dermis and Subcutis

VI

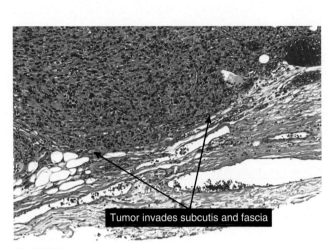

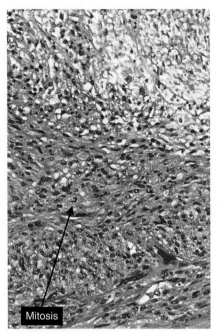

Fig. VIC1b.f

Fig. VIC1b.g

Fig. VIC1b.f. *Malignant fibrous histiocytoma, medium power.* This highly cellular tumor may show zones of spindled cells or, as seen here, large epithelioid cells with obvious nuclear atypia and pleomorphism.

Fig. VIC1b.g. *Malignant fibrous histiocytoma, high power.* The atypical cells may have multiple nucleoli. Mitoses as well as atypical mitoses are easily identified.

Dermatofibrosarcoma Protuberans With Sarcomatoid Change

See Figs. VIC1b.h–k.

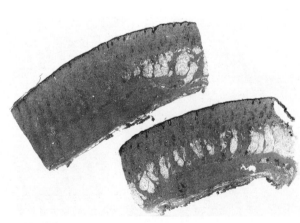

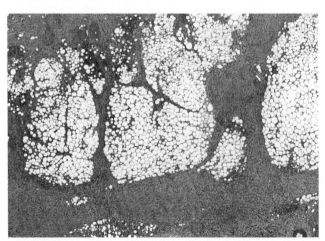

Fig. VIC1b.h

Fig. VIC1b.i

Fig. VIC1b.h. *Dermatofibrosarcoma protuberans with sarcomatoid change, low power.* A bulky tumor that extensively involves the subcutaneous fat and the fascia.

Fig. VIC1b.i. *Dermatofibrosarcoma protuberans with sarcomatoid change, low power.* Extensive honeycombing of the fat.

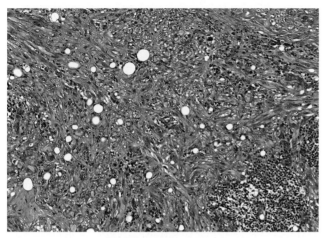

Fig. VIC1b.j

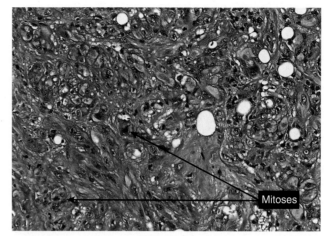

Fig. VIC1b.k

Fig. VIC1b.j. *Dermatofibrosarcoma protuberans with sarcomatoid change, low power.* A very cellular and somewhat storiform proliferation.

Fig. VIC1b.k. *Dermatofibrosarcoma protuberans with Sarcomatoid change, low power.* Severe atypia and frequent mitoses.

VIC1c Lesions With Myxoid Changes

Localized myxoid lesions may present clinically as cysts, but they lack an epithelial lining and represent localized lesions of fibroblasts characterized by overproduction of mostly nonfibrillary matrix materials.

Mucocele

See Figs. VIC1c.a,b.

Digital Mucous Cyst

See Clin. Fig. VIC1c.a and Figs. VIC1c.c,d.

Cutaneous Myxoma

See Figs. VIC1c.e–g.

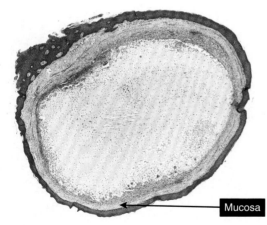

Fig. VIC1c.a

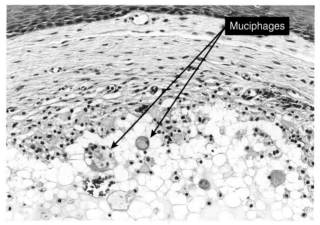

Fig. VIC1c.b

Fig. VIC1c.a. *Mucocele, low power.* Within the submucosa there is a cystic structure filled with amorphous material. Minor salivary glands are seen in the lower portion of this biopsy.

Fig. VIC1c.b. *Mucocele, medium power.* This lesion has no true cyst wall but the apparent "wall" is composed of a fibroblastic response. There are also numerous macrophages which have engulfed the mucinous material (muciphages).

VI Tumors and Cysts of the Dermis and Subcutis

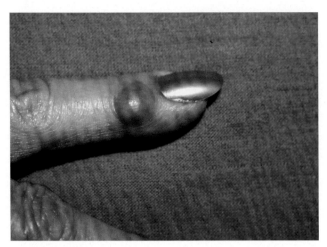

Clin. Fig. VIC1c.a

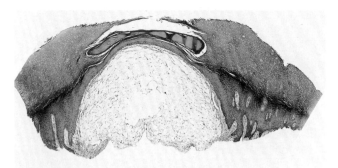

Fig. VIC1c.c

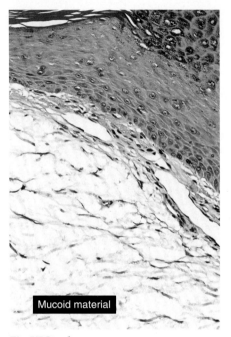

Mucoid material

Fig. VIC1c.d

Clin. Fig. VIC1c.a. *Digital mucous cyst.* This asymptomatic nodule could be excised if desired.

Fig. VIC1c.c. *Digital mucous cyst, low power.* This biopsy of acral skin shows a dome-shaped lesion created by an expanded papillary dermis. The overlying stratum corneum shows a focus of crusting.

Fig. VIC1c.d. *Digital mucous cyst, medium power.* The pale-staining area is composed of glycosaminoglycans which can be high-lighted using alcian blue or colloidal iron stains. There are scattered small fibroblasts. The adjacent epidermis shows mild hyperplasia.

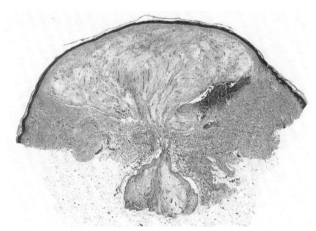

Fig. VIC1c.e

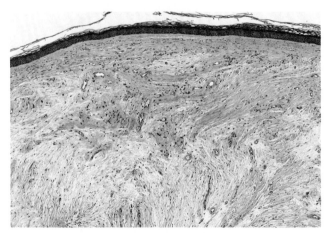

Fig. VIC1c.f

Fig. VIC1c.e. *Cutaneous myxoma, low power.* There is a symmetrical pale-staining area within the upper and mid dermis. The overlying epidermis shows an effaced rete ridge architecture.

Fig. VIC1c.f. *Cutaneous myxoma, medium power.* The nonencapsulated area within the dermis is hypocellular with a bluish, mucinous background representing the myxoid matrix.

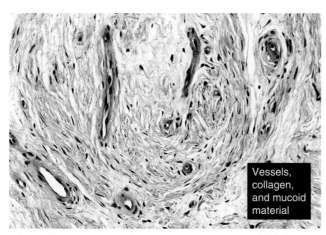

Vessels, collagen, and mucoid material

Fig. VIC1c.g

Fig. VIC1c.g. *Cutaneous myxoma, high power.* There are scattered bland-appearing fibroblasts and small mature vascular channels embedded in the bluish mucinous matrix.

Conditions to consider in the differential diagnosis:

fibrohistiocytic tumors
   benign fibrous histiocytoma (dermatofibroma)
   cellular dermatofibroma
   aneurysmal fibrous histiocytoma
   juvenile xanthogranuloma, spindle cell variant
   progressive nodular histiocytoma (deep fibrous
      type)
   plexiform fibrohistiocytic tumor
   atypical fibroxanthoma
fibrous tumors
   fibrous papule (angiofibroma)
   hypertrophic scar, keloid
   dermatofibrosarcoma protuberans
sarcomas
   malignant fibrous histiocytoma
   angiomatoid fibrous histiocytoma
   synovial sarcoma
fibromatoses
   desmoid tumor
   recurrent infantile digital fibromatosis
   juvenile hyaline fibromatosis
fibromas
   fibroma of tendon sheath
   follicular fibroma
   acquired digital fibroma
   elastofibroma
   dermatomyofibroma
giant cell tumors
   giant cell fibroblastoma
   giant cell tumor of tendon sheath
proliferative lesions of the fascia
   nodular fasciitis
   cranial fasciitis of childhood

myxoid spindle cell lesions
   cutaneous myxoma
   digital mucous cyst
   mucocele of oral mucosa

VIC2 Schwannian/Neural Spindle Cell Tumors

These tumors are composed of elongated, narrow spindle cells that tend to have serpentine S-shaped nuclei, and to be arranged in "wavy" fiber bundles. Immunohistochemistry for S100 is useful, but not specific.

Neurofibromas

CLINICAL SUMMARY. Extraneural sporadic cutaneous neurofibromas (111) (ESCNs) (the common sporadic neurofibromas) are soft, polypoid, skin-colored or slightly tan, and small (rarely larger than a centimeter in diameter). They usually arise in adulthood. The presence of more than a few cutaneous neurofibromas raises the possibility of neurofibromatosis, and should prompt an evaluation for other confirmatory stigmata. Diffuse neurofibromas are usually larger and are highly infiltrative, and have a somewhat greater chance of being associated with neurofibromatosis. Plexiform neurofibromas are more likely than not to be associated with NF-1.

HISTOPATHOLOGY. Most examples of ESCN are faintly eosinophilic, and are circumscribed but not encapsulated: they are extraneural. Thin spindle cells with elongated, wavy nuclei are regularly spaced among thin, wavy collagenous strands. The strands are either closely spaced (homogeneous pattern) or loosely spaced in a clear matrix (loose pattern). The two patterns are often intermixed in a single lesion. Rarely, ESCNs are composed of widely spaced spindle and stellate cells in a myxoid matrix. The regular spacing of adnexa is preserved in cutaneous neurofibromas. Entrapped small nerves occasionally are enlarged and hypercellular. Tactoid (tactile corpuscle-like) bodies and pigmented dendritic melanocytes are most uncommon. These tumors are essentially the same as those that occur in von Recklinghausen neurofibromatosis.

Neurofibromatosis

See Clin. Fig. VIC2.a and Figs. VIC2.d–g.

Schwannoma (Neurilemmoma)

CLINICAL SUMMARY. These benign, Schwann cell neoplasms present as solitary, skin-colored tumors along the course of peripheral or cranial nerves (112). Their usual size is between 2 and 4 cm and their usual location is the head or the flexor aspect of the extremities. When small,

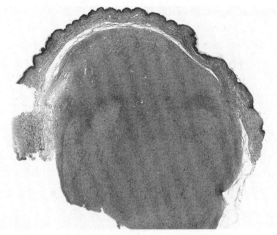

Fig. VIC2.a

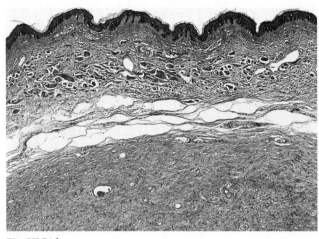

Fig. VIC2.b

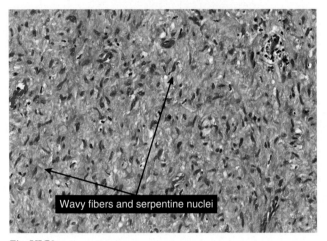

Wavy fibers and serpentine nuclei

Fig. VIC2.c

Fig. VIC2.a. *Neurofibroma, low power.* There is a dome-shaped, nonencapsulated neoplasm within the dermis.

Fig. VIC2.b. *Neurofibroma, medium power.* The lesion is composed of elongate, spindled cells which are embedded in an eosinophilic matrix. In the center of this photomicrograph, there is a structure resembling a small cutaneous nerve.

Fig. VIC2.c. *Neurofibroma, high power.* The nuclei are elongate and S-shaped or serpentine, with tapered ends, and they are embedded in an eosinophilic matrix made up of "wavy" fibers. Mast cells are frequently seen in neural tumors.

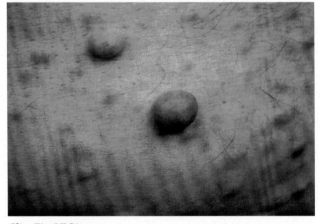

Clin. Fig. VIC2.a

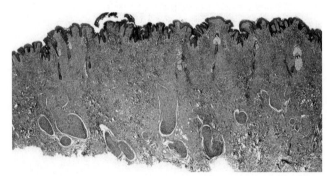

Fig. VIC2.d

Clin. Fig. VIC2.a. *Neurofibromatosis.* A 51-year-old man presented with axillary freckling, cafe au lait macules and generalized soft pigmented and flesh colored papules and nodules with "button-hole" compression (soft, compressible centers).

Fig. VIC2.d. *Plexiform neurofibroma, low power.* This plaque-like lesion shows multiple nodular aggregates embedded in an eosinophilic background.

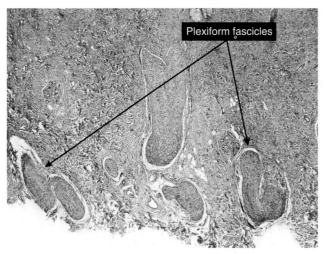

Fig. VIC2.e

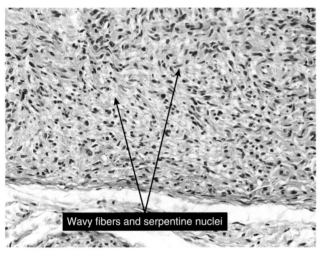

Fig. VIC2.g

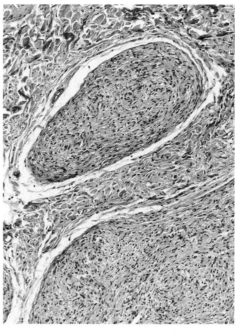

Fig. VIC2.f

Fig. VIC2.e. *Plexiform neurofibroma, medium power.* There are plexiform tangles of neural tissue with slight retraction from the background matrix. The background matrix shows typical changes of a neurofibroma.

Fig. VIC2.f. *Plexiform neurofibroma, medium power.* The plexiform tangles resemble large nerves. The background shows spindled cells in an eosinophilic matrix.

Fig. VIC2.g. *Plexiform neurofibroma, high power.* Close inspection of the nodular aggregates reveal wavy spindled cells with small uniform nuclei. There are scattered mast cells.

most schwannomas are asymptomatic, but pain, localized to the tumor or radiating along the nerve of origin, can be a complaint.

HISTOPATHOLOGY. Schwannomas are intraneural and symmetrically expansile. They are confined by the perineurium of the nerve of origin and displace and compress the endoneurial matrix. Most of the symmetrically bundled nerve fibers of the nerve of origin are displaced eccentrically between the tumor and the perineurium. Two variant patterns, namely Antoni A and Antoni B types, have been described. In the Antoni type A tissue, uniform spindle cells are arranged back to back, and each cell is outlined by delicate, rigid reticular fibers (basement membranes). The cells tend to cluster in stacks, and the respective nuclei tend to form palisades. Two neighboring palisades, the intervening cytoplasms of Schwann cells, and associated reticular fibers, all constitute a Verocay body. In Antoni type B tissue, files of elongated Schwann cells, arranged end to end, and individual Schwann cells are loosely spaced in a clear, watery matrix. Clusters of dilated, congested vessels with hyalinized walls, thrombi, and subendothelial collections of foam cells are represented in both Antoni A and Antoni B tissue. Cystic changes, extravasated erythrocytes, and hemosiderin deposits are variable features.

Palisaded Encapsulated Neuroma

See Figs. VIC2.k–m.

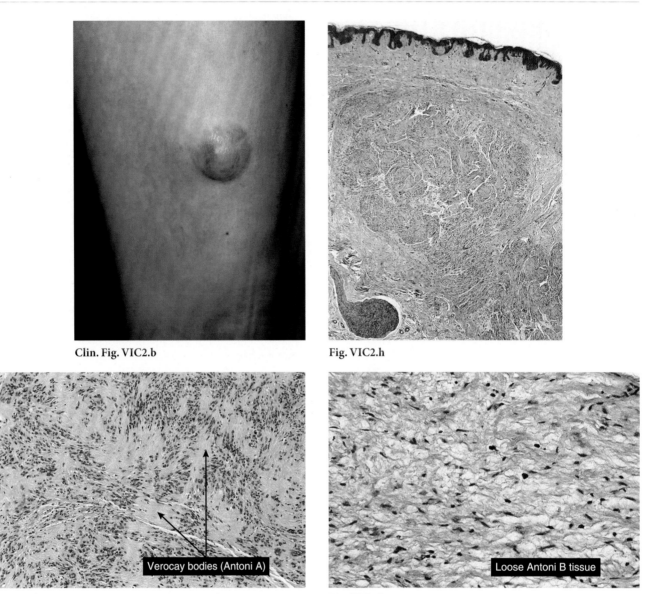

Clin. Fig. VIC2.b

Fig. VIC2.h

Fig. VIC2.i

Fig. VIC2.j

Clin. Fig. VIC2.b. *Schwannoma.* A reasonably symmetrical firm nodule that grew slowly on the thigh since childhood in a 48-year-old woman.

Fig. VIC2.h. *Schwannoma (neurilemmoma), low power.* Within the dermis there is a relatively well-circumscribed, but nonencapsulated cellular neoplasm. The overlying epidermis is unremarkable.

Fig. VIC2.i. *Schwannoma (neurilemmoma), medium power.* In this area of the neurilemmoma the Antoni type A tissue shows Verocay body formation where the nuclei of the spindle cells are aligned in parallel arrays.

Fig. VIC2.j. *Schwannoma (neurilemmoma), medium power.* In the Antoni type B tissue, Schwann cells are loosely spaced in a clear, watery matrix.

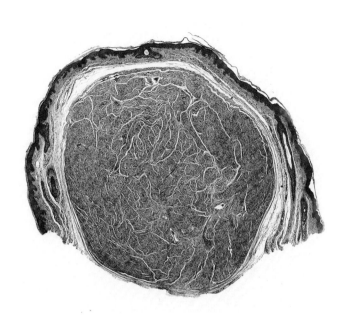

Fig. VIC2.k

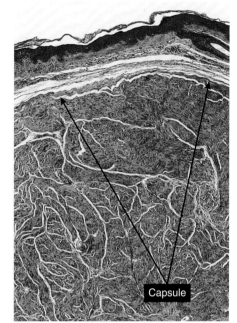

Capsule

Fig. VIC2.l

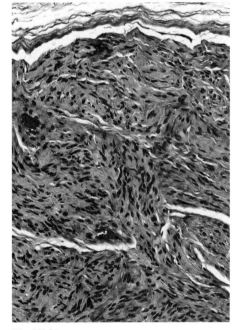

Fig. VIC2.m

Fig. VIC2.k. *Palisaded encapsulated neuroma, low power.* Within the superficial dermis there is a well-circumscribed nodular tumor.

Fig. VIC2.l. *Palisaded encapsulated neuroma, medium power.* This well-circumscribed tumor is surrounded by a thin zone of fibrous connective tissue but despite its name does not always form a true capsule. The tumor is composed of interlacing bundles of neural tissue.

Fig. VIC2.m. *Palisaded encapsulated neuroma, high power.* These bundles are composed of elongate spindled cells which are wavy in appearance. Significant atypia or mitotic activity is not seen. The capsule may stain with epithelial membrane antigen (EMA).

Accessory Digit

See Figs. VIC2.n–p.

Conditions to consider in the differential diagnosis:

neurofibromas
    sporadic cutaneous neurofibroma (common neurofibroma)
    extraneural (common neurofibroma)
    intraneural neurofibroma
    pacinian neurofibroma
neurofibromatosis
    plexiform neurofibroma
    diffuse neurofibroma
nerve sheath tumors
    fibrolamellar nerve sheath tumor
    storiform nerve sheath tumor
      (perineurioma)

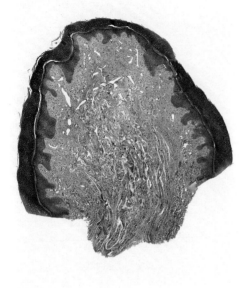

Fig. VIC2.n

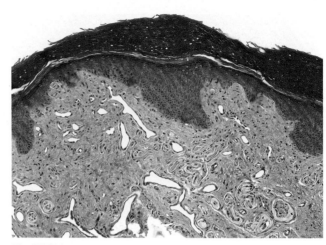

Fig. VIC2.o

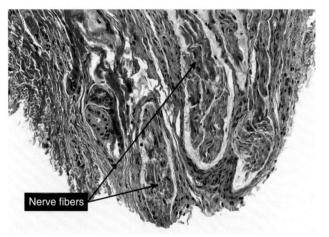

Nerve fibers

Fig. VIC2.p

Fig. VIC2.n. *Accessory digit, low power.* This dome-shaped lesion of acral skin shows mild epidermal hyperplasia.

Fig. VIC2.o. *Accessory digit, low power.* There is increased cellularity and vascularity in the dermis.

Fig. VIC2.p. *Accessory digit, medium power.* At the base of this lesion there are haphazardly arranged bundles of neural tissue.

mature (myxoid) neurothekeoma, nerve sheath myxoma
granular cell nerve sheath tumor (granular cell tumor/schwannoma)
plexiform granular cell nerve sheath tumor
malignant granular cell tumor
extraneural neuromas
traumatic neuroma
intraneural neuromas
palisaded and encapsulated neuroma (PEN)
intraneural plexiform neuroma
mucosal neuroma syndrome
linear cutaneous neuroma
neurilemmomas (schwannomas)
typical schwannoma

cellular schwannoma
atypical schwannoma
transformed (borderline) schwannoma
epithelioid schwannoma
glandular schwannoma
plexiform schwannoma
infiltrating fascicular schwannoma of infancy
malignant schwannomas, intraneural or extraneural
malignant nerve sheath tumor
psammomatous malignant schwannoma
epithelioid malignant schwannoma
miscellaneous
impingement neurofasciitis (Morton neuroma)
accessory digit
ganglioneuroma

VIC3 Spindle Cell Tumors of Muscle

Smooth muscle cells have more abundant cytoplasm than fibroblasts or Schwann cells. The cytoplasm is trichrome positive, and reacts with muscle markers—desmin, muscle-specific actin. The nuclei tend to have blunt ends. In neoplasms, the cells tend to be arranged in whorled bundles.

Leiomyomas

CLINICAL SUMMARY. Five types of leiomyomas of the skin (113) are: (1) multiple piloleiomyomas and (2) solitary piloleiomyomas, both arising from arrectores pilorum muscles; (3) solitary genital leiomyomas, arising from the dartoic, vulvar, or mammillary muscles; (4) solitary angioleiomyomas, arising from the muscles of veins; and (5) leiomyomas with additional mesenchymal elements.

Multiple piloleiomyomas, by far the most common type of leiomyoma, are small, firm, red or brown intradermal nodules arranged in a group or in a linear pattern. Often, two or more areas are affected. Usually, but not always, the lesions are tender and give rise spontaneously to occasional attacks of pain. *Solitary piloleiomyomas* are intradermal nodules that are usually larger than those of multiple piloleiomyomas, measuring up to 2 cm in diameter. Most of them are tender and also occasionally painful. *Solitary genital leiomyomas* are located on the scrotum, the labia majora, or, rarely, the nipples. Their location is

intradermal. In contrast to the other leiomyomas, most genital leiomyomas are asymptomatic. *Solitary angioleiomyomas* are usually subcutaneous. Pain and tenderness are evoked by most, but not all, angioleiomyomas.

HISTOPATHOLOGY. Piloleiomyomas, whether multiple or solitary, and genital leiomyomas are similar in histologic appearance. They are poorly demarcated and are composed of interlacing bundles of smooth muscle fibers within which varying amounts of collagen bundles are intermingled. The muscle fibers composing the smooth muscle bundles are generally straight, with little or no waviness; they contain centrally located, thin, very long, blunt-edged, "eel-like" nuclei. *Angioleiomyomas* differ from the other types of leiomyomas in that they are encapsulated and contain numerous vessels, with only small amounts of collagen as a rule. The numerous veins that are present vary in size and have muscular walls of varying thickness. On this basis, angioleiomyomas have been subdivided into a capillary or solid type, a cavernous type, and a venous type. In the capillary type, the vascular channels are numerous but small.

Smooth Muscle Hamartoma

See Clin. Fig. VIC3.b and Figs. VIC3.g–i.

Leiomyosarcoma

See Figs. VIC3.j–m.

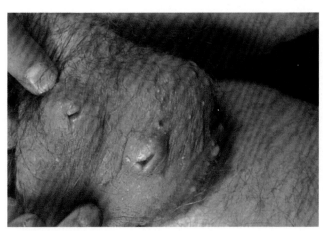

Clin. Fig. VIC3.a

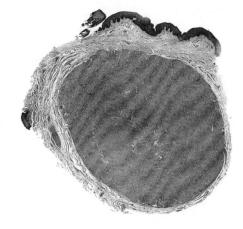

Fig. VIC3.a

Clin. Fig. VIC3.a. *Multiple scrotal leiomyomas.* A 60-year-old man presented with multiple asymptomatic flesh-colored nodules over the scrotum.

Fig. VIC3.a. *Scrotal Leiomyoma, low power.* Within the dermis there is a poorly circumscribed neoplasm which has replaced the pre-existing adnexal structures. The neoplasm is composed of interlacing bundles of eosinophilic material. (*continues*)

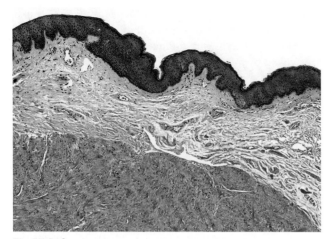

Fig. VIC3.b

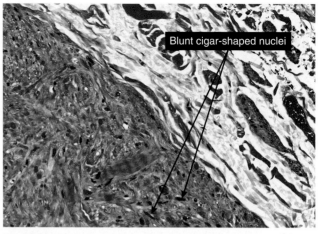

Fig. VIC3.c

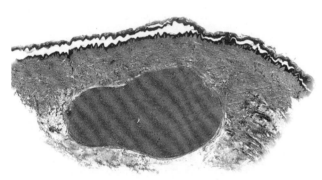

Fig. VIC3.d

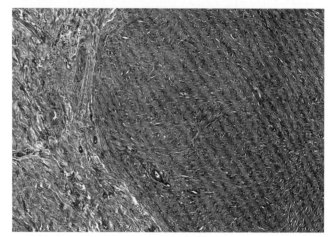

Fig. VIC3.e

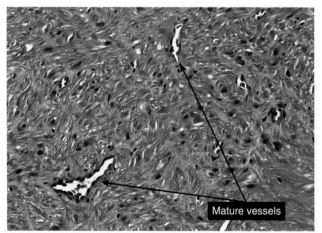

Fig. VIC3.f

Fig. VIC3.b. *Scrotal Leiomyoma, medium power.* At this magnification there are interwoven bundles of spindle cells, many perpendicular to one another. The nuclei are small and bland.

Fig. VIC3.c. *Scrotal Leiomyoma, high power.* The nuclei of smooth muscle are elongate with blunt ends (cigar-shaped). Perinuclear vacuolization is frequently seen in smooth muscle cells.

Fig. VIC3.d. *Angioleiomyoma, low power.* There is a well-circumscribed nodule within the deep dermis or subcutaneous fat. Unlike piloleiomyoma, the lesion is sharply separated from the surrounding normal tissue.

Fig. VIC3.e. *Angioleiomyoma, medium power.* There are only a few dilated vascular channels within this proliferation of smooth muscle.

Fig. VIC3.f. *Angioleiomyoma, high power.* The nuclei are elongate with blunt ends and there may be perinuclear vacuolization.

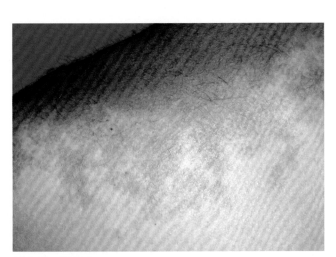

Clin. Fig. VIC3.b

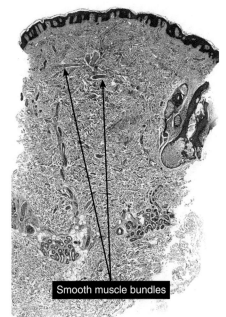

Smooth muscle bundles

Fig. VIC3.g

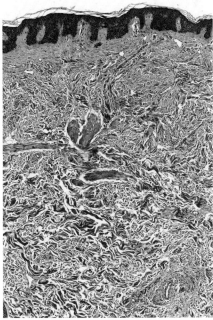

Fig. VIC3.h

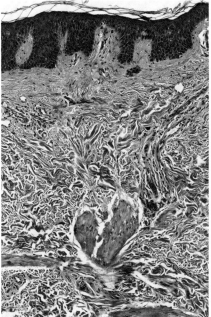

Fig. VIC3.i

Clin. Fig. VIC3.b. *Becker nevus.* This tan patch with feathery borders and terminal hairs became most evident during puberty. Histologically, there is often an associated smooth muscle hamartoma.

Fig. VIC3.g. *Becker nevus/smooth muscle hamartoma, low power.* The epidermis is slightly hyperplastic. Within the dermis there is an increased number of smooth muscle bundles. The smooth muscle bundles do not form a solid aggregate as they do in a leiomyoma.

Fig. VIC3.h. *Becker nevus/smooth muscle hamartoma, medium power.* The bundles of smooth muscle are separated from one another by intervening normal collagen.

Fig. VIC3.i. *Becker nevus/smooth muscle hamartoma, medium power.* The overlying epidermis shows slightly elongate rete ridges and diffuse basal layer hyperpigmentation. There are scattered small melanocytes without formation of nests.

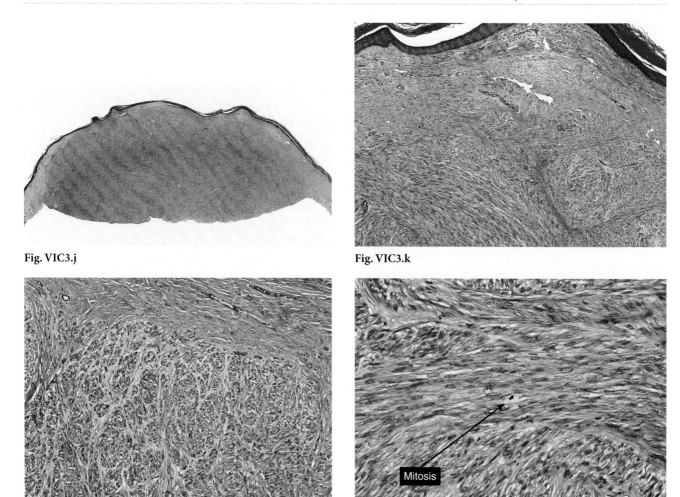

Fig. VIC3.j

Fig. VIC3.k

Fig. VIC3.l

Fig. VIC3.m

Fig. VIC3.j. *Leiomyosarcoma, low power.* The dermis has been replaced by a highly cellular spindle cell neoplasm. There is no association with the overlying epidermis. This superficial tumor should have an excellent prognosis.

Fig. VIC3.k. *Leiomyosarcoma, medium power.* The tumor has an infiltrative border.

Fig. VIC3.l. *Leiomyosarcoma, medium power.* The neoplasm is composed of spindled cells which form interlocking bundles, a similar pattern to what was seen in a leiomyoma. However, even at this power, the lesion is more cellular (more nuclei are visible).

Fig. VIC3.m. *Leiomyosarcoma, high power.* The individual cells are large and spindled in form. The nuclei are atypical and mitotic figures are requisite for the diagnosis. The nuclei in this case show the typical cigar shape that is seen in the benign leiomyoma, but this is not always the case. The differential diagnosis includes malignant melanoma, squamous cell carcinoma, and atypical fibroxanthoma. Generally, immunoperoxidase stains are required for definitive diagnosis. An immunoperoxidase stain for smooth muscle actin was positive, and stains for S-100 protein, high– and low–molecular-weight keratins as well as histiocyte markers were negative in this tumor.

Conditions to consider in the differential diagnosis:

leiomyoma
angioleiomyoma
superficial leiomyosarcoma
infantile myofibromatosis
solitary myofibroma

dermatomyofibroma
benign mixed mesodermal proliferations
malignant mesenchymal tumors of uncertain
    origin
smooth muscle hamartoma
rhabdomyosarcoma

VIC4 | Melanocytic Spindle Cell Tumors

Melanocytic spindle cell tumors may have many attributes of schwannian tumors described above. S100 is positive, and HMB45 is often negative in the spindle cell melanomas. Diagnosis of melanoma then depends on recognizing melanocytic differentiation—pigment synthesis, or a characteristic intraepidermal *in situ* or microinvasive component.

Desmoplastic Melanoma

CLINICAL SUMMARY. Desmoplastic melanoma (114) presents attributes of melanocytic, fibroblastic, and Schwannian differentiation, often mixed within a single lesion. Desmoplasia is most often observed in a spindle cell VGP of lentigo maligna melanoma or acral lentiginous melanoma. The clinical presentation is therefore that of the *in situ* or microinvasive RGP component. However, desmoplastic changes are occasionally seen in tumors with rounded or undifferentiated melanoma cells. Although the reported survival rate for desmoplastic melanoma is poor, this is because many of the cases reported in the earlier literature had already recurred at the time the diagnoses were made. However, the probability of survival is relatively good for prospectively diagnosed and definitively treated desmoplastic melanoma, because, despite the considerable thickness of many of these lesions, the prognostically important mitotic rate and tumor-infiltrating lymphocyte responses are often favorable. "Mixed" desmoplastic melanomas, which by definition have a >10% component of epithelial differentiation,

have a significantly worse prognosis; in a recent study 5 of 23 mixed but none of 17 pure desmoplastic melanomas had positive sentinel nodes (115).

HISTOPATHOLOGY. The collagen in pure desmoplastic melanoma is arranged as delicate fibrils that extend among the tumor cells and separate them from one another. In mixed tumors there is a component of >10% of the tumor in which the cells, which may be spindled or epithelioid, are in continuity with each other in nests, fascicles or sheets. The tumor cells in desmoplastic areas are typically spindle-shaped and tend not to exhibit high-grade nuclear atypia. The mitotic rate is often very low or even zero. A characteristic feature is the presence of clusters of tumor-infiltrating lymphocytes within the tumor. The cells tend to be arranged in "wavy" fiber bundles which may recall the "schwannian" patterns of neurofibromas, neurotized nevi, and malignant schwannomas, and may lead to diagnostic error. Because the melanoma cells are usually elongated and amelanotic and are embedded in a markedly fibrotic stroma, the tumors may simulate a fibromatosis or a fibrohistiocytic lesion. Staining with S-100 or Sox10 antibody usually marks many of the spindle-shaped cells, indicating that they are not fibroblastic. The HMB-45 and Melan-A antigens are not usually demonstrable in desmoplastic melanomas, although they will often react with the epithelial component of "mixed" desmoplastic melanomas (116). The most convincing evidence that many of the tumors are melanomas may come from examination of the overlying

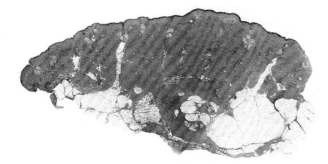

Fig. VIC4.a

Fig. VIC4.a. *Desmoplastic melanoma, low power.* There is a spindle cell proliferation throughout the dermis. It is associated with increased collagen production, a feature which may suggest a diagnosis of a dermatofibroma or a fibromatosis.

Fig. VIC4.b. *Desmoplastic melanoma, medium power.* These lesions are generally not diagnosed early and therefore most lesions are relatively thick extending to the deep reticular dermis or subcutaneous fat. (*continues*)

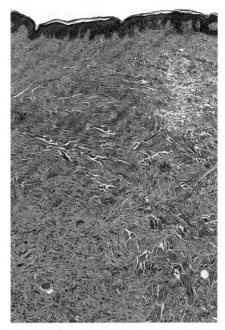

Fig. VIC4.b

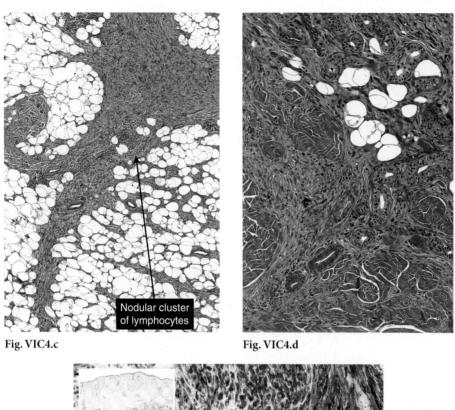

Fig. VIC4.c

Fig. VIC4.d

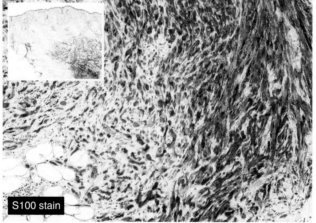

Fig. VIC4.e

Fig. VIC4.c. *Desmoplastic melanoma, high power.* The spindle cells are haphazardly arranged and scattered cells show enlarged hyperchromatic nuclei. Nodular clusters of lymphocytes are commonly present.

Fig. VIC4.d. *Desmoplastic melanoma, high power.* Desmoplastic melanoma may mimic a neural tumor and it frequently shows neurotropism with spindle cells extending in and around small cutaneous nerves. The neurotropism is frequently associated with a lymphocytic infiltrate.

Fig. VIC4.e. *Desmoplastic melanoma, S100 stain.* An S100 stain highlights neoplastic spindle cells infiltrating deep reticular dermis and fat. Note the partially "pure" pattern of single cells at the bottom left of the image, and the epithelial pattern of sheets of cells at the top right.

intraepidermal component, where diagnostic changes of microinvasive or *in situ* melanoma may be seen, usually of the lentigo maligna, acral or mucosal lentiginous types. Electron microscopy may or may not demonstrate melanosomes, often after prolonged searching, and is of little or no diagnostic utility.

Conditions to consider in the differential diagnosis:

desmoplastic melanoma, including amelanotic
cellular blue nevus, amelanotic
blue nevus, amelanotic
desmoplastic Spitz nevus
spindle cell metastatic melanoma

VIC5 | Tumors and Proliferations of Angiogenic Cells

There is a dermal proliferation of vascular endothelium. CD31 and Factor VIII staining may be helpful in demonstrating endothelial differentiation. D2-40 is a specific marker for lymphatic endothelium (117). The many variants of benign hemangiomas and lymphangiomas should be carefully considered in the differential diagnosis of Kaposi sarcoma and angiosarcoma.

Pyogenic Granuloma (Lobular Capillary Hemangioma)

CLINICAL SUMMARY. Pyogenic granuloma (118) is a common proliferative lesion that often occurs shortly

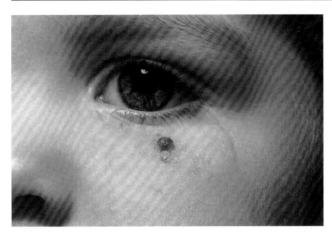

Clin. Fig. VIC5.a

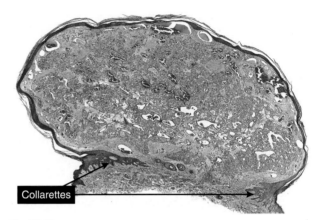

Collarettes

Fig. VIC5.a

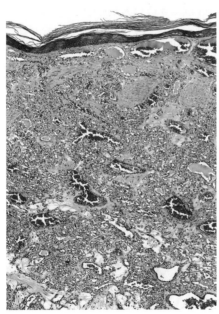

Fig. VIC5.b

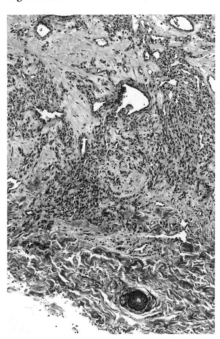

Fig. VIC5.c

Clin. Fig. VIC5.a. *Pyogenic granuloma.* A child suddenly developed a single dark red bleeding papule.

Fig. VIC5.a. *Pyogenic granuloma, low power.* Pyogenic granulomas show a dome-shaped nodular architecture which sits above the level of the skin surface. The epidermis shows a flattened effaced rete ridge architecture.

Fig. VIC5.b. *Pyogenic granuloma, medium power.* At the edge of the neoplasm, the epidermis focally extends underneath the vascular proliferation forming a collaret.

Fig. VIC5.c. *Pyogenic granuloma, medium power.* There are lobular aggregates of small mature vascular channels filled with erythrocytes. These aggregates are separated by a fibrous stroma in long-standing lesions. This intervening stroma can be very edematous and mucinous in early lesions.

after a minor injury or infection of the skin. Typically, the lesion grows rapidly for a few weeks before stabilizing as an elevated, bright red papule, usually not more than 1 to 2 cm in size; it then may persist indefinitely unless destroyed. Recurrence after surgery or cautery is not rare. Pyogenic granuloma most often affects children or young adults of either gender, but the age range is wide; the hands, fingers, and face, especially the lips and gums, are the most common sites. Pyogenic granuloma of the gingiva in pregnancy (epulis of pregnancy) is a special subgroup. A rare and alarming event is the development of multiple satellite angiomatous lesions at and around the site of a previously destroyed pyogenic granuloma.

HISTOPATHOLOGY. The typical lesion presents as a polypoid mass of angiomatous tissue protruding above the surrounding skin, and often constricted at its base by a collaret of acanthotic epidermis. An intact flattened epidermis may cover the entire lesion, but surface erosions are common. In ulcerated lesions a superficial inflammatory cell reaction can give rise to an appearance suggestive of granulation tissue, but inflammation is usually slight in the deeper part of the lesion and may be absent when the epidermis is intact. The angiomatous tissue tends to occur in discrete masses or lobules, and is composed of a variably dilated network of blood-filled capillary vessels and groups of poorly canalized vascular tufts. Mitotic activity varies and can be prominent. Feeding vessels often extend into the adjacent dermis and rare lesions show a deep component in the reticular dermis.

Intravascular Papillary Endothelial Hyperplasia (Masson's Hemangioendotheliome Vegetant Intravasculaire)

CLINICAL SUMMARY. This not uncommon condition is an unusual endothelial proliferation in an organizing thrombus that can be misdiagnosed as angiosarcoma (119). The lesion arises primarily within a venous channel or secondarily within a preceding angioma or some type of vascular anomaly, including hemorrhoids, or extravascularly in association with a hematoma. The lesions are almost always solitary, arising in the skin, subcutaneous tissue, or even muscle with the head and neck region, and the upper extremities, especially the fingers the most common sites. Primary lesions are usually tender nodules less than 2 cm in size, whereas secondary lesions occur because some preceding vascular abnormality increases in size.

HISTOPATHOLOGY. Often, low-power examination allows recognition of the intravascular nature of the process in a single thin-walled vein or as part of a preceding angiomatous condition. Extravascular lesions fail to reveal a blood vessel wall despite serial sectioning. The main lesion consists of a mass of anastomosing vascular channels with a variable degree of intraluminal papillary projections. The stroma consists of hyalinized eosinophilic material that may merge with uncanalized thrombus remnants. The infiltrating vascular channels show enlarged and prominent endothelial cells that may be "heaped up" to give rise to intraluminal prominences, but atypia and mitotic activity are slight.

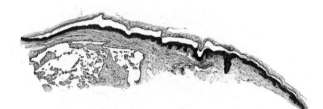

Fig. VIC5.d

Fig. VIC5.d. *Intravascular papillary endothelial hyperplasia, low power.* There are several dilated cystic spaces which show papillary fronds within the lumen of the channels.

Fig. VIC5.e. *Intravascular papillary endothelial hyperplasia, medium power.* The cystic spaces as well as the papillary fronds are all lined by a single layer of endothelial cells. Because of the papillary nature the fronds appear as small islands floating within a pond. The endothelial cells fail to reveal cytologic atypia. Residual thrombus material may be visible.

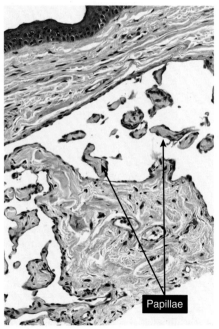

Fig. VIC5.e

Stasis Dermatitis With Vascular Proliferation (Acroangiodermatitis, Pseudo-Kaposi Sarcoma)

CLINICAL SUMMARY. Patients with long-standing venous insufficiency and lower-extremity edema may develop pruritic, erythematous, scaly papules and plaques on the lower legs, often in association with brown pigmentation and hair loss.

HISTOPATHOLOGY. The epidermis is hyperkeratotic with areas of parakeratosis, acanthosis, and focal spongiosis. There is a superficial, perivascular lymphohistiocytic infiltrate that surrounds plump, thickened capillaries and venules. The superficial dermal vessels may be arranged in lobular aggregates. The proliferation may be florid, mimicking Kaposi sarcoma (acroangiodermatitis) (120). The reticular dermis is often fibrotic. Hemosiderin is usually present superficially but may be identified about the deep vascular plexus as well.

Kaposi Sarcoma

CLINICAL SUMMARY. Kaposi sarcoma (121,122) can be classified into four groups. *Classic Kaposi sarcoma* is rare, affecting mainly patients of Eastern European and Mediterranean origin, and occurs in male patients over the age of 50 with the slow development of angiomatous nodules and plaques on the lower extremities. *Kaposi sarcoma in Africa* is very common with a higher proportion of young people affected, and with a more aggressive disease manifested by widespread tumors, deep infiltrative or elevated fungating lesions, and bone involvement. *AIDS-associated Kaposi sarcoma* occurs especially in active homosexuals. The clinical features differ from the classic disease in the more rapid evolution of the lesions, their atypical distribution affecting the trunk, and a greater tendency to mucosal involvement. *Kaposi sarcoma associated with iatrogenic immunosuppression* occurs in the context of organ transplantation-related immunosuppression, and may regress on discontinuation of the therapy. Kaposi sarcoma is associated with immune dysregulation associated with HHV8 infection leading to production of cytokines that induce activation of endothelial cells leading to spindle cell formation and angiogenesis. The process may spread to multiple sites through spread of virally-infected cells. The early lesions appear to be reactive polyclonal proliferations that can progress over time to frankly malignant sarcomatous lesions (65). Whether this lesion qualifies as a true sarcoma is a matter of debate. The term "HHV8–associated vascular proliferation" has been proposed as a synonym (123).

The histologic spectrum can be divided into stages roughly corresponding to the clinical type of lesion: early and late macules, plaques, nodules, and aggressive late lesions.

HISTOPATHOLOGY. In early macules there is usually a patchy, sparse, upper dermal perivascular infiltrate

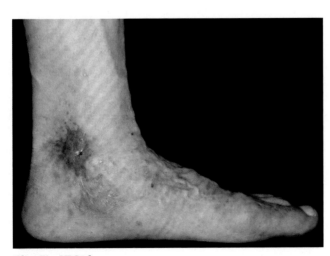

Clin. Fig. VIC5.b

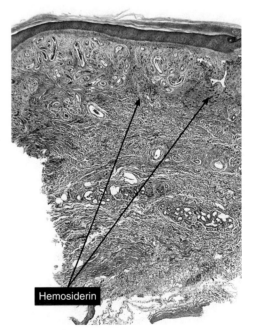

Fig. VIC5.f

Clin. Fig. VIC5.b. *Stasis dermatitis.* An indurated, brawny, asymmetrical scaly plaque on the lower extremity in a 48-year-old man with a history of long-standing varicose veins.

Fig. VIC5.f. *Stasis dermatitis with vascular proliferation, low power.* Within the superficial dermis there is a proliferation of vascular channels associated with dermal pigment deposition. (*continues*)

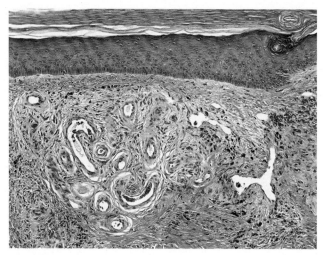

Fig. VIC5.g

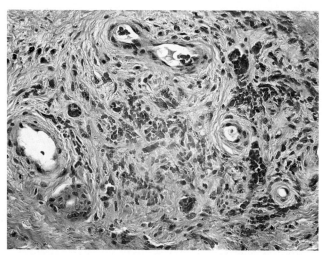

Fig. VIC5.h

Fig. VIC5.g. *Stasis dermatitis with vascular proliferation, medium power.* The vascular channels are mature and have thick walls. They form clusters within the superficial dermis. There is prominent pigment surrounding these vascular channels secondary to hemosiderin deposition. The overlying epidermis may or may not show spongiotic changes.

Fig. VIC5.h. *Stasis dermatitis with vascular proliferation, high power.* Surrounding the small vascular channels is extravasation of erythrocytes.

consisting of lymphocytes and plasma cells. Narrow cords of cells, with evidence of luminal differentiation, are insinuated between collagen bundles. Usually a few dilated irregular or angulated lymphatic-like spaces lined by delicate endothelial cells are also present. Vessels with "jagged" outlines tending to separate collagen bundles are especially characteristic. Normal adnexal structures and pre-existing blood vessels often protrude into newly formed blood vessels, a finding known as the "promontory sign." In late macular lesions there is a more extensive infiltrate of vessels in the dermis, with "jagged" vessels and with cords of thicker-walled vessels similar to those in granulation tissue. At this stage, red blood cell extravasation and siderophages may be encountered (see IIIA1c).

In the plaque stage a diffuse infiltrate of small blood vessels extends through most parts of the dermis and tends to displace collagen. The vessels vary in morphology, some occurring as poorly canalized cords, some as blood-containing ovoid vessels, and some having lymphatic-like features. Loosely distributed spindle cells, arranged in short fascicles, are also encountered. Intracytoplasmic hyaline globules, seen more often in lesions from patients with AIDS, may be found in areas of denser infiltrate.

In the tumor stage, well-defined nodules composed of vascular spaces and spindle cells replace dermal collagen. These tumor nodules tend to be compartmentalized by dense bands of fibrocollagenous tissue. Dilated lymphatic spaces can also be seen between tumor aggregates. The characteristic feature is a honeycomb-like network of blood-filled spaces or slits, closely associated with interweaving spindle cells. The presence of a closely set honeycomb-like pattern of "back-to-back" vascular spaces is an important diagnostic feature of Kaposi sarcoma. In the vascular spaces of pyogenic granuloma and most angiomas, the endothelial cells of the capillary walls are more prominent and the vessels are set farther apart by intervening stroma. Blood pigment–containing macrophages are nearly always prominent adjacent to the nodules, especially in lesions at dependent sites. The spindle cells in the nodules are elongated and fusiform with a well-defined cytoplasm. Their nuclei are ovoid and somewhat flattened with finely granular chromatin in the long axis of the cells. Nucleoli are generally inconspicuous and nuclear atypia is absent or slight. Mitosis is infrequent. Prominent and consistent positivity for CD34 is seen in the spindle cell population.

Aggressive late stage "infiltrating" lesions, mostly in African Kaposi sarcoma, show a more obviously sarcomatous character with reduction or loss of the vascular component. The spindle cells demonstrate a greater degree of cytologic atypia with regard to size, shape, and nuclear features, with mitosis becoming frequent. In such lesions, phagocytozed erythrocytes and the presence of hyaline globules may provide clues about the tumor's origin.

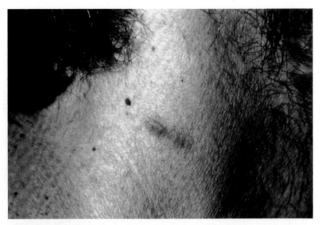

Clin. Fig. VIC5.c

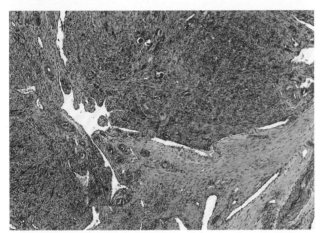

Fig. VIC5.j

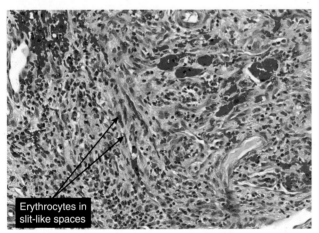

Erythrocytes in
slit-like spaces

Fig. VIC5.l

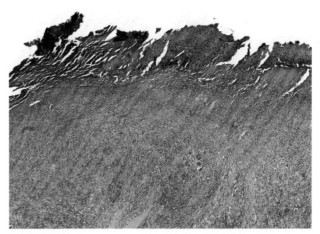

Fig. VIC5.i

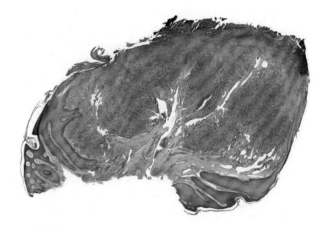

Fig. VIC5.k

Clin. Fig. VIC5.c. *Kaposi sarcoma, plaque and early nodule.* An HIV-positive man developed an elongated erythematous nodule.

Fig. VIC5.i. *Kaposi sarcoma, nodular type, low power.* In nodular (tumor stage) Kaposi sarcoma there is a mass of spindle cells within the dermis. This lesion is ulcerated.

Fig. VIC5.j. *Kaposi sarcoma, medium power.* The spindle cells fail to reveal an organized pattern. The tumor is highly cellular and occasionally the hemorrhage can be seen at scanning magnification.

Fig. VIC5.k. *Kaposi sarcoma, high power.* The spindled cells show enlarged nuclei and erythrocytes are seen between tumor cells. Occasionally, one can identify intracytoplasmic pink droplets (not shown).

Fig. VIC5.l. *Kaposi sarcoma, high power.* An infiltrate of plasma cells is frequently seen in Kaposi sarcoma. Red cells are present in slit-like spaces between the tumor cells and interstitially. HHV-8 staining (not shown) is helpful in establishing the diagnosis.

Diffuse Dermal Angiomatosis

CLINICAL SUMMARY. Diffuse dermal angiomatosis is a reactive vascular proliferation under the larger category of reactive angioendotheliomatosis (124). While this latter category generally implies an intraluminal proliferation of endothelial cells, diffuse dermal angiomatosis characteristically is a proliferation of vessels within the dermis. It was initially described in patients with severe atherosclerotic disease (125), however it is also associated with arteriovenous

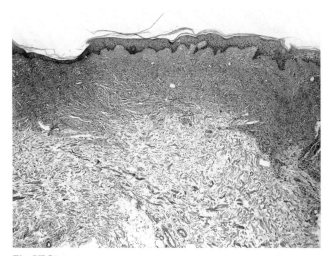

Fig. VIC5.m

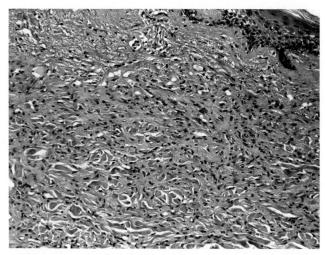

Fig. VIC5.n

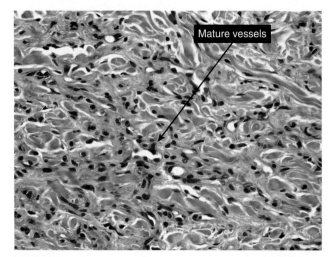

Mature vessels

Fig. VIC5.o

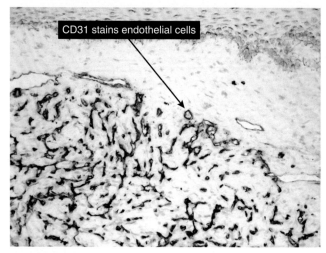

CD31 stains endothelial cells

Fig. VIC5.p

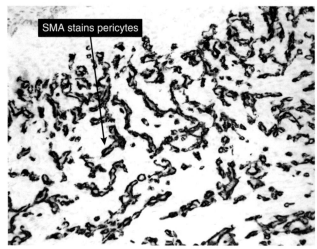

SMA stains pericytes

Fig. VIC5.q

Fig. VIC5.m. *Diffuse dermal angiomatosis, low power.* There is a cellular proliferation in the papillary and upper reticular dermis which is not associated with the overlying epidermis.

Fig. VIC5.n. *Diffuse dermal angiomatosis, medium power.* The cellular areas are composed of numerous spindle cells.

Fig. VIC5.o. *Diffuse dermal angiomatosis, high power.* The spindle cells are small and bland in appearance. They form small vascular channels.

Fig. VIC5.p. *Diffuse dermal angiomatosis, medium power, CD31 immunoperoxidase stain.* CD31 highlights the spindle cells as well as the formation of small vascular channels.

Fig. VIC5.q. *Diffuse dermal angiomatosis, medium power, smooth muscle actin immunoperoxidase stain.* A stain for smooth muscle actin highlights the pericyte component of the spindle cell proliferation.

fistulas of hemodialysis and anticardiolipin antibodies. Patients present with firm violaceous or hyperpigmented plaques. Lesions of the extremities are more common than those on axial areas. The lesions may be painful and frequently ulcerate. In patients who have severe atherosclerotic disease, bypass grafting to correct the vascular insufficiency may lead to resolution of the ulcers. The vascular proliferation seen in diffuse dermal angiomatosis is hypothesized to be secondary to ischemia, which may induce vascular endothelial growth factor or endothelial cell hyperplasia produced by small thrombi.

HISTOPATHOLOGY. Within the upper and mid-dermis there is a highly cellular proliferation of small bland-appearing spindle cells which upon close inspection form vascular spaces which contain erythrocytes (126). There may be a sparse mononuclear cell infiltrate. The spindle cells stain positively with endothelial markers CD31 and CD34. Smooth muscle actin is also strongly positive in the associated pericyte layer of spindle cells. Unlike angiosarcoma, the spindle cells are bland and lack cytologic atypia. Additionally, the vascular channels are well formed allowing one to eliminate the possibilities of angiosarcoma and Kaposi sarcoma. HHV8 staining has been described in lesions not judged to represent Kaposi sarcoma. Acroangiodermatitis, which can be associated with venous insufficiency, also shows well-formed channels. However, this entity shows associated dermal fibrosis, mixed inflammation, and extravasation of erythrocytes frequently with hemosiderin deposition.

Cutaneous Angiosarcoma

CLINICAL SUMMARY. Most angiosarcomas of the skin (127) arise in the following clinical settings: (1) angiosarcoma of the face and scalp in the elderly, (2) angiosarcoma (lymphangiosarcoma) secondary to chronic lymphedema, and (3) angiosarcoma as a complication of chronic radiodermatitis or arising from the effects of severe skin trauma or ulceration. In a 2011 study of 98 cases from a single institution, tumors were classified histologically as vasoformative (44%), spindled (21%), epithelioid (16%), and mixed (18%). The median time to death was 2.1 years, with vasoformative tumors having a somewhat less rapid progression of disease (128).

Angiosarcoma of the scalp and face of the elderly is almost invariably a fatal tumor that usually arises as seemingly innocuous erythematous or bruise-like lesions on the scalp or middle and upper face with predilection for men. Subsequent plaques, nodules, or ulcerations develop; metastasis to nodes or internal organs usually arises as a late complication with many patients dying as a result of extensive local disease. Angiosarcoma following lymphedema (postmastectomy lymphangiosarcoma or the Stewart–Treves syndrome) presents in women who have had severe long-standing lymphedema of the arm following

breast surgery, but has also been described in men and from causes other than cancer surgery, including congenital lymphedema and tropical lymphedema due to filaria. The prognosis despite radical surgery is extremely poor. Postirradiation angiosarcoma may arise in the skin after radiotherapy for internal cancer. The most common sites are the breast or chest wall and the lower abdomen after therapy for breast or gynecologic cancer.

HISTOPATHOLOGY. Usually the tumor extends well beyond the limits of the apparent clinical lesion. As a rule, the tumor shows varied differentiation in different biopsies, even within different fields in a single biopsy. In well-differentiated areas, irregular anastomosing vascular channels lined by a single layer of somewhat enlarged endothelial cells permeate between collagen bundles. Isolation and enclosure of collagen bundles, figuratively referred to as "dissection of collagen," is a characteristic feature. Nuclear atypia is always present and may be slight to moderate, but occasional large hyperchromatic cells may be encountered. At this stage the vascular lumens are generally bloodless, but they may contain free-lying shed malignant cells. In less well-differentiated areas endothelial cells increase in size and number, forming intraluminal papillary projections where there is enhanced mitotic activity. In poorly differentiated areas, solid sheets of large pleomorphic cells with little or no evidence of luminal differentiation, can resemble metastatic carcinoma or melanoma. Focally, areas showing epithelioid cells are not uncommon. Other areas may simulate a poorly differentiated spindle cell sarcoma. Interstitial hemorrhage and widely dilated blood-filled spaces may sometimes develop.

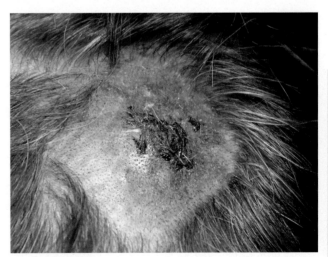

Clin. Fig. VIC5.d

Clin. Fig. VIC5.d. *Cutaneous angiosarcoma*. A 66-year-old man with a 5-month history of a multinodular ulcerated and bleeding tumor arising in a plaque-like hemorrhagic background in the skin of the scalp. (*continues*)

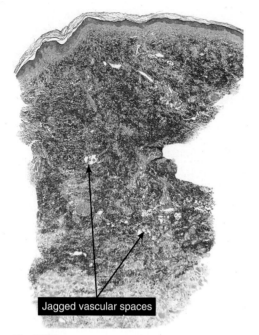

Fig. VIC5.r

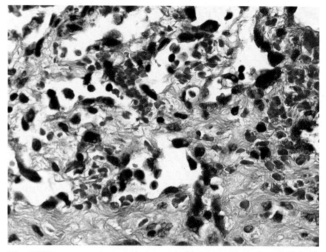

Fig. VIC5.s

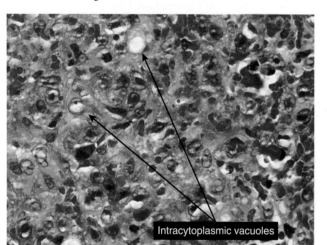

Fig. VIC5.t

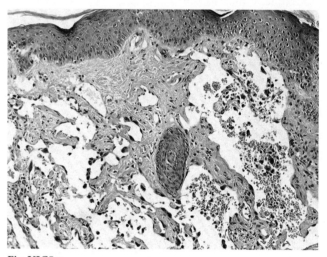

Fig. VIC5.u

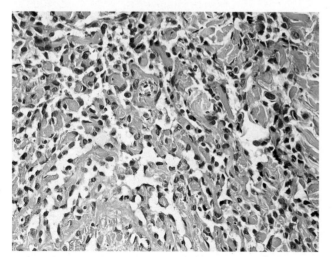

Fig. VIC5.v

Fig. VIC5.r. *Cutaneous angiosarcoma, low power.* The architecture of the dermis is replaced by hemorrhagic tissue within which subtle jagged spaces can be seen.

Fig. VIC5.s. *Cutaneous angiosarcoma, high power.* Jagged spaces containing erythrocytes and lined by plump, hyperchromatic endothelial cells. This pattern of dissection throughout the reticular dermal collagen is typical of angiosarcoma.

Fig. VIC5.t. *Cutaneous angiosarcoma, high power.* A population of more epithelioid angiosarcoma cells, with intracytoplasmic vacuoles as a clue to endothelial differentiation.

Fig. VIC5.u. *Cutaneous angiosarcoma, high power.* Another example, with jagged spaces lined by atypical endothelial cells.

Fig. VIC5.v. *Cutaneous angiosarcoma, high power.* A characteristic pattern of infiltration among reticular dermis collagen fibers.

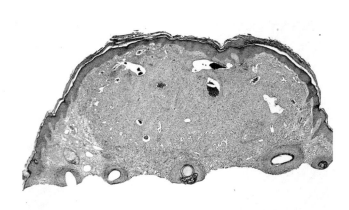

Fig. VIC5.w

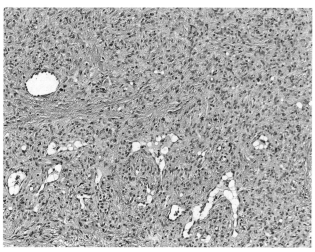

Fig. VIC5.x

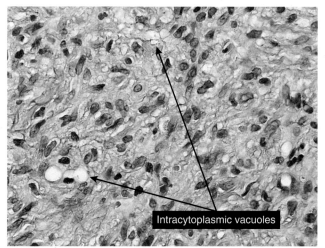

Intracytoplasmic vacuoles

Fig. VIC5.y

Fig. VIC5.w. *Epithelioid hemangioendothelioma, low power.* There is a relatively well circumscribed but nonencapsulated dome-shaped lesion within the dermis. The epidermis is uninvolved and shows an effaced rete ridge pattern.

Fig. VIC5.x. *Epithelioid hemangioendothelioma, medium power.* The neoplasm is composed of a solid sheet of uniform, bland-appearing cells associated with small dilated vascular channels which contain erythrocytes.

Fig. VIC5.y. *Epithelioid hemangioendothelioma, high power.* The cells contain an abundance of cytoplasm and show intracytoplasmic vacuoles. There may be scattered erythrocytes between the cells, with interstitial hemorrhage. Although significant cytologic atypia is not present, these lesions may have an uncertain prognosis.

Cutaneous Epithelioid Angiomatous Nodule/ Epithelioid Hemangioendothelioma

Cutaneous epithelioid angiomatous nodule is an uncommon vascular proliferation, which presents histologically as a well-circumscribed, mainly unilobular, solid proliferation of endothelial cells with prominent epithelioid features. The cytoplasm is abundant and eosinophilic, and many of the neoplastic cells contain prominent vacuoles. Inflammatory infiltrates are variable. There may be overlap with epithelioid hemangioendothelioma which is a low-grade malignancy, however all the cases reported to date have followed a benign course (129).

Targetoid Hemosiderotic Hemangioma (Hobnail Hemangioma)

CLINICAL SUMMARY. Targetoid hemosiderotic hemangioma is a benign acquired vascular lesion that presents as a macule with central papule or solitary macule on the trunk or extremities of young- to middle-aged adults (130,131). It can have a varied clinical appearance, mimicking a melanocytic nevus, particularly a dysplastic nevus, dermatofibroma, Kaposi sarcoma, or even a melanoma. Though not present in the majority of cases, the "classic" clinical morphology is that of a pale, erythematous, or ecchymotic ring measuring 1 to 2 cm with a central red, violaceous, or brown papule measuring 2 to 3 mm, resulting in a targetoid appearance. It is believed to represent a reactive vascular ectasia rather than a true neoplasm, and trauma may be a predisposing factor. A history of waxing and waning with respect to size and color is common, and a changing morphology with the menstrual cycle has been reported.

HISTOPATHOLOGY. The histologic appearance may also mimic malignant conditions such as Kaposi sarcoma

VI Tumors and Cysts of the Dermis and Subcutis

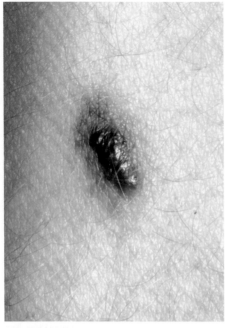

Clin. Fig. VIC5.e

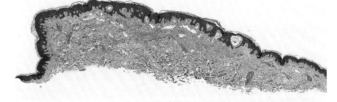

Fig. VIC5.z

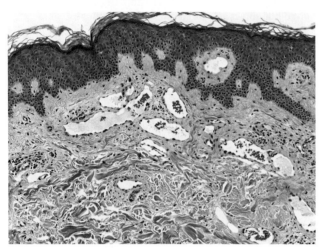

Fig. VIC5.za

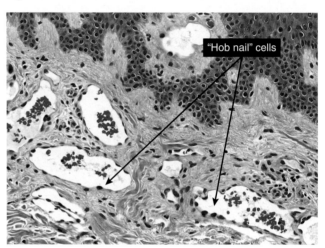

Fig. VIC5.zb

Clin. Fig. VIC5.e. *Targetoid hemosiderotic hemangioma.* Note the violaceous papule (the bull's eye) surrounded by an erythematous halo.

Fig. VIC5.z. *Targetoid hemosiderotic hemangioma, low power.* Dilated blood vessels are present in the upper dermis. In the reticular dermis, vessels are often flatter and extend interstitially, resulting in a wedge-shaped architecture. Extravasated red blood cells are present around vessels.

Fig. VIC5.za. *Targetoid hemosiderotic hemangioma, medium power.* Somewhat flattened vessels dissect between collagen in the reticular dermis. There is an inflammatory component made up mostly of lymphocytes. Red blood cell extravasation can be extensive, and later lesions will show hemosiderin within macrophages, not seen here.

Fig. VIC5.zb. *Targetoid hemosiderotic hemangioma, high power.* Dilated vascular channels are characteristically lined by hobnail endothelial cells with nuclei that protrude into the lumen.

or angiosarcoma. Telangiectatic blood-filled vessels are present in the papillary dermis or superficial reticular dermis, becoming flattened vascular spaces that dissect between collagen bundles with deeper, wedge-shaped extension into the reticular dermis and thus potentially mimicking angiosarcoma. The endothelial cells lining the vessels are bland, but may have rounded nuclei which project into vascular lumina and resemble hobnails, hence the alternate designation for this lesion. Superficial vessels may also contain fibrin thrombi and papillary projections. Vascular channels in the deeper dermis are often irregular and jagged, with subtle lumina lined by low endothelial cells. Extravasated red blood cells may be present and prominent, and later lesions will often show hemosiderin-laden macrophages. A lymphocytic inflammatory infiltrate can be seen.

Conditions to be considered in the differential diagnosis:

> Angiosarcoma
> Kaposi sarcoma
> Acroangiodermatitis
> Other forms of angioendotheliomatosis

Angiokeratoma

See Clin. Fig. VIC5.f and Figs. VIC5.zc,zd.

Arteriovenous Hemangioma

See Figs. VIC5.ze,zf.

Cavernous Hemangioma

See Figs. VIC5.zg,zh.

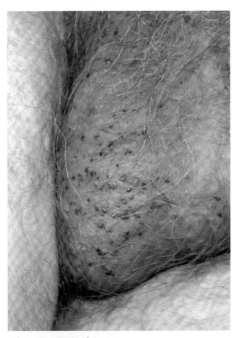

Clin. Fig. VIC5.f

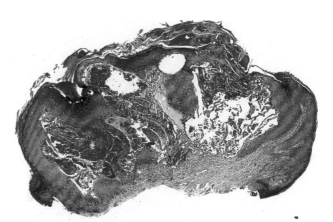

Fig. VIC5.zc

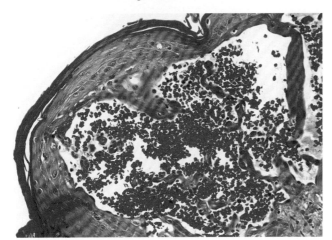

Fig. VIC5.zd

Clin. Fig. VIC5.f. *Angiokeratoma.* These small purplish papules are commonly found on the scrotum.

Fig. VIC5.zc. *Angiokeratoma, low power.* There is a vascular proliferation predominantly within the papillary dermis. The associated epidermis is hyperplastic and appears to encircle the vascular channels.

Fig. VIC5.zd. *Angiokeratoma, medium power.* The vascular channels are thin walled and lined by mature endothelial cells. They are filled with erythrocytes. The hyperplastic epithelium surrounds these vascular channels and occasionally it may appear that the vascular channels are within the epithelium.

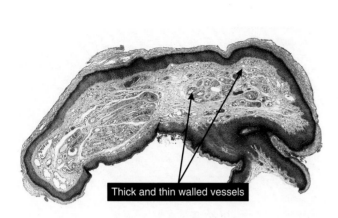

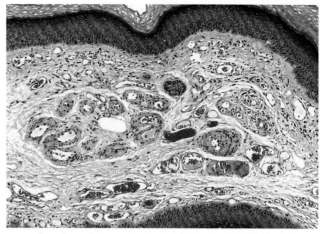

Fig. VIC5.ze

Fig. VIC5.zf

Fig. VIC5.ze. *Arteriovenous hemangioma, low power.* There is a well-circumscribed vascular proliferation within the superficial dermis.

Fig. VIC5.zf. *Arteriovenous hemangioma, medium power.* The vascular proliferation is composed of mature thick- and thin-walled vascular channels filled with erythrocytes.

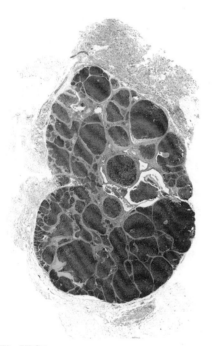

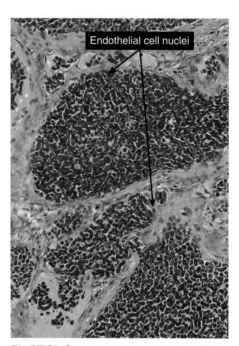

Fig. VIC5.zg

Fig. VIC5.zh

Fig. VIC5.zg. *Cavernous hemangioma, low power.* Within the deep dermis and subcutaneous tissue there is a proliferation of vascular channels filled with erythrocytes. All cavernous hemangiomas are not as well circumscribed as this example.

Fig. VIC5.zh. *Cavernous hemangioma, medium power.* The vascular channels show thin-walled endothelial cells without atypia. The channels are filled with erythrocytes.

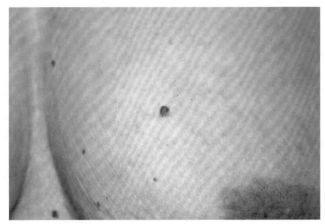

Clin. Fig. VIC5.g

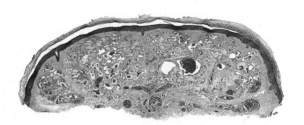

Fig. VIC5.zi

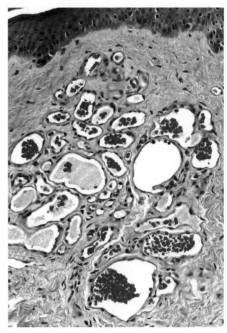

Fig. VIC5.zj

Clin. Fig. VIC5.g. *Cherry hemangioma.* A 66-year-old woman had a 5-year history of small symmetrical red papules on the chest.

Fig. VIC5.zi. *Cherry hemangioma, low power.* This dome-shaped papular lesion shows a vascular proliferation within the superficial dermis.

Fig. VIC5.zj. *Cherry hemangioma, medium power.* There is a proliferation of thin-walled mature vascular channels filled with erythrocytes. The associated stroma may be edematous or fibrotic.

Cherry Hemangioma

See Clin. Fig. VIC5.g and Figs. VIC5.zi,zj.

Microvenular Hemangioma

These benign acquired lesions typically occur as small, enlarging lesions often on the forearm or leg in an adult. Clinically, they are purple to red lesions usually considered to be hemangiomas. Histologically, there are irregular, branching venules with inconspicuous lumina. There is no cytologic atypia (132).

Cutaneous Lymphangioma

See Clin. Fig. VIC5.h and Figs. VIC5.zn,zo.

Venous Lake

See Clin. Fig. VIC5.i and Figs. VIC5.zp,zq.

Glomangioma

See Clin. Fig. VIC5.j and Figs. VIC5.zr–zt.

Glomus Tumor

See Figs. VIC5.zu–zw.

Conditions to consider in the differential diagnosis:

hyperplasias
   intravascular papillary endothelial hyperplasia
   reactive angioendotheliomatosis
   angiolymphoid hyperplasia with eosinophilia
angiomas
   juvenile hemangioendothelioma (strawberry nevus)
   cherry hemangioma
   glomeruloid hemangioma
   tufted angioma (angioblastoma)
   angiokeratoma
   cavernous hemangioma
   sinusoidal hemangioma
   verrucous hemangioma
   microvenular hemangioma
   targetoid hemosiderotic (hobnail) hemangioma
   cirsoid aneurysm (A-V hemangioma)
   epithelioid hemangioma

VI

Tumors and Cysts of the Dermis and Subcutis

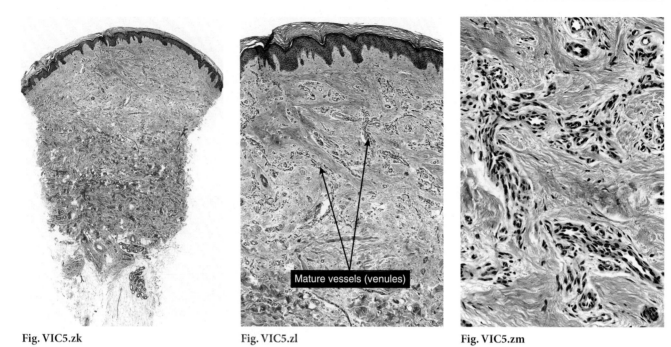

Fig. VIC5.zk   **Fig. VIC5.zl**   **Fig. VIC5.zm**

Fig. VIC5.zk. *Microvenular hemangioma, low power.* At scanning magnification there is increased cellularity throughout the reticular dermis.

Fig. VIC5.zl. *Microvenular hemangioma, medium power.* There is a proliferation of small venules throughout the reticular dermis without formation of lobular aggregates. No large vascular spaces are seen.

Fig. VIC5.zm. *Microvenular hemangioma, high power.* The vessels are all mature small venules without atypia. There is an associated fibrotic stroma.

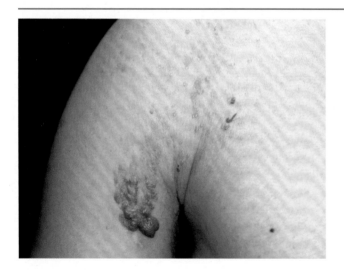

Clin. Fig. VIC5.h

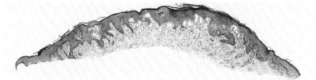

Fig. VIC5.zn

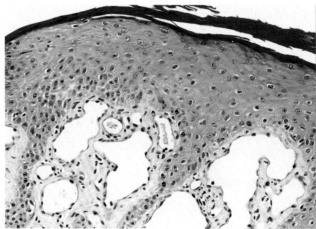

Fig. VIC5.zo

Clin. Fig. VIC5.h. *Cutaneous lymphangioma ("lymphangioma circumscriptum").* A 19-year-old man had a 10-year history of multiple papules filled with clear fluid, sometimes slightly tinged with blood.

Fig. VIC5.zn. *Cutaneous lymphangioma ("lymphangioma circumscriptum"), low power.* There are multiple dilated vascular channels within the papillary dermis extending into the superficial reticular dermis.

Fig. VIC5.zo. *Cutaneous lymphangioma, medium power.* In the papillary dermis these vascular channels are lined by a thin wall consisting only of endothelial cells. Amorphous material may be seen within the lumen. Erythrocytes, however, are not present within the vascular channels.

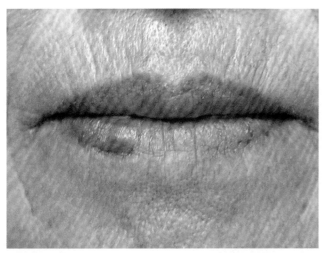

Clin. Fig. VIC5.i

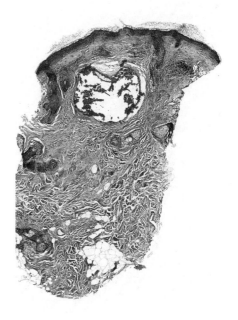

Fig. VIC5.zp

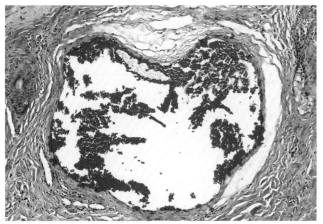

Fig. VIC5.zq

Clin. Fig. VIC5.i. *Venous lake.* A 67-year-old woman has an easily compressible blood-filled cystic papule on the lower lip, which refills promptly after compression.

Fig. VIC5.zp. *Venous lake, low power.* In the superficial dermis there is a vascular dilatation composed of solitary or occasionally few dilated vascular spaces.

Fig. VIC5.zq. *Venous lake, medium power.* The dilated vascular channel is lined by a thin endothelial wall with a few pericytes.

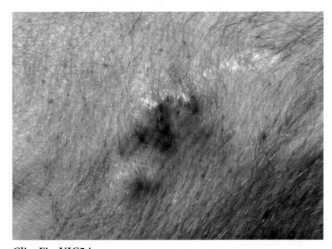

Clin. Fig. VIC5.j

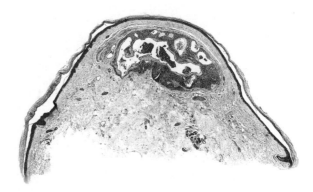

Fig. VIC5.zr

Clin. Fig. VIC5.j. *Glomangioma.* These compressible, purplish nodules on the extremity can be inherited in an autosomal dominant fashion.

Fig. VIC5.zr. *Glomangioma, low power.* In the deep reticular dermis there is a neoplasm composed of multiple cystic-like spaces lined by a thickened wall. (*continues*)

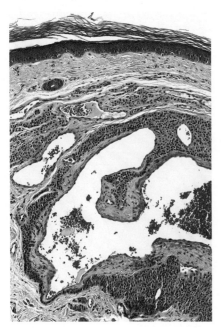

Fig. VIC5.zs

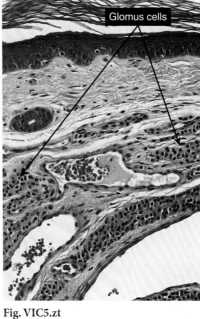

Fig. VIC5.zt

Fig. VIC5.zs. *Glomangioma, medium power.* The cystic spaces are lined by several layers of small cuboidal cells.

Fig. VIC5.zt. *Glomangioma, medium power.* Another area of the glomangioma showing cystic spaces lined by cuboidal glomus cells. The individual cells are monotonously bland and lack cytologic atypia. Erythrocytes may be seen in the cavernous spaces.

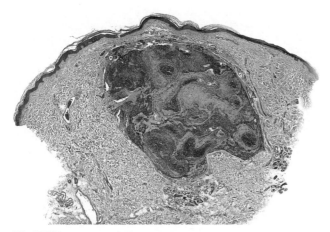

Fig. VIC5.zu

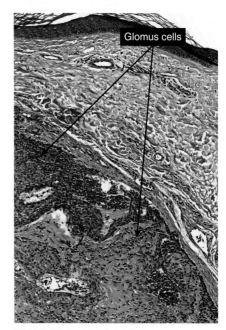

Fig. VIC5.zv

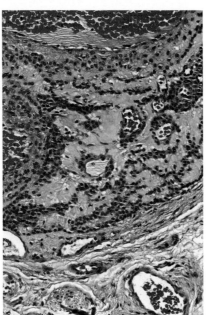

Fig. VIC5.zw

Fig. VIC5.zu. *Glomus tumor, low power.* This biopsy shows a cellular tumor in the deep dermis. In contrast to a glomangioma, fewer vascular channels are seen, and glomus cells in sheets are the predominant feature.

Fig. VIC5.zv. *Glomus tumor, high power.* There are both thin cords and solid areas of tumor composed of uniform cuboidal cells with small round nuclei.

Fig. VIC5.zw. *Glomus tumor, high power.* The tumor is composed of uniform cuboidal cells with small round nuclei.

pyogenic granuloma
bacillary angiomatosis
lymphangiomas
cavernous lymphangioma and cystic hygroma
lymphangioma circumscriptum
progressive lymphangioma (benign lymphangioen-
dothelioma)
lymphangiomatosis
telangiectases
hereditary hemorrhagic telangiectasia
spider nevus
venous lakes
vascular malformations
angioma serpiginosum
glomus tumors
glomus tumor, glomangioma, glomangiomyoma
infiltrating glomus tumor
glomangiosarcoma
vascular lipomas
angiomyolipoma
angiolipoma
angiosarcomas
cutaneous angiosarcoma
epithelioid angiosarcoma
Kaposi sarcoma
Kaposi sarcoma simulants (see also angiomas)
aneurysmal fibrous histiocytoma
spindle cell hemangioendothelioma
Kaposi-like infantile hemangioendothelioma
acroangiodermatitis (pseudo-Kaposi sarcoma)
multinucleate cell angiohistiocytoma
hemangioendotheliomas
epithelioid hemangioendothelioma
retiform hemangioendothelioma
malignant endovascular papillary angioendotheli-
oma (Dabska tumor)
spindle cell hemangioendothelioma
Kaposi-like infantile hemangioendothelioma
other vascular tumors
diffuse dermal angioendotheliomatosis
angiomatosis
hemangiopericytoma
intravascular lymphoma (malignant angioendotheliomatosis)

VIC6 **Tumors of Adipose Tissue**

Most tumors of adipose tissue occur in the subcutis or
deeper soft tissues, but some may involve the skin. The
lesional cells may range from mature adipocytes indistinguishable from those of mature fat in typical lipomas,
to more or less undifferentiated round cells or pleomorphic cells in the high-grade liposarcomas. Nevus
lipomatosus superficialis is a lipomatous neoplastic or
hamartomatous disorder that primarily involves the
skin (133).

Nevus Lipomatosus Superficialis

CLINICAL SUMMARY. Nevus lipomatosus superficialis is
a fairly uncommon lesion which may present as groups of
soft, flattened papules or nodules that have smooth or wrinkled surfaces and are skin-colored or pale yellow. Characteristically, the lesions are linearly distributed on one hip or
buttock (nevus lipomatosus superficialis of Hoffman and
Zurhelle), from where they may overlap onto the adjacent
skin of the back or the upper thigh. Other areas, such as the
thorax or the abdomen, are only rarely affected. The lesions
may be present at birth or may begin in infancy (nevus
angiolipomatosus of Howell), in which case the replacement of hypoplastic dermis may cause pseudotumorous
yellow protrusions and be associated with skeletal and
other malformations, but they develop most commonly
during the first two decades of life and occasionally later.
Multiple lesions may coalesce. Solitary lesions may be diagnosed as nevus lipomatosus superficialis, or as solitary,
baglike, soft fibromas or polypoid fibrolipomas. The rather
common presence of fat cells within long-standing intradermal melanocytic nevi represents an involutionary phenomenon and not a nevus lipomatosus.

HISTOPATHOLOGY. Groups and strands of fat cells are
found embedded among the collagen bundles of the dermis, often as high as the papillary dermis. The proportion
of fatty tissue varies greatly. In cases with only small
deposits, the fat cells are apt to be situated in small foci
around the subpapillary vessels. In instances with relatively large amounts of fat, the fat lobules are irregularly
distributed throughout the dermis, and the boundary
between the dermis and the hypoderm is ill-defined or
lost. The fat cells may all be mature, but in some instances
an occasional small, incompletely lipidized cell may be
observed. Aside from the presence of fat cells, the dermis
may be entirely normal, but in some instances the density
of the collagen bundles, the number of fibroblasts, and the
vascularity are greater than in normal skin.

Lipoma

By definition, lipomas contain mature adipocytes as a principal component. They tend to be located in the subcutis
and surrounded by a thin connective tissue capsule and are
composed, often entirely, of normal fat cells that are indistinguishable from the fat cells in the subcutaneous tissue.

Angiolipoma

Angiolipomas usually occur as encapsulated subcutaneous
lesions. As a rule, they arise in young adults. The forearm
is the single most common location for this tumor, which
is more often multifocal than solitary. They are often tender or painful. Inapparent at the gross level, angiolipomas
microscopically show sharp encapsulation, numerous
small-caliber vascular channels containing characteristic

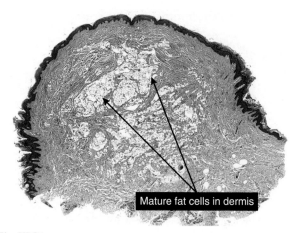

Fig. VIC6.a

Mature fat cells in dermis

Fig. VIC6.a. *Nevus lipomatosus superficialis, low power.* Mature adipose tissue extends up into the reticular dermis. There is no associated inflammatory reaction.

Fig. VIC6.b. *Nevus lipomatosus superficialis, medium power.* Mature adipocytes are seen in the superficial and mid reticular dermis.

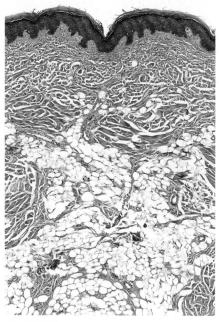

Fig. VIC6.b

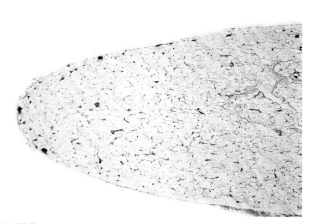

Fig. VIC6.c

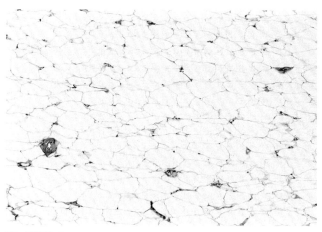

Fig. VIC6.d

Fig. VIC6.c. *Lipoma, low power.* This circumscribed neoplasm shows a very thin fibrous capsule. Lipomas reside in the subcutaneous fat. At scanning magnification, the lesion is hypocellular.

Fig. VIC6.d. *Lipoma, high power.* A lipoma is composed of uniform adipocytes which are approximately of equal size. The small nucleus is pushed to the side of the cell and is barely visible.

microthrombi, and variable amounts of mature adipose tissue. The degree of vascularity is quite variable, ranging from only a few small angiomatous foci to lesions with a predominance of dense vascular and stromal tissue.

Spindle Cell Lipoma

Clinically, the tumor is a slowly growing, painless nodule centered in the dermis or subcutis and exhibiting a predilection for the posterior neck and shoulder girdle region in men in their sixth decade. Although the lesion is well circumscribed histologically, it is seldom encapsulated. It is comprised of mature fat cells and uniform, slender spindle cells within a mucinous matrix. Spindle cell lipoma is polymorphous as a result of variations in cellularity, collagen content, and the ratio of spindle cells to mature adipocytes.

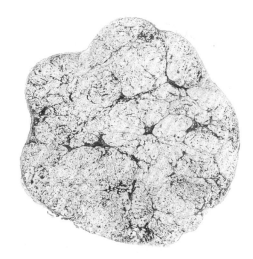

Fig. VIC6.e

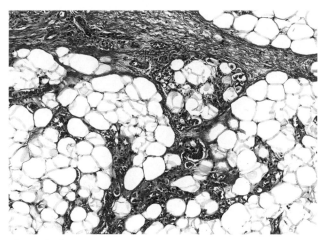

Fig. VIC6.f

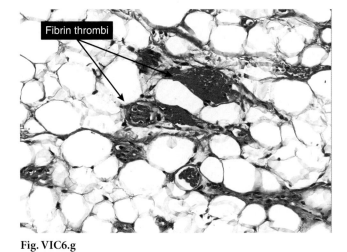

Fig. VIC6.g

Fig. VIC6.e. *Angiolipoma, low power.* Similar to a lipoma, an angiolipoma is a well-circumscribed subcutaneous mass with a very thin fibrous capsule. However, in contrast, this lesion is more cellular than the one seen in Figure VIC6.c.

Fig. VIC6.f. *Angiolipoma, medium power.* The increased cellularity in angiolipomas is secondary to a proliferation of small mature vascular channels filled with erythrocytes and fibrin thrombi.

Fig. VIC6.g. *Angiolipoma, high power.* Multiple fibrin thrombi are frequently found in the small vessels of an angiolipoma.

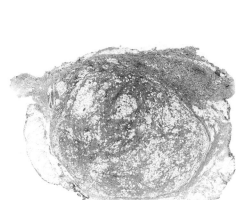

Fig. VIC6.h

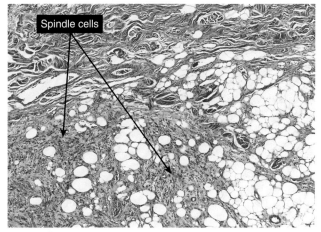

Fig. VIC6.i

Fig. VIC6.h. *Spindle cell lipoma, low power.* At scanning magnification this tumor is composed of cellular areas as well as hypocellular areas.

Fig. VIC6.i. *Spindle cell lipoma, medium power.* The hypocellular areas are mature adipocytes. In the hypercellular areas there is a proliferation of bland-appearing spindle cells. (*continues*)

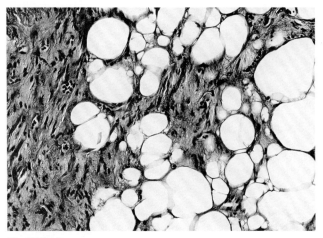

Fig. VIC6.j

Fig. VIC6.j. *Spindle cell lipoma, high power.* The spindle cells are wavy in appearance but lack cytologic atypia. The associated stroma is frequently mucinous and there are scattered mast cells.

Pleomorphic Lipoma

CLINICAL SUMMARY. Like spindle cell lipomas, the great majority of pleomorphic lipomas are solitary tumors of the shoulder girdle and neck in men in the fifth to seventh decade. The lesion presents as a slowly growing, well-circumscribed dermal or subcutaneous mass grossly resembling an ordinary lipoma. Despite occasional lipoblast-like cells and atypical mitotic figures, local excision should be curative.

DIFFERENTIAL DIAGNOSIS. No single feature confirms the diagnosis of pleomorphic lipoma and excludes liposarcoma. Only a multivariate analysis leads to the correct diagnosis, and such an analysis should consider (1) the age and sex of the patient, (2) anatomic location, (3) size, (4) epicenter of growth (deep or superficial), (5) degree of local invasion, and (6) histologic appearance. Liposarcomas differ from pleomorphic lipomas by their infiltrative growth, greater cellularity, more nuclear atypicality including atypical mitoses, more numerous multivacuolated lipoblasts, prominent necrosis, and absence of thick collagen bundles. Floret-type giant cells are rarely seen in liposarcomas, and then only in small numbers.

Liposarcoma

Liposarcomas are large tumors of the deep subcutis or deeper soft tissue. As such, they rarely come to the attention of the dermatopathologist.

Conditions to consider in the differential diagnosis:

lipomas
spindle cell lipoma
pleomorphic lipoma
chondroid lipoma
angiolipoma

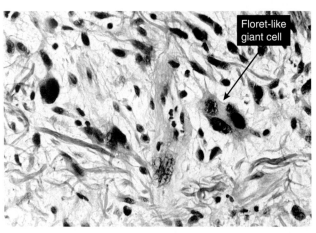

Fig. VIC6.k

Fig. VIC6.k. *Pleomorphic lipoma, high power.* These are usually subcutaneous tumors. Mature and immature fat cells are situated singly and in groups in a mucinous stroma traversed by dense collagen bundles. Characteristic multinucleated giant cells, found in most but not all cases, exhibit multiple, marginally placed, and often overlapping hyperchromatic nuclei within an eosinophilic cytoplasm. This peculiar arrangement is not unlike that of the petals of a small flower, and these giant cells are therefore referred to as *floret-type giant cells.*

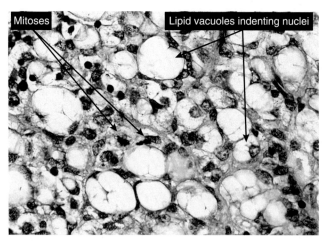

Fig. VIC6.l

Fig. VIC6.l. *Liposarcoma, round cell type, high power.* This is a large, poorly circumscribed tumor without a defined capsule. Although in some areas one can identify adipocytes, other areas are very cellular. Admixed with the adipocytes are larger cells with large hyperchromatic nuclei many of which contain vacuoles many of which indent the nucleus, creating a delicate scalloping of the nuclear membrane (monovacuolar and multivacuolar lipoblasts). Mitotic figures are also seen.

liposarcomas
   well-differentiated
   atypical lipomatous tumor
   myxoid
   round cell
   pleomorphic
miscellaneous
   hibernoma
   benign lipoblastoma
   nevus lipomatosus superficialis

VIC7 | Tumors of Cartilaginous Tissue

Most tumors of cartilaginous tissue occur in the bones and joints or in the deep soft tissues, but some may involve the skin. The lesional cells may range from mature chondrocytes indistinguishable from those of mature cartilage in an enchondroma, to more or less undifferentiated round cells or pleomorphic cells in a high-grade chondrosarcoma. Because of their location, these tumors come to the attention of the dermatopathologist only rarely.

Conditions to consider in the differential diagnosis:

   chondroid lipoma
   soft tissue chondroma
   chondrosarcoma

VIC8 | Tumors of Osseous Tissue

Metaplastic ossification, disturbances of calcium metabolism, and presumably other poorly-understood mechanisms including hereditary abnormalities may lead to local areas of calcification and also to focal or diffuse ossification in the dermis.

Albright's Hereditary Osteodystrophy and Osteoma Cutis

In Albright's hereditary osteodystrophy (AHO), multiple areas of subcutaneous or intracutaneous ossification are often encountered (134). These may be present at birth or may arise later in life, and have no definite area of predilection. The areas may be small or large (5 cm). Those located in the skin may cause ulceration, and bony spicules may be extruded through the ulcer. In addition to cutaneous and subcutaneous osteomas, bone formation may be observed in some cases along fascial planes. AHO includes the syndromes of pseudohypoparathyroidism and pseudopseudohypoparathyroidism. Patients with AHO have short stature, round facies, and multiple skeletal abnormalities, such as curvature of the radius and shortening of some of the metacarpal bones. As a result of this shortening, some knuckles are absent when the fists are clenched, and depressions or dimples are apparent there instead. This important diagnostic sign is referred to as the Albright dimpling sign. Additional manifestations include basal ganglia calcification and mental retardation. The mode of inheritance is dominant, possibly X-linked dominant.

The term *osteoma cutis* is applied to cases of primary cutaneous ossification in which there is no evidence of AHO in either the patients or their families. The lesions may present as a solitary or even multiple tumor-like lesions. Clinically inapparent incidental small foci of ossification are commonly seen within the dermis or stroma in other lesions, such as melanocytic nevi or acne scars. The possibility of AHO should be seriously considered in patients with extensive foci of ossification.

HISTOPATHOLOGY. Spicules of bone of various sizes may be found within the dermis or in the subcutaneous tissue. The bone contains fairly numerous osteocytes as well as cement lines that may be accentuated in polarized light. In addition, there are osteoblasts along the surface of the spicules and often, osteoclasts in Howship lacunae. The spicules of bone may enclose, either partially or completely, areas of mature fat cells, representing establishment of a medullary cavity. Hematopoietic elements are observed rarely among the fat cells. The histologic findings in osteoma cutis are the same as in primary cutaneous ossification occurring in conjunction with Albright's hereditary osteodystrophy.

Conditions to consider in the differential diagnosis:

   Albright's hereditary osteodystrophy
   osteoma cutis
   metaplastic ossification
   subungual exostosis

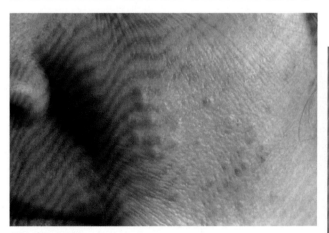

Clin. Fig. VIC8

Clin. Fig. VIC8. *Multiple cutaneous osteomas.* A 50-year-old woman developed multiple 2–3 mm flesh-colored and slightly erythematous firm papules on the cheeks. (*continues*)

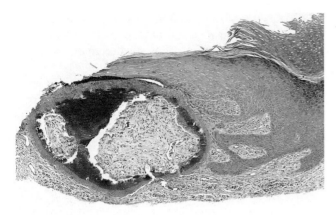

Fig. VIC8.a

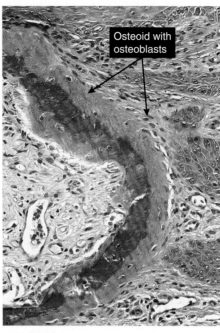

Osteoid with osteoblasts

Fig. VIC8.a. *Osteoma cutis, low power.* Within the superficial dermis there is a well-circumscribed zone of eosinophilic to purplish material.

Fig. VIC8.b. *Osteoma cutis, medium power.* Eosinophilic bone shows numerous osteocytes. There is an associated fibrovascular stroma.

Fig. VIC8.b

 CYSTS OF THE DERMIS AND SUBCUTIS

1. Pilar Differentiation
2. Eccrine and Similar Differentiation
3. Apocrine Differentiation

A cyst is a space lined by epithelium; its contents are usually a product of its lining. Some cysts are inclusion or retention cysts of normal structures (hair follicle-related cysts). Others are benign neoplasms. Some malignant neoplasms may be cystic. These tend to be larger and asymmetric, with a poorly circumscribed and infiltrative border. Their epithelial lining is proliferative, with cytologic atypia.

VID1 **Pilar Differentiation**

Cystic proliferations are present in the dermis, these show spaces surrounded by epithelium of follicular origin and differentiation. Keratin is usually seen in the cystic cavity. Associated cells may be sparse or may include lymphocytes and plasma cells.

Epidermal or Infundibular Cyst

CLINICAL SUMMARY. Epidermal cysts (135) are slowly growing, elevated, round, firm, intradermal or subcutaneous tumors that cease growing after having reached 1 to 5 cm in diameter. Most epidermal cysts arise spontaneously in hair-bearing areas most commonly on the face, scalp, neck, and trunk, but occasionally on the palms or soles and occasionally as a result of trauma. Usually a patient has only one or a few epidermal cysts, rarely many. In Gardner syndrome, numerous epidermal cysts occur, especially on the scalp and face.

HISTOPATHOLOGY. Epidermal cysts have a wall composed of true epidermis, as seen on the skin surface and in the infundibulum of hair follicles, the infundibulum being the uppermost part of the hair follicle that extends down to the entry of the sebaceous duct. In young epidermal cysts, several layers of squamous and granular cells can usually be recognized. In older epidermal cysts, the wall often is markedly atrophic, either in some areas or in the entire cyst, and may consist of only one or two rows of greatly flattened cells. The cyst is filled with horny material arranged in laminated layers. When an epidermal cyst ruptures and the contents of the cyst are released into the dermis, a considerable foreign-body reaction with numerous multinucleated giant cells results, forming a *keratin granuloma*. The foreign-body reaction usually causes disintegration of the cyst wall. However, it may lead to a pseudoepitheliomatous proliferation in remnants of the cyst wall, simulating a squamous cell carcinoma. Most epidermal cysts are thought to be retention cysts derived from hair follicles; *epidermal inclusion cysts (EICs)* are less common but may be seen at sites of injury where included epithelium forms into a cyst. For general purposes, the noncommittal term "epidermal cyst" is the most appropriate.

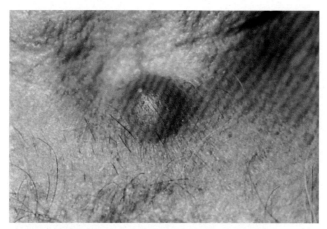

Clin. Fig. VID1.a

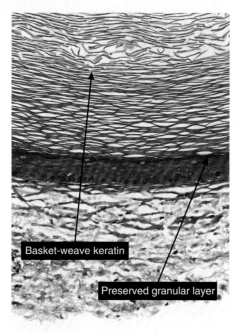

Basket-weave keratin

Preserved granular layer

Fig. VID1.b

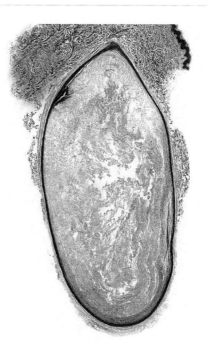

Fig. VID1.a

Clin. Fig. VID1.a. *Epidermal cyst.* An elderly man presented with a firm slowly enlarging asymptomatic flesh-colored nodule on the cheek.

Fig. VID1.a. *Epidermal cyst, low power.* Within the dermis there is a well-circumscribed cystic structure filled with laminated keratin.

Fig. VID1.b. *Epidermal cyst, high power.* The wall of the cyst is composed of mature squamous epithelium with formation of a granular cell layer. The contents of the cyst are composed of laminated ("basket-weave") orthokeratin.

Trichilemmal (Pilar) Cyst

Trichilemmal cysts are also known, especially in surgical terminology, as "sebaceous cysts," however they do not exhibit sebaceous differentiation. They are derived as retention cysts from the lower part of the hair follicle where the hair sheath or "trichilemmal" keratinizes abruptly without an interposed granular layer. The keratin is compact rather than basket weave as in an epidermal cyst.

Steatocystoma

See Clin. Fig. VID1.b and Figs. VID1.e–g.

Vellus Hair Cyst

See Figs. VID1.h,i.

Conditions to consider in the differential diagnosis:

epidermal cyst
milia
trichilemmal cyst
steatocystoma multiplex
pigmented follicular cyst
dermoid cyst
bronchogenic and thyroglossal duct cysts
eruptive vellus hair cyst
pilar sheath acanthoma
dilated pore of Winer

VI Tumors and Cysts of the Dermis and Subcutis

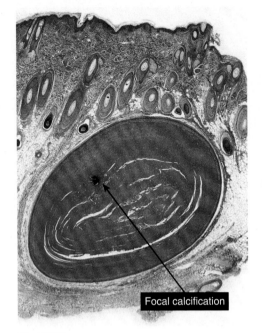

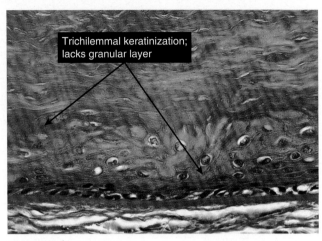

Fig. VID1.c   **Fig. VID1.d**

Fig. VID1.c. *Trichilemmal (pilar) cyst, low power.* In this scalp biopsy there is a well-circumscribed cystic structure in the subcutaneous fat. Focal calcification is present; this is a common incidental finding.

Fig. VID1.d. *Trichilemmal (pilar) cyst, high power.* The wall of the cyst is composed of mature squamous epithelium which shows keratinization without formation of a granular layer.

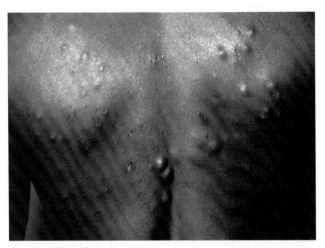

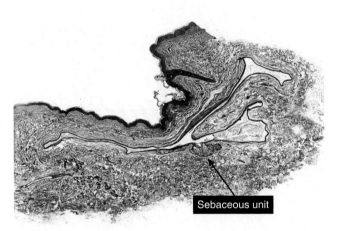

Clin. Fig. VID1.b   **Fig. VID1.e**

Clin. Fig. VID1.b. *Steatocystoma multiplex.* This uncommon autosomal dominant disorder results in the development of multiple, sebum-draining, dermal cysts.

Fig. VID1.e. *Steatocystoma, low power.* Steatocystoma may show a solitary cystic space or a multiloculated appearance with numerous infoldings of the cyst wall.

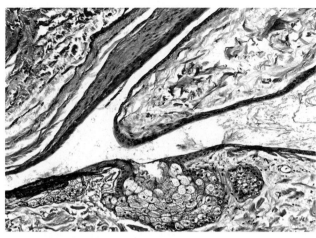

Fig. VID1.f

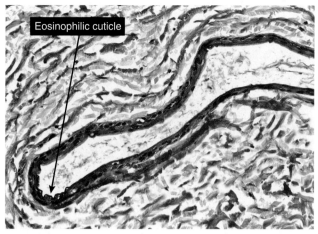

Fig. VID1.g

Fig. VID1.f. *Steatocystoma, medium power.* Mature sebaceous lobules are seen arising from the wall of the cyst.

Fig. VID1.g. *Steatocystoma, high power.* The epithelial wall of the steatocystoma shows a corrugated luminal surface associated with an eosinophilic cuticle.

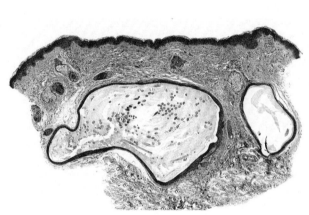

Fig. VID1.h

Fig. VID1.i

Fig. VID1.h. *Vellus hair cyst, low power.* The wall of this cyst is lined by mature squamous epithelium. There may be formation of a granular cell layer, changes indistinguishable from the lining of an epidermal inclusion cyst.

Fig. VID1.i. *Vellus hair cyst, medium power.* There are numerous small (vellus) hair shafts within the cavity of the cyst.

VID2 Eccrine and Similar Differentiation

Cystic proliferations are present in the dermis, these show spaces surrounded by eccrine epithelium (small dark epithelial cells). The epithelium of ciliated and bronchogenic cysts is not eccrine but may resemble that of an eccrine cyst. Eccrine hidrocystoma is the prototype (136).

Eccrine Hidrocystoma

CLINICAL SUMMARY. In this condition, usually one lesion, but occasionally several, and rarely numerous lesions are present on the face. The lesions are small, translucent, cystic nodules 1 to 3 mm in diameter that often have a bluish hue. In some patients with numerous lesions, the number of cysts increases in warm weather and decreases during winter.

HISTOPATHOLOGY. Eccrine hidrocystoma shows a single cystic cavity located in the dermis. The cyst wall usually shows two layers of small, cuboidal epithelial cells. In some areas, only a single layer of flattened epithelial cells can be seen, their flattened nuclei extending parallel

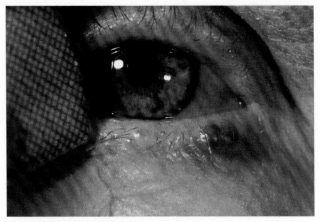

Clin. Fig. VID2

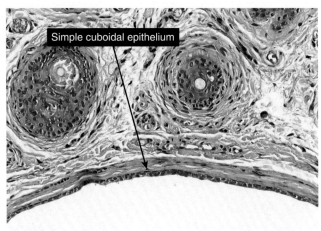

Fig. VID2.a

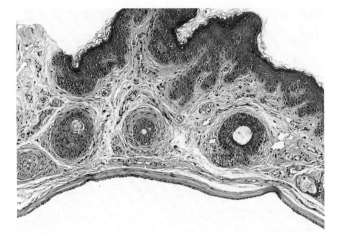

Fig. VID2.b

Simple cuboidal epithelium

Fig. VID2.c

> **Clin. Fig. VID2.** *Eccrine hidrocystoma.* An elderly woman developed compressible blue translucent papules on the lower eyelid.
>
> **Fig. VID2.a.** *Eccrine hidrocystoma, low power.* Multiple sections of a thin-walled cystic structure.
>
> **Fig. VID2.b.** *Eccrine hidrocystoma, low power.* The cyst is located within the dermis and may be empty as here or may be filled with amorphous material.
>
> **Fig. VID2.c.** *Eccrine hidrocystoma, high power.* The wall of the cystic structure is composed of simple cuboidal cells.

to the cyst wall. Small papillary projections extending into the cavity of the cyst are observed only rarely. Eccrine secretory tubules and ducts are often located below the cyst and in close approximation to it, and, on serial sections, one may find an eccrine duct leading into the cyst from below. However, no connection can be found between the cyst and the epidermis.

Median Raphe Cyst

See Figs. VID2.d,e.

Bronchogenic Cyst

The most common location for these very uncommon lesions is the suprasternal notch and presternal area, followed by the neck, and scapula. Histologic findings include a ciliated pseudostratified epithelial lining with the presence of smooth muscle cells, goblet cells and occasionally cartilage (137).

Cutaneous Endometriosis

See Figs. VID2.i–k.

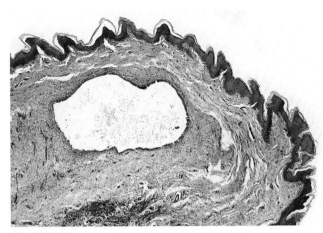

Fig. VID2.d

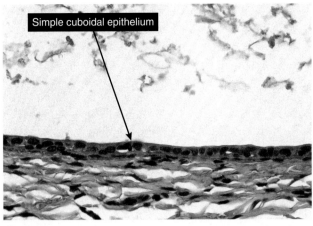

Fig. VID2.e

Fig. VID2.d. *Median raphe cyst of the penis, low power.* Within the superficial dermis there is a solitary cystic structure.

Fig. VID2.e. *Median raphe cyst of the penis, high power.* The wall of the cyst is frequently composed of pseudostratified columnar epithelium or, as seen here, only 1–2 layers of cells may be present, resembling an eccrine hidrocystoma.

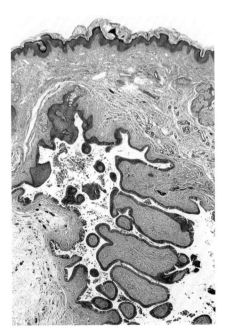

Fig. VID2.f

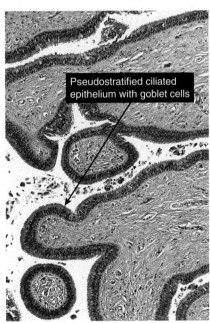

Fig. VID2.g

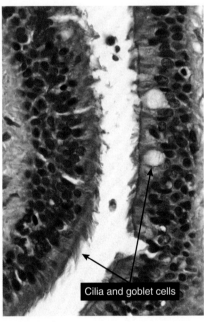

Fig. VID2.h

Fig. VID2.f. *Bronchogenic cyst, low power.* Within the dermis there is a solitary cyst with a slightly papilliferous wall.

Fig. VID2.g. *Bronchogenic cyst, medium power.* The projections are lined by pseudostratified columnar epithelium. There is a fibrotic stroma which may contain smooth muscle.

Fig. VID2.h. *Bronchogenic cyst, high power.* The pseudostratified columnar epithelial wall shows numerous cilia extending into the lumen. Goblet cells are also present.

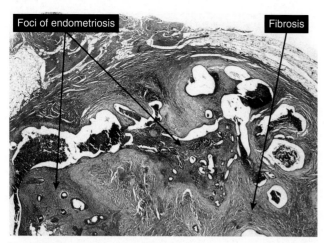

Foci of endometriosis   Fibrosis

Fig. VID2.i

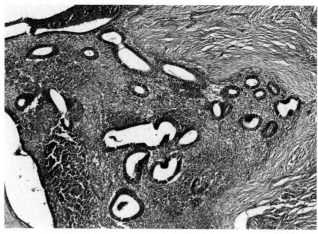

Fig. VID2.j

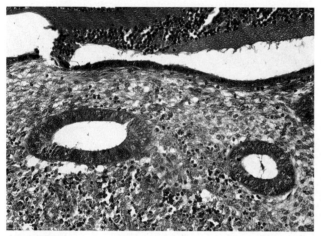

Fig. VID2.k

Fig. VID2.i. *Cutaneous endometriosis, low power.* This well-circumscribed nodular tumor-like lesion is present in the deep dermis and subcutaneous fat. It is composed of two elements, glandular structures and a prominent stroma, embedded in dense fibrous tissue.

Fig. VID2.j. *Cutaneous endometriosis, medium power.* Numerous glandular structures are embedded in a well vascularized and hypercellular stroma. In some areas, as on the right side of this photomicrograph, the stroma is fibrotic.

Fig. VID2.k. *Cutaneous endometriosis, high power.* The glandular component and the associated specialized and here focally hemorrhagic stroma resemble uterine endometrium during the phases of the menstrual cycle.

Conditions to consider in the differential diagnosis:

> eccrine hidrocystoma
> cutaneous ciliated cyst
> bronchogenic and thyroglossal duct cysts
> median raphe cyst of the penis
> cutaneous endometriosis

VID3 Apocrine Differentiation

Cystic proliferations are present in the dermis; these show spaces surrounded by apocrine epithelium (large pink cells with decapitation secretion). There may be lymphocytes and plasma cells (syringocystadenoma). Apocrine hidrocystoma (138) and hidradenoma papilliferum are prototypic (139).

Apocrine Hidrocystoma

CLINICAL SUMMARY. Apocrine hidrocystoma presents as a solitary translucent cystic nodule, between 3 and 15 mm in diameter. The lesion may be skin-colored, or may have a blue hue resembling a blue nevus. The usual

location is on the face, but also on the ears, scalp, chest, or shoulders. Multiple apocrine hidrocystomas are rare.

HISTOPATHOLOGY. The dermis contains one or several large cystic spaces into which papillary projections often extend. The inner surface of the wall and the papillary projections are lined by a row of secretory cells of variable height showing "decapitation" secretion indicative of apocrine secretion. There is an outer layer of elongated myoepithelial cells, their long axes running parallel to the cyst wall.

Hidradenoma Papilliferum

CLINICAL SUMMARY. Hidradenoma papilliferum occurs only in women, usually on the labia majora or in the perineal or perianal region. The tumor is covered by normal skin and measures only a few millimeters in diameter. Malignant changes are extremely rare.

HISTOPATHOLOGY. The tumor represents an adenoma with apocrine differentiation. It is located in the dermis, is

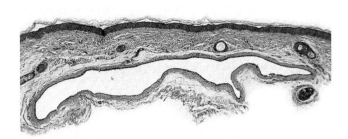

Fig. VID3.a

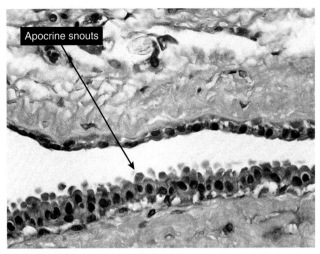

Fig. VID3.b

Fig. VID3.a. *Apocrine hidrocystoma, low power.* Within the dermis there is a well-circumscribed cystic structure.

Fig. VID3.b. *Apocrine hidrocystoma, high power.* The wall of this cystic structure is composed of one or more layers of bland-appearing cuboidal cells. The cells show decapitation secretion manifested by small droplets of cytoplasm on their luminal surface.

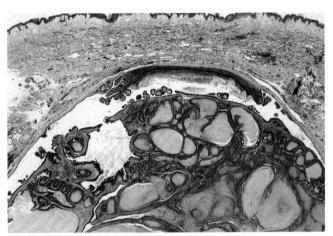

Fig. VID3.c

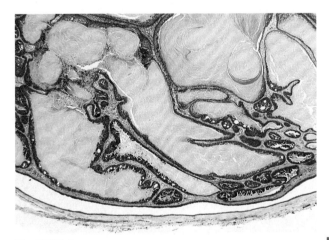

Fig. VID3.d

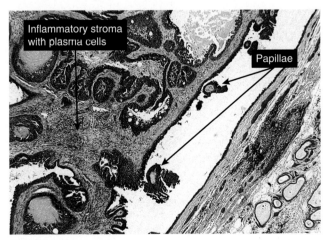

Fig. VID3.e

Fig. VID3.c. *Hidradenoma papilliferum, low power.* This well-circumscribed neoplasm has a thin surrounding fibrous capsule.

Fig. VID3.d. *Hidradenoma papilliferum, low power.* There are multiple papillary folds and cystic spaces.

Fig. VID3.e. *Hidradenoma papilliferum, medium power.* There are numerous papillary projections which extend into the cystic spaces. The lesional cells facing the lumen show evidence of decapitation secretion.

well circumscribed, is surrounded by a fibrous capsule, and has no connection with the overlying epidermis. Some tumors have a peripheral epithelial wall with areas of keratinization. Within the tumor, there are tubular and cystic structures. Papillary folds project into the cystic spaces. Usually, the lumina are surrounded by a double layer of cells consisting of a luminal layer of secretory cells and of an outer layer of small cuboidal cells with deeply basophilic nuclei. These are myoepithelial cells. The lumina are lined occasionally with only a single row of columnar cells, which show an oval, pale-staining nucleus located near the base, a faintly eosinophilic cytoplasm, and active decapitation secretion as seen in the secretory cells of apocrine glands.

Conditions to consider in the differential diagnosis:

hidradenoma papilliferum
syringocystadenoma papilliferum
apocrine hidrocystoma

References

1. Hallermann C, Niermann C, Fischer RJ, et al. Survival data for 299 patients with primary cutaneous lymphomas: a monocentre study. *Acta Derm Venereol* 2011;91(5):521–525.

2. Bogle MA, Riddle CC, Triana EM, et al. Primary cutaneous B-cell lymphoma. *J Am Acad Dermatol* 2005;53(3):479–484.

3. Garcia CF, Weiss LM, Warnke RA, et al. Cutaneous follicular lymphoma. *Am J Surg Pathol* 1986;10:454.

4. Willemze R, Santucci M, Swerdlow SH, et al. Primary cutaneous follicle centre lymphoma. In: Elder DE, Massi D, Scolyer RW, Willemze R, eds. *WHO Classification of Skin Tumours*. 4th ed. Lyon: IARC; 2018:258–259.

5. Kempf W, Burg G, Ralfkier E, et al. Cutaneous marginal zone lymphoma. In: LeBoit PE, Burg G, Weedon D, Sarasin A, eds. *World Health Organization Classification of Tumours. Pathology and Genetics of Skin Tumours*. Lyon: IARC Press; 2006:194–195.

6. Pimpinelli N, Kerl H, Berti E, et al. Cutaneous follicular center cell lymphoma. In: LeBoit PE, Burg G, Weedon D, Sarasin A, eds. *World Health Organization Classification of Tumours. Pathology and Genetics of Skin Tumours*. Lyon: IARC Press; 2006:196–197.

7. Swerdlow SH, Kurrer M, Bernengo M, et al. Cutaneous involvement in primary cutaneous B-cell lymphoma. In: LeBoit PE, Burg G, Weedon D, Sarasin A, eds. *World Health Organization Classification of Tumours. Pathology and Genetics of Skin Tumours*. Lyon: IARC Press; 2006:204–206.

8. Burg G, Kempf W, Jaffe ES, et al. Cutaneous diffuse large B-cell lymphoma. In: LeBoit PE, Burg G, Weedon D, Sarasin A, eds. *World Health Organization Classification of Tumours. Pathology and Genetics of Skin Tumours*. Lyon: IARC Press; 2006:198–199.

9. Kempf W, Duncan LM, Swerdlow SH, et al. Primary cutaneous marginal zone (MALT) lymphoma. In: Elder DE, Massi D, Scolyer RW, Willemze R, eds. *WHO Classification of Skin Tumours*. 4th ed. Lyon: IARC; 2018:256–257.

10. Burg G, Kazakov DV, Kempf W, et al. Mycosis fungoides. In: LeBoit PE, Burg G, Weedon D, Sarasin A, eds. *World Health Organization Classification of Tumours. Pathology and Genetics of Skin Tumours*. Lyon: IARC Press; 2006:198–199.

11. Smolle J, Torne R, Soyer HP, et al. Immunohistochemical classification of cutaneous pseudolymphomas: delineation of distinct patterns. *J Cutan Pathol* 1990;17:149–159.

12. Bergman R, Khamaysi K, Khamaysi Z, et al. A study of histologic and immunophenotypical staining patterns in cutaneous lymphoid hyperplasia. *J Am Acad Dermatol* 2011;65(1):112–124.

13. Wong KF, Chan JK, Li LP, et al. Primary cutaneous plasmacytoma: report of two cases and review of the literature. *Am J Dermatopathol* 1994;16:392–397.

14. Kois JM, Sexton FM, Lookingbill DP. Cutaneous manifestations of multiple myeloma. *Arch Dermatol* 1991;127:69–74.

15. Rongioletti F, Patterson JW, Rebora A. The histological and pathogenetic spectrum of cutaneous disease in monoclonal gammopathies. *J Cutan Pathol* 2008;35(8):705–721. Review.

16. Ratner D, Nelson BR, Brown MD, et al. Merkel cell carcinoma. *J Am Acad Dermatol* 1993;29:143–156.

17. Allen PJ, Bowne WB, Jaques DP, et al. Merkel cell carcinoma: prognosis and treatment of patients from a single institution. *J Clin Oncol* 2005;23:2300–2309.

18. Chang Y, Moore PS. Merkel cell carcinoma: a virus-induced human cancer. *Annu Rev Pathol* 2011;7:123–144.

19. Frierson HF Jr, Cooper PH. Prognostic factors in squamous cell carcinoma of the lower lip. *Hum Pathol* 1986;17:346–354.

20. Murphy GF, Beer TW, Cerio R, et al. Squamous cell carcinoma. In: Elder DE, Massi D, Scolyer RA, Willemze R, eds. *WHO Classification of Skin Tumours*. 4th ed. Lyon: IARC; 2018: 35–45.

21. Karaa A, Khachemoune A. Keratoacanthoma: a tumor in search of a classification. *Int J Dermatol* 2007;46(7):671–678.

22. Chu EY, Wanat KA, Miller CJ, et al. Diverse cutaneous side effects associated with BRAF inhibitor therapy: a clinicopathologic study. *J Am Acad Dermatol* 2012;67(6):1265–1272.

23. Lever WF. Inverted follicular keratosis is an irritated seborrheic keratosis. *Am J Dermatopathol* 1983;5:474.

24. Battistella M, Peltre B, Cribier B. Composite tumors associating trichoblastoma and benign epidermal/follicular neoplasm: another proof of the follicular nature of inverted follicular keratosis. *J Cutan Pathol* 2010;37(10):1057–1063.

25. El-Khoury J, Kibbi AG, Abbas O. Mucocutaneous pseudoepitheliomatous hyperplasia: a review. *Am J Dermatopathol* 2012;34(2):165–175.

26. Brownstein MH, Arluk DJ. Proliferating trichilemmal cyst: a simulant of squamous cell carcinoma. *Cancer* 1981;48:1207–1214.

27. Satyaprakash AK, Sheehan DJ, Sangüeza OP. Proliferating trichilemmal tumors: a review of the literature. *Dermatol Surg* 2007;33(9):1102–1108. Review.

28. Requena L, Crowson AN, Kaddu S, et al. Proliferating trichilemmal tumor. In: Elder DE, Massi D, Scolyer RA, Willemze R, eds. *WHO Classification of Skin Tumours*. 4th ed. Lyon: IARC; 2018:196–197.

29. Rowland Payne CME, Wilkinson JD, McKee PH, et al. Nodular prurigo: a clinicopathological study of 46 patients. *Br J Dermatol* 1985;113:431–439.

30. Johansson O, Liang Y, Emtestam L. Increased nerve growth factor- and tyrosine kinase A-like immunoreactivities in prurigo nodularis skin—an exploration of the cause of neurohyperplasia. *Arch Dermatol Res* 2002;293:614–619.

31. Mentrikoski MJ, Wick MR. Immunohistochemical distinction of primary sweat gland carcinoma and metastatic breast

carcinoma: can it always be accomplished reliably? *Am J Clin Pathol* 2015;143(3):430–436.

32. Xu X, Chu AY, Pasha TL, et al. Immunoprofile of MITF, tyrosinase, Melan-A, and MAGE-1 in HMB45-negative melanomas. *Am J Surg Pathol* 2002;26:82–87.

33. Murphy GF, Elder DE. Benign melanocytic tumors. In: Murphy GF, Elder DE, eds. *Nonmelanocytic Tumors of the Skin*. Washington, DC: Armed Forces Institute of Pathology; 1990:9.

34. Elder DE, Murphy GF. *Melanocytic Tumors of the Skin*. Washington, DC: Armed Forces Institute of Pathology; 2009.

35. Bastian BC, de la Fouchardiere A, Elder DE, et al. Genomic landscape of melanoma. In: Elder DE, Massi D, Scolyer RA, Willemze R, eds. *WHO Classification of Skin Tumours*. 4th ed. Lyon: IARC; 2018:72–75.

36. Kopf AW, Morrill SD, Silberberg I. Broad spectrum of leukoderma acquisitum centrifugum. *Arch Dermatol* 1965;92:14–33.

37. Weyant GW, Chung CG, Helm KF. Halo nevus: review of the literature and clinicopathologic findings. *Int J Dermatol* 2015;54(10):e433–e435.

38. Moon KR, Choi YD, Kim JM, et al. Genetic alterations in primary acral melanoma and acral melanocytic nevus in Korea: common mutated genes show distinct cytomorphological features. *J Invest Dermatol* 2018;138(4):933–945.

39. Rodriguez HA, Ackerman LV. Cellular blue nevus. Clinicopathologic study of forty-five cases. *Cancer* 1968;21:393–405.

40. Luzar B, Calonje E. Deep penetrating nevus: a review. *Arch Pathol Lab Med* 2011;135(3):321–326. Review.

41. Magro CM, Crowson AN, Mihm MC Jr, et al. The dermal-based borderline melanocytic tumor: a categorical approach. *J Am Acad Dermatol* 2010;62(3):469–479.

42. Barnhill RL, Cerroni L, Cook M, et al. State of the art, nomenclature, and points of consensus and controversy concerning benign melanocytic lesions: outcome of an international workshop. *Adv Anat Pathol* 2010;17(2):73–90.

43. Paniago-Pereira C, Maize JC, Ackerman AB. Nevus of large spindle and/or epithelioid cells: Spitz's nevus. *Arch Dermatol* 1978;114:1811–1823.

44. Barnhill RL. The Spitzoid lesion: rethinking Spitz tumors, atypical variants, 'Spitzoid melanoma' and risk assessment. *Mod Pathol* 2006;19(Suppl 2):S21–S33.

45. Smith KJ, Barett TL, Skelton HG, et al. Spindle cell and epithelioid cell nevi with atypia and metastasis (malignant Spitz tumor). *Am J Surg Pathol* 1989;13:931–939.

46. Bastian BC, Olshen AB, LeBoit PE, et al. Classifying melanocytic tumors based on DNA copy number changes. *Am J Pathol* 2003;163:1765–1770.

47. van Dijk MC, Bernsen MR, Ruiter DJ. Analysis of mutations in B-RAF, N-RAS, and H-RAS Genes in the differential diagnosis of Spitz nevus and spitzoid melanoma. *Am J Surg Pathol* 2005; 29:1145–1151.

48. Cerroni L, Barnhill R, Elder D, et al. Melanocytic tumors of uncertain malignant potential: results of a tutorial held at the XXIX Symposium of the International Society of Dermatopathology in Graz, October 2008. *Am J Surg Pathol* 2010;34(3):314–326.

49. Gammon B, Beilfuss B, Guitart J, et al. Enhanced detection of spitzoid melanomas using fluorescence in situ hybridization with 9p21 as an adjunctive probe. *Am J Surg Pathol* 2012; 36(1):81–88.

50. Broekaert SM, Roy R, Okamoto I, et al. Genetic and morphologic features for melanoma classification. *Pigment Cell Melanoma Res* 2010;23(6):763–770.

51. Viros A, Fridlyand J, Bauer J, et al. Improving melanoma classification by integrating genetic and morphologic features. *PLoS Med* 2008;5(6):e120.

52. Levene A. On the histological diagnosis and prognosis of malignant melanoma. *J Clin Pathol* 1980;33:101–124.

53. Schmoeckel C, Castro CE, Braun-Falco O. Nevoid malignant melanoma. *Arch Dermatol Res* 1985;277:362–369.

54. Abernethy JL, Soyer HP, Kerl H, et al. Epidermotropic metastatic malignant melanoma simulating melanoma in situ: a report of 10 examples from two patients. *Am J Dermatopathol* 1994;18:1140–1149.

55. Bahrami S, Cheng L, Wang M, et al. Clonal relationships between epidermotropic metastatic melanomas and their primary lesions: a loss of heterozygosity and X-chromosome inactivation-based analysis. *Mod Pathol* 2007;20(8): 821–827.

56. Stratakis CA, Kirschner LS, Carney JA. Clinical and molecular features of the Carney complex: diagnostic criteria and recommendations for patient evaluation. *J Clin Endocrinol Metab* 2001;86:4041–4046.

57. Zembowicz A, Carney JA, Mihm MC. Pigmented epithelioid melanocytoma: a low-grade melanocytic tumor with metastatic potential indistinguishable from animal-type melanoma and epithelioid blue nevus. *Am J Surg Pathol* 2004;28:31–40.

58. Zembowicz A, Knoepp SM, Bei T, et al. Loss of expression of protein kinase a regulatory subunit 1alpha in pigmented epithelioid melanocytoma but not in melanoma or other melanocytic lesions. *Am J Surg Pathol* 2007;31(11):1764–1775.

59. Zembowicz A, Calonje E, Mihm MC Jr. Pigmented epithelioid melanocytoma. In: Elder DE, Massi D, Scolyer RW, Willemze R, eds. *WHO Classification of Skin Tumours*. 4th ed. Lyon: IARC; 2018:297–298.

60. Berk DR, LaBuz E, Dadras SS, et al. Melanoma and melanocytic tumors of uncertain malignant potential in children, adolescents and young adults—the Stanford experience 1995–2008. *Pediatr Dermatol* 2010;27:244–254.

61. Plaza JA, Ortega PF, Stockman DL, et al. Value of p63 and podoplanin(D2-40) immunoreactivity in the distinction between primary cutaneous tumors and adenocarcinomas metastatic to the skin: a clinicopathologic and immunohistochemical study of 79 cases. *J Cutan Pathol* 2010;37(4):403–410.

62. Mambo NC. Eccrine spiradenoma: clinical and pathologic study of 49 tumors. *J Cutan Pathol* 1983;10:312–320.

63. Massoumi R, Paus R. Cylindromatosis and the CYLD gene: new lessons on the molecular principles of epithelial growth control. *Bioessays* 2007;29(12):1203–1214. Review.

64. Sangueza OP, Cassarino DS, Glusac EJ, et al. Poroma. In: Elder DE, Massi D, Scolyer RA, Willemze R, eds. *WHO Classification of Skin Tumours*. 4th ed. Lyon: IARC; 2018:185.

65. Sangueza OP, Cassarino DS, Glusac EJ, et al. Syringoma. In: Elder DE, Massi D, Scolyer RA, Willemze R, eds. *WHO Classification of Skin Tumours*. 4th ed. Lyon: IARC; 2018:184.

66. Haupt HM, Stern JB, Berlin SJ. Immunohistochemistry in the differential diagnosis of nodular hidradenoma and glomus tumor. *Am J Dermatopathol* 1992;14:310–314.

67. Nandeesh B, Rajalakshmi T. A study of histopathologic spectrum of nodular hidradenoma. *Am J Dermatopathol* 2012;34(5): 461–470.

68. Sangueza OP, Cassarino DS, Glusac EJ, et al. Mixed tumor. In: Elder DE, Massi D, Scolyer RA, Willemze R, eds. *WHO classification of Skin Tumours*. 4th ed. Lyon: IARC; 2018:193.

69. Leboit P, Sexton M. Microcystic adnexal carcinoma of the skin: a reappraisal of the differentiation and differential diagnosis of an under-recognized neoplasm. *J Am Acad Dermatol* 1993;29: 609–618.

70. Kazakov DV, Argenyi ZB, Brenn T, et al. Mucinous carcinoma. In: Elder DE, Massi D, Scolyer RA, Willemze R, eds. *WHO Classification of Skin Tumours*. 4th ed. Lyon: IARC; 2018:166–167.

71. Kao GF, Graham JH, Helwig EB. Aggressive digital papillary adenocarcinoma. *Arch Dermatol* 1984;120:1612.

72. Kao GF, Helwig EB, Graham JH. Aggressive digital papillary adenoma and adenocarcinoma: a clinicopathological study of 57 patients, with histochemical, immunopathological and ultrastructural observations. *J Cutan Pathol* 1987;14: 129–146.

73. Hsu HC, Ho CY, Chen CH, et al. Aggressive digital papillary adenocarcinoma: a review. *Clin Exp Dermatol* 2010;35(2): 113–119. Review.

74. Umbert P, Winkelmann RK. Tubular apocrine adenoma. *J Cutan Pathol* 1976;3:75–87.

75. Vanatta PR, Bangert JL, Freeman RG. Syringocystadenoma papilliferum: a plasmacytotropic tumor. *Am J Surg Pathol* 1985;9:678–683.

76. Kazakov DV, Requena L, Kutzner H, et al. Morphologic diversity of syringocystadenocarcinoma papilliferum based on a clinicopathologic study of 6 cases and review of the literature. *Am J Dermatopathol* 2010;32(4):340–347. Review.

77. Headington JT. Tumors of the hair follicle: a review. *Am J Pathol* 1976;85:479–514.

78. Brownstein MH, Shapiro L. Desmoplastic trichoepithelioma. *Cancer* 1977;40:2979–2986.

79. Kallioinen M, Twoani M-L, Dammert K, et al. Desmoplastic trichoepithelioma: clinicopathologic features and immunohistochemical study of basement membrane proteins, laminin and type IV collagen. *Br J Dermatol* 1984;111:571–577.

80. Takei Y, Fukushiro S, Ackerman AB. Criteria for histologic differentiation of desmoplastic trichoepithelioma (sclerosing epithelial hamartoma) from morphea-like basal cell carcinoma. *Am J Dermatopathol* 1985;7(3):207–221.

81. Palmirotta R, Savonarola A, Ludovici G, et al. Association between Birt Hogg Dube syndrome and cancer predisposition. *Anticancer Res* 2010;30(3):751–757. Review.

82. Headington JT. Tumors of the hair follicle. A review. *Am J Pathol* 1976;85:480–505.

83. Ackerman AB, de Viragh PA, Chongchitnant N. *Neoplasms With Follicular Differentiation*. Philadelphia, PA: Lea & Febiger; 1993:359–420.

84. Schirren CG, Rutten A, Kaudewitz P, et al. Trichoblastoma and basal cell carcinoma are neoplasms with follicular differentiation sharing the same profile of cytokeratin intermediate filaments. *Am J Dermatopathol* 1997;19(4):314–350.

85. Prioleau PG, Santa Cruz DJ. Sebaceous gland neoplasia. *J Cutan Pathol* 1984;11:396–414.

86. Shalin SC, Lyle S, Calonje E, et al. Sebaceous neoplasia and the Muir Torre syndrome: important connections with clinical implications. *Histopathology* 2010;56(1):133–147. Review.

87. Ringel E, Moschella S. Primary histiocytic dermatoses. *Arch Dermatol* 1985;121(12):1531–1541. Review.

88. Newman B, Hu W, Nigro K, et al. Aggressive histiocytic disorders that can involve the skin. *J Am Acad Dermatol* 2007;56(2): 302–316.

89. Tajirian AL, Malik MK, Robinson-Bostom L, et al. Multicentric reticulohistiocytosis. *Clin Dermatol* 2006;24(6):486–492. Review.

90. Sangüeza OP, Salmon JK, White CR Jr, et al. Juvenile xanthogranuloma: a clinical, histopathologic, and immunohistochemical study. *J Cutan Pathol* 1995;22:327–335.

91. Zelger B, Cerio R, Soyer HP, et al. Reticulohistiocytoma and multicentric reticulohistiocytosis: histopathologic and immunophenotypic distinct entities. *Am J Dermatopathol* 1994;16: 577–584.

92. Paulli M, Berti E, Rosso R, et al. CD30/Ki-1–positive lymphoproliferative disorders of the skin: clinicopathologic correlation and statistical analysis of 86 cases. A multicentric study from the European Organization for Research and Treatment of Cancer Cutaneous Lymphoma Project Group. *J Clin Oncol* 1995;13: 1343–1354.

93. Karp DL, Horn TD. Lymphomatoid papulosis. *J Am Acad Dermatol* 1994;30:379–395.

94. Willemze R, Kadin ME, Kempf W, et al. Primary cutaneous CD 30+ T cell lymphoproliferative disorders. In: Elder DE, Massi D, Scolyer RW, Willemze R, eds. *WHO Classification of Skin Tumours*. 4th ed. Lyon: IARC; 2018:236–239.

95. Klco JM, Welch JS, Nguyen TT, et al. State of the art in myeloid sarcoma. *Int J Lab Hematol* 2011;33(6):555–565.

96. Willemze R, Battistella M, Duncan LM, et al. Primary cutaneous diffuse large B cell lymphoma, leg type. In: Elder DE, Massi D, Scolyer RW, Willemze R, eds. *WHO Classification of Skin Tumours*. 4th ed. Lyon: IARC; 2018:260–261.

97. Akin C. Clonality and molecular pathogenesis of mastocytosis. *Acta Haematol* 2005;114:61–69.

98. Chase DR, Enzinger FM. Epithelioid sarcoma: diagnosis, prognostic indicators, and treatment. *Am J Surg Pathol* 1985;9: 241–263.

99. Armah HB, Parwani AV. Epithelioid sarcoma. *Arch Pathol Lab Med* 2009;133(5):814–819. Review.

100. Lazar A, Argenyi ZB. Granular cell tumour. In: Elder DE, Massi D, Scolyer RA, Willemze R, eds. *WHO Classification of Skin Tumours*. 4th ed. Lyon: IARC; 2018:364.

101. Kanitakis J, Schmitt D, Thivolet J. Immunohistologic study of cellular populations of histiocytofibromas ("dermatofibromas"). *J Cutan Pathol* 1984;11:88–94.

102. Colome-Grimmer MI, Evans HL. Metastasizing cellular dermatofibroma. A report of two cases. *Am J Surg Pathol* 1996; 20(11):1361–1367.

103. Tetzlaff MT, Xu X, Elder DE, et al. Angiomatoid Spitz nevus: a clinicopathological study of six cases and a review of the literature. *J Cutan Pathol* 2009;36(4):471–476. Review.

104. Zelger B, Sidoroff A, Stanzl U, et al. Deep penetrating dermatofibroma versus dermatofibrosarcoma protuberans. *Am J Surg Pathol* 1994;18:677–686.

105. Llombart B, Monteagudo C, Sanmartín O, et al. Dermatofibrosarcoma protuberans: a clinicopathological, immunohistochemical, genetic (COL1A1-PDGFB), and therapeutic study of low-grade versus high-grade (fibrosarcomatous) tumors. *J Am Acad Dermatol* 2011;65(3):564–575.

106. Ogawa R. Keloid and hypertrophic scars are the result of chronic inflammation in the reticular dermis. *Int J Mol Sci* 2017;18(3):E606.

107. Cupp JS, Miller MA, Montgomery KD, et al. Translocation and expression of CSF1 in pigmented villonodular synovitis,

107 (cont.) tenosynovial giant cell tumor, rheumatoid arthritis and other reactive synovitides. *Am J Surg Pathol* 2007;31(6):970–976.

108. Ehrenstein V, Andersen SL, Qazi I, et al. Tenosynovial giant cell tumor: incidence, prevalence, patient characteristics, and recurrence. A registry-based cohort study in Denmark. *J Rheumatol* 2017;44(10):1476–1483.

109. Somerhausen NS, Fletcher CD. Diffuse-type giant cell tumor: clinicopathologic and immunohistochemical analysis of 50 cases with extraarticular disease. *Am J Surg Pathol* 2000;24(4):479–492.

110. Fretzin DFJ, Helwig EB. Atypical fibroxanthoma of the skin. *Cancer* 1973;31:1541–1552.

111. Reed RJ, Harkin JC. *Supplement: Tumors of the Peripheral Nervous System. 2nd series, Fasc. 3.* Washington, DC: Armed Forces Institute of Pathology; 1983.

112. Hajdu SI. Schwannomas. *Mod Pathol* 1995;8:109–115.

113. Fisher WC, Helwig EB. Leiomyomas of the skin. *Arch Dermatol* 1963;88:510–520.

114. Carlson JA, Dickersin GR, Sober AJ, et al. Desmoplastic neurotropic melanoma: a clinicopathologic analysis of 28 cases. *Cancer* 1995;75:478–494.

115. George E, McClain SE, Slingluff CL, et al. Subclassification of desmoplastic melanoma: pure and mixed variants have significantly different capacities for lymph node metastasis. *J Cutan Pathol* 2009;36(4):425–432.

116. Kucher C, Zhang PJ, Pasha T, et al. Expression of Melan-A and Ki-67 in desmoplastic melanoma and desmoplastic nevi. *Am J Dermatopathol* 2004;26:452–457.

117. Fukunaga M. Expression of D2-40 in lymphatic endothelium of normal tissues and in vascular tumours. *Histopathology* 2005;46(4):396–402.

118. Patrice SJ, Wiss K, Mulliken JB. Pyogenic granuloma (lobular capillary hemangioma): a clinicopathologic study of 178 cases. *Pediatr Dermatol* 1994;8:267–276.

119. Hashimoto H, Daimaru Y, Enjoji M. Intravascular papillary endothelial hyperplasia. A clinicopathologic study of 91 cases. *Am J Dermatopathol* 1983;5:539–546.

120. Rao B, Unis M, Poulos E. Acroangiodermatitis: a study of ten cases. *Int J Dermatol* 1994;33:179–183.

121. Chor PJ, Santa Cruz DJ. Kaposi's sarcoma: a clinicopathologic review and differential diagnosis. *J Cutan Pathol* 1992;19:6–20.

122. Ensoli B, Sgadari C, Barillari G, et al. Biology of Kaposi's sarcoma. *Eur J Cancer* 2001;37:1251–1269.

123. Grayson W, Landman G. Kaposi sarcoma. In: Elder DE, Massi D, Scolyer RW, Willemze R, eds. *WHO Classification of Skin Tumours.* 4th ed. Lyon: IARC; 2018:341–343.

124. Krell JM, Sanchez RL, Solomon AR. Diffuse dermal angiomatosis: a variant of reactive cutaneous angioendotheliomatosis. *J Cutan Pathol* 1994;21(4):363–370.

125. Kim S, Elenitsas R, James WD, Diffuse dermal angiomatosis: a variant of reactive angioendotheliomatosis associated with peripheral vascular atherosclerosis. *Arch Dermatol* 2002;138(4):456–458.

126. Rongioletti F, Rebora A. Cutaneous reactive angiomatoses: patterns and classification of reactive vascular proliferation. *J Am Acad Dermatol* 2003;49(5):887–896.

127. Mark RJ, Tron LM, Sercarz J, et al. Angiosarcoma of the head and neck: The UCLA experience 1955 through 1990. *Arch Otolaryngol Head Neck Surg* 1993;119:973–978.

128. Shon W, Jenkins SM, Ross DT, et al. Angiosarcoma: a study of 98 cases with immunohistochemical evaluation of TLE3, a recently described marker of potential taxane responsiveness. *J Cutan Pathol* 2011;38(12):961–966.

129. Sangüeza OP, Walsh SN, Sheehan DJ, et al. Cutaneous epithelioid angiomatous nodule: a case series and proposed classification. *Am J Dermatopathol* 2008;30(1):16–20.

130. Santa Cruz DJ, Aronberg J. Targetoid hemosiderotic hemangioma. *J Am Acad Dermatol* 1988;19:550–558.

131. Mentzel T, Partanen TA, Kutzner H. Hobnail hemangioma ("targetoid hemosiderotic hemangioma"): clinicopathologic and immunohistochemical analysis of 62 cases. *J Cutan Pathol* 1999;26:279–286.

132. Hunt SJ, Santa Cruz DJ, Barr RJ. Microvenular hemangioma. *J Cutan Pathol* 1991;18(4):235–240.

133. Dotz W, Prioleau PG. Nevus lipomatosus cutaneus superficialis: a light and electron microscopic study. *Arch Dermatol* 1984;120:376–379.

134. Brook CG, Valman HG. Osteoma cutis and Albright's hereditary osteodystrophy. *Br J Dermatol* 1971;85:471–475.

135. McGavran MH, Binnington B. Keratinous cysts of the skin. *Arch Dermatol* 1966;94:499–508.

136. Sperling LC, Sakas EL. Eccrine hidrocystomas. *J Am Acad Dermatol* 1982;7:763–770.

137. Zvulunov A, Amichai B, Grunwald MH, et al. Cutaneous bronchogenic cyst: delineation of a poorly recognized lesion. *Pediatr Dermatol* 1998;15(4):277–281. Review.

138. Smith JD, Chernosky ME. Apocrine hidrocystoma (cystadenoma). *Arch Dermatol* 1974;109:700–702.

139. Meeker HJ, Neubecker RD, Helwig EG. Hidradenoma papilliferum. *Am J Clin Pathol* 1962;37:182–195.

Inflammatory and Other Disorders of Skin Appendages

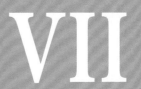

VII

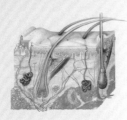

The hair, sebaceous glands, eccrine glands, apocrine glands and nails may be involved in inflammatory processes (e.g., hidradenitis, folliculitis). Some neoplasms may masquerade as inflammatory processes.

VIIA   PATHOLOGY INVOLVING HAIR FOLLICLES

Acne and related conditions present as dilatation of follicles which are filled with keratin, sebum, and bacteria (1). Inflammatory processes may present as alopecia, or as follicular localization of inflammatory rashes. A classic division is into scarring (cicatricial) and nonscarring (noncicatricial) alopecia (2,3). Cicatricial alopecia may be either primary (i.e., a disease specifically targeting the hair follicle) or secondary (i.e., a disease that secondarily involves hair follicles). Potential causes of secondary cicatricial alopecia of the scalp include trauma, burns, radiation dermatitis, malignancies, sarcoidosis, scleroderma, necrobiosis lipoidica, tuberculosis, and infection, involving the follicle nonspecifically, and covered in other relevant sections of this book. Primary cicatricial alopecia includes disorders in which follicular and sebaceous epithelium is destroyed and replaced by fibrous tissue (follicular scarring). The destruction includes the bulge zone in the isthmus, which is the locus of follicular stem cells. In contrast, in noncicatricial alopecia the follicular epithelium is preserved and the hair loss is potentially reversible (1). A proposed simplified classification has been offered, which starts with a diffuse versus patchy clinical presentation, and then relies on follicular size (miniaturization) and phase (catagen/telogen count). Clinicopathologic correlation is also very important. Evaluation of most alopecias can be achieved best from transverse sectioning of punch biopsy material (a 4-mm punch is recommended) (4), combined with vertical sections in the HoVert technique, which can aid in the diagnosis of scarring alopecias (5). Diminution of follicular size, most effectively measured by assessment of hair shaft diameter, can be obtained with relative simplicity using an optical micrometer. Because this approach allows assessment of all follicles in the specimen, direct counting of anagen, telogen, and catagen follicles can be undertaken and the percentages of each obtained.

1. Scant Inflammation
2. Lymphocytes Predominant
3. With Eosinophils Present
4. Neutrophils Prominent
5. Plasma Cells Prominent
6. Fibrosing and Suppurative Follicular Disorders

VIIA1   Scant Inflammation

There is follicular alteration with a sparse infiltrate of cells, mainly lymphocytes. Androgenetic alopecia (AGA) and trichotillomania are important examples. These conditions may result in nonscarring alopecia, in which the number of follicles is normal, at least in the early stages of hair loss (see Table VII.1).

Androgenetic Alopecia

CLINICAL SUMMARY. The expression of AGA frequently has a familial and probably genetic inheritance pattern. Hair shafts become progressively finer and shorter (miniaturization), with clinically apparent alopecia occurring only as a later event. In men this process is characterized early on by bitemporal recession and/or vertex thinning, progressing in more severe cases to involve the entire crown of the scalp. This process can also occur in women, although less frequently and with a pattern distinguished by thinning over the crown with retention of the frontal hairline. In women, AGA is of lesser severity so that significant balding is quite unusual.

HISTOPATHOLOGY. Reduction of follicular size in AGA appears to be randomized, so that, initially, normal-size follicles coexist with an increased number of smaller ones within each follicular unit. Ultimately, follicular miniaturization becomes more persistent and obvious. Associated with this reduction in follicular size, there is an increase in the percentage of regressing follicles which may present as telogen hairs (normal club pattern), catagen hairs, and telogen germinal units (telogen epithelial remnants). Lymphocytic inflammation may be present around superficial blood vessels (6). Peri-infundibular fibroplasia may be seen, ultimately leading to focal follicular scarring and a reduction in the density of follicles, though typically the cause of alopecia is clinically apparent at this point and is infrequently biopsied. The diminution of follicles leads to a substantial increase in the number of fibrous streamers (a.k.a. stelae) in the deeper dermis and subcutaneous tissue.

Trichotillomania

CLINICAL SUMMARY. Compulsive avulsion of hair shafts leads to zones of thin, ragged, broken stubble on the affected scalp. If the damage is done in localized fashion it can occasionally mimic alopecia areata. Follicular breakage and loss may occasionally be associated with evidence of external damage to the scalp by erosions, crusts, or lichen simplex chronicus (7).

HISTOPATHOLOGY. The most important findings in biopsy specimens are an increase in catagen and telogen hairs (up to 75%), pigment casts, evidence of traumatized hair bulbs, and trichomalacia (a distorted hair shaft within a follicle) (8). Occasionally, follicles may be identified still in anagen but empty because of hair shaft avulsion. Follicles can show considerable distortion of the bulbar epithelium and sometimes conspicuous peribulbar hemorrhage. Hair shaft avulsion may deposit melanin pigment in the hair papilla and peribulbar connective tissue. Pigment casts may be identified in the isthmus or infundibulum. Trichomalacia is commonly seen in trichotillomania but can also be seen in alopecia areata. Longitudinal splitting

TABLE VII.1. Nonscarring Alopecia (Normal Follicular Density)

	Clinical Pattern	Degree of Miniaturization (0–+++)	Telogen Count	Inflammation	Other Histo Features
Hereditary/ androgenetic alopecia (AGA)	Males—thinning of vertex, crown, bitemporal Females—thinning of crown, retention of frontal hairline	++	16.8% avg.	Lymphocytic; superficial perivascular (37% of cases)	May have superficial perifollicular fibrosis
Alopecia areata (AA)	Round bald patches, diffuse absence of scalp hair (*totalis*), diffuse absence of scalp and body hair (*universalis*). May see exclamation point hairs	+++	27% avg.; >50% favors AA	Lymphocytic; peribulbar ("swarm of bees") around terminal hairs (acute) and miniaturized hairs (chronic, recurrent)	Nanogen hairs, pigment casts, melanin pigment deposition in fibrous tracts, intra- and intercellular edema of matrix keratinocytes
Telogen effluvium: acute	Diffuse thinning	None	>15%—suggestive >20%—presumptive >25%—definitive (usually not >50%)	Absent	May resemble normal scalp if in resolution
Telogen effluvium: chronic	Diffuse thinning	None	11% avg.	Absent	Often resembles normal scalp
Trichotillomania	Patchy or diffuse. Hairs of irregular length, broken hairs	None	Elevated (>15%)	Absent	Distorted hair anatomy, empty/torn away anagen hairs, trichomalacia, pigment casts, peribulbar hemorrhage

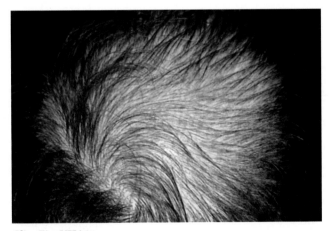

Clin. Fig. VIIA1.a

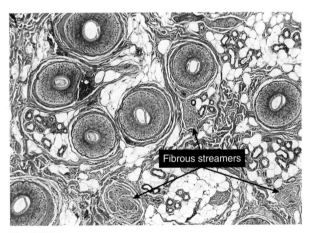

Fig. VIIA1.a

Clin. Fig. VIIA1.a. *Androgenetic alopecia.* Affected hairs undergo a shortened anagen phase resulting in a gradual transformation of terminal hairs to vellus-like hairs.

Fig. VIIA1.a. *Androgenetic alopecia, medium power, horizontal section.* Within the superficial subcutis, one sees the lower segment of terminal anagen follicles and an increased number of fibrous streamers. (*continues*)

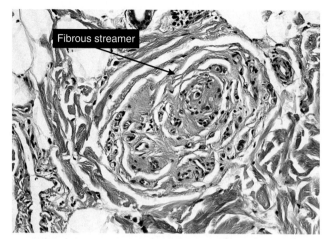

Fig. VIIA1.b

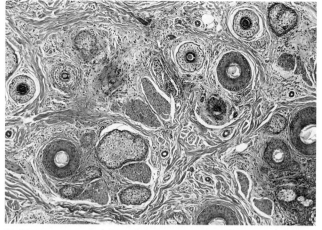

Fig. VIIA1.c

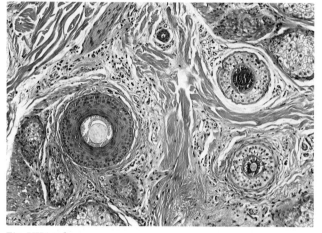

Fig. VIIA1.d

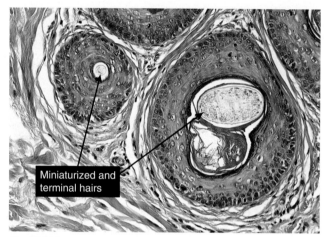

Fig. VIIA1.e

Fig. VIIA1.b. *Androgenetic alopecia, high power, horizontal section.* A streamer is characterized by a concentric arrangement of loose fibrovascular tissue resembling a collapsed fibrous sheath. Streamers result from shortening of follicles, either from follicular miniaturization or an increased percentage of follicles in the resting (telogen) phase.

Fig. VIIA1.c. *Androgenetic alopecia, medium power, horizontal section.* Early in the course of this disorder the density of follicles remains normal. There is great variation in follicular size, with an increased number of indeterminate and vellus follicles. An increase in the percentage of catagen and telogen follicles can sometimes be seen.

Fig. VIIA1.d. *Androgenetic alopecia, medium power, horizontal section.* Higher magnification reveals hair shafts of varying diameter. The hair shaft of terminal hairs measures >0.06 mm and that of vellus hairs measures <0.03 mm, while the thickness of indeterminate hairs is between these two. All three are seen in this cross-section taken just below the level of the isthmus (the inner root sheath is fully keratinized, but still intact).

Fig. VIIA1.e. *Androgenetic alopecia, high power, horizontal section.* A miniaturized hair resides next to a terminal hair at the level of the infundibulum.

of a hair shaft with blood cells sandwiched in between has been called the "hamburger sign" (9). These various injuries to the bulbar portions of follicles are not accompanied by significant inflammatory infiltrates. Trichotillomania is not associated with miniaturization of follicles or with

deep perifollicular infiltrates, features that usually serve to differentiate it from alopecia areata. Histologic findings in early traction alopecia are said to be identical with those of trichotillomania, but fewer follicles are involved, the changes are less dramatic, and vellus hairs are preserved.

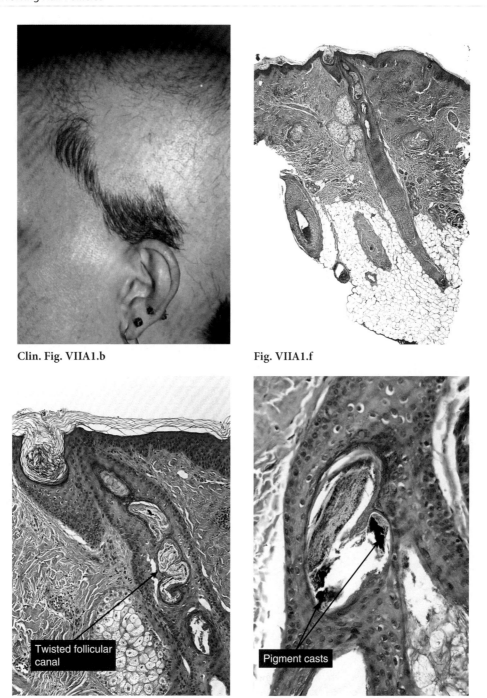

Clin. Fig. VIIA1.b

Fig. VIIA1.f

Fig. VIIA1.g

Fig. VIIA1.h

Clin. Fig. VIIA1.b. *Trichotillomania.* "Plucking" of hairs by a middle-aged female with a delusional disorder resulted in well-demarcated patches of alopecia in a diffuse distribution.

Fig. VIIA1.f. *Trichotillomania, low power.* At scanning magnification there is a normal number of hair follicles per cross-section.

Fig. VIIA1.g. *Trichotillomania, medium power.* One frequently sees distortion of the hair follicle, as manifested here by the twisted contour of the follicular canal.

Fig. VIIA1.h. *Trichotillomania, high power.* A characteristic finding in trichotillomania is the presence of pigment casts (clumps of pigment) which are present in the follicular canal. (*continues*)

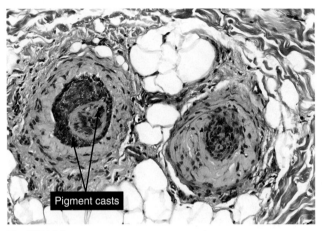

Fig. VIIA1.i

Fig. VIIA1.i. *Trichotillomania, high power.* Brown pigment casts in a cross-section.

Telogen Effluvium

CLINICAL SUMMARY. Telogen effluvium represents the increased or excessive shedding of hair in the telogen phase of the growth cycle. Telogen effluvium has multiple precipitating causes and associated conditions, which may cause hair thinning by eliciting changes in the length of the anagen period of growth, prematurely sending follicles into telogen. Plucked or shed telogen hairs have a club-like appearance at the bottom of the shaft, and are therefore often known as "club hairs."

HISTOPATHOLOGY. Acute telogen effluvium is characterized by dramatic shedding which typically occurs 2 to 3 months after an insult, such as high fever, surgery, general anesthesia, crash diet, traumatic accident, psychological stress, thyroid dysfunction, and drugs, which prematurely sends anagen hairs into catagen and then telogen. Shedding does not occur until the follicle re-enters the anagen phase and the new hair shaft pushes out the old hair shaft, so that a late biopsy of acute telogen effluvium may show nearly 100% anagen phase follicles (1).

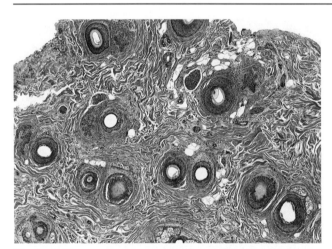

Fig. VIIA1.j

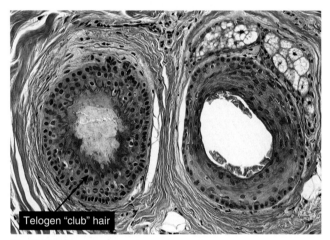

Fig. VIIA1.k

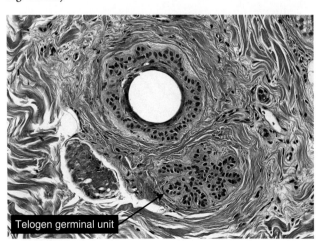

Fig. VIIA1.l

Fig. VIIA1.j. *Telogen effluvium, low power, horizontal section.* At scanning magnification there is a normal density of terminal follicles. An increased percentage of catagen and telogen follicles, as is seen in the early phases, is best appreciated at or just below the level of the isthmus. Inflammation is not seen here or deeper within the fat.

Fig. VIIA1.k. *Telogen effluvium, high power, horizontal section.* A telogen (club) hair, on the left, is readily identifiable by a hair shaft which fills the follicular canal and merges with the outer root sheath via an eosinophilic zone, a consequence of trichilemmal keratinization.

Fig. VIIA1.l. *Telogen effluvium, medium power, horizontal section.* The irregular island of basaloid epithelium represents a telogen germinal unit, an epithelial remnant of a telogen follicle. Such structures may be increased in telogen effluvium.

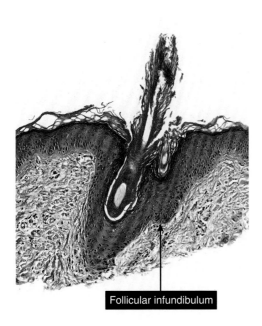
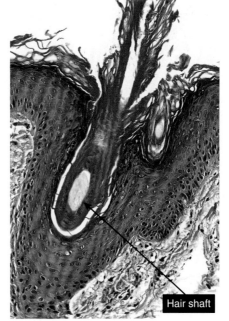

Follicular infundibulum

Hair shaft

Fig. VIIA1.m

Fig. VIIA1.n

Fig. VIIA1.m. *Keratosis pilaris, low power.* In the center of this biopsy is the edge of a hair follicle which is manifested by an invagination of epithelium (infundibulum). This is associated with marked hyperkeratosis of the follicular orifice.

Fig. VIIA1.n. *Keratosis pilaris, medium power.* The follicular epithelium and the adjacent epidermis are mildly acanthotic. The characteristic hyperkeratotic scale may be both ortho- and parakeratotic. There is only minimal inflammation in the surrounding dermis.

Telogen effluvium does not have significant inflammatory infiltrates, nor should there be evidence of diminution of follicular and hair shaft size, unless telogen effluvium occurs in patients with established AGA (10). A proportion of telogen follicles in the range of 15% to 25% is considered to be abnormal and suggests the likely presence of telogen effluvium. If a biopsy is obtained in the stages of recovery, the biopsy may be entirely normal (11), which is also often the case in patients with chronic telogen effluvium.

Keratosis Pilaris

Keratosis pilaris (KP) is a common inherited disorder of follicular hyperkeratosis, which is characterized by small, follicular keratotic papules that may have surrounding erythema, most commonly affecting the extensor aspects of the upper arms, upper legs, and buttocks. The small papules impart a stippled appearance to the skin resembling gooseflesh (12).

Scurvy

CLINICAL SUMMARY. The earliest symptom of scurvy, occurring only after many weeks of deficient intake of vitamin C, is fatigue. Cutaneous findings include follicular hyperkeratosis, perifollicular hemorrhages, ecchymoses, xerosis, leg edema, poor wound healing, and bent or coiled body hairs. Gum abnormalities include gingival swelling, purplish discoloration, and hemorrhages. Pain in the back and joints is common, sometimes accompanied

by obvious soft tissue and hemorrhage. Syncope and sudden death may occur. Anemia is frequent, while leukopenia occurs less commonly. Treatment with vitamin C results in rapid improvement (13).

HISTOPATHOLOGY. Follicular hyperkeratosis and perifollicular erythrocyte extravasation without an accompanying vasculopathy are characteristic. Extensive extravasations are usually associated with deposits of hemosiderin within and outside of macrophages. A coiled hair may emanate from the dilated follicular orifice (14).

Conditions to consider in the differential diagnosis:

Follicular maturation disorders
 androgenetic alopecia
 telogen effluvium
 trichotillomania
 scurvy
 vitamin A deficiency (phrynoderma)
Follicular keratinization disorders
 keratosis pilaris
 lichen spinulosus
 trichorrhexis invaginata (Netherton syndrome)
 trichostasis spinulosa
 acne vulgaris
 Favre–Racouchot syndrome (nodular elastosis with cysts and comedones)
 nevus comedonicus
 Bazex syndrome (follicular atrophoderma)

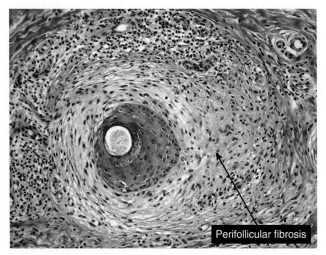

Fig. VIIA1.o

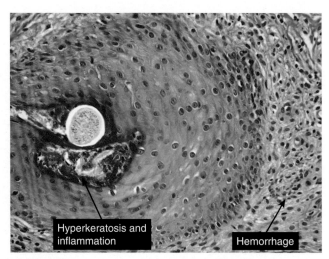

Fig. VIIA1.p

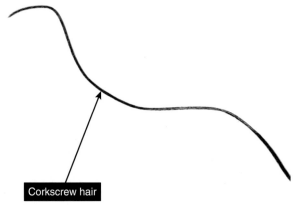

Fig. VIIA1.q

Fig. VIIA1.o. *Scurvy, medium power.* A horizontally sectioned biopsy from the leg shows a terminal follicle with eccentric placement of the hair shaft and focal thinning of the outer root sheath epithelium. There is perifollicular fibrosis, a lymphocytic infiltrate, and extravasated red blood cells to the right of the follicle.

Fig. VIIA1.p. *Scurvy, medium power.* In another section, the follicular canal is distorted and shows hyperkeratosis and a few neutrophils. Extravasated red blood cells are present in the surrounding stroma.

Fig. VIIA1.q. *Scurvy.* A plucked leg hair from the same patient shows the characteristic corkscrew morphology.

VIIA2 | Lymphocytes Predominant

There is follicular alteration with an inflammatory infiltrate mainly of lymphocytes. Conditions associated with inflammation may in many instances result in scarring alopecia in which hairs are lost and replaced by fibrosis (see Table VII.2).

Alopecia Areata

CLINICAL SUMMARY. Alopecia areata, considered likely to be an autoimmune disease, is characterized by complete or nearly complete absence of hair in one or more circumscribed areas of the scalp (15). Inflammatory change is not clinically obvious, and the follicular openings are preserved. Complete scalp involvement (alopecia totalis), or complete or nearly complete loss of body hair (alopecia universalis) can occur. Involvement of the eyebrows and eyelashes and a pitted defect in the nail plates are additional features of this condition. The majority of patients undergo spontaneous resolution, but a few

patients have permanent hair loss. In the areas of active hair shedding, a short, fractured hair shaft that tapers toward the scalp may be identified—the characteristic "exclamation point" hair.

HISTOPATHOLOGY. The critical diagnostic pathologic sign is lymphocytic infiltrates in the peribulbar area of anagen follicles, or follicles in early catagen (16). Lymphocytes may be seen sparsely infiltrating the matrix epithelium of follicles still in anagen. The lymphocytic infiltrates are present around the receding epithelial remnant of catagen hairs but also in the area of the collapsing follicular sheaths. Follicles diminish in size rapidly and become miniaturized, and as a result are identified more superficially in the dermis (17). Diminutive anagen follicles may be quite numerous, resulting in a higher proportion of miniaturized follicles than is seen in AGA, and often approaching 100% (18). In severe alopecia universalis and totalis of long duration (a decade or more), functional follicular structures may be diminished in number and some

TABLE VII.2. Scarring Alopecia (Decreased Follicular Density)

	Clinical Pattern	Inflammation Type	Site of Follicular Inflammation	Other Histo Features	Elastic Stain (VVG)
Lichen planopilaris (LPP) (and variants)	Irregularly shaped patches of hair loss scattered over the scalp. Perifollicular erythema and scale.	Lymphocytic	Isthmus and lower infundibulum; lichenoid/ interface with occasional colloid bodies. Sometimes interfollicular epidermis involved (~lichen planus).	Hypergranulosis of infundibula. Cleft between follicular epithelium and dermis—often. Perivascular and perieccrine inflammation absent.	Wedge-shaped scar (VVG negative) involving upper one-third of the follicle.
Discoid lupus erythematosus (DLE)	Classic lesions show alopecic areas with erythema, atrophy, dilated and plugged infundibula. May have central hypopigmentation.	Lymphoplasmacytic	Typically involves infundibulum but may involve entire follicle; interface vacuolar or lichenoid; colloid bodies less common than LPP. Epidermal involvement more common than LPP.	Superficial and deep perivascular and perieccrine inflammation. Dermal mucin is often increased. Epidermis may show thickened basement membrane zone (PAS+).	Broad scar throughout the dermis with destruction of perifollicular elastic sheath.
Central centrifugal cicatricial alopecia (CCCA)	Area of alopecia centered on the crown or vertex; progresses centrifugally.	Lymphocytic	Lower infundibulum and isthmus, without interface alteration.	Early finding is premature desquamation of the inner root sheath. Eccentric thinning of the outer root sheath and concentric lamellar fibrosis ensues.	Broad fibrous tracts outlined by an intact elastic sheath. Also, thickened elastic fibers throughout, due to "recoil" of the dermis.
Folliculitis decalvans	Multifocal pustules or larger alopecic patch on the crown with erythema, pustules, and crusting at the periphery.	Neutrophilic and lymphocytic	Intrafollicular and perifollicular involving the infundibulum and isthmus.	Resembles a bacterial folliculitis (may represent inflammatory stage of CCCA).	N/A
Acne keloidalis	Papules, pustules, and small areas of alopecia involving the posterior neck and occiput. In advanced cases, keloidal plaques form.	Lymphoplasmacytic (neutrophils if a pustule is biopsied)	Lower infundibulum and isthmus.	As follicles are destroyed, hair shaft fragments may serve as a stimulus for fibrosis.	N/A
Dissecting scalp cellulitis	Firm and fluctuant nodules, with areas of purulent drainage, primarily over the crown and vertex.	Lymphocytic, neutrophilic, and plasmacytic	Initially, perifollicular inflammation in the lower dermis and subcutaneous fat. Later, superficial parts of follicle are affected.	Early on, alopecia is due to conversion to catagen/ telogen hairs. Later, follicles are destroyed; granulation tissue, sinus tracts, and fibrosis develop. Sebaceous glands destroyed late.	N/A

VVG, Verhoef Van Gieson.

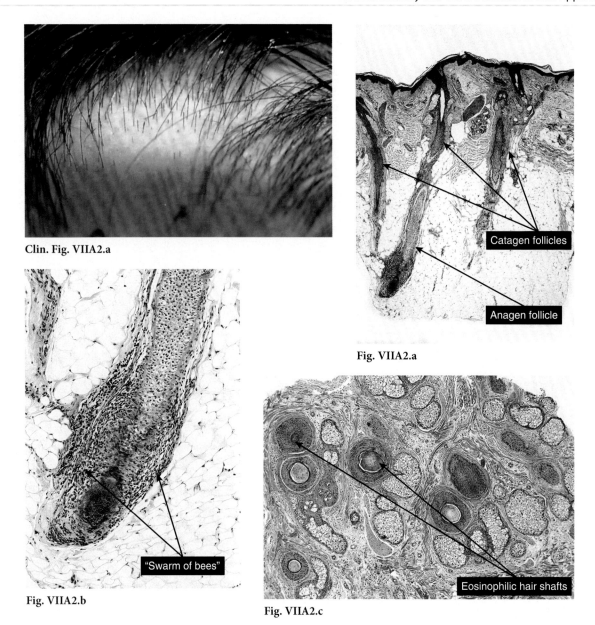

Clin. Fig. VIIA2.a

Fig. VIIA2.a

Fig. VIIA2.b

Fig. VIIA2.c

Clin. Fig. VIIA2.a. *Alopecia areata.* Well-circumscribed patch of alopecia with "exclamation" (!) hairs (tapering at proximal end) at the periphery typically responds to intralesional corticosteroids.

Fig. VIIA2.a. *Alopecia areata, low power, vertical section.* There are three catagen follicles, as indicated by a prominent eosinophilic cuticle. Beneath one of the catagen follicles there is a terminal anagen follicle with perifollicular inflammation within the subcutis. Catagen follicles are infrequently seen on vertical sectioning unless increased in number.

Fig. VIIA2.b. *Alopecia areata, high power, vertical section.* A dense lymphocytic infiltrate ("swarm of bees") hugs the bulb of the terminal anagen follicle seen in the previous figure.

Fig. VIIA2.c. *Alopecia areata, low power, horizontal section.* Most of the hairs present in this figure show varying degrees of eosinophilic change of the hair shaft, indicating that they are in various stages of transition from catagen to telogen hairs. At this level of sectioning, the lymphocytes are not present and the differential diagnosis would include telogen effluvium.

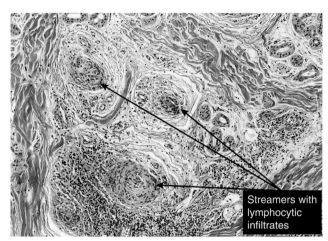

Fig. VIIA2.d

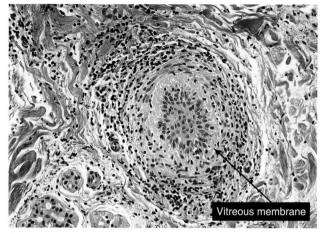

Fig. VIIA2.e

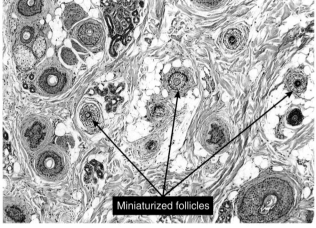

Fig. VIIA2.f

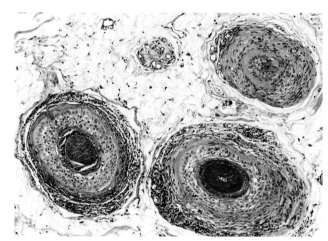

Fig. VIIA2.g

Fig. VIIA2.d. *Alopecia areata, medium power, horizontal section.* The increased percentage of resting follicles is reflected by the numerous streamers seen near the dermal–subcutaneous junction. A lymphoid infiltrate is apparent, concentrated about the streamers.

Fig. VIIA2.e. *Alopecia areata, high power, horizontal section.* Perifollicular lymphocytes can be seen affecting catagen and telogen follicles as they retreat upward into the dermis. The eosinophilic vitreous membrane is characteristic of this catagen follicle.

Fig. VIIA2.f. *Alopecia areata, low power, horizontal section.* In long-standing alopecia areata, there is an increased number of catagen and telogen follicles. In addition, follicular miniaturization is common.

Fig. VIIA2.g. *Alopecia areata, medium power, horizontal section.* Peribulbar lymphocytic inflammation is easily seen on horizontal sections within the subcutis. Since all of the follicles in the biopsy specimen can be visualized on horizontal sections, an increased number of streamers and catagen follicles can be easily assessed.

scarring of the follicular sheaths may be identified. Dilated follicular infundibula, which on horizontal sectioning bears resemblance to Swiss cheese, is another helpful clue in alopecia areata (19).

Lichen Planopilaris

CLINICAL SUMMARY. Lichen planopilaris (LPP) is follicular involvement by lichen planus. This type of lichen planus predominantly affects the scalp. Initially, there may be only follicular papules or perifollicular erythema; however, with progressive hair loss irregularly shaped atrophic patches of scarring alopecia develop on the scalp (20). The axillae and the pubic region may also be affected and the alopecia in these areas may be cicatricial. The association of scarring alopecia of the scalp and hyperkeratotic follicular papules on the trunk and extremities is known as Graham-Little syndrome. LPP may also coexist with typical lichen planus lesions on skin, mucous membranes, or nails.

Frontal fibrosing alopecia (FFA) is a variant of LPP that occurs in a band over the frontal scalp, typically in postmenopausal females (21). The characteristic histologic findings also involve vellus hair follicles on the face, clinically presenting as small papules (22).

HISTOPATHOLOGY. Most early lesions of LPP have a focally dense, band-like perifollicular lymphocytic infiltrate at the level of the lower infundibulum and the isthmus, where the hair "bulge" is located (23). The inferior segment of the hair follicle is spared. Vacuolar changes of the basal layer of the outer root sheath and necrotic keratinocytes are often seen. In addition, orthokeratosis and follicular plugging are observed. A few biopsies will exhibit simultaneous involvement of the interfollicular epidermis by lichen planus. In more developed lesions, perifollicular fibrosis and epithelial atrophy at the level of the infundibulum and isthmus are characteristic findings. Damage to the hair bulge, the site where stem cells of the hair follicle reside, results in permanent scarring alopecia (24). As in all scarring alopecias, sebaceous glands are lost. Distinction between LPP and FFA is not reliably possible by histopathology and should be based on clinicopathologic correlation (25). End-stage LPP will have vertically oriented fibrotic tracts containing clumps of degenerated elastic fibers replacing the destroyed hair follicles. This histologic picture in which no visible hair follicles remain resembles pseudopelade of Brocq.

Central Centrifugal Cicatricial Alopecia

CLINICAL SUMMARY. Central centrifugal cicatricial alopecia (CCCA) is a unifying concept that has been proposed to reflect the overlap of types of scarring alopecia that share clinical and histologic features (26). CCCA encompasses types of permanent hair loss which have in common the following features: alopecia centered on the crown or vertex of the scalp; fairly symmetrical expansion with the most active areas at the periphery; progressive chronic disease with eventual "burnout"; and clinical and microscopic evidence of inflammation in these active sites (27).

HISTOPATHOLOGY. CCCA displays all of the following histologic features: eccentric thinning of the outer root sheath epithelium, most prominent at the level of the isthmus and lower infundibulum, associated with close apposition of the hair shaft and follicular contents to the dermis; concentric lamellar fibroplasia ("onion skin" fibrosis); and chronic inflammation composed of lymphocytes and plasma cells surrounding the zone of fibroplasia (28). Eventually the hair shaft migrates into the dermis, inciting granulomatous inflammation and additional epithelial destruction. Finally, the follicle is replaced by a vertical band of connective tissue, resulting in a "follicular scar." Singly, these histologic features may be found in other types of scarring alopecia.

CCCA may also show one of three histologic patterns of disease: follicular degeneration syndrome, pseudopelade pattern (a "modern" use of the term, not pseudopelade of Brocq), and folliculitis decalvans (29). For instance, African-American patients with CCCA who display characteristics of the follicular degeneration syndrome pattern tend to show premature desquamation of the inner root sheath (30,31). A characteristic histologic feature of the folliculitis decalvans pattern is folliculocentric neutrophilic inflammation, typically seen if a pustule from the expanding margin is biopsied.

Discoid Lupus Erythematosus of the Scalp

As discussed in Section IIIH4, discoid lupus is characterized clinically by well-demarcated, erythematous, slightly infiltrated, "discoid" plaques that often have adherent thick scales and follicular plugging. The lesions are often limited to the face, where the malar areas and the nose are predominantly affected. In addition, the scalp, ears, oral mucosa, and vermilion border of the lips may be involved. The histologic findings include hyperkeratosis with follicular and sometimes eccrine duct plugging. Parakeratosis is not conspicuous, and may be absent. In the epidermis, there is thinning and flattening of the stratum malpighii, interface change with vacuolar degeneration of basal cells, dyskeratosis, and squamotization of basilar keratinocytes. The basement membrane is thickened and tortuous. In the dermis, there is a predominantly lymphocytic infiltrate (often with plasma cells), arranged along the dermal–epidermal junction, around blood vessels, hair follicles, and eccrine coils, and in an interstitial pattern often into the deep reticular dermis, with interstitial mucin deposition, edema, vasodilatation, and slight extravasation of erythrocytes. CD123 + plasmacytoid dendritic cells may be present in clusters and can serve as a helpful though not pathognomonic marker (32). There may be extension of the inflammatory infiltrate into the subcutis.

Follicular Mucinosis and Alopecia Mucinosa

Follicular mucinosis (FM) can be seen in childhood but is more common in adults. It may occur in three settings: a primary idiopathic form, a form associated with malignancy, and a form secondary to inflammatory conditions. The histologic hallmark is accumulation of mucin in the follicular epithelium (33). When FM affects terminal hair-bearing areas and is associated with hair loss, the term alopecia mucinosa (AM) is often used.

The possibility of mycosis fungoides should always be considered when a diagnosis of FM/AM is contemplated. It has been said that an isolated patch in the head or neck area is much more likely to be FM than mycosis fungoides,

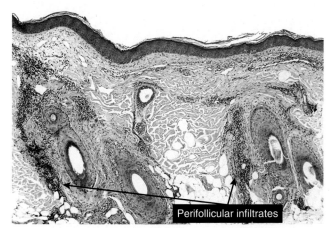

Fig. VIIA2.h

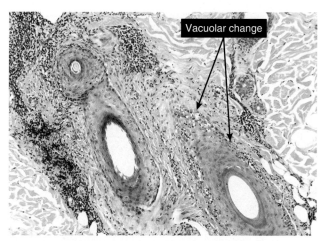

Fig. VIIA2.i

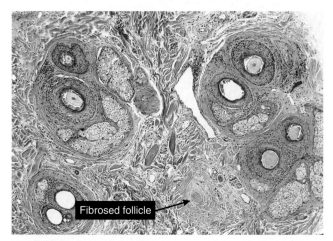

Fig. VIIA2.j

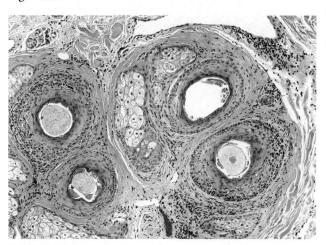

Fig. VIIA2.k

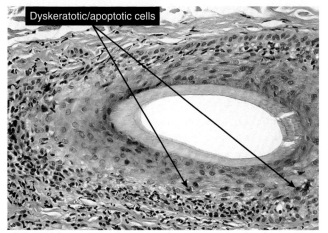

Fig. VIIA2.l

Fig. VIIA2.h. *Lichen planopilaris, low power, vertical section.* A dense, mostly perifollicular lymphoid infiltrate affecting predominantly the isthmus and lower infundibulum is seen on scanning magnification. The interfollicular epidermis, which is best visualized on vertical sections, is largely unaffected.

Fig. VIIA2.i. *Lichen planopilaris, medium power, vertical section.* The lymphocytic infiltrate is associated with vacuolar alteration of the outer layers of the follicular epithelium.

Fig. VIIA2.j. *Lichen planopilaris, low power, horizontal section.* Follicular loss (i.e., scarring) is best identified on horizontal sections. A perifollicular lymphoid infiltrate is also apparent.

Fig. VIIA2.k. *Lichen planopilaris, medium power, horizontal section.* At the level of the isthmus, vacuolar change, perifollicular fibrosis, and inflammation are most prominent.

Fig. VIIA2.l. *Lichen planopilaris, high power, horizontal section.* The lymphocytic infiltrate is associated with blurring of the interface between the follicular epithelium and dermis, keratinocyte vacuolization, and dyskeratosis/apoptosis.

Inflammatory and Other Disorders of Skin Appendages

VII

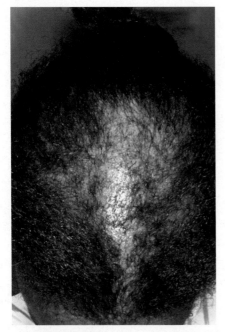

Clin. Fig. VIIA2.b

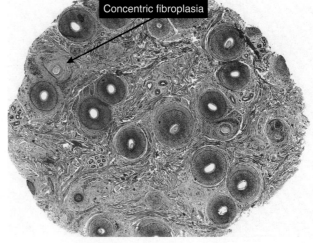

Fig. VIIA2.m

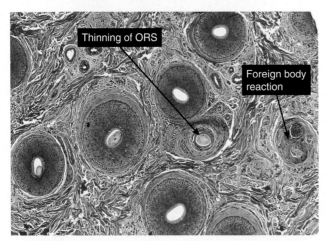

Fig. VIIA2.n

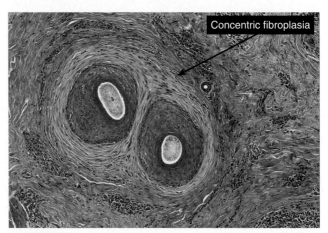

Fig. VIIA2.o

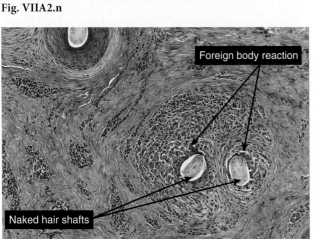

Fig. VIIA2.p

Clin. Fig. VIIA2.b. *Central centrifugal cicatricial alopecia.* This condition occurs most commonly in African-Americans and affects the crown and vertex of the scalp. Hair loss is permanent.

Fig. VIIA2.m,n. *Central centrifugal cicatricial alopecia, transverse section.* In the upper dermis, the affected follicles show eccentric thinning of the outer root sheath (ORS) epithelium and perifollicular fibrosis manifested by concentric lamellar fibroplasia. There is lymphoplasmacytic inflammation peripheral to the fibrosis. Sebaceous glands, normally seen at this level, are notably absent.

Fig. VIIA2.o. *Central centrifugal cicatricial alopecia, transverse section.* The affected follicles show early perifollicular fibrosis with some mononuclear inflammation.

Fig. VIIA2.p. *Central centrifugal cicatricial alopecia, transverse section.* The follicular epithelium may be completely destroyed, resulting in naked hair shafts which incite a granulomatous response.

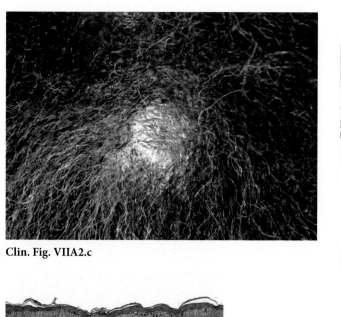

Clin. Fig. VIIA2.c

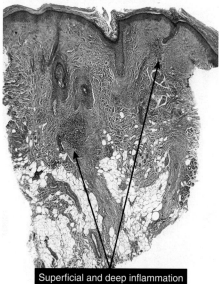

Superficial and deep inflammation

Fig. VIIA2.q

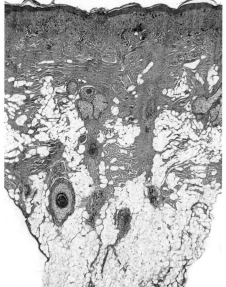

Fig. VIIA2.r

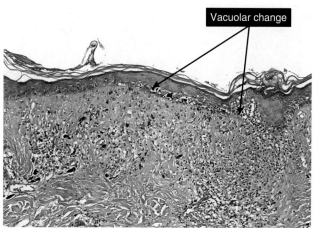

Vacuolar change

Fig. VIIA2.s

Clin. Fig. VIIA2.c. *Discoid lupus erythematosus.* The inflammation in this hyperpigmented plaque with follicular plugging led to permanent hair loss.

Fig. VIIA2.q. *Discoid lupus erythematosus of the scalp, low power.* A superficial and deep often quite prominent perivascular and perifollicular inflammatory infiltrate is seen at low magnification.

Fig. VIIA2.r. *Discoid lupus erythematosus, low power.* In some examples, as here, the infiltrate can be quite sparse. The number of hair follicles is diminished at scanning magnification.

Fig. VIIA2.s. *Discoid lupus erythematosus, medium power.* As in other forms of lupus erythematosus, the epidermis reveals atrophy, vacuolar alteration, and an interface dermatitis. This superficial infiltrate is composed primarily of lymphocytes and there is prominent pigment incontinence. (*continues*)

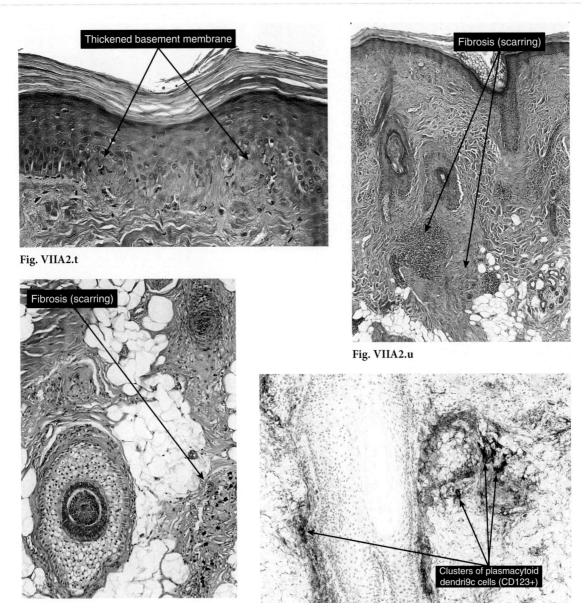

Fig. VIIA2.t. *Discoid lupus erythematosus, high power.* Close examination of the epidermis reveals hyper-keratosis and thickening of the basement membrane zone. Pigment-laden macrophages are seen in the papillary dermis.

Fig. VIIA2.u. *Discoid lupus erythematosus, medium power.* The perifollicular infiltrate is associated with eventual scarring and fibrosis at the site of hair follicles.

Fig. VIIA2.v. *Discoid lupus erythematosus, medium power.* Pigment-laden macrophages may be seen in the subcutaneous fat at the site of previous hair follicles. However, this finding is not specific to this diagnosis and can be seen in other forms of alopecia.

Fig. VIIA2.w. CD123 staining demonstrates clustering of plasmacytoid dendritic cells in the dermis adjacent to a follicle in a discoid lesion of the scalp.

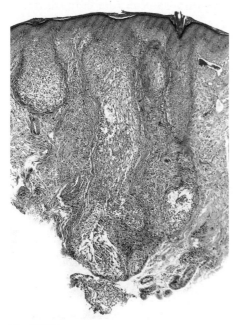

Fig. VIIA2.x

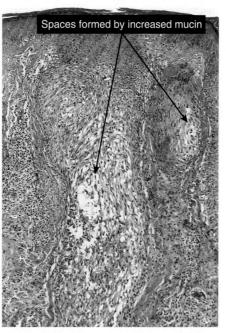

Spaces formed by increased mucin

Fig. VIIA2.y

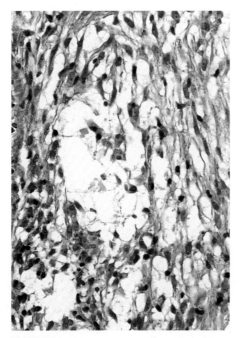

Fig. VIIA2.z

Fig. VIIA2.x. *Follicular mucinosis, low power.* At scanning magnification, the follicular epithelium appears widened by multiple clear spaces. The overlying epidermis is uninvolved.

Fig. VIIA2.y. *Alopecia mucinosa, medium power.* The follicular keratinocytes are pale and in many areas are separated from adjacent keratinocytes. There is a surrounding perivascular and perifollicular lymphoid infiltrate.

Fig. VIIA2.z. *Alopecia mucinosa, high power.* The follicular epithelium appears clear because of extensive deposition of acid mucopolysaccharide. The epithelium is also infiltrated by small lymphoid cells which lack significant cytologic atypia. The acid mucopolysaccharide can be demonstrated using alcian blue or colloidal iron stains. The predominant component is hyaluronic acid which can be removed by digestion with hyaluronidase.

that younger patients are more likely to have FM with spontaneous remission, and older patients are more likely to develop mycosis fungoides, and that none of the clinicopathologic features of FM or mycosis fungoides (including monoclonality) are without overlap (34).

Rosacea

CLINICAL SUMMARY. Rosacea is a very common condition characterized by transient or persistent central facial erythema, dilated blood vessels, and often papules and pustules. Rosacea can be classified into four broad subtypes: erythematotelangiectatic (ETR), papulopustular (PPR), phymatous (characterized by thickening, e.g., rhinophyma, otophyma), and ocular (e.g., blepharitis, conjunctivitis) (35).

HISTOPATHOLOGY. The histologic features of rosacea include perivascular and perifollicular lymphocytic inflammation, telangiectatic blood vessels, prominent dermatoheliosis, and often Demodex mites within the infundibulum of hair follicles. Granulomatous rosacea will additionally have a histiocytic infiltrate, often arranged in small collections amid the lymphocytic inflammation. In a detailed study, histopathologic findings associated with severity of rosacea differed according to subtype. The intensity of perifollicular lymphohistiocytic inflammation and the presence of a follicular inflammatory reaction were dependent on the severity of rosacea in both the ETR and the PPR subtypes, with the intensity of inflammatory reactions being higher in the PPR subtype (36).

Conditions to consider in the differential diagnosis:

alopecia areata
discoid lupus erythematosus
alopecia mucinosa/follicular mucinosis
folliculotropic mycosis fungoides
lichen planopilaris
Fox–Fordyce disease
syringolymphoid hyperplasia with alopecia
lichen striatus
chronic folliculitis
rosacea
perioral dermatitis
disseminate and recurrent infundibular folliculitis
acne varioliformis (acne necrotica)

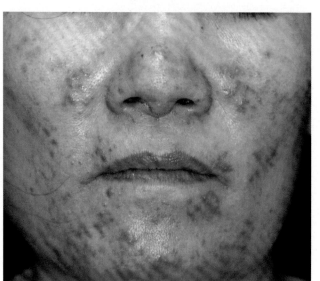

Clin. Fig. VIIA2.d

Clin. Fig. VIIA2.d. *Rosacea, papulopustular subtype.* A 52-year-old woman has erythematous papulopustular lesions on the face. The biopsy showed many Demodex mites within the follicles.

Fig. VIIA2.za. *Rosacea, low power.* This biopsy from facial skin reveals prominent sebaceous glands, a lymphoid infiltrate, and telangiectasia.

Fig. VIIA2.zb. *Rosacea, high power.* The infiltrate may be perivascular, interstitial, and perifollicular.

Fig. VIIA2.zc. *Rosacea, high power.* Here the infiltrate is vaguely granulomatous.

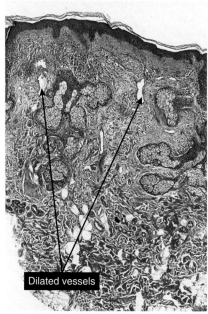

Dilated vessels

Fig. VIIA2.za

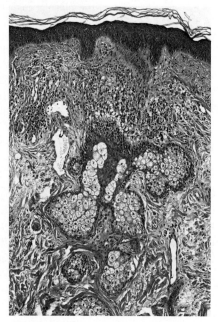

Fig. VIIA2.zb

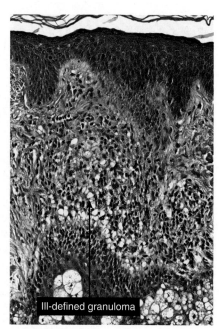

Ill-defined granuloma

Fig. VIIA2.zc

VIIA3 With Prominent Eosinophils

Eosinophils are prominent in the infiltrate and may infiltrate the follicular structures. Eosinophilic pustular folliculitis is prototypic (37).

Eosinophilic Pustular Folliculitis

CLINICAL SUMMARY. This condition demonstrates broad patches of itchy follicular papules and pustules involving particularly the face, trunk, and arms (38).

The involved areas may take on various configurations including circinate, and there may be central healing and peripheral spread. The condition occurs in adults, most often in Japan (Ofuji disease), in infants and also in patients with HIV infection or another immunosuppressive state (39). Extrafollicular lesions with involvement of both palms and soles, and scarring alopecia through scalp involvement may occur. Moderate leukocytosis and eosinophilia in the peripheral blood are also present.

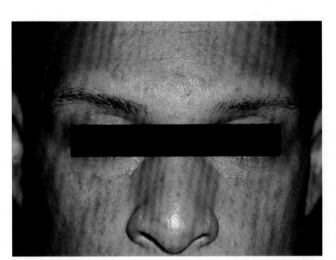

Clin. Fig. VIIA3

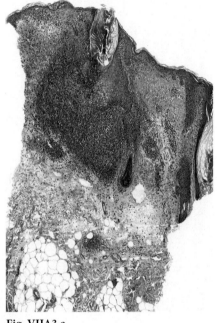

Fig. VIIA3.a

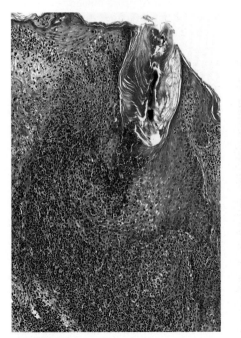

Fig. VIIA3.b

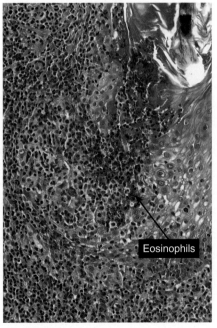

Eosinophils

Fig. VIIA3.c

Clin. Fig. VIIA3. *Eosinophilic pustular folliculitis.* Pruritic erythematous papules commonly seen on the face of HIV-infected patients characterize this recalcitrant condition.

Fig. VIIA3.a. *Eosinophilic pustular folliculitis, low power.* In the center of this punch biopsy, a hair follicle shows an intense inflammatory infiltrate involving the upper half of the follicular epithelium.

Fig. VIIA3.b. *Eosinophilic pustular folliculitis, medium power.* The infiltrate involves the follicular epithelium, sebaceous ducts and lobules, and the surrounding dermis.

Fig. VIIA3.c. *Eosinophilic pustular folliculitis, high power.* The infiltrate is composed predominantly of neutrophils and numerous eosinophils.

HISTOPATHOLOGY. Involved follicles may have spongiotic change with exocytosis extending from the sebaceous gland and its duct throughout the infundibular zone (40). Lymphocytes with some eosinophils migrate into the epidermis initially in a somewhat diffuse pattern, but micropustular aggregation develops and the ultimate lesion is an infundibular eosinophilic pustule (41). The epidermis adjacent to the follicle may be involved with eosinophilic microabscess formation. In the adjacent dermis, there are perivascular infiltrates of lymphocytes and numerous eosinophils.

Conditions to consider in the differential diagnosis:

eosinophilic pustular folliculitis
erythema toxicum neonatorum
Ofuji syndrome
fungal folliculitis

VIIA4 Neutrophils Prominent

There is a follicular inflammatory infiltrate containing neutrophils, which may result in disruption of the follicle. Furuncle is prototypic (42).

Acute Deep Folliculitis (Furuncle)

CLINICAL SUMMARY. A furuncle is caused by staphylococci and consists of a tender, red, perifollicular swelling terminating in the discharge of pus and of a necrotic plug.

HISTOPATHOLOGY. A furuncle has an area of perifollicular necrosis containing fibrinoid material and many neutrophils. At the deep end of the necrotic plug, in the subcutaneous tissue, is a large abscess. A Gram stain reveals small clusters of staphylococci in the center of the abscess.

Tinea Capitis

See also IC1, VIIA5.

This term refers to dermatophyte fungal infections occurring in the scalp and involving hairs. The involvement can be "endothrix" (within the hair shaft) or "ectothrix" (encircling the hair shaft).

Majocchi Granuloma

CLINICAL SUMMARY. Occasionally, *Trichophyton rubrum* causes a papular folliculitis, often arising in areas

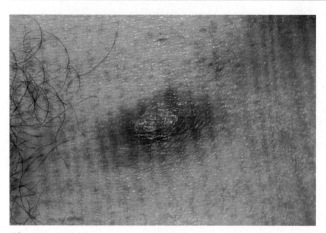

Clin. Fig. VIIA4

Clin. Fig. VIIA4. *Furuncle.* An inflamed tender nodule represents the acute stage of a furuncle caused by *Staphylococcal aureus.*

Fig. VIIA4.a. *Acute folliculitis.* Scanning magnification is essentially indistinguishable from eosinophilic pustular folliculitis. The hair follicle shows intense infiltration of its epithelium by an acute inflammatory cell reaction. There is a surrounding perivascular infiltrate.

Fig. VIIA4.b. *Acute folliculitis, high power.* The infiltrate within the follicular epithelium is composed predominantly of neutrophils. Eosinophils may be seen but not to the extent that they are present in eosinophilic pustular folliculitis. There are yeast forms consistent with Pityrosporum organisms which are generally saprophytic but may be etiologic in some cases.

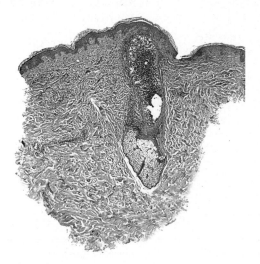

Fig. VIIA4.a

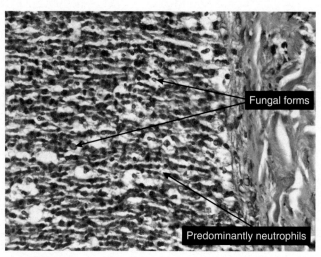

Fig. VIIA4.b

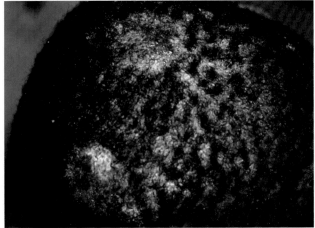

Clin. Fig. VIIA4.b

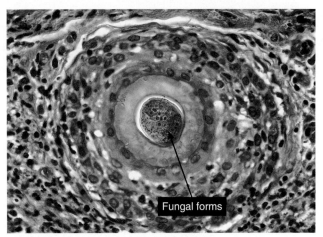

Fig. VIIA4.c

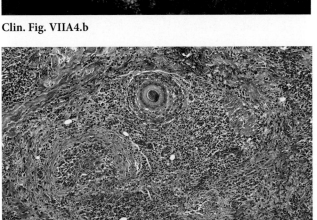

Fig. VIIA4.d

Fungal forms

Fig. VIIA4.e

Clin. Fig. VIIA4.b. *Tinea capitis.* Scaly patches with associated hair loss is a common presentation of tinea capitis in African-American children.

Fig. VIIA4.c. *Tinea capitis, low power, horizontal section.* The extensive inflammation in this case has led to follicular destruction and scarring.

Fig. VIIA4.d. *Tinea capitis, medium power, horizontal section.* The dense inflammatory infiltrate contains mixed cell types.

Fig. VIIA4.e. *Tinea capitis, high power, horizontal section.* Neutrophils and other inflammatory cells surround this small follicle. Fungal elements are present within the hair shaft.

of superficial dermatophyte infection ("ringworm") that is characterized by annular scaly erythematous patches. "Majocchi granuloma" is seen most commonly on the legs in association with an infection of the soles, particularly in women who shave their legs (43) or in patients in whom a tinea infection was treated with potent topical corticosteroids.

HISTOPATHOLOGY. Sections show a nodular folliculitis and perifolliculitis forming an abscess in the dermis. On staining with PAS or methenamine silver, numerous

hyphae and spores are seen within hairs and hair follicles and sometimes in the inflammatory infiltrate of the dermis. The fungal elements reach the dermis through a break in the follicular wall. The dermal infiltrate shows lymphocytes, macrophages, and scattered multinucleated giant cells around and within an area of central necrosis and occasionally also suppuration.

Herpes Simplex Viral Folliculitis

Viral folliculitis can be caused by both herpes simplex virus and varicella-zoster virus, though varicella-zoster

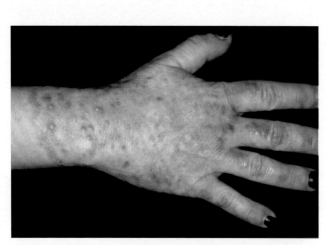

Clin. Fig. VIIA4.c

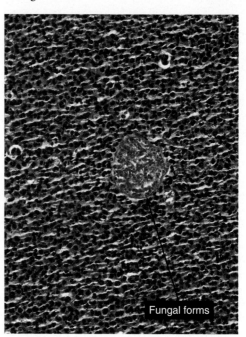

Follicular derived pustule

Fig. VIIA4.f

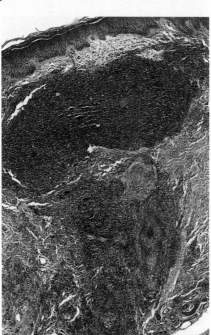

Fig. VIIA4.g

Fungal forms

Fig. VIIA4.h

Clin. Fig. VIIA4.c. *Majocchi granuloma.* KOH scraping of these scaly papules within an annular plaque confirmed the diagnosis.

Fig. VIIA4.f. *Majocchi granuloma, low power.* Scanning magnification reveals an abscess in the superficial dermis.

Fig. VIIA4.g. *Majocchi granuloma, medium power.* Beneath this abscess, the hair follicles show an intense inflammatory reaction.

Fig. VIIA4.h. *Majocchi granuloma, high power.* Upon close examination of the hair shaft on the H&E stained sections, one can identify pale blue–staining fungal hyphae within the hair shaft.

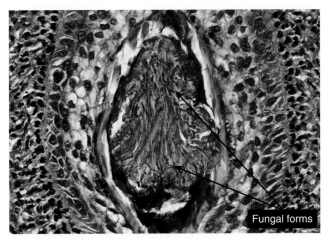

Fig. VIIA4.i

Fig. VIIA4.i. *Majocchi granuloma, high power.* PAS stain reveals multiple organisms which have replaced a fragment of hair shaft embedded in a sea of neutrophils (abscess).

more commonly involves follicles (44,45). In early lesions, herpes folliculitis presents as lymphocytic folliculitis which may be devoid of epithelial changes considered to be diagnostic of herpes virus infections. Exclusive involvement of follicles is not uncommon in zoster.

Conditions to consider in the differential diagnosis:

superficial folliculitis
  acute bacterial folliculitis
  Impetigo Bockhart
  Pseudomonas folliculitis
  acne vulgaris
deep folliculitis
  furuncle, carbuncle
  folliculitis barbae, decalvans
  pseudofolliculitis of the beard
  pyoderma gangrenosum
follicular occlusion disorders
  dissecting cellulitis/perifolliculitis capitis abscedens
    et suffodiens
  hidradenitis suppurativa
  acne conglobata
fungal folliculitis
  Majocchi granuloma (T. rubrum)
  favus (T. schoenleinii)
  alopecia of secondary syphilis
  Pityrosporum folliculitis
  viral folliculitis
  acne fulminans

VIIA5 | Plasma Cells Prominent

Plasma cells are seen in abundance in the infiltrate. In most instances they are admixed with lymphocytes. Acne keloidalis is prototypic.

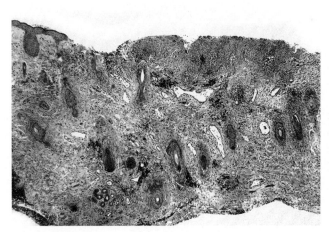

Fig. VIIA4.j

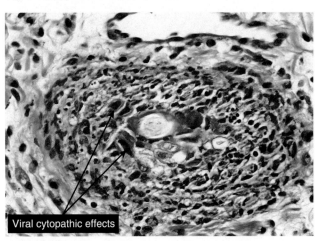

Fig. VIIA4.k

Fig. VIIA4.j. *Herpes simplex viral folliculitis, low power.* Scanning magnification reveals epidermal ulceration and a perivascular and perifollicular inflammatory infiltrate which is generally mixed, including both acute and chronic inflammatory cells. Early lesions often show a lymphocytic folliculitis without epidermal changes.

Fig. VIIA4.k. *Herpes simplex viral folliculitis, high power.* The follicular epithelium shows extensive necrosis and destruction associated with an inflammatory infiltrate that contains many neutrophils. Follicular keratinocytes show peripheral rimming of nuclear chromatin and may show multinucleation. These changes may also be seen in the overlying epidermis.

Folliculitis (Acne) Keloidalis Nuchae

CLINICAL SUMMARY. Folliculitis keloidalis nuchae represents a chronic folliculitis on the nape of the neck in men that causes hypertrophic scarring (46). In early cases, there are follicular papules, pustules, and occasionally abscesses. The lesions are replaced gradually by indurated fibrous nodules and sometimes plaques (47).

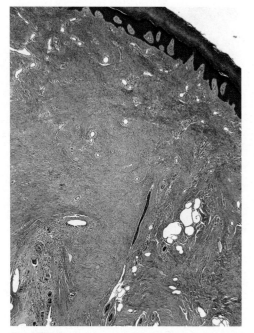

Fig. VIIA5.a

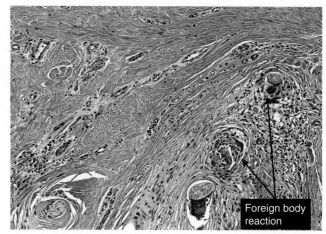

Fig. VIIA5.b

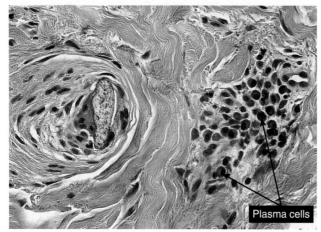

Fig. VIIA5.c

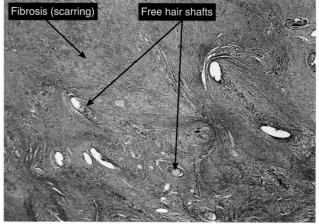

Fig. VIIA5.d

Fig. VIIA5.a. *Acne keloidalis nuchae, low power.* Several hair shafts are seen within the deep dermis surrounded by chronic inflammation and extensive scarring.

Fig. VIIA5.b. *Acne keloidalis nuchae, medium power.* The dermis becomes fibrotic secondary to chronic inflammation. Free hair shafts are surrounded by granulomatous inflammation.

Fig. VIIA5.c. *Acne keloidalis nuchae, high power.* A portion of a hair shaft is being engulfed by a multinucleated giant cell. The infiltrate also contains numerous plasma cells.

Fig. VIIA5.d. *Acne keloidalis nuchae, medium power.* In a late lesion, free hair shafts have incited chronic inflammation leading to dense fibrosis in the dermis.

HISTOPATHOLOGY. Deep folliculitis progresses to follicular destruction and dermal fibrosis. Late-stage lesions show extensive fibrosis and scarring, only sometimes with keloidal collagen.

Tinea Capitis

See also IC1, VIIA4.

Plasma cells may be quite prominent in the infiltrate associated with tinea capitis, which can clinically mimic many causes of scarring alopecia, including folliculitis, chronic furuncles, folliculitis decalvans, dissecting scalp cellulitis, discoid lupus erythematosus, and traction alopecia, as well as eczema and psoriasis (48).

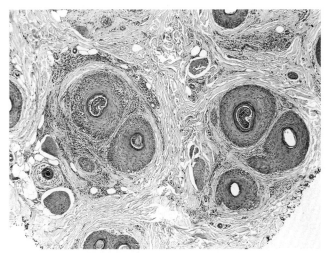

Fig. VIIA5.e

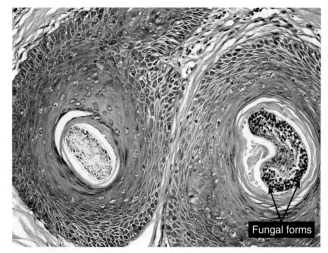

Fungal forms

Fig. VIIA5.f

Fig. VIIA5.e. *Tinea capitis, low power, horizontal section.* The infiltrate in this example is perifollicular and interstitial, and is composed predominantly of lymphocytes and plasma cells.

Fig. VIIA5.f. *Tinea capitis, high power, horizontal section.* This PAS-stained section highlights the fungal spores and hyphae in cross-section that characterize this endothrix infection with *Trichophyton tonsurans.* Horizontal sections demonstrate that not every follicle is involved.

Conditions to consider in the differential diagnosis:

acne keloidalis
fungal folliculitis
alopecia of secondary syphilis

VIIA6 Fibrosing and Suppurative Follicular Disorders

There is extensive fibrosis of the dermis, often with keratin tunnels of follicular origin, and with embedded hairs with associated foreign-body inflammation. Neutrophils and plasma cells are seen in abundance in the infiltrate, in addition to lymphocytes.

Follicular Occlusion Triad (Hidradenitis Suppurativa, Acne Conglobata, and Perifolliculitis Capitis Abscedens et Suffodiens)

CLINICAL SUMMARY. The three diseases included in the follicular occlusion triad are similar. Quite frequently, two or three of the diseases are encountered in the same patient. All three diseases represent a chronic, recurrent, deep-seated folliculitis resulting in abscesses and followed by the formation of sinus tracts and scarring. In *hidradenitis suppurativa,* the axillary and anogenital regions are primarily affected (49). In acute lesions there are red, tender nodules that become fluctuant and heal after discharging pus. In chronic cases, deep-seated abscesses lead to the discharge of pus through sinus tracts, resulting in severe scarring. *Acne conglobata* occurs mainly on the back, buttocks, and chest and only rarely on the face or the extremities. In addition to comedones, fluctuant nodules discharging pus or a mucoid material occur, as well as deep-seated abscesses that discharge through interconnecting sinus tracts. In *perifolliculitis capitis abscedens et suffodiens,* which involves the scalp and neck, nodules and abscesses as described above occur in the scalp, also known as *dissecting cellulitis of the scalp* (50,51). *Pilonidal sinus* is often also considered to be a part of this group of disorders ("follicular occlusion tetrad").

HISTOPATHOLOGY. Early lesions show follicular hyperkeratosis with plugging and dilatation of the follicle. The follicular epithelium may proliferate or may be destroyed. At first there is little inflammation, but eventually a perifolliculitis develops with an extensive deep reticular dermal or subcutaneous infiltrate composed of neutrophils, lymphocytes, and histiocytes. Abscess formation results and leads to the destruction first of the pilosebaceous structures and later of other cutaneous appendages. Apocrine glands in hidradenitis suppurativa of the axillae or groin regions may be secondarily involved by the inflammatory process. In response to this destruction, granulation tissue containing lymphoid and plasma cells, and foreign-body giant cells related to fragments of keratin and to embedded hairs, infiltrate the area near the remnants of hair follicles. As the abscesses extend deeper into the subcutaneous tissue, draining sinus tracts develop that are lined with epidermis. In areas of healing, there is extensive fibrosis.

Hidradenitis Suppurativa

See Clin. Fig. VIIA6.a and Figs. VIIA6.a–d.

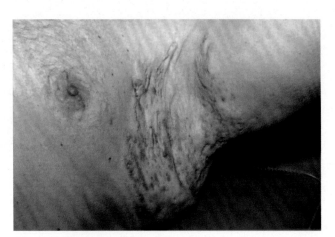

Clin. Fig. VIIA6.a

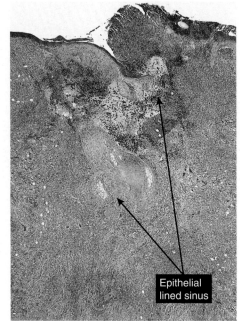
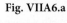

Fig. VIIA6.a

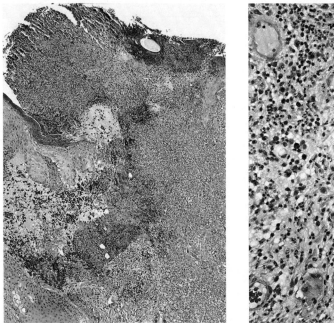

Fig. VIIA6.b

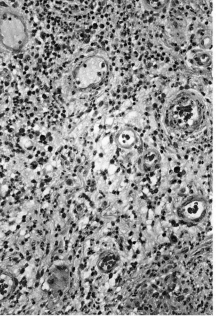

Fig. VIIA6.c

Clin. Fig. VIIA6.a. *Hidradenitis suppurativa.* Draining sinus tracts were present in the axillae, characteristic of hidradenitis suppurativa.

Fig. VIIA6.a. *Hidradenitis suppurativa, low power.* There is an area of epidermal ulceration associated with an invagination of epithelium. There is a dense inflammatory reaction throughout the dermis.

Fig. VIIA6.b. *Hidradenitis suppurativa, medium power.* At the edge of the ulceration the epithelium shows hyperplasia. The infiltrate is intense and frequently forms abscesses composed of neutrophils.

Fig. VIIA6.c. *Hidradenitis suppurativa, high power.* The dermis, as seen here, may show granulation tissue–like changes with a mixed acute and chronic inflammatory infiltrate. One may also see extensive fibrosis and granulomatous inflammation, changes which may be indistinguishable from a ruptured epidermal cyst.

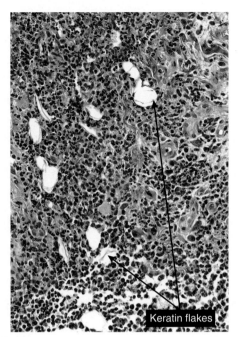

Fig. VIIA6.d

Fig. VIIA6.d. *Hidradenitis suppurativa, high power.* There may be flakes of keratin (often gray in color as here), eliciting a neutrophilic and often a granulomatous response.

Dissecting Cellulitis of the Scalp

See Figs. VIIA6.e–g.

Folliculitis Decalvans

CLINICAL SUMMARY. In folliculitis decalvans, scattered through the scalp are slowly enlarging, bald, atrophic areas with follicular pustules at their peripheries (52). In some instances, other hairy areas, such as the beard and pubic regions, the axillae, eyebrows, and eyelashes, are also involved. It may represent a highly inflammatory stage of CCCA with pustules, erythema, crusting, and bacterial superinfection.

HISTOPATHOLOGY. As in the other forms of chronic deep folliculitis, folliculitis keloidalis nuchae, and folliculitis barbae, in early lesions there is a perifollicular infiltrate composed largely of neutrophils but also containing lymphoid cells, histiocytes, and plasma cells (53). The infiltrate develops into a perifollicular abscess leading to destruction of the hair and hair follicles. Often, foreign-body giant cells are present around remnants of hair follicles, and particles of keratin may be located near the giant cells. As healing takes place, fibrosis is observed. If

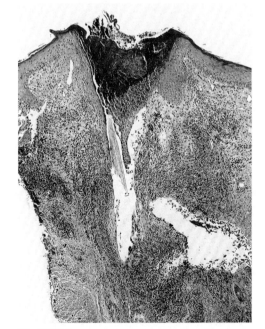

Fig. VIIA6.e

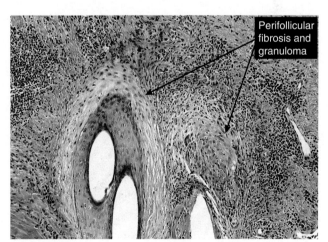

Fig. VIIA6.f

Fig. VIIA6.e. *Dissecting cellulitis of the scalp, low power.* Early lesions may show follicular plugging with acute perifollicular inflammation. Eventually the follicle is destroyed and replaced by dense mixed inflammation. The appearances are indistinguishable from hidradenitis suppurativa.

Fig. VIIA6.f. *Dissecting cellulitis of the scalp, medium power.* Perifollicular fibrosis ensues and is accompanied by granulomatous inflammation to follicular contents. Advanced lesions may show sinus tract formation. (*continues*)

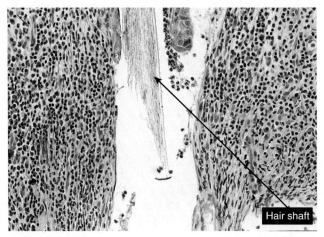

Fig. VIIA6.g

Fig. VIIA6.g. *Dissecting cellulitis of the scalp, high power.* The follicular epithelium is almost completely destroyed, leaving the hair shaft exposed to the dermis and a mixed infiltrate of neutrophils, lymphocytes, histiocytes, and plasma cells.

there is hypertrophic scar formation, as in folliculitis keloidalis nuchae, numerous thick bundles of sclerotic collagen are present.

Conditions to consider in the differential diagnosis:

    acne keloidalis
follicular occlusion disorders
    pilonidal sinus
    hidradenitis suppurativa
    acne conglobata
    perifolliculitis capitis abscedens et suffodiens
    (dissecting cellulitis of the scalp)
deep folliculitis
    folliculitis barbae, decalvans

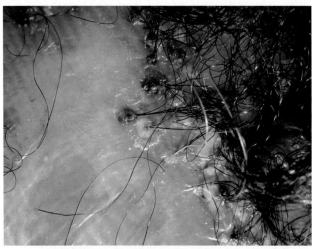

Clin. Fig. VIIA6.b

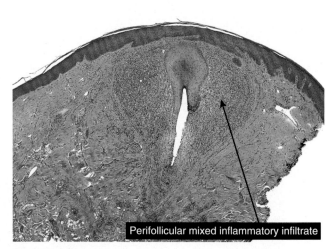

Fig. VIIA6.h

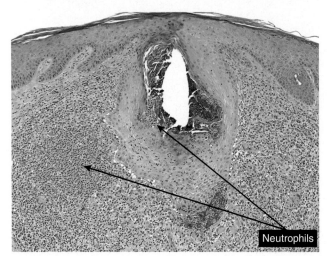

Fig. VIIA6.i

Clin. Fig. VIIA6.b. *Folliculitis decalvans.* An area of scarring alopecia in a middle-aged man, associated with a hyperkeratotic scale-crust with follicular hyperkeratosis and erythema, and follicular pustules.

Fig. VIIA6.h. *Folliculitis decalvans, medium power, vertical section.* Early lesions show a follicular-based pustule with perifollicular inflammation composed predominantly of neutrophils, with chronic inflammatory cells as well.

Fig. VIIA6.i. *Folliculitis decalvans, low power, vertical section.* A later lesion shows destruction of the follicle with a perifollicular microabscess and fibrosis in the surrounding dermis.

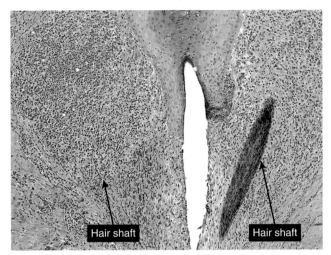

Fig. VIIA6.j

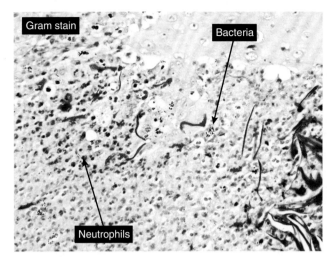

Fig. VIIA6.k

Fig. VIIA6.j. *Folliculitis decalvans, high power, vertical section.* As the hair shaft and follicular keratin come in contact with the dermis, chronic and granulomatous inflammation ensues.

Fig. VIIA6.k. *Folliculitis decalvans, high power, Gram stain.* Pustular lesions may develop as a consequence of bacterial superinfection. The Gram stain shows clusters of gram-positive cocci amid the perifollicular neutrophils.

VIIB PATHOLOGY INVOLVING SWEAT GLANDS

The sebaceous glands, eccrine glands, and apocrine glands may be involved in inflammatory processes (hidradenitis).

1. Scant Inflammation
2. Lymphocytes Predominant

2a. With Plasma Cells
2b. With Eosinophils
2c. Neutrophils Predominant

VIIB1 Scant Inflammation

Sweat glands are abnormal in size or number, but there is little or no inflammation.

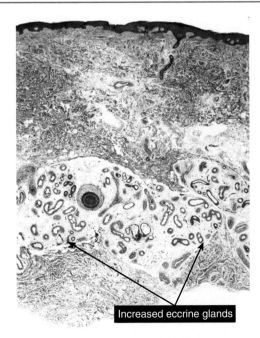

Fig. VIIB1.a

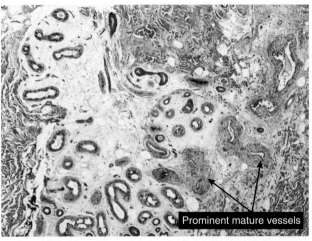

Fig. VIIB1.b

Fig. VIIB1.a. *Eccrine angiomatous hamartoma, low power.* In the deep dermis, there is an increased number of eccrine glands in a mucinous stroma.

Fig. VIIB1.b. *Eccrine angiomatous hamartoma, medium power.* The eccrine glands may be dilated, as seen here; there is an increased number of mature vascular channels.

Eccrine Nevus

CLINICAL SUMMARY. Eccrine nevi are very rare. They may show a circumscribed area of hyperhidrosis, a solitary sweat-discharging pore, or papular lesions in a linear arrangement (54). In the so-called eccrine angiomatous hamartoma, there may be one or several nodules or a solitary large plaque. The lesions are generally present on an extremity at birth. Hyperhidrosis and/or pain may be apparent.

HISTOPATHOLOGY. Eccrine nevi show an increase in the size of the eccrine coil or in both the size and the number of coils. In other cases, there is ductal hyperplasia consisting of thickening of the walls and dilatation of the lumina. Eccrine angiomatous hamartomas show increased numbers of eccrine structures with numerous surrounding or intermingled capillary channels. These hamartomas may also contain fatty tissue and pilar structures.

Conditions to consider in the differential diagnosis:

> argyria
> syringosquamous metaplasia
> eccrine nevus
> eccrine angiomatous hamartoma
> coma blister

VIIB2 Lymphocytes Predominant

There is a predominantly lymphocytic infiltrate in and around the sweat glands. Lichen striatus is a prototypic example (55).

Lichen Striatus

CLINICAL SUMMARY. This fairly uncommon dermatitis occurs as a rule in children. It presents as a unilateral eruption along Blaschko lines (56) on the extremities, trunk, or neck as either a continuous or an interrupted band composed of minute, slightly raised, erythematous papules, which may have a scaly surface. The lesions appear suddenly and usually involute within a year. They are occasionally pruritic.

HISTOPATHOLOGY. Although the histologic picture is highly variable, there is usually a superficial perivascular inflammatory infiltrate of lymphocytes admixed with a variable number of histiocytes (57). Plasma cells and eosinophils are rare. Focally, in the papillary dermis, the infiltrate may have a band-like distribution with extension into the lower portion of the epidermis, with vacuolar alteration of the basal layer and necrotic keratinocytes. Additional epidermal changes consist of spongiosis and intracellular edema often associated with exocytosis of lymphocytes and focal parakeratosis. Less frequently, there are scattered necrotic/apoptotic keratinocytes in the spinous layer as well as subcorneal spongiotic vesicles filled with Langerhans cells. A very distinctive feature is the presence of an inflammatory infiltrate in the reticular dermis around hair follicles and eccrine glands.

Conditions to consider in the differential diagnosis:

> lupus erythematosus
> syringolymphoid hyperplasia with alopecia
> lichen striatus
> erythema annulare centrifugum
> erythema chronicum migrans

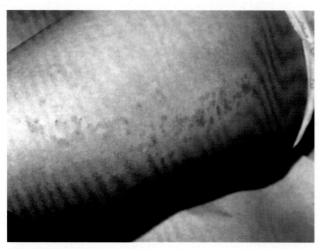

Clin. Fig. VIIB2

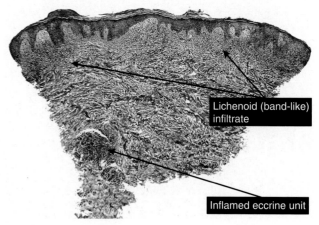

Fig. VIIB2.a

Clin. Fig. VIIB2. *Lichen striatus.* A linear eruption of erythematous papules suddenly appeared on the thigh of a girl.

Fig. VIIB2.a. *Lichen striatus, low power.* There is a patchy band-like infiltrate in the papillary dermis. A sweat gland unit in the lower left is infiltrated by inflammatory cells.

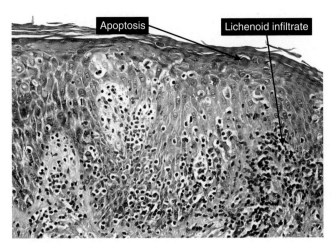

Fig. VIIB2.b

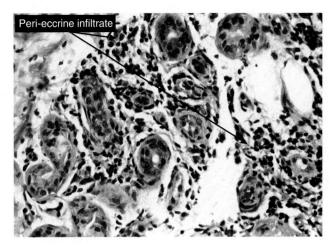

Fig. VIIB2.c

Fig. VIIB2.b. *Lichen striatus, medium power.* There is lymphocytic exocytosis into the epidermis, associated with only mild spongiosis.

Fig. VIIB2.c. *Lichen striatus, high power.* A perieccrine lymphocytic infiltrate is a characteristic feature of lichen striatus.

VIIB2a With Plasma Cells

There is a predominantly lymphocytic infiltrate in and around the sweat glands. Plasma cells are also present as a minority population.

Lupus Erythematosus

See additional discussion in IIIH.4.

HISTOPATHOLOGY. In lupus, the inflammatory infiltrate in the dermis is usually lymphocytic with or without

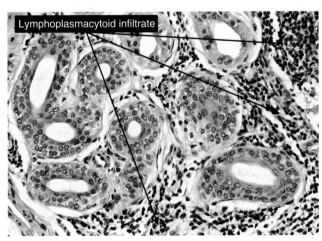

Fig. VIIB2a

Fig. VIIB2a. *Lupus erythematosus, high power.* A perieccrine infiltrate composed predominantly of lymphocytes with or without a few plasma cells suggests a diagnosis of lupus erythematosus. Annular erythemas may also produce a perieccrine lymphocytic infiltrate.

an admixture of plasma cells (58,59). Its distribution is a clue to the diagnosis of lupus. Lymphocytic and plasmacytic inflammation around eccrine coils is a characteristic finding. In hair-bearing areas, there is a similar infiltrate located around hair follicles and the sebaceous glands. Frequently, there are hydropic changes in the basal layer of the hair follicles, which may be of diagnostic value in the absence of dermal–epidermal changes. By impinging on pilosebaceous units, the infiltrate causes their gradual atrophy and disappearance. A patchy inflammatory infiltrate also may be present in the upper dermis in an interstitial pattern and occasionally, the infiltrate extends into the subcutaneous fat.

Conditions to consider in the differential diagnosis:

> lupus erythematosus
> secondary syphilis
> cheilitis glandularis
> erythema chronicum migrans

VIIB2b With Eosinophils

There is an inflammatory infiltrate with lymphocytes and eosinophils in and around the sweat glands (60).

Arthropod Assault Reaction

See Figs. VIIB2b.a,b.

Conditions to consider in the differential diagnosis:

> arthropod assault reaction
> insect bite reaction
> drug reaction
> dermal allergic eruption

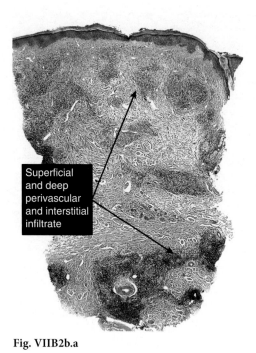

Superficial and deep perivascular and interstitial infiltrate

Fig. VIIB2b.a

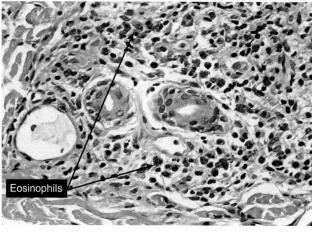

Eosinophils

Fig. VIIB2b.b

Fig. VIIB2b.a. *Arthropod assault reaction, low power.* Bite/sting reactions may reveal a superficial and deep inflammatory reaction that is perivascular, periadnexal, and interstitial.

Fig. VIIB2b.b. *Arthropod assault reaction, high power.* The inflammatory reaction is present around eccrine glands. Generally, there are numerous eosinophils, a clue to the diagnosis.

VIIB2c Neutrophils Predominant

There is an inflammatory infiltrate with neutrophils in and around the sweat glands.

Neutrophilic Eccrine Hidradenitis

CLINICAL SUMMARY. This condition may present with erythematous, often acral, papules and plaques several days after cytoreductive chemotherapy for hematologic malignancy, likely representing a reaction to a cytotoxic drug (e.g., cytarabine) in the sweat gland (61). The description of cases occurring before the diagnosis of the malignancy, of cases in individuals treated with granulocyte colony-stimulating factor, and in patients with other malignancies, suggests that neutrophilic eccrine hidradenitis (NEH) may be related to Sweet syndrome as a part of the spectrum of neutrophilic diseases (see also VC2). The cutaneous lesions of NEH may be single or multiple and characteristically present as infiltrated or edematous papules or plaques of variable size, which may be asymptomatic or painful, and may resemble lesions of Sweet syndrome. The lesions are usually erythematous, or may be pigmented or purpuric. There are typically no epidermal changes; however, pustules may occasionally occur. A subset of NEH that occurs in healthy children and young adults, *palmoplantar hidradenitis*, has been reported under many names and demonstrates painful erythematous papules and nodules on the palms and soles. The pathogenesis is unclear, but the condition is benign and self-limited.

HISTOPATHOLOGY. There is variable infiltration of the eccrine coil by neutrophils and lymphocytes with necrosis of secretory epithelium (62). Individual cells or whole coils show increased cytoplasmic eosinophilia, degeneration of nuclei, and loss of integrity of cell walls.

Idiopathic Recurrent Palmoplantar Hidradenitis

CLINICAL SUMMARY. Idiopathic recurrent palmoplantar hidradenitis has been reported under many names and is an entity that is histologically indistinguishable from NEH. Idiopathic palmoplantar hidradenitis occurs primarily in children and presents as multiple tender erythematous nodules on the palms, soles, or both (63). It occurs in otherwise healthy patients. There is a slight predominance in females, and the mean age of onset is 6 years (64). Some patients have an associated low-grade fever. In most cases, the lesions spontaneously resolve in approximately 3 weeks, but may recur. Unlike NEH, there is no association with chemotherapy use and/or leukemia. The etiology is unknown but some authors have speculated the possibility of moisture and/or trauma-producing rupture of eccrine glands and subsequently inciting a neutrophil-rich inflammatory process. There have been a few reports of similar clinical lesions that have been associated with infections including *Pseudomonas* (65), *Serratia*, *Enterobacter*, *Staphylococcus*, *Nocardia*, and HIV. *Pseudomonas*-associated lesions on the soles due to children wading in a community pool with a gritty floor have been termed *Pseudomonas* hot-foot syndrome (59).

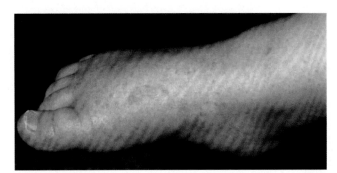

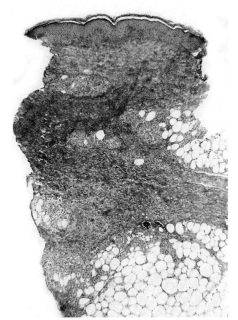

Clin. Fig. VIIB2c

Fig. VIIB2c.a

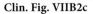

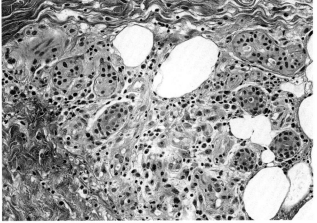

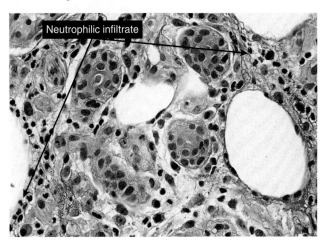

Neutrophilic infiltrate

Fig. VIIB2c.b

Fig. VIIB2c.c

Clin. Fig. VIIB2c. *Neutrophilic eccrine hidradenitis.* A young child with acute lymphocytic leukemia developed erythematous papules and plaques while on maintenance chemotherapy.

Fig. VIIB2c.a. *Neutrophilic eccrine hidradenitis, low power.* There is a sparse, perivascular and perieccrine infiltrate which is seen predominantly at the dermal–subcutaneous junction.

Fig. VIIB2c.b. *Neutrophilic eccrine hidradenitis, medium power.* Upon closer inspection the inflammatory infiltrate is found to be predominantly around eccrine coils at the dermal–subcutaneous junction.

Fig. VIIB2c.c. *Neutrophilic eccrine hidradenitis, high power.* The infiltrate is mixed but contains neutrophils. The eccrine ducts show focal pallor consistent with early necrosis.

HISTOPATHOLOGY. The epidermis is essentially unremarkable. Within the dermis is a moderately intense neutrophilic infiltrate that shows preferential involvement of eccrine coils in the deep dermis (66). Neutrophils can also be seen perivascularly and interstitially in the dermis and focally in the subcutaneous tissue. Neutrophils can be seen within the eccrine epithelium and there may be associated degeneration and/or necrosis of the epithelium.

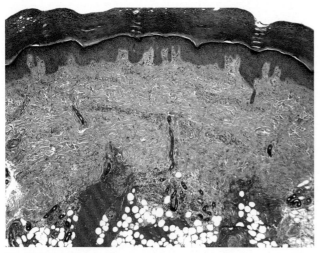

Fig. VIIB2c.d

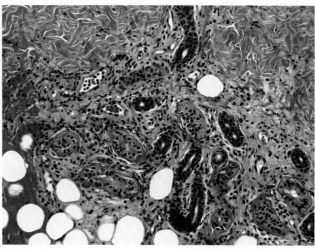

Fig. VIIB2c.e

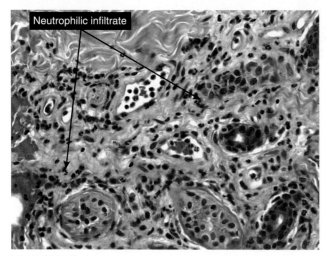

Neutrophilic infiltrate

Fig. VIIB2c.f

Fig. VIIB2c.d. *Idiopathic recurrent palmoplantar hidradenitis, low power.* There is sparse superficial and deep inflammatory infiltrate which is perivascular, perieccrine, and focally interstitial.

Fig. VIIB2c.e. *Idiopathic recurrent palmoplantar hidradenitis, high power.* The neutrophilic infiltrate concentrates around eccrine coils and may be seen within the eccrine epithelium.

Fig. VIIB2c.f. *Idiopathic recurrent palmoplantar hidradenitis, high power.* The infiltrate is composed almost exclusively of neutrophils.

Vasculitis and/or leukocytoclasia is not seen. Special stains for infectious organisms are typically negative. The differential diagnosis includes other neutrophil-rich dermal inflammatory processes, such as an early lesion of Sweet syndrome. This latter entity shows a more intense neutrophilic infiltrate associated with prominent papillary dermal edema. Urticaria should also be considered, however urticaria will reveal eosinophils and lymphocytes in addition to neutrophils. The histopathology is indistinguishable from the chemotherapy-associated NEH.

Conditions to consider in the differential diagnosis:

insect bite reactions
neutrophilic eccrine hidradenitis
idiopathic recurrent palmoplantar hidradenitis
urticaria
Sweet syndrome
infectious etiologies with bacteria, atypical mycobacteria, and fungi

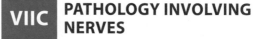

VIIC PATHOLOGY INVOLVING NERVES

Specific inflammatory involvement of nerves is uncommon in dermatopathology.

1. Lymphocytic Infiltrates
2. Mixed Inflammatory Infiltrates
3. Neoplastic Infiltrates

VIIC1 Lymphocytic Infiltrates

Neurotropic spread of neoplasms, especially neurotropic melanoma, may be associated with a dense lymphocytic infiltrate that may tend to obscure a subtle infiltrate of neoplastic spindle cells. Any of the infections listed below may present as a pure (or predominant) lymphocytic neuritis.

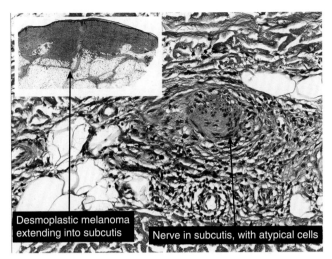

Fig. VIIC1

Fig. VIIC1. *Neurotropic melanoma, high power (see also Fig. VIIC3).* The presence of a lymphocytic infiltrate can call attention to nerve involvement in a melanoma (inset).

Conditions to consider in the differential diagnosis:

> neurotropic melanoma
> leprosy
> polyneuritis
> leprosy
> erythema chronicum migrans
> arthropod bite reaction

VIIC2 | Mixed Inflammatory Infiltrates

There is a mixed inflammatory infiltrate involving nerves.

Nerve Involvement in Leprosy

CLINICAL SUMMARY. Nerve involvement can be demonstrated in most lesions of leprosy (67), but is most prominent in the tuberculoid type (TT). In the various patterns of leprosy, the major peripheral nerves often undergo parallel pathologies. The inflammation is similar, and the same classification system is applied. However, the density of acid-fast bacilli is often a logarithm higher than in the nearby skin. The skin lesions of TT leprosy are scanty, dry, erythematous, hypopigmented papules or plaques with sharply defined edges. Anesthesia is prominent (except on the face). Thickened local peripheral nerves may be found. The lesions heal rapidly with therapy.

HISTOPATHOLOGY. Primary TT leprosy has large epithelioid cells arranged in compact granulomas along with neurovascular bundles, with dense peripheral lymphocyte accumulation. Langhans giant cells are typically absent. Dermal nerves may be absent (obliterated) or surrounded and eroded by dense lymphocyte cuffs. Acid-fast bacilli are rarely found, even in nerves. A second pattern of TT leprosy is found in certain reactional states.

Erythema Chronicum Migrans With Nerve Involvement

See Figs. VIIC2.c,d.

Arthropod Bite Reaction With Nerve Involvement

See Fig. VIIC2.e.

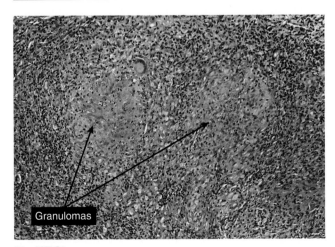

Fig. VIIC2.a

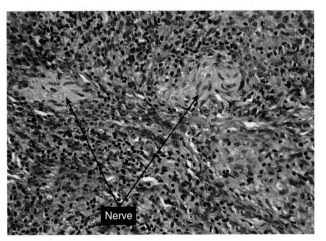

Fig. VIIC2.b

Fig. VIIC2.a. *Tuberculoid leprosy, medium power.* Within the dermis there is an intense granulomatous infiltrate.

Fig. VIIC2.b. *Tuberculoid leprosy, high power.* This granulomatous inflammation surrounds small cutaneous nerves.

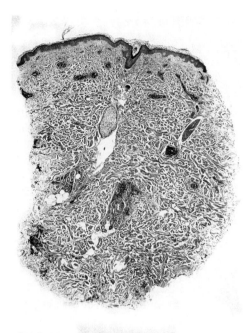

Fig. VIIC2.c

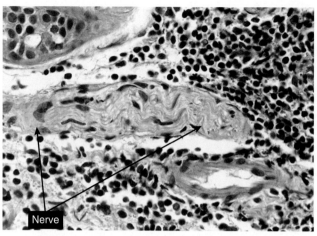

Fig. VIIC2.d

Fig. VIIC2.c. *Erythema chronicum migrans, low power.* There is a superficial and deep perivascular and periadnexal infiltrate without a significant interstitial component.

Fig. VIIC2.d. *Erythema chronicum migrans, high power.* This infiltrate which is composed predominantly of lymphocytes and occasional plasma cells (not shown), may surround small nerves as well as eccrine units.

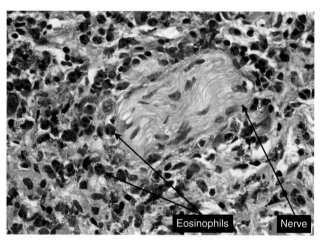

Fig. VIIC2.e

Fig. VIIC2.e. *Arthropod bite reaction, high power.* The inflammatory infiltrate of a bite reaction, which is rich in eosinophils, may also show perineural involvement.

Conditions to consider in the differential diagnosis:

  leprosy
  erythema chronicum migrans
  arthropod bite reaction

VIIC3 | Neoplastic Infiltrates

Many neoplasms may occasionally involve nerves. The involvement by carcinomas (basal cell, squamous cell, metastatic) is commonly in the perineural space, while involvement by neurotropic melanoma tends to occupy the endoneurium and be associated with a dense lymphocytic infiltrate that may tend to obscure a subtle infiltrate of neoplastic spindle cells.

Neurotropic Melanoma

CLINICAL SUMMARY. Neurotropic melanoma is defined as a melanoma that invades nerves. Usually, there are no specific clinical stigmata of nerve involvement, but occasionally pain or paresthesias may be reported by the patient. Neurotropism in a primary melanoma is associated with increased risk for local recurrence, even after standard "definitive" therapy, and also with increased mortality.

HISTOPATHOLOGY. Neurotropism is often seen in a desmoplastic melanoma (68). There are fascicles of neoplastic spindle cells that have invaded cutaneous nerves, usually in a spindle-cell vertical component with fibrosis. However, some neurotropic melanomas lack these latter features of desmoplastic melanoma. Many of these are spindle-cell tumorigenic melanomas of acral lentiginous or lentigo maligna type, but some are composed of epithelioid cells. Although the neoplastic cells in the nerves are often highly atypical, in some cases the involvement may be subtle because the malignant cells may be sparsely distributed within the endoneurium of the nerve. In some cases, the presence of a lymphocytic infiltrate in the nerve may draw attention to the neoplastic involvement.

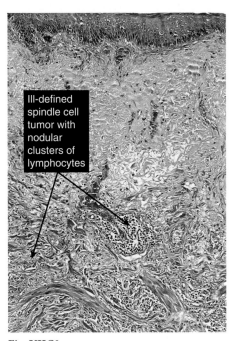

Fig. VIIC3.a

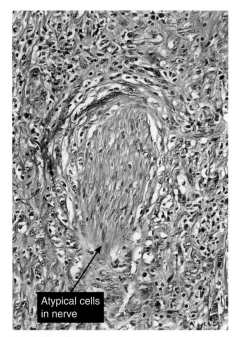

Fig. VIIC3.b

Fig. VIIC3.a. *Desmoplastic and neurotropic melanoma, medium power.* In the middermis there is a subtle proliferation of spindle cells associated with a lymphoid infiltrate.

Fig. VIIC3.b. *Neurotropism in a melanoma, high power.* Involvement of nerves may be quite subtle, as here. The lymphocytic infiltrate is a marker that may draw attention to the involved nerves. In this case the neoplastic cells are within the nerve (endoneurial invasion) rather than around it (perineural). These lesions have a higher incidence of local recurrence because of the nerve involvement.

Conditions to consider in the differential diagnosis:

> neurotropic melanoma
> neurotropic carcinomas and other tumors

VIID PATHOLOGY OF THE NAILS

Several inflammatory dermatoses more often seen elsewhere in the skin may present incidentally or exclusively in the nails. The reaction patterns have overlapping features with those seen in other areas of the cutaneous surface, but also have histologic features distinct to the nail unit.

1. Lymphocytic Infiltrates
2. Lymphocytes With Neutrophils
3. Vesiculobullous Diseases
4. Parasitic Infestations

VIID1 Lymphocytic Infiltrates

There is an increased number of lymphocytes in the nail bed and matrix. They may be arranged in a perivascular or diffuse pattern, and may be confined to the dermis, or may involve the epithelium in a lichenoid, spongiotic, or other pattern.

Acral Lentiginous Melanoma

The periphery of an *in situ* component of acral lentiginous melanoma may mimic a lymphocytic infiltrate, because brisk infiltrating lymphocytes in a lichenoid

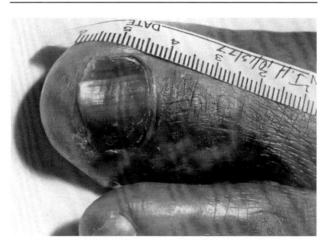

Clin. Fig. VIID1

Clin. Fig. VIID1. *Subungual acral lentiginous melanoma.* There is a very broad and variegated pigmented lesion which extends from the nail to the surrounding skin. This extension of pigmentation from the nail to the skin is termed Hutchinson sign. (*continues*)

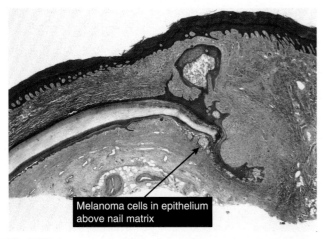

Fig. VIID1.a

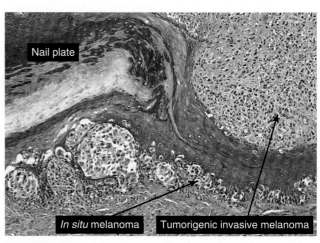

Fig. VIID1.b

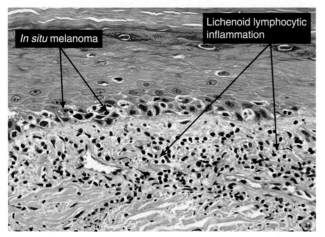

Fig. VIID1.c

Fig. VIID1.a. *Subungual acral lentiginous melanoma, low power.* This excisional biopsy of the nail unit shows only subtle changes at the dermal–epithelial junction of the nail matrix at scanning magnification.

Fig. VIID1.b. *Subungual acral lentiginous melanoma, medium power.* At this magnification one can identify variably sized collections of atypical melanocytes at the dermal–epithelial interface of the nail matrix, focally forming dermal collections in the upper right hand corner of this photomicrograph. There is an associated mild lymphoid infiltrate.

Fig. VIID1.c. *Acral lentiginous melanoma, high power.* In this field, the predominant feature is a diffuse lymphocytic infiltrate in the papillary dermis and basal epithelium, occasionally so prominently as to obscure subtle involvement of the epidermis by *in situ* melanoma.

pattern may obscure the lesional neoplastic melanocytes in focal areas of the lesion, especially when viewed at low power.

Conditions to consider in the differential diagnosis:

    spongiotic dermatitis
    lichen planus
    acral lentiginous melanoma

VIID2 | Lymphocytes With Neutrophils

Neutrophils may be present in the dermis in acute infections and in gangrenous necrosis. As in the skin proper, neutrophils in the nail plate should suggest fungus infection, or may be indicative of psoriasis or a related condition (69).

Onychomycosis

CLINICAL SUMMARY. Fungal infection of the nails may be the most common nail disorder (70). There are four main types: distal lateral subungual onychomycosis, proximal subungual onychomycosis, white superficial onychomycosis, and candidal onychomycosis. Distal lateral subungual onychomycosis is the most common form and is usually caused by *T. rubrum*. The fungus initially invades the hyponychium and lateral nail folds, causing yellowing, onycholysis, and eventual subungual hyperkeratosis. It is important to remember that onychomycosis may coexist with other dermatoses, such as nail unit psoriasis (71,72), or nail unit tumors.

HISTOPATHOLOGY. Most commonly, onychomycosis is diagnosed histologically by a nail clipping. Biopsy of the nail plate often reveals hyperkeratosis. A fungal stain such as PAS or GMS should be performed on all nail biopsies. This stain reveals fungal organisms that are usually located in the ventral aspect of the nail plate. When specimens include soft tissue from the nail unit, the nail bed epidermis shows acanthosis, spongiosis, and exocytosis of lymphocytes and histiocytes. In proximal subungual onychomycosis, infection initially involves the area of the proximal nail fold. Superficial white onychomycosis is

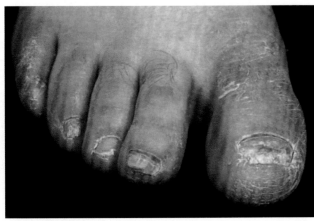

Clin. Fig. VIID2

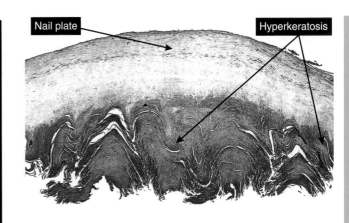

Nail plate

Hyperkeratosis

Fig. VIID2.a

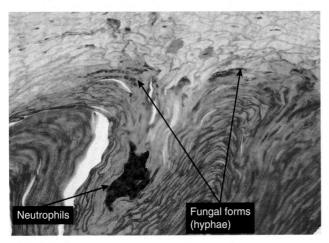

Neutrophils

Fungal forms
(hyphae)

Fig. VIID2.b

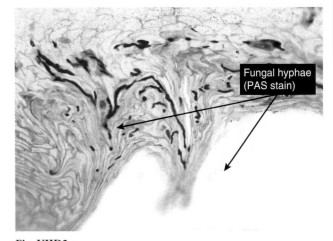

Fungal hyphae
(PAS stain)

Fig. VIID2.c

Clin. Fig. VIID2. *Onychomycosis.* Chronic infection with *Trichophyton rubrum* resulted in thickened, yellowish nails with subungual debris.

Fig. VIID2.a. *Onychomycosis, low power.* This photomicrograph shows a nail plate composed of laminated keratin. The ventral surface shows a papillomatous architecture with parakeratin. No nail bed or nail matrix is seen in this biopsy.

Fig. VIID2.b. *Onychomycosis, high power.* Within the orthokeratotic and parakeratotic scale there are focal collections of neutrophils. Hyphae can be seen on H&E-stained sections but this is quite difficult without special stains.

Fig. VIID2.c. *Onychomycosis, high power, PAS stain.* PAS stains reveal septate hyphae within the thickened keratin layer.

often caused by *Trichophyton mentagrophytes*, located on the superficial nail plate only. In HIV-infected persons, superficial white onychomycosis is usually caused by *T. rubrum. Candida* may involve the nail plate and nail bed in patients with chronic mucocutaneous candidiasis and in HIV-infected patients.

Conditions to consider in the differential diagnosis:

psoriasis
tinea unguium, onychomycosis

VIID3 Vesiculobullous Diseases

Vesiculobullous disease more commonly seen elsewhere in the skin may also involve the nails. Darier disease commonly involves the nail with characteristic clinical findings that are not often biopsied.

Darier Disease

CLINICAL SUMMARY. Nail changes usually occur in association with other clinical findings. Rarely, involvement may be limited to the nail alone. Nail changes may occur in the proximal nail fold, matrix, nail bed, and hyponychium. Involvement of the nail matrix in Darier–White disease is usually located in the distal lunula. The nails have characteristic changes of V-shaped nicking, linear striations, onycholysis, and subungual keratotic reaction. The nails in Darier disease have been described as "candy cane nails," referring to the alternating areas of red and white stripes (alternating longitudinal erythronychia and longitudinal leukonychia). See clinical image in Clinical Figure IVD1.b.

HISTOPATHOLOGY. The proximal nail fold may show keratotic papules that are histologically similar to those of acrokeratosis verruciformis of Hopf. However, in addition to papillary epidermal hyperplasia, focal areas of suprabasilar acantholysis may be seen. Histologically, the leukonychia is due to foci of persistent parakeratosis in the lower nail plate related to the usual histology of Darier–White disease of the distal matrix (73).

Conditions to consider in the differential diagnosis:

  Darier disease
  pemphigus
  erythema multiforme
  toxic epidermal necrolysis
  epidermolysis bullosa
  bullous pemphigoid

VIID4 | Parasitic Infestations

Scabies is an example of a parasitic infection that may involve the nails (74).

Scabies

CLINICAL SUMMARY AND HISTOPATHOLOGY. *Sarcoptes scabiei* may involve the nail unit. Organisms are often present in distal subungual hyperkeratotic debris found in the hyponychium and may be a cause of persistent epidemics of scabies (75). Norwegian scabies may cause severe involvement of the nail folds.

Conditions to consider in the differential diagnosis:

  scabies
  Norwegian scabies

References

1. Ioffreda MD. Inflammatory diseases of hair follicles, sweat glands, and cartilage. In: Elder D, Elenitsas R, Jaworsky C, et al. *Lever's Histopathology of the Skin*. 8th ed. Philadelphia, PA: Lippincott-Raven Publishers; 2008.
2. Kolivras A, Thompson C. Primary scalp alopecia: new histopathological tools, new concepts and a practical guide to diagnosis. *J Cutan Pathol* 2017;44(1):53–69.
3. Stefanato CM. Histopathology of alopecia: a clinicopathological approach to diagnosis. *Histopathol* 2010;56(1):24–38.
4. Whiting DA. Diagnostic and predictive value of horizontal sections of scalp biopsy specimens in male pattern androgenetic alopecia. *J Am Acad Dermatol* 1993;28:755–763.
5. Nguyen JV, Hudacek K, Whitten JA, et al. The HoVert technique: a novel method for the sectioning of alopecia biopsies. *J Cutan Pathol* 2011;38:401–406.
6. Jaworsky C, Kligman AM, Murphy GF. Characterization of inflammatory infiltrates in male pattern alopecia: implications for pathogenesis. *Brit J Dermatol* 1992;127:239–246.
7. Muylaert BPB, Trindade MT, Michalany AO, et al. Lichen simplex chronicus on the scalp: exuberant clinical, dermoscopic, and histopathological findings. *An Bras Dermatol* 2018;93:108–110.
8. Hautmann G, Hercogova J, Lotti T. Trichotillomania. *J Am Acad Dermatol* 2002;46(6):807–821; quiz 822–826.
9. Royer MC, Sperling LC. Splitting hairs: the 'hamburger sign' in trichotillomania. *J Cutan Pathol* 2006;33 Suppl 2:63–64.
10. Headington JT. Telogen effluvium. New concepts and review. *Arch Dermatol* 1993;129:356–363.
11. Sperling LL, Lupton GP. Histopathology of non-scarring alopecia. *J Cutan Pathol* 1995;22:97–114.
12. Hwang S, Schwartz RA. Keratosis pilaris: a common follicular hyperkeratosis. *Cutis* 2008;82(3):177–180. Review.
13. Hirschmann JV, Raugi GJ. Adult scurvy. *J Am Acad Dermatol* 1999;41(6):895–906.
14. Magro C, Crowson AN, Mihm MC. Cutaneous manifestations of nutritional deficiency states and gastrointestinal disease. In: Elder DE, Elenitsas R, Rosenbach M, et al., eds. *Lever's Histopathology of the Skin*. 11th ed. Philadelphia, PA: Wolters Kluwer.
15. Strazzulla LC, Wang EHC, Avila L, et al. Alopecia areata: disease characteristics, clinical evaluation, and new perspectives on pathogenesis. *J Am Acad Dermatol* 2018;78(1):1–12.
16. Headington JT. The histopathology of alopecia areata. *J Invest Dermatol* 1991;96:69S–70S.
17. Whiting DA. Histopathologic features of alopecia areata: a new look. *Arch Dermatol* 2003;139:1555–1559.
18. Yadav D, Khandpur S, Ramam M, et al. Utility of horizontal sections of scalp biopsies in differentiating between androgenetic alopecia and alopecia areata. *Dermatol* 2018;234:137–147.
19. Muller CS, El Shabrawi-Caelen L. 'Follicular Swiss cheese' pattern—another histopathologic clue to alopecia areata. *J Cutan Pathol* 2011;38(2):185.
20. Assouly P, Reygagne P. Lichen planopilaris: update on diagnosis and treatment. *Semin Cutan Med Surg* 2009;28(1):3–10.
21. Kossard S, Lee MS, Wilkinson B. Postmenopausal frontal fibrosing alopecia: a frontal variant of lichen planopilaris. *J Am Acad Dermatol* 1997;36:59–66.
22. Donati A, Molina L, Doche I, et al. Facial papules in frontal fibrosing alopecia: evidence of vellus follicle involvement. *Arch Dermatol* 2011;147(12):1424–1427.
23. Tandon YK, Somani N, Cevasco NC, et al. A histologic review of 27 patients with lichen planopilaris. *J Am Acad Dermatol* 2008;59(1):91–98.
24. Harries MJ, Jimenez F, Izeta A, et al. Lichen planopilaris and frontal fibrosing alopecia as model epithelial stem cell diseases. *Trends Mol Med* 2018;24:435–448.
25. Gálvez-Canseco A, Sperling L. Lichen planopilaris and frontal fibrosing alopecia cannot be differentiated by histopathology. *J Cutan Pathol* 2018;45(5):313–317.
26. Sperling LC. Scarring alopecia and the dermatopathologist. *J Cutan Pathol* 2001;28:333–342.

27. Callender VD, Onwudiwe O. Prevalence and etiology of central centrifugal cicatricial alopecia. *Arch Dermatol* 2011;147(8): 972–974.

28. Whiting DA, Olsen EA. Central centrifugal cicatricial alopecia. *Dermatol Ther* 2008;21(4):268–278.

29. Sperling LC, Solomon AR, Whiting DA. A new look at scarring alopecia. *Arch Dermatol* 2000;136:235–242.

30. Sperling LC. Premature desquamation of the inner root sheath is still a useful concept! *J Cutan Pathol* 2007;34(10):809–810.

31. Tan T. Guitart J, Gerami P, et al. Premature desquamation of the inner root sheath in noninflamed hair follicles as a specific marker for central centrifugal cicatricial alopecia. *Am J Dermatopathol* 2019;41(5):350–354.

32. Fening K, Parekh V, McKay K. CD123 immunohistochemistry for plasmacytoid dendritic cells is useful in the diagnosis of scarring alopecia. *J Cutan Pathol* 2016;43(8):643–648.

33. Anderson BE, Mackley CL, Helm KF. Alopecia mucinosa: report of a case and review. *J Cutan Med Surg* 2003;7:124–128.

34. Hooper KK, Smoller BR, Brown JA. Idiopathic follicular mucinosis or mycosis fungoides? classification and diagnostic challenges. *Cutis* 2015;95(6):E9–E14.

35. Crawford GH, Pelle MT, James WD, et al. Rosacea: I. Etiology, pathogenesis, and subtype classification. *J Am Acad Dermatol* 2004;51:327–341; quiz 342–344.

36. Lee WJ, Jung JM, Lee YJ, et al. Histopathological analysis of 226 patients with rosacea according to rosacea subtype and severity. *Am J Dermatopathol* 2016;38(5):347–352.

37. Nervi SJ, Schwartz RA, Dmochowski M, et al. Eosinophilic pustular folliculitis: a 40-year retrospect. *J Am Acad Dermatol* 2006; 55:285–289.

38. Nomura T, Katoh M, Yamamoto Y, et al. Eosinophilic pustular folliculitis: a proposal of diagnostic and therapeutic algorithms. *J Dermatol* 2016;43(11):1301–1306.

39. Piantanida EW, Turiansky GW, Kenner JR, et al. HIV-associated eosinophilic folliculitis: diagnosis by transverse histologic sections. *J Am Acad Dermatol* 1998;38:124–126.

40. Lankerani L, Thompson R. Eosinophilic pustular folliculitis: case report and review of the literature. *Cutis* 2010;86(4):190–194.

41. Scavo S, Magro G, Caltabiano R. Erythematous and edematous eruption of the face. Eosinophilic pustular folliculitis. *Intl J Dermatol* 2010; 49(9):975–977.

42. Pinkus H. Furuncle. *J Cutan Pathol* 1979;6:517–518.

43. Mikhail GR. Trichophyton rubrum granuloma. *Int J Dermatol* 1970;9:41–46.

44. Boer A, Herder N, Winter K, et al. Herpes folliculitis: clinical, histopathological, and molecular pathologic observations. *Brit J Dermatol* 2006;154(4):743–746.

45. Oon HH, Lim KS, Chong WS, et al. Erythematous and edematous eruption of the face. Herpes folliculitis. *Int J Dermatol* 2010;49(9):973–974.

46. Quarles FN, Brody H, Badreshia S, et al. Acne keloidalis nuchae. *Dermatol Ther* 2007;20(3):128–132.

47. Shapero J, Shapero H. Acne keloidalis nuchae is scar and keloid formation secondary to mechanically induced folliculitis. *J Cutan Med Surg* 2011;15(4):238–240.

48. Mirmirani P, Willey A, Chamlin S, et al. Tinea capitis mimicking cicatricial alopecia: what host and dermatophyte factors lead to this unusual clinical presentation? *J Am Acad Dermatol* 2009; 60(3):490–495.

49. Jemec GB. Clinical practice. Hidradenitis suppurativa. *N Engl J Med* 2012;366(2):158–164.

50. Scheinfeld NS. A case of dissecting cellulitis and a review of the literature. *Dermatol Online J* 2003;9(1):8.

51. Branisteanu DE, Molodoi A, Ciobanu D, et al. The importance of histopathologic aspects in the diagnosis of dissecting cellulitis of the scalp. *Roman J Morphol Embryol* 2009;50(4):719–724.

52. Powell JJ, Dawber RPR, Gatter K. Folliculitis decalvans including tufted folliculitis: clinical, histological and therapeutic findings. *Br J Dermatol* 1999;140:328–333.

53. Chiarini C, Torchia D, Bianchi B, et al. Immunopathogenesis of folliculitis decalvans: clues in early lesions. *Amer J Clin Pathol* 2008;130(4):526–534.

54. Chen J, Sun JF, Zeng XS, et al. Mucinous eccrine nevus: a case report and literature review. *Amer J Dermatopathol* 2009;31(4): 387–390.

55. Zhang Y, Mc Nutt NS. Lichen striatus. Histological, immunohistochemical and ultrastructural study of 37 cases. *J Cut Pathol* 2001;28:65–71.

56. Muller CS, Schmaltz R, Vogt T, et al. Lichen striatus and blaschkitis: reappraisal of the concept of blaschkolinear dermatoses. *Brit J Dermatol* 2011;164(2):257–262.

57. Gianotti R, Restano L, Grimalt R, et al. Lichen striatus—a chameleon: an histopathological and immunohistological study of forty-one cases. *J Cutan Pathol* 1995;22:18–22.

58. Tsokos GC. Systemic lupus erythematosus. *N Engl J Med* 2011; 365(22):2110–2121.

59. Fu SM, Deshmukh US, Gaskin F. Pathogenesis of systemic lupus erythematosus revisited 2011: end organ resistance to damage, autoantibody initiation and diversification, and HLA-DR. *J Autoimmun* 2011;37(2):104–112.

60. Miteva M, Elsner P, Ziemer M. A histopathologic study of arthropod bite reactions in 20 patients highlights relevant adnexal involvement. *J Cutan Pathol* 2009;36(1):26–33.

61. Harrist TJ, Fine JD, Berman RS, et al. Neutrophilic hidradenitis: a distinctive type of neutrophilic dermatosis associated with myelogenous leukemia and chemotherapy. *Arch Dermatol* 1982;118:263–266.

62. Grillo E, Vano-Galvan S, Gonzalez C, et al. Letter: neutrophilic eccrine hidradenitis with atypical findings. *Dermatol Online J* 2011;17(9):14.

63. Stahr BJ, Cooper PH, Caputo RV. Idiopathic plantar hidradenitis: a neutrophilic eccrine hidradenitis occurring primarily in children. *J Cutan Pathol* 1994;21:289–296.

64. Lee WJ, Kim CH, Chang SE, et al. Generalized idiopathic neutrophilic eccrine hidradenitis in childhood. *Int J Dermatol* 2010;49(1):75–78.

65. Fiorillo L, Zucker M, Sawyer D, et al. The pseudomonas hot-foot syndrome. *N Engl J Med* 2001;345:335–338.

66. Shih IH, Huang YH, Yang CH, et al. Childhood neutrophilic eccrine hidradenitis: a clinicopathologic and immunohistochemical study of 10 patients. *J Am Acad Dermatol* 2005;52: 963–966.

67. Ridley DS, Ridley MJ. The classification of nerves is modified by delayed recognition of M. leprae. *Int J Lepr* 1986;54:596–606.

68. Chen JY, Hruby G, Scolyer RA, et al. Desmoplastic neurotropic melanoma: a clinicopathologic analysis of 128 cases. *Cancer* 2008;113(10):2770–2778.

69. Kouskoukis CE, Scher RK, Ackerman AB. What histologic finding distinguishes onychomycosis and psoriasis? *Am J Dermatopathol* 1983;5:501–503.

70. Singal A, Khanna D. Onychomycosis: diagnosis and management. *Indian J Dermatol Venereol Leprol* 2011;77(6):659–672.

71. Tabassum S, Rahman A, Awan S, et al. Factors associated with onychomycosis in nail psoriasis: a multicenter study in Pakistan. *Int J Dermatol* 2019;58(6):672–678.

72. Chaowattanapanit S, Pattanaprichakul P, Leeyaphan C, et al. Coexistence of fungal infections in psoriatic nails and their correlation with severity of nail psoriasis. *Indian Dermatol Online J* 2018;9(5):314–317.

73. Zaias N, Ackerman AB. The nail in Darier-White disease. *Arch Dermatol* 1973;107:193–199.

74. Scher RK. Subungual scabies. *Am J Dermatopathol* 1983;5: 187–189.

75. Nakamura E, Taniguchi H, Ohtaki N. A case of crusted scabies with a bullous pemphigoid-like eruption and nail involvement. *J Dermatol* 2006;33(3):196–201.

Disorders of the Subcutis

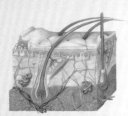

The reactions in the subcutis are mostly inflammatory (panniculitis), although tumors of the subcutis do occur, including metastases from other sites. Pathologic conditions arising in the dermis may extend to the subcutis. The conditions can be classified according to their septal or lobular location, and the presence or absence of vasculitis (1). Even though all panniculitides are somewhat mixed because the inflammatory infiltrate involves both the septa and lobules, the differential diagnosis between a mostly septal and a mostly lobular panniculitis is usually straightforward at scanning magnification (2). In a report of findings in a series of 55 panniculitis cases there was considerable clinical overlap. Biopsy findings were described. A definite panniculitis diagnosis was made in 53 cases including erythema nodosum (28 cases), leukocytoclastic vasculitis (7 cases), nodular vasculitis (4 cases), superficial thrombophlebitis (2 cases), eosinophilic panniculitis (3 cases), infection-related panniculitis (5 cases), and 1 case each of erythema nodosum leprosum, lupus panniculitis, pancreatic fat necrosis and acne conglobata with 2 cases remaining unclassified. Histologically, "predominantly septal" and "mixed panniculitis" were the chief inflammatory patterns in erythema nodosum cases, while mixed panniculitis was seen in most leukocytoclastic vasculitis cases and predominantly lobular and mixed panniculitis in nodular vasculitis cases (3).

vasculitis may present as a component of systemic vasculitic syndromes such as rheumatoid vasculitis or antineutrophil cytoplasmic antibody (ANCA)–associated primary vasculitic syndromes (4). ANCA-related vasculitides commonly involve the skin in addition to other organs and present as severe necrotizing vasculitis affecting small-sized vessels. They include granulomatosis with polyangiitis (GPA, formerly called Wegener granulomatosis), eosinophilic granulomatosis with polyangiitis (EGPA, formerly called Churg–Strauss syndrome), and microscopic polyangiitis (MPA) (5). Systemic polyarteritis nodosa frequently may present first in the skin, and demonstration of multiorgan involvement, particularly in the kidneys, heart, and liver, is necessary to make the distinction.

HISTOPATHOLOGY. The morphology is that of vasculitis anywhere, with vessel wall damage often resulting in pink "fibrinoid change," and a neutrophilic infiltrate with leukocytoclasia. A biopsy diagnosis of vasculitis must be correlated with clinical history, physical and laboratory findings, and/or angiographic features to arrive at specific diagnosis (6). Diagnosis of any individual case therefore depends on clinicopathologic correlation (7). Vasculitis extending deep into the reticular dermis or subcutaneous tissue seems to be associated more often with systemic disease such as malignancy or connective tissue disease (8).

VIIIA SUBCUTANEOUS VASCULITIS AND VASCULOPATHY (SEPTAL OR LOBULAR)

True vasculitis is defined by the presence of necrosis and inflammation in vessel walls. Other forms of vasculopathy include thrombosis and thrombophlebitis, fibrointimal hyperplasia, calcification, and neoplastic infiltration of vessel walls.

1. Neutrophilic Vasculitis
2. Lymphocytic "Vasculitis"
3. Granulomatous "Vasculitis"

VIIIA1 Neutrophilic Vasculitis

Neutrophils and disrupted nuclei are present in the wall of the vessel, with associated eosinophilic "fibrinoid" necrosis.

Cutaneous/Subcutaneous Polyarteritis Nodosa (See also Section VB3 and Table VIII.1)

CLINICAL SUMMARY. Cutaneous polyarteritis nodosa is a vasculitis involving arteries and arterioles of the septa of the dermis or subcutaneous fat with few or relatively minor systemic manifestations, such as fever, malaise, myalgias, arthralgias, and neuropathy. Cutaneous

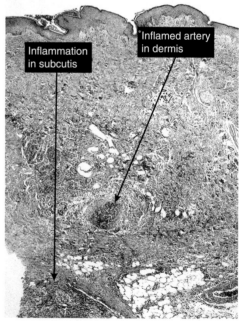

Fig. VIIIA1.a

Fig. VIIIA1.a. *Subcutaneous polyarteritis nodosa, low power.* In the deep reticular dermis extending into the superficial subcutaneous tissue there is an intense perivascular inflammatory reaction. Even at scanning magnification one can identify an intense infiltrate of a medium-sized vessel.

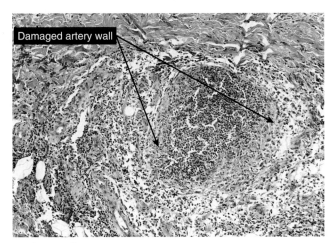

Fig. VIIIA1.b

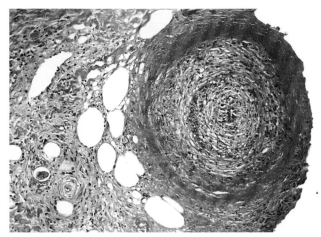

Fig. VIIIA1.c

Fig. VIIIA1.b. *Subcutaneous polyarteritis nodosa, medium power.* This medium-sized artery shows extensive infiltration and destruction of the vessel by a neutrophilic infiltrate.

Fig. VIIIA1.c. *Subcutaneous polyarteritis nodosa, medium power.* Another medium-sized artery in the subcutaneous fat shows luminal obliteration, a mixed acute and chronic inflammatory infiltrate within the wall, and hemorrhage and fibrin surrounding the vessel.

It is important but sometimes difficult to distinguish between superficial thrombophlebitis and arteritis. Veins in the lower legs may have a compact concentric smooth muscle pattern with a round lumen and an intimal elastic fiber proliferation that may mimic the characteristic features of arteries; however elastic fibers are prominent between the bundles of smooth muscle in vein walls, while being sparse in the medial muscular layer in arteries (9).

Conditions to consider in the differential diagnosis:

> leukocytoclastic vasculitis
> subcutaneous polyarteritis nodosa
> superficial migratory thrombophlebitis
> erythema nodosum leprosum

VIIIA2 Lymphocytic "Vasculitis"

The concept of "lymphocytic vasculitis" is a controversial one. Many disorders characterized by lymphocytes within the walls of vessels are best classified as lymphocytic infiltrates. The term "vasculitis" may be appropriate when there is vessel wall damage, as in nodular vasculitis, even in the absence of neutrophils and "fibrinoid" changes (10). Other situations in which this may occur include cutaneous lymphomas such as angiocentric T-cell lymphoma, connective tissue disease vasculitis, particularly lupus vasculitis, and Behçet disease. Lichenoid lymphocytic vasculitis with lymphocytic fibrinoid necrosis of small vessels has been said to be associated with inflammatory dermatoses such as pityriasis lichenoides, graft-versus-host disease, herpetic dermatitis, chilblains and

perniosis, lupus erythematosus, lichenoid drug eruptions, and Degos disease (11). In this pattern, lymphocytic fibrinoid necrosis of small vessels is found in combination with extravasated red blood cells (purpura) and a lichenoid or vacuolar interface lymphocytic dermatitis.

Conditions to consider in the differential diagnosis:

> nodular vasculitis
> perniosis (see Section VB2)
> angiocentric lymphomas

VIIIA3 Granulomatous "Vasculitis"

The inflammatory infiltrate in the vessel walls is composed of mixed cells including more or less epithelioid histiocytes, and giant cells. Other cell types including lymphocytes and plasma cells, and sometimes neutrophils and eosinophils, are also commonly present.

Erythema Induratum (Nodular Vasculitis)

CLINICAL SUMMARY. The lesions of erythema induratum (12,13), also known as "nodular vasculitis," consist of painless but somewhat tender, deep-seated, circumscribed, nodular, subcutaneous infiltrations of the lower legs, especially on the calves. Gradually, the infiltrations extend toward the surface, forming blue-red plaques that can ulcerate before healing with atrophy and scarring. Recurrences are common and often are precipitated by the onset of cold weather. Women are more commonly affected than men. Many cases are associated with detectable sequences of *Mycobacterium tuberculosis* in lesional tissue by PCR, with a prevalence that varies geographically, perhaps related to the prevalence of tuberculosis in the community (14,15). "Nodular vasculitis" has been proposed as a term for those cases with erythema induratum–like lesions that were not associated with tuberculosis.

HISTOPATHOLOGY.   In contrast to erythema nodosum that is mainly a septal panniculitis, erythema induratum (nodular vasculitis) initially is mainly a lobular panniculitis characterized by inflammation and necrosis of the fat lobule with relatively less involvement of the structures of the septa. It is controversial whether vasculitis should be required as a necessary diagnostic feature, but nevertheless some form of vasculitis is present in most cases (16). The fat necrosis elicits granulomatous inflammation. Epithelioid cells and giant cells and/or lymphocytes and plasma cells form broad zones of inflammation surrounding the necrosis and extending between the fat cells but also can form well-delimited granulomas of the tuberculoid type. Ziehl–Neelsen stains are negative for mycobacteria. Vascular changes are typically extensive and severe. The walls of small and medium-sized arteries and veins are infiltrated by a dense lymphoid or granulomatous inflammatory infiltrate, associated with endothelial swelling and edema of the vessel walls, fibrous thickening of the intima and, often, thrombosis of the lumen. Compromise of the lumen produces ischemic and caseous fat necrosis, which when extensive may lead to involvement of the overlying dermis and ulceration. In the necrotic fat there may be fat cysts, with surrounding amorphous, finely granular, eosinophilic material containing some pyknotic nuclei. Later lesions contain many foamy histiocytes surrounding the areas of fat necrosis.

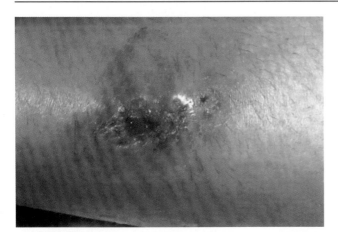

Clin. Fig. VIIIA3

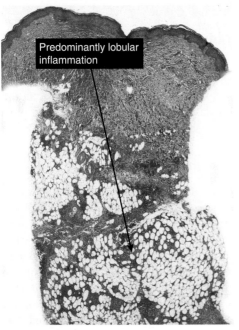

Fig. VIIIA3.a

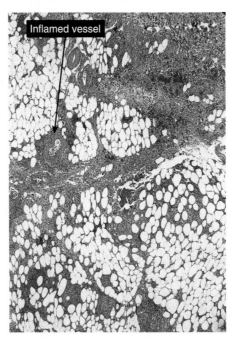

Fig. VIIIA3.b

Clin. Fig. VIIIA3.   *Erythema induratum.* A young female presented with a tender ulcerated nodule in the left pretibial area (more typically the calf is involved). Cultures for tuberculosis were negative.

Fig. VIIIA3.a.   *Erythema induratum/nodular vasculitis, low power.* There is inflammation involving the subcutaneous lobules with little or no inflammation in the overlying epidermis and dermis.

Fig. VIIIA3.b.   *Erythema induratum/nodular vasculitis, medium power.* This is a predominantly lobular panniculitis with less intense involvement of the subcutaneous septa.

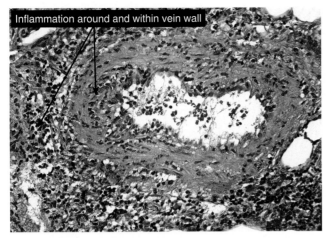

Fig. VIIIA3.c

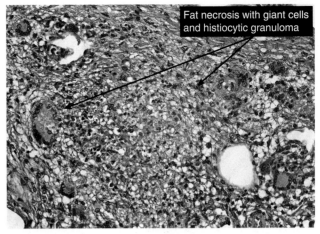

Fig. VIIIA3.d

Fig. VIIIA3.c. *Erythema induratum/nodular vasculitis, high power.* This vein shows a moderately intense lymphoid infiltrate surrounding the vessel and also involving the wall of the vessel. Thickening of the intima and luminal thrombosis (not seen here) may also be present.

Fig. VIIIA3.d. *Erythema induratum/nodular vasculitis, high power.* The infiltrate in the subcutaneous fat is frequently granulomatous composed of histiocytes and giant cells as well as a mixed inflammatory infiltrate.

Conditions to consider in the differential diagnosis:

erythema induratum/nodular vasculitis
erythema nodosum leprosum (type 2 leprosy reaction)
Wegener granulomatosis
Churg–Strauss vasculitis
Crohn disease
giant cell arteritis

 SEPTAL PANNICULITIS WITHOUT VASCULITIS

The inflammation is mainly confined to the septa, although there may be some lobular involvement.

1. Septal Panniculitis, Lymphocytes and Mixed Infiltrates
2. Septal Panniculitis, Granulomatous
3. Septal Panniculitis, Sclerotic

VIIIB1 | **Septal Panniculitis, Lymphocytes and Mixed Infiltrates**

The inflammation predominantly involves the subcutaneous septa, although there may be "spillover" into the fat lobules. The infiltrate is mainly lymphocytic although other cells can be found including plasma cells and acute inflammatory cells.

Erythema Nodosum

CLINICAL SUMMARY. Although the causes of erythema nodosum (17) are multiple and cannot always be determined, streptococcal infection is the most common. Other associations include medications, sarcoidosis, pregnancy, inflammatory bowel disease, vaccination, autoimmune disease, malignancy, and miscellaneous/idiopathic (18). In the *acute form* of erythema nodosum, there is a sudden appearance of tender, bright red or dusky red–purple nodules that only slightly elevate the level of the skin surface and have a strong predilection for the anterior surfaces of the lower legs, although they also may occur elsewhere, but mostly on dependent regions. The lesions do not ulcerate and generally involute within a few weeks, while new lesions may intermittently appear for several months. The lesions are tender and warm, and the acute disease often is accompanied by fever, malaise, leukocytosis, and arthropathy. Focal hemorrhages are common and can cause the lesions to resemble bruises (*erythema contusiforme*). The *chronic form* of erythema nodosum may last from a few months to a few years and is also known as *erythema nodosum migrans* or subacute nodular migratory panniculitis. There are one or several red, slightly tender subcutaneous nodules that are found, usually unilaterally, on the lower leg. Most of the patients are women with a solitary lesion and a recent history of sore throat and arthralgia. The nodules enlarge by peripheral extension into plaques, often with central clearing.

Erythema nodosum–like lesions have been described in patients on BRAF inhibitor therapy; however the histologic features have included vasculitis and neutrophilic lobular panniculitis, in addition to septal panniculitis (19).

HISTOPATHOLOGY. In early acute lesions there is edema of the subcutaneous septa with a lymphohistiocytic

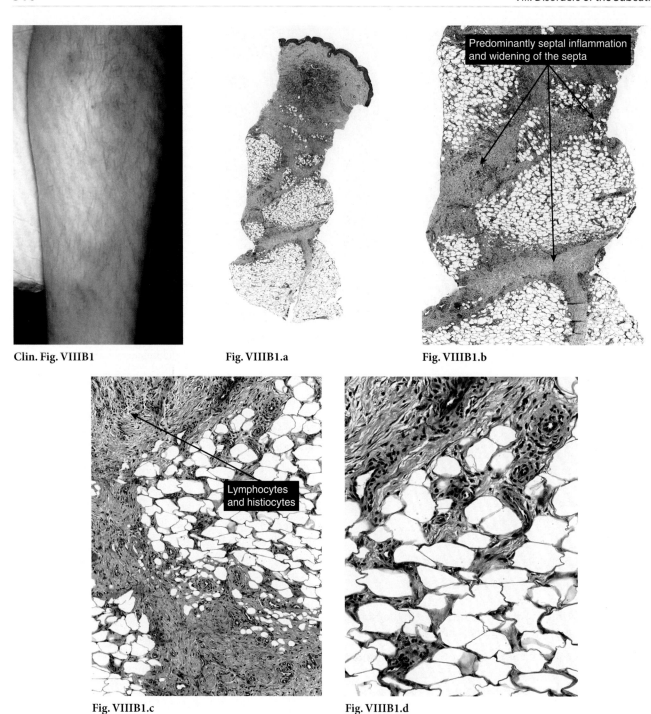

Clin. Fig. VIIIB1   **Fig. VIIIB1.a**   **Fig. VIIIB1.b**

Predominantly septal inflammation and widening of the septa

Lymphocytes and histiocytes

Fig. VIIIB1.c   **Fig. VIIIB1.d**

Clin. Fig. VIIIB1. *Erythema nodosum.* Tender erythematous nodules on the shins is a classic presentation.

Fig. VIIIB1.a. *Erythema nodosum, low power.* Scanning magnification reveals thickening of the fibrous septa.

Fig. VIIIB1.b. *Erythema nodosum, medium power.* The septa are edematous and fibrotic. There is a mixed inflammatory infiltrate in this midstage lesion which begins to extend into the adjacent fat lobules.

Fig. VIIIB1.c. *Erythema nodosum, high power.* Vasculitis is absent. The septa are fibrotic.

Fig. VIIIB1.d. *Erythema nodosum, high power.* Lymphocytes and histiocytes are present in the expanded septa.

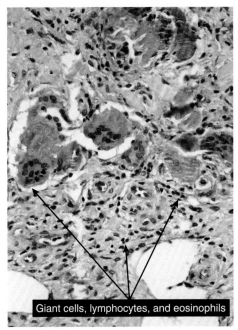

Fig. VIIIB1.e

Fig. VIIIB1.e. *Erythema nodosum, high power.* Giant cells, lymphocytes, and occasionally eosinophils and neutrophils may also be present.

infiltrate, having a slight admixture of neutrophils and eosinophils. Focal fibrin deposition and extravasation of erythrocytes occur frequently. Often the inflammation is most intense at the periphery of the edematous septa and extends into the periphery of the fat lobules between individual fat cells in a lace-like fashion without prominent necrosis of the fat. Clusters of macrophages around small blood vessels, or a slit-like space, occur in early lesions and are known as Miescher radial nodules. The degree of vascular involvement is variable, but usually falls short of true vasculitis. Later acute lesions show widening of the septa, often with fibrosis and with inflammation at the periphery of the fat lobules. Neutrophils usually are absent and there are more macrophages in the infiltrate. Macrophages at the edges of the fat lobules have a "foam-cell" appearance from phagocytosed lipid. Loosely formed granulomas comprised of macrophages and giant cells, without lipid deposition, are more frequent in late lesions compared to the early ones. The oldest lesions have septal widening and fibrosis with a decrease in all of the inflammatory cells, except for a few persisting at the periphery of the fat lobules.

In chronic erythema nodosum, the histologic findings are generally the same as those of the late stages of acute erythema nodosum. However, granuloma and lipogranuloma formation often is more pronounced. There is vascular proliferation and thickening of the endothelium with extravasation of erythrocytes.

Conditions to consider in the differential diagnosis:

erythema nodosum and variants
Crohn disease
morphea

VIIIB2 **Septal Panniculitis, Granulomatous**

Subcutaneous granulomas may present as ill-defined collections of epithelioid histiocytes, as well-formed epithelioid cell granulomas, and as palisading granulomas in which histiocytes are radially arranged around areas of necrosis or necrobiosis. Most of the conditions in this list may also present as mixed lobular/septal panniculitis (see **VIIIC.5**).

Subcutaneous Granuloma Annulare

CLINICAL SUMMARY. In this disorder, subcutaneous nodules occur, especially in children, either alone or in association with intradermal lesions (20). The subcutaneous nodules clinically resemble rheumatoid nodules, although there is a greater tendency to occur on the legs and feet, and there is no history of arthritis. A very rare, deep, destructive form of granuloma annulare has also been described. This lesion might also be considered in the section on mixed septal and lobular involvement (Section VIIID6).

HISTOPATHOLOGY. The subcutaneous nodules of granuloma annulare usually show large foci of palisaded histiocytes surrounding areas of degenerated collagen and prominent mucin with a pale appearance (21); however, biopsies in which mucin was not apparent or the central area appeared more fibrinoid have also been reported. The histopathologic differential diagnosis includes rheumatoid nodule, necrobiosis lipoidica, and epithelioid sarcoma (22). Especially in the pediatric population, it is important to consider subcutaneous granuloma annulare before making a diagnosis of rheumatoid nodule.

Conditions to consider in the differential diagnosis:

palisaded granulomas
    subcutaneous granuloma annulare
    rheumatoid nodules
sarcoidosis
lichen scrofulosorum
Crohn disease
subcutaneous infections
    syphilis
    tuberculosis

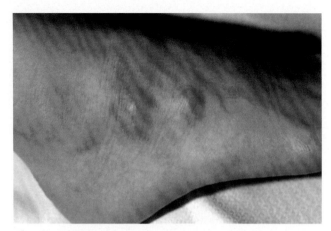

Clin. Fig. VIIIB2

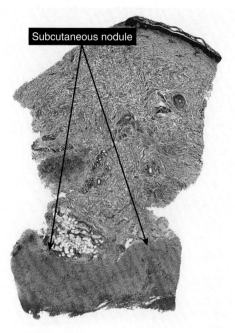

Subcutaneous nodule

Fig. VIIIB2.a

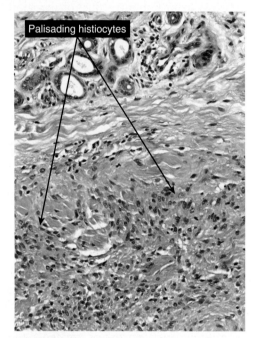

Palisading histiocytes

Fig. VIIIB2.b

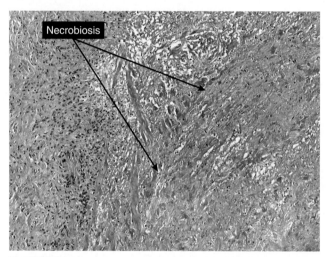

Necrobiosis

Fig. VIIIB2.c

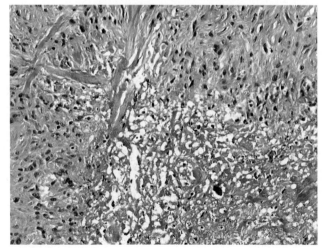

Fig. VIIIB2.d

Clin. Fig. VIIIB2. *Subcutaneous granuloma annulare.* Subcutaneous nodules in an annular distribution developed on a child's dorsal foot.

Fig. VIIIB2.a. *Subcutaneous granuloma annulare, low power.* The septum of the subcutaneous fat has been replaced by inflammation and altered connective tissue.

Fig. VIIIB2.b. *Subcutaneous granuloma annulare, medium power.* In the subcutaneous septum, there is palisaded granulomatous inflammation.

Fig. VIIIB2.c,d. *Subcutaneous granuloma annulare, high power.* The altered (necrobiotic) collagen is surrounded by a palisade of histiocytes as well as fibrosis.

TABLE VIII.1. Selected Panniculitides

Lesion Attribute	Erythema Nodosum	Erythema Induratum	Polyarteritis Nodosa	Sarcoidosis	Granuloma Annulare
Clinical	Nodules on shins, tender	Nodules on calves, tender	Preferentially on lower extremity	Nodules wide distribution	Nodules wide distribution
Ulceration	No	Possible	Possible	No	No
Distribution	Septal	Lobular	Mixed	Mixed	Mixed
Vasculitis	No	Large and small, veins and arteries	Large vessels, arteries	No	No
Histology	Neutrophils, histiocytes	Fat necrosis, histiocytes	Tissue necrosis, neutrophils	Noncaseating granulomas	Palisading histiocytes, necrobiosis
Section	VIIIB1	VIIIA3	VIIIA1	VIIIC7	VIIIB7

VIIIB3 Septal Panniculitis, Sclerotic

Sclerosis of the panniculitis may begin as a septal process and extend into the lobules.

Scleroderma and Morphea

CLINICAL SUMMARY. See also VF1. Morphea is also known as localized scleroderma, and is differentiated from systemic sclerosis based on the absence of sclerodactyly, Raynaud phenomenon, and nailfold capillary changes (23,24). Many patients with morphea have systemic manifestations, such as malaise, fatigue, arthralgias, and myalgias, and positive autoantibody serologies. The pathogenesis of morphea is not understood at this time, but ultimately results in an imbalance of collagen production and destruction.

HISTOPATHOLOGY. Changes in the subcutis are prominent in both scleroderma and morphea. The inflammatory infiltrate involving the subcutaneous fat in morphea is often much more pronounced than that in the dermis. It consists of lymphocytes and plasma cells, and extends upward toward the eccrine glands. Trabeculae subdividing the subcutaneous fat are thickened by an inflammatory infiltrate and deposition of new collagen. Large areas of subcutaneous fat are replaced by newly formed collagen composed of fine, wavy fibers. Vascular changes in the early inflammatory stage may consist of endothelial swelling and edema of the walls of the vessels. In the late sclerotic stage, as seen in the center of old morphea lesions, the inflammatory infiltrate has disappeared almost completely, except in some areas of the subcutis. The fascia and striated muscles underlying lesions of morphea may be affected in the linear, segmental, subcutaneous, and generalized types, showing fibrosis and sclerosis similar to that seen in subcutaneous tissue. The muscle fibers appear vacuolated and separated from one another by edema and focal collections of inflammatory cells. Aggregates of calcium may also be seen in the late stage within areas of sclerotic, homogeneous collagen of the subcutaneous tissue.

In early lesions of systemic scleroderma, the inflammatory reaction is less pronounced than in morphea. The vascular changes in early lesions are slight, as in morphea. In contrast, in the late stage, systemic scleroderma shows more pronounced vascular changes than morphea, particularly in the subcutis. These changes include a paucity of blood vessels, thickening and hyalinization of their walls, and narrowing of the lumen.

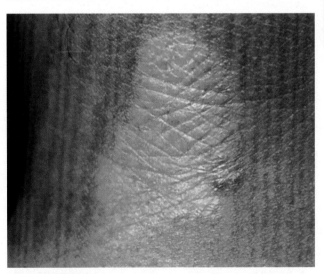

Clin. Fig. VIIIB3

Clin. Fig. VIIIB3. *Morphea.* This indurated plaque with an ivory color represents the plaque type of this disease. (*continues*)

VIII Disorders of the Subcutis

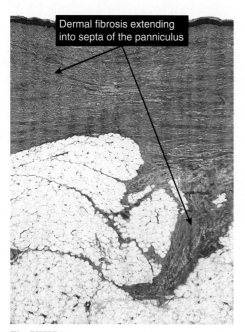

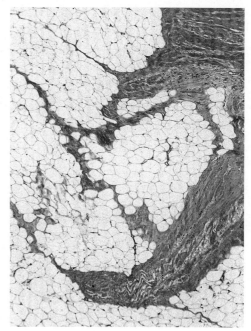

Fig. VIIIB3.a   **Fig. VIIIB3.b**

Fig. VIIIB3.a. *Scleroderma/morphea, low power.* In the later stage of this disease, adnexal structures are absent and inflammation is minimal. The reticular dermal collagen is sclerotic and extends into the subcutaneous fat forming thickened, hyalinized collagen within the septa. At this later stage, there is little or no inflammation.

Fig. VIIIB3.b. *Scleroderma/morphea, medium power.* The sclerotic subcutaneous septa lack the granulomatous inflammation which is seen in later stages of erythema nodosum.

Conditions to consider in the differential diagnosis:

    scleroderma, morphea
    eosinophilic fasciitis
    ischemic liposclerosis
    lipodermatosclerosis
    toxins

 LOBULAR PANNICULITIS WITHOUT VASCULITIS

The inflammation is mainly confined to the lobules, although there may be some septal involvement.

1. Lobular Panniculitis, Lymphocytes Predominant
2. Lobular Panniculitis, Lymphocytes and Plasma Cells
3. Lobular Panniculitis, Neutrophilic
4. Lobular Panniculitis, Eosinophils Prominent
5. Lobular Panniculitis, Histiocytes Prominent
6. Lobular Panniculitis, Mixed With Foam Cells
7. Lobular Panniculitis, Granulomatous
8. Lobular Panniculitis, Crystal Deposits, Calcifications
9. Lobular Panniculitis, Necrosis Prominent
10. Lobular Panniculitis, Embryonic Fat Pattern
11. Lobular Panniculitis, Miscellaneous

VIIIC1 **Lobular Panniculitis, Lymphocytes Predominant**

Lymphocytes are the primary infiltrating cells.

Lupus Erythematosus Panniculitis

CLINICAL SUMMARY. In patients with chronic cutaneous lupus erythematosus, the lesions can be deep and can involve the panniculus either alone or accompanied by dermal lesions, constituting lupus erythematosus panniculitis (LEP) (25). The patients can have either chronic discoid lupus erythematosus or systemic lupus erythematosus. Most commonly, the skin lesions are firm, indurated subcutaneous nodules and plaques that tend to involve the skin of the trunk and proximal extremities, particularly the lateral aspects of the upper arms, thighs, and buttocks. The overlying skin shows no specific changes. The lesions are painful and have a tendency to ulcerate and to heal leaving depressed scars. When the overlying skin is involved there is a loss of hair, erythema, poikiloderma, and epidermal atrophy. The patients may present with localized depressions of lipoatrophy alone. The term "lupus profundus" has been used both for lupus panniculitis and also for discoid lupus erythematosus lesions that involve the dermis and extend deeply into the subcutis.

HISTOPATHOLOGY. In histologic sections there is a deep lymphocytic infiltrate in the fat lobules and in the septa. Lymphoid aggregates, nodules, and germinal centers are common. Usually there is mucinous edema of the septa and of the overlying dermis. The dermis can have a superficial and deep perivascular lymphocytic infiltrate with plasma cells or all of the changes of lesions of discoid lupus erythematosus may be present. A distinctive feature is the so-called "hyaline necrosis" of the fat, in which portions of the fat lobule have lost nuclear staining of the fat cells and there is an accumulation of fibrin and other proteins in a homogeneous eosinophilic matrix between residual fat cells and extracellular fat globules. Blood vessels are infiltrated by lymphoid cells and can have restriction of their lumen diameter. Calcification may be present in older lesions.

The differential diagnosis includes subcutaneous panniculitis-like T-cell lymphoma (SPTCL). Features helpful in making this distinction included the presence of involvement of the epidermis, lymphoid follicles with

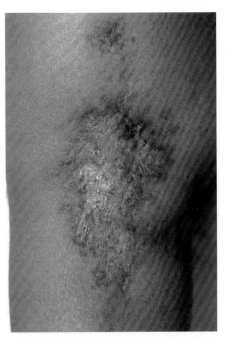

Clin. Fig. VIIIC1

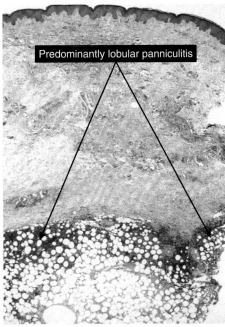

Fig. VIIIC1.a

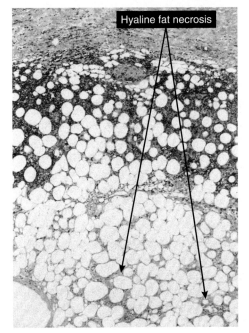

Fig. VIIIC1.b

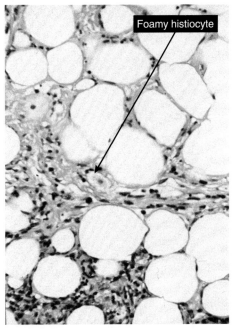

Fig. VIIIC1.c

Clin. Fig. VIIIC1. *Lupus panniculitis.* A patient with discoid lupus erythematosus developed an indurated subcutaneous area with postinflammatory hyper/hypopigmentation on the lateral thigh.

Fig. VIIIC1.a. *Lupus panniculitis, low power.* An intense inflammatory infiltrate is present at the dermal–subcutaneous junction, extending into the adipose tissue in an interstitial pattern. (C. Jaworsky.)

Fig. VIIIC1.b. *Lupus panniculitis, medium power.* The inflammatory infiltrate outlines individual adipocytes, creating a lace-like pattern. (C. Jaworsky.)

Fig. VIIIC1.c. *Lupus panniculitis, high power.* Foam cells indicate adipocyte injury. Note also the hyaline matrix between adipocytes ("hyaline fat necrosis"). (C. Jaworsky.)

VIII Disorders of the Subcutis

reactive germinal centers, mixed cell infiltrate with prominent plasma cells, clusters of B lymphocytes, and polyclonal TCR–gamma gene rearrangements in LEP (26). Ki-67 "hot spots" in SPTCL have been described as a helpful discriminatory feature (27). Monoclonal gene rearrangements have been described in rare cases, and clear distinction between these entities may require observation over time in some difficult cases (28).

Conditions to consider in the differential diagnosis:

lupus panniculitis lupus profundus
nodular vasculitis/erythema induratum, inapparent vasculitis
poststeroid panniculitis
subcutaneous lymphoma–leukemia

VIIIC2 | Lobular Panniculitis, Lymphocytes and Plasma Cells

Lymphocytes and plasma cells are the primary infiltrating cells. These conditions are more likely to present as primarily septal or as mixed panniculitis (see Sections **VIIIB3** and **VIIIC1**).

Conditions to consider in the differential diagnosis:

lupus profundus
scleroderma

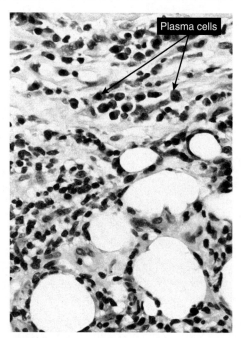
Plasma cells

Fig. VIIIC2.a

Fig. VIIIC2.a. *Lupus panniculitis, high power.* A lymphoplasmacytic infiltrate splays collagen bundles and adipocytes (see also VIIIC1). (C. Jaworsky.)

VIIIC3 | Lobular Panniculitis, Neutrophilic

Lymphocytes and neutrophils are the primary infiltrating cells. The conditions listed below are more likely to present as a mixed lobular and septal panniculitis (see Section VIIID1), and may also involve the dermis. In some cases with pancreatic enzyme panniculitis, possibly with early lesions, biopsies of subcutaneous nodules show only a nonspecific pattern of a necrotizing panniculitis with a neutrophilic inflammatory response. If there is no necrosis and if other entities can be ruled out, and in an appropriate clinical setting, the diagnosis for a neutrophilic panniculitis may be subcutaneous Sweet syndrome (29).

Conditions to consider in the differential diagnosis:

infection (cellulitis)
necrotizing fasciitis
ruptured follicles and cysts
pancreatic fat necrosis
traumatic panniculitis
subcutaneous Sweet syndrome

VIIIC4 | Lobular Panniculitis, Eosinophils Prominent

Lymphocytes and eosinophils are the primary infiltrating cells. The conditions listed below are more likely to present as a mixed lobular and septal panniculitis (**see Section VIIID3**), and may also involve the dermis.

Conditions to consider in the differential diagnosis:

eosinophilic fasciitis
eosinophilic panniculitis
arthropod assault reactions
parasites
hypersensitivity reactions
Wells syndrome

VIIIC5 | Lobular Panniculitis, Histiocytes Prominent

Lymphocytes and histiocytes are the primary infiltrating cells. The conditions listed below are more likely to present as a mixed lobular and septal panniculitis (see also Section VIIID4).

Cytophagic Histiocytic Panniculitis

CLINICAL SUMMARY. Cytophagic histiocytic panniculitis (CHP) (30,31) is a frequently fatal systemic disease that is characterized by recurrent, widely distributed, painful subcutaneous nodules associated with malaise and fever. It is often associated with hemophagocytic lymphohistiocytosis (HLH), and also may be associated with malignancy, including SPTCL (32). The nodules can be hemorrhagic and may ulcerate. Hepatosplenomegaly, pancytopenia, and progressive liver dysfunction develop in most cases. The patients may follow a long chronic course or the disease can be fulminant. The patients usually die a hemorrhagic death due to depletion of blood coagulation factors. In some patients, the disease seems limited to the skin and subcutaneous tissue and follows a more benign course. Some of these cases may be virally associated.

In most instances, the cytophagic panniculitis is the result of a malignant lymphoma in which the abnormal lymphocyte population has stimulated benign macrophages to engage in fulminant hemophagocytosis. Lymphoma may or may not be evident in any given biopsy of skin and/or subcutaneous tissue. The NK cell marker CD56 is an important marker for distinguishing two major patterns of subcutaneous lymphomas with features of cytotoxic T cell and natural killer (NK)/T-cell lymphomas. CD56-negative cases tend to be mainly in the younger age group and have systemic subcutaneous nodules without ulceration, with subcutaneous invasion by medium-sized lymphoma cells, scattered erythrophagocytosis, patchy necrosis, and little tumor invasion in the superficial dermis, and a somewhat better prognosis. CD56-positive cases tend to have systemic ulcerative skin tumors composed of pleomorphic lymphoma cells with massive necrosis and little erythrophagocytosis, involving the subcutis and also often the whole dermis, with a relatively poor prognosis (33). There is overlap between this condition and HLH (34), however most patients with HLH do not have CHP (35).

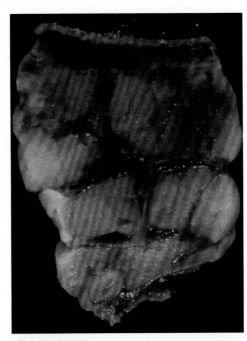

Clin. Fig. VIIIC5

Clin. Fig. VIIIC5. *Cytophagic histiocytic panniculitis.* This cross-sectioned skin nodule shows both septal and lobular infiltration and hemorrhage. Note also the dermal hemorrhage. (N.S. McNutt, A. Moreno, F. Contreras.)

Fig. VIIIC5.a. *Cytophagic histiocytic panniculitis, medium power.* There is hemorrhagic necrosis of the fat, with an infiltrate of lymphocytes and macrophages. (N.S. McNutt, A. Moreno, F. Contreras.)

Fig. VIIIC5.b. *Cytophagic histiocytic panniculitis, high power.* Macrophages and multinucleated cells ingest lymphocytes and erythrocytes to form so-called "bean-bag cells." (N.S. McNutt, A. Moreno, F. Contreras.)

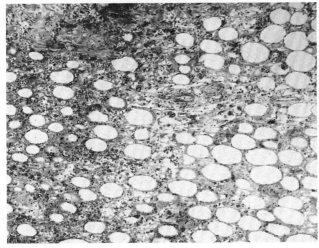

Fig. VIIIC5.a

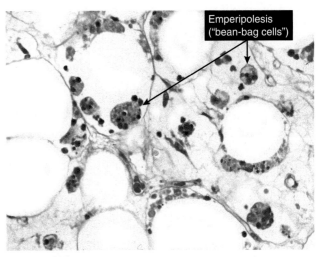

Fig. VIIIC5.b

VIII Disorders of the Subcutis

HISTOPATHOLOGY. A deep biopsy usually shows both subcutaneous and dermal nodules composed of macrophages and a mixed inflammatory infiltrate. In the subcutis the inflammation is both septal and lobular. Often there is necrosis and hemorrhage. The nuclei of the macrophages are without significant atypia. In some areas the macrophages become so engorged by phagocytosis of erythrocytes, lymphocytes, and cell fragments (termed "emperipolesis") that they have been named "bean bag cells." In some patients, early lesions contain a rather dense infiltrate of small lymphocytes and only focal areas with cytophagic histiocytes. Overt lymphoma may not be evident in biopsies of early-stage lesions, or ever. The involvement of other organs by similar cytophagic macrophages leads to diffuse infiltration of liver, bone marrow, spleen, lymph nodes, myocardium, lungs, and gastrointestinal tract. The cytophagic macrophages can deplete almost all of the bone marrow elements.

Conditions to consider in the differential diagnosis:

cytophagic histiocytic panniculitis
Rosai–Dorfman disease
subcutaneous histiocytoid Sweet syndrome
atypical mycobacteria
lepromatous leprosy
sarcoidosis

VIIIC6 Lobular Panniculitis, Mixed With Foam Cells

Lymphocytes, plasma cells, and a variety of infiltrating cells can be seen including giant cells and foamy histiocytes.

Relapsing Febrile Nodular Nonsuppurative Panniculitis

CLINICAL SUMMARY. The term Weber–Christian disease has been applied to cases of predominantly lobular panniculitis with a lymphohistiocytic infiltrate. This is a diagnosis of exclusion. It is made much less frequently now than it was in the past, due to the greater power of current laboratory testing to reveal LEP, AAT deficiency panniculitis, histiocytic cytophagic panniculitis, or infectious etiologies in cases that might previously have been classified as Weber–Christian disease. The classical clinical description is of a disease characterized by the appearance of crops of tender nodules and plaques in the subcutaneous fat, usually in association with mild fever. The lower extremities are favored sites, but lesions can occur also on the trunk, the upper extremities, and rarely on the face. The lesions may ulcerate; as they involute, they leave depressions in the skin surface. The overlying skin usually shows no involvement other than mild erythema. In general, the prognosis is good, with the attacks gradually becoming less severe and ultimately ceasing. The name

Weber–Christian disease has been used in such a general fashion that the term has lost its meaning beyond being a clinical syndrome with nodular panniculitis for which the etiology has not yet been determined (35).

HISTOPATHOLOGY. The histopathologic appearance itself is not sufficiently specific to exclude the other diseases mentioned above. The classical description is that of a lobular panniculitis that evolves through three phases. The first phase is acute inflammation of the fat lobules with degeneration of fat cells accompanied by an infiltrate of neutrophils, lymphocytes, and macrophages. Neutrophils may predominate, but abscesses do not occur. In the second phase, after the lesions have been present for several days, the infiltrate is discretely localized to the fat lobules and consists mainly of foamy macrophages, usually also with a few lymphocytes and plasma cells. The foam cells can be large and often some of them are multinucleated. Foamy macrophages replace the fat lobules and extracellular lipid masses ("microcysts") result from lysis of the fat. In some cases, the lesions perforate the skin surface and discharge a sterile, oily liquid. The third phase, in clinical lesions that are depressed and indurated, shows many fibroblasts and scattered lymphocytes and a few plasma cells that have replaced the fat; dense fibrosis results.

Systemic lesions that may be seen in this setting include involvement of the mesenteric and omental fat; involvement of intravisceral adipose tissue, causing focal necrosis in liver or spleen; involvement of the bone marrow; and accumulation of large amounts of oily fluid in either the peritoneal or pleural cavity.

Conditions to consider in the differential diagnosis:

alpha-1-antitrypsin deficiency panniculitis
Weber–Christian disease

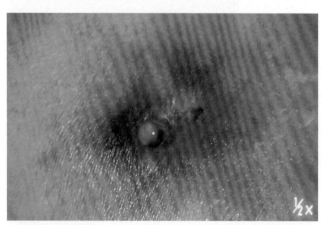

Clin. Fig. VIIIC6

Clin. Fig. VIIIC6. *Nodular panniculitis.* An indurated nodule on the leg has developed a perforation and drains a turbid, sterile, oily fluid with necrotic tissue. (N.S. McNutt, A. Moreno, F. Contreras.)

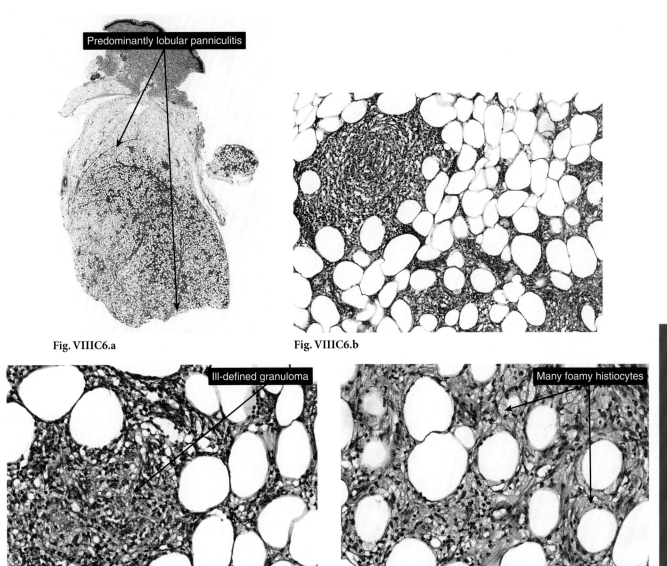

Fig. VIIIC6.a

Fig. VIIIC6.b

Fig. VIIIC6.c

Fig. VIIIC6.d

Fig. VIIIC6.a. *Lobular panniculitis, low power.* A dense lymphocytic infiltrate is sharply localized to the fat lobules without vasculitis.

Fig. VIIIC6.b. *Lobular panniculitis, high power.* The infiltrate is composed mainly of lymphocytes and macrophages with variable numbers of neutrophils.

Fig. VIIIC6.c. *Lobular panniculitis, high power.* An ill-defined granuloma is present. There is no vasculitis. Infection should be ruled out.

Fig. VIIIC6.d. *Lobular panniculitis, later lesion, medium power.* The fat is necrotic and has been extensively replaced by lipid-laden macrophages or "foam cells." There is no more specific diagnosis that can be applied to this histologic appearance than "lobular panniculitis, NOS." Clinicopathologic correlation and laboratory investigation may allow for a more specific diagnosis to be made.

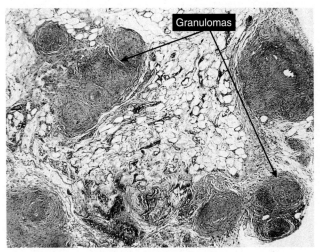

Fig. VIIIC7.a

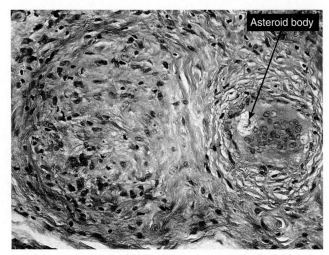

Fig. VIIIC7.b

Fig. VIIIC7.a. *Subcutaneous sarcoidosis, low power.* Within the subcutaneous fat, there are multiple granulomas with minimal necrosis.

Fig. VIIIC7.b. *Subcutaneous sarcoidosis, medium power.* The granulomas are well formed, composed of epithelioid histiocytes and giant cells with a sprinkling of lymphocytes. An asteroid body is present in one giant cell.

panniculitis, NOS
traumatic fat necrosis
cold panniculitis
injection granuloma
factitious panniculitis
necrobiotic xanthogranuloma with paraproteinemia

VIIIC7 Lobular Panniculitis, Granulomatous

Lymphocytes and histiocytes are the primary infiltrating cells. Except for erythema induratum, discussed in Section VIIIA.3 because it is usually associated with evident vasculitis, most of the conditions in this list may more usually present as mixed lobular/septal panniculitis (see Section VIIIC.5).

Subcutaneous Sarcoidosis

Sarcoidosis may present as a subcutaneous nodule, characterized as in other sites by noncaseating epithelioid cell granulomas, usually with only slight associated lymphocytic inflammation. The diagnosis should be based on exclusion of other granulomatous disorders, especially infection, with clinicopathologic correlation.

Conditions to consider in the differential diagnosis:

palisaded granulomas
subcutaneous granuloma annulare/pseudorheumatoid nodule
rheumatoid nodules
erythema induratum/nodular vasculitis (if vasculitis is inapparent)

subcutaneous sarcoidosis
tuberculosis
Crohn disease
epithelioid sarcoma

VIIIC8 Lobular Panniculitis, Crystal Deposits, Calcifications

Crystalline deposits derived from free fatty acids or other precipitated salts are present in the fat lobules.

Subcutaneous Fat Necrosis of the Newborn

CLINICAL SUMMARY. Subcutaneous fat necrosis of the newborn usually occurs in premature or full-term infants, often in the past after delivery with forceps (36), or after a history of fetal distress (37). Indurated nodules and plaques appear in the subcutis a few days after birth. Rarely, in cases with numerous nodules, the lesions may discharge a caseous material. The patient's health generally is good and the nodules resolve spontaneously after a few weeks or months.

HISTOPATHOLOGY. Focal areas of fat necrosis are present in the fat lobules and are infiltrated by macrophages and foreign-body giant cells. The fat deposits in the macrophages and giant cells contain crystalline fat, which forms needle-shaped clefts in a radial arrangement. Calcium deposits usually are scattered in the necrotic fat. An important histologic differential diagnosis is sclerema

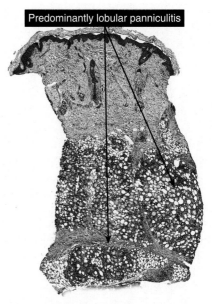

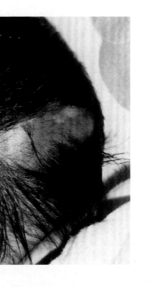

Clin. Fig. VIIIC8.a

Fig. VIIIC8.a

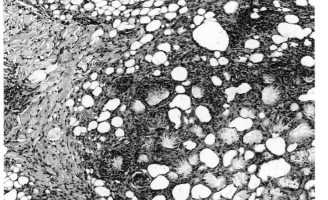

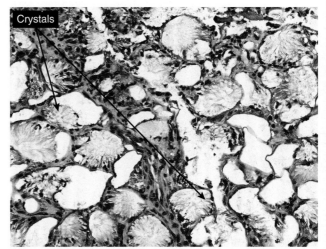

Fig. VIIIC8.b

Fig. VIIIC8.c

Clin. Fig. VIIIC8.a. *Subcutaneous fat necrosis of the newborn.* A healthy full-term infant developed an indurated plaque with alopecia on the scalp, an unusual presentation. (P. Honig.)

Fig. VIIIC8.a. *Subcutaneous fat necrosis of the newborn, low power.* Scanning magnification reveals a predominantly lobular panniculitis. The overlying epidermis and dermis show almost no inflammation.

Fig. VIIIC8.b. *Subcutaneous fat necrosis of the newborn, medium power.* Within the subcutaneous lobules there is a lymphoid infiltrate associated with large giant cells. Occasionally, as seen here, they may be numerous.

Fig. VIIIC8.c. *Subcutaneous fat necrosis of the newborn, high power.* The giant cells show numerous needle-shaped clefts in a radial array, a characteristic finding in this disease.

neonatorum, which shows less inflammation than subcutaneous fat necrosis of the newborn, and occurs in severely ill infants.

Calcifying Panniculitis (Calciphylaxis)

See also Section VB.

CLINICAL SUMMARY. Calciphylaxis (also known as calcific uremic arteriolopathy) is an uncommon complication usually associated with chronic renal failure, although nonuremic cases are becoming more frequently diagnosed. Other associations include female gender, diabetes mellitus, obesity, and autoimmune conditions such as lupus, antiphospholipid antibody syndrome, temporal arteritis, rheumatoid arthritis, end-stage liver disease, and hypoalbuminemia (38). Painful violaceous lesions that may be indurated often develop in areas of livedo reticularis on the trunk and extremities and can rapidly progress to form bullae, ulcers, eschars, and gangrene. The prognosis is extremely poor, especially for proximal disease, even with aggressive treatment. Fulminant sepsis may develop from infection of necrotic or gangrenous tissue.

HISTOPATHOLOGY. The principal histologic findings include: calcification of soft tissue (including perieccrine calcification) and small vessels; intimal proliferation of small vessels, often resulting in luminal narrowing; usually fibrin thrombi in small vessels; and frequent ischemic necrosis of skin and subcutis. The small vessels involved by this process cannot be identified as either arterial or venous. Small-vessel vasculitic changes may also be seen in some cases. Foreign-body giant cell reaction to calcium and mixed inflammatory cell infiltrates that are neutrophil rich may be seen. The relationships between the calcification and thrombosis, and the ischemic necrosis in calciphylaxis are unclear. Some similar cases have been described with subcutaneous thrombotic vasculopathy but without calcification, and may represent an early stage or a related lesion (39). Although vascular calcification is common in uremic patients, calciphylaxis is rare. Alterations in calcium and phosphate balance, perhaps in association with transformation of vascular smooth muscle cells into osteoblast-like phenotypes, and also with hypercoagulability, are considered to be involved in the pathogenesis of calciphylaxis (43). Although they are relatively nonspecific when considered in isolation, the cited histopathologic features allow for the diagnosis of this potentially lethal disorder when seen in combination, particularly if detailed clinical data also are available (40). However, skin biopsy may lack sensitivity for various reasons, and calciphylaxis is considered to be predominantly a clinical diagnosis. In a patient with end-stage renal disease presenting with painful, erythematous, livedoid skin changes on adipose-rich areas, the diagnosis is calciphylaxis until proven otherwise (43).

Conditions to consider in the differential diagnosis:

sclerema neonatorum
subcutaneous fat necrosis of the newborn
gout
oxalosis
calcifying panniculitis

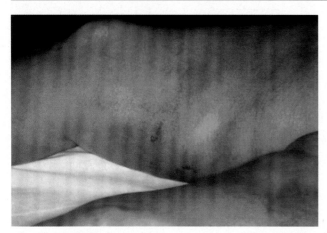
Clin. Fig. VIIIC8.b

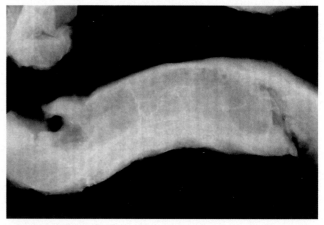
Clin. Fig. VIIIC8.c

Clin. Fig. VIIIC8.b. *Calcifying panniculitis.* This patient with hyperparathyroidism developed erythematous, hemorrhagic, indurated plaques that were cold to touch. (N.S. McNutt, A. Moreno, F. Contreras.)

Clin. Fig. VIIIC8.c. *Calciphylaxis.* An x-ray of a skin biopsy from a patient with calciphylaxis reveals linear calcifications in vessel walls.

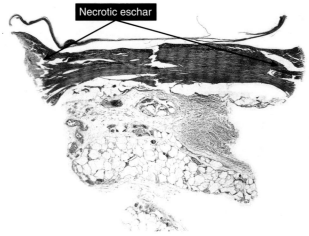

Fig. VIIIC8.d

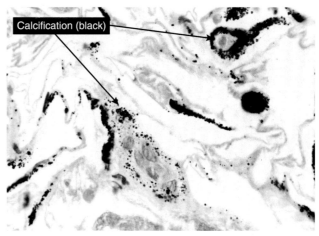

Fig. VIIIC8.e

Fig. VIIIC8.f

Fig. VIIIC8.g

Fig. VIIIC8.d. *Calcifying panniculitis, low power.* Although the subcutis appears relatively unaffected at low power, gangrenous necrosis of the epidermis and dermis suggests vascular injury at a deeper level.

Fig. VIIIC8.e. *Calcifying panniculitis, high power.* In addition to lipomembranous change, small vessels within the subcutis are seen to contain basophilic granular material consistent with calcium within their walls.

Fig. VIIIC8.f. *Calcifying panniculitis, medium power, von Kossa stain.* The material stains positive for calcium, and is localized primarily to the media of small vessels in the subcutis.

Fig. VIIIC8.g. *Calcifying panniculitis, high power, von Kossa stain.* Granular amorphous material characteristic of calcium is primarily deposited within the media of small vessels between individual adipocytes.

VIII Disorders of the Subcutis

VIIIC9 Lobular Panniculitis, Necrosis Prominent

There is fat necrosis with a resulting infiltrate that is mixed.

Subcutaneous Nodular Fat Necrosis in Pancreatic Disease

CLINICAL SUMMARY. In patients with pancreatitis or pancreatic neoplasms, the release of lipase enzymes into the blood can lead to nodules of fat necrosis in the subcutis

(41). The pretibial region is the most common site of the nodules, but they may occur on the thighs, buttocks, and elsewhere. The nodules usually are tender and red and may be fluctuant, but they only rarely discharge oily fluid through fistulae. Abdominal pain is present in most cases of pancreatitis but may be absent in pancreatic carcinoma when the nodules appear. Arthralgia in the ankles is a common early symptom.

HISTOPATHOLOGY. The histologic appearance of the subcutaneous nodules in pancreatic disease is characteristic

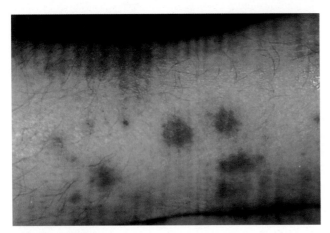

Clin. Fig. VIIIC9

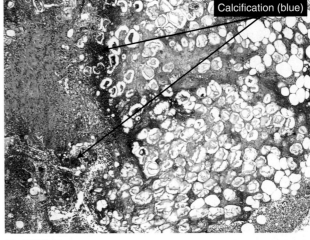

Fig. VIIIC9.a

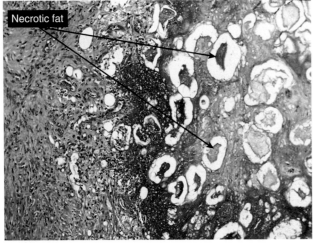

Fig. VIIIC9.b

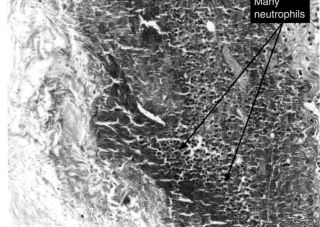

Fig. VIIIC9.c

Clin. Fig. VIIIC9. *Pancreatic panniculitis.* Erythematous nodules appear most commonly on the lower legs. (N.S. McNutt, A. Moreno, F. Contreras.)

Fig. VIIIC9.a. *Pancreatic panniculitis, low power.* Calcification forms granular basophilic material. Focal hemorrhage is frequent. (N.S. McNutt, A. Moreno, F. Contreras.)

Fig. VIIIC9.b. *Pancreatic panniculitis, high power.* Necrotic fat cells contain eosinophilic deposits of partially hydrolyzed fat. (N.S. McNutt, A. Moreno, F. Contreras.)

Fig. VIIIC9.c. *Pancreatic panniculitis, high power.* Many neutrophils are present at the margin of the zone of calcification and fat necrosis.

---

in most instances. In the foci of fat necrosis, there are ghost-like fat cells having thick, faintly stained cell peripheries and no nuclear staining. Calcification forms basophilic granules in the cytoplasm of the necrotic fat cells, and sometimes lamellar deposits around individual fat cells or patchy basophilic deposits at the periphery of the fat necrosis. A polymorphous infiltrate surrounds the foci of fat necrosis and consists of neutrophils, lymphoid cells, macrophages, foam cells, and foreign-body giant cells. There can be extensive hemorrhage into the lesions. Older lesions have fibrosis and hemosiderin deposition in addition to the inflammatory infiltrates. In some cases of pancreatic enzyme panniculitis, possibly with early lesions, biopsies of subcutaneous nodules show only a nonspecific pattern of a necrotizing panniculitis with a neutrophilic inflammatory response.

Conditions to consider in the differential diagnosis:

pancreatic panniculitis
erythema induratum, inapparent vasculitis

necrobiotic xanthogranuloma with paraproteinemia
gummatous syphilis
infarct
abscess

VIIIC10 Lobular Panniculitis, Embryonic Fat Pattern

Due to atrophy or to failure of normal morphogenesis, immature small fat cells are present in the lobules.

Localized Lipoatrophy and Lipodystrophy

CLINICAL SUMMARY. Both localized lipoatrophy (42,43) and lipodystrophy can have lesions with a similar clinical appearance; however, lipoatrophy usually involves one or several circumscribed, round, depressed areas, from one to several centimeters in diameter. In contrast, lipodystrophy produces the loss of large areas of subcutaneous fat. Most cases of lipodystrophy are of the cephalothoracic type and involve the face, neck, upper extremities, and upper trunk. The condition may be of genetic or acquired

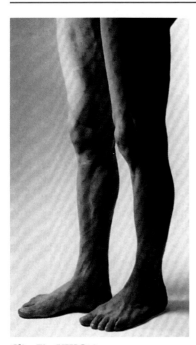

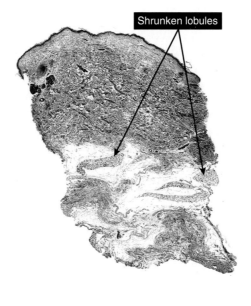

Shrunken lobules

Clin. Fig. VIIIC10. *Lipoatrophy.* Insulin resistance and hypertriglyceridemia were present in this middle-aged male who presented with loss of subcutaneous fat leading to the appearance of hypertrophic muscles.

Fig. VIIIC10.a. *Lipoatrophy, low power.* At this magnification the subcutaneous fat appears fibrotic and the lobules appear shrunken and hypercellular.

Fig. VIIIC10.b. *Lipoatrophy, high power.* The individual adipocytes are small and the fat is not truly hypercellular but appears such because the individual nuclei are closer to one another.

Fig. VIIIC10.c. *Lipoatrophy, high power.* The fat cells are reduced in size.

Clin. Fig. VIIIC10   Fig. VIIIC10.a

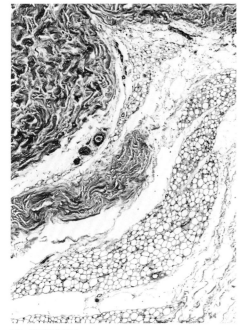

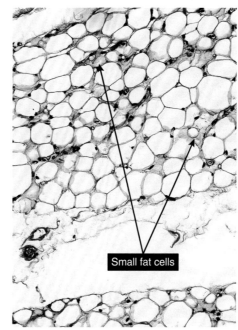

Small fat cells

Fig. VIIIC10.b   Fig. VIIIC10.c

Disorders of the Subcutis

VIII

pathogenesis. Acquired lipodystrophy may occur with diabetes and with glomerulonephritis, and also may be drug induced or related to insulin resistance, hypertriglyceridemia, or hepatic steatosis. Lipoatrophic panniculitis also occurs in connective tissue panniculitis, following subcutaneous corticosteroid injection, and in HIV-associated lipodystrophy.

HISTOPATHOLOGY. Lesions of lipodystrophy are described with total loss of the subcutaneous fat producing dermis adjacent to fascia. However, localized lipoatrophy has been described as having two types: inflammatory and noninflammatory or "involutional" types. In the inflammatory type, multiple lesions are common and have a lymphocytic infiltrate around the blood vessels and scattered diffusely in the fat lobules. Areas of fat necrosis can be present with infiltration by macrophages. In the involutional type, usually there is only a solitary lesion that exhibits a decrease in size of the individual adipocytes. They are separated from each other by abundant eosinophilic, hyaline material, or in some instances by mucoid material.

Conditions to consider in the differential diagnosis:

  lipoatrophy
  lipodystrophy

VIIIC11 Lobular Panniculitis, Lipomembranous

Lymphocytes, plasma cells, and a variety of infiltrating cells can be seen including giant cells and histiocytes.

Lipomembranous Change or Lipomembranous Panniculitis

CLINICAL SUMMARY. Patients with severe stasis, diabetes, and other causes of arterial vascular insufficiency to the lower legs can develop indurated plaques in the subcutis. They are depressed and painful, but rarely ulcerate (44).

HISTOPATHOLOGY. The lesions are defined microscopically by the presence of lipomembranes around fat deposits or "cysts" (1,45). Biopsies deep into the fat show a lobular panniculitis with focal macrophage infiltration and fibrosis around the shrunken lobules. At the border of the lobules with the septa there are fat cysts that are lined by a thin eosinophilic layer of protein that has fine, feathery projections into the fat cavity. This layer is called a lipomembrane and is positive on PAS and elastic-tissue stains. Early lesions have focal areas of fat necrosis, such as those produced by partial ischemia. Lipomembranous change has been found also in LEP and in morphea.

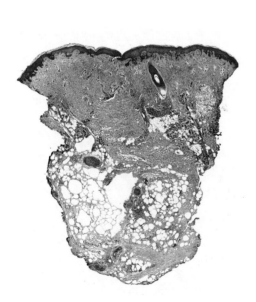

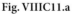

Fig. VIIIC11.a

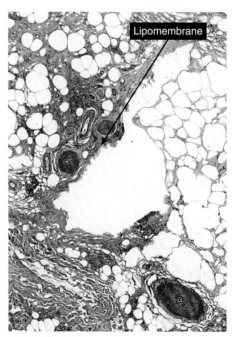

Fig. VIIIC11.b

Fig. VIIIC11.a. *Lipomembranous panniculitis, low power.* The subcutaneous tissue shows fibrosis of both septa and lobules with cystic space formation, associated with a mild chronic inflammatory infiltrate.

Fig. VIIIC11.b. *Lipomembranous panniculitis, medium power.* Within the fat one can see variably sized cystic structures which are surrounded by eosinophilic material.

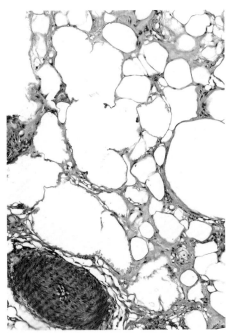
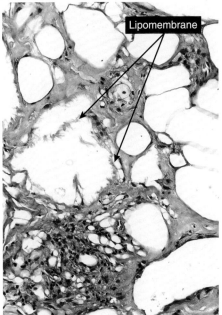

Lipomembrane

Fig. VIIIC11.c   **Fig. VIIIC11.d**

Fig. VIIIC11.c. *Lipomembranous panniculitis, medium power.* The fat cells vary in size and shape.

Fig. VIIIC11.d. *Lipomembranous panniculitis, high power.* The cysts are surrounded by feathery eosinophilic material which is frequently positive with PAS stains.

Conditions to consider in the differential diagnosis:

lipomembranous panniculitis
lipogranulomatosis of Rothmann–Makai
granulomatous panniculitis in light-chain disease
early stages of pyoderma gangrenosum
necrobiotic xanthogranuloma
lipodermatosclerosis

VIIID   MIXED LOBULAR AND SEPTAL PANNICULITIS

Neoplastic infiltrates and inflammation due to trauma or infection do not respect anatomic compartments of the subcutis.

1. With Hemorrhage or Sclerosis
2. With Many Neutrophils
3. With Many Eosinophils
4. With Many Lymphocytes
5. With Cytophagic Histiocytes
6. With Granulomas

VIIID1   With Hemorrhage or Sclerosis

Inflammation due to trauma is likely to be associated with hemorrhage, neutrophilic inflammation, and sclerosis in late lesions.

Panniculitis due to Physical or Chemical Agents

CLINICAL SUMMARY. Trauma may be due to physical injury or chemical injury, such as that produced by injection of noxious substances. Physical injury can be produced by blunt pressure or impact, cold (46) or excessive heat, or electrical injury. All of these factors can produce firm nodules in the subcutaneous fat. Surreptitious injections of noxious substances can produce bizarre clinical and histologic patterns of lesions. Insulin injections, often on the thigh and lower abdomen, can result in subcutaneous lesions. Meperidine hydrochloride or Demerol and pentazocine or Talwin injections are known to produce traumatic panniculitis. The introduction of oily substances such as paraffin or silicone for cosmetic effects can produce a panniculitis (47). Mentally ill persons and drug addicts may purposely or inadvertently inject themselves with foreign substances, such as feces or milk, sometimes used to dilute or cut narcotics (48). These various physical or chemical traumas lead to indurated subcutaneous nodules that may undergo liquefaction, ulcerate, and discharge pus or a thick oily fluid. Healing leaves depressed scars. Lesions produced by extreme cold may include nodules or plaques that appear from 1 to 3 days after exposure and subside spontaneously within 2 weeks. Excessive heat and electrical injury usually are accompanied by ulceration and eschar formation.

HISTOPATHOLOGY. The injection of various toxic agents will produce a variable histologic picture of acute

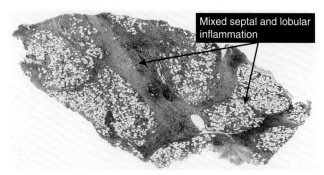

Mixed septal and lobular inflammation

Fig. VIIID1.a

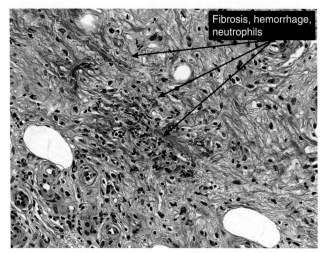

Fibrosis, hemorrhage, neutrophils

Fig. VIIID1.c

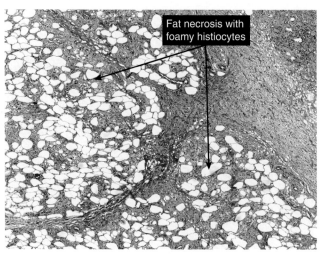

Fat necrosis with foamy histiocytes

Fig. VIIID1.b

Fig. VIIID1.a. *Traumatic panniculitis, low power.* There is extensive fibrosis, with inflammation involving lobules and septa.

Fig. VIIID1.b. *Traumatic panniculitis, medium power.* In addition to fibrosis, there is a mild mixed infiltrate composed of lymphocytes, and foamy histiocytes.

Fig. VIIID1.c. *Traumatic panniculitis, medium power.* A focus of hemorrhage with a small cluster of neutrophils is present.

inflammation, with aggregation of neutrophils and focal fat necrosis with hemorrhage. Older lesions have infiltrates of lymphocytes and macrophages with fibrosis. Vasculitis usually is absent. Polarized light may reveal foreign material in injection sites. The injection of oily liquids leads to the formation of many pockets of fatty material "fat cysts," often with a surrounding fibrous reaction containing foamy macrophages, that produces a "Swiss-cheese appearance" after the fat is extracted during routine histologic processing. Trauma due to cold injury initially has an infiltrate of lymphocytes and macrophages near the blood vessels of the deep plexus at the junction of dermis and subcutis. Such changes have also been described in perniosis. Biopsies at the third day, the height of the reaction, show rupture of the fat cells with fat pockets in the tissue surrounded by an infiltrate of lymphocytes, macrophages, neutrophils, and occasional eosinophils.

Conditions to consider in the differential diagnosis:

> traumatic panniculitis (including postsurgical)
> cold panniculitis
> injections including factitial panniculitis
> blunt trauma: sclerosing lipogranuloma
> scleroderma/morphea
> lipodermatosclerosis

VIIID2 With Many Neutrophils

Neutrophilic inflammation diffusely involves the subcutis and extends along fascial planes.

Necrotizing Fasciitis

CLINICAL SUMMARY. Necrotizing fasciitis (NF) is caused most commonly by group A beta-hemolytic streptococci, and it typically presents with rapidly spreading erythema and pain (49). In a case series of uncommon synchronous multifocal NF of the extremities, Vibrio species were the most common, while others were Aeromonas spp., group A β-hemolytic streptococcus, and coagulase-negative staphylococcus (50). The erythema is more ill-defined than that of erysipelas and progresses to painless ulceration and necrosis along fascial planes. Whereas erysipelas involves the more superficial layers of the skin, fasciitis extends more deeply into the subcutaneous tissues. Although virtually all cases of erysipelas are caused by beta-hemolytic streptococci, primarily group A, the list of causative agents of cellulitis/fasciitis is much more extensive (51).

HISTOPATHOLOGY. The histologic picture is characterized by acute and chronic inflammation with necrosis.

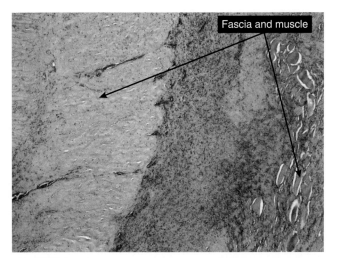

Fig. VIIID2.a

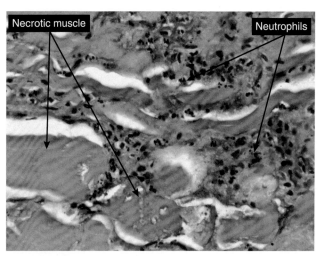

Fig. VIIID2.b

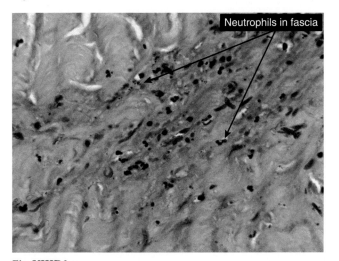

Fig. VIIID2.c

Fig. VIIID2.a. *Necrotizing fasciitis, low power.* Necrosis of muscle and fascia in a patient with a staphylococcal infection complicating a hysterectomy.

Fig. VIIID2.b. *Necrotizing fasciitis, high power.* Necrotic muscle infiltrated by degenerating neutrophils.

Fig. VIIID2.c. *Necrotizing fasciitis, high power.* Fascia with focal edema and neutrophils. Presence of neutrophils in the fascia is compatible with this diagnosis in an appropriate clinical setting, even in the absence of necrosis in a particular biopsy specimen.

Often there is thrombosis of blood vessels as the result of damage to vessel walls from the inflammatory process. The key feature in distinguishing NF from a less-threatening superficial cellulitis is the location of the inflammation. In the former, the inflammation involves the subcutaneous fat, fascia, and muscle in addition to the dermis. A biopsy may be submitted at the time of surgical debridement for frozen section examination; however more often the presumptive diagnosis is made clinical and an urgently preformed debridement specimen is received for routine histologic evaluation. In an appropriate setting, the presence of edema and neutrophils in these deep locations supports the diagnosis. Frank necrosis may not be demonstrable, and bacteria are frequently not evident in an initial biopsy.

Alpha-1-Antitrypsin Deficiency–Associated Panniculitis

AATD is an autosomal codominant genetic condition characterized by decreased concentration and activity of alpha-1 antitrypsin (AAT) in blood and body tissues (52). AAT is an acute-phase glycoprotein that inhibits neutrophil proteases such as elastase. Severe AATD predisposes to chronic obstructive pulmonary disease and liver disease. Systemic vasculitis and neutrophilic panniculitis are less frequent associations.

CLINICAL SUMMARY. Panniculitis associated with AATD is extremely rare, with fewer than 50 reported cases in a recent review (40). The classical disease presentation is as recurrent erythematous subcutaneous nodules on the trunk and proximal extremities that frequently develop discrete or "punched-out" ulcers draining characteristic oily material and heal with atrophic scarring. The lesions are sometimes preceded by trauma.

HISTOPATHOLOGY. In a review of five cases, lobular panniculitis was seen in four cases, and septal widening in four cases. Neutrophils were the predominant inflammatory

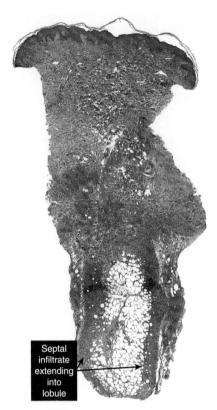

Fig. VIIID2.d

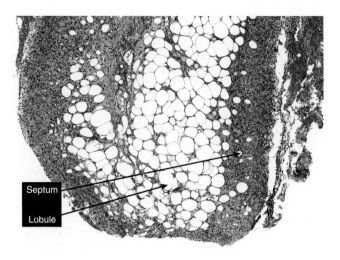

Fig. VIIID2.e

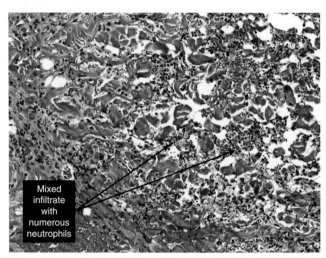

Fig. VIIID2.f

Fig. VIIID2.d. *Alpha-1-antitrypsin deficiency–associated panniculitis.* A mixed lobular and septal inflammatory infiltrate.

Fig. VIIID2.e. *Alpha-1-antitrypsin deficiency–associated panniculitis.* Inflammatory cells extending from the septa into the lobule. Lymphocytes and histiocytes predominate in this field.

Fig. VIIID2.f. *Alpha-1-antitrypsin deficiency–associated panniculitis.* In the lower dermis there is an infiltrate containing many neutrophils.

cells, seen in all five cases. Lipophagic change and fat necrosis were seen in all specimens, while granuloma formation was seen in four of them (40).

Conditions to consider in the differential diagnosis:

necrotizing fasciitis (bacterial infection)
abscesses
North American blastomycosis
pyoderma gangrenosum (involves dermis also)
ecthyma gangrenosum
alpha-1-antitrypsin deficiency
infection (cellulitis)
dissecting cellulitis of the scalp (perifolliculitis capitis abscedens et suffodiens)
hidradenitis suppurativa
ruptured follicles and cysts

VIIID3 With Many Eosinophils

Few to many eosinophils are present in subcutaneous lobules and septa.

Eosinophilic Fasciitis (Shulman Syndrome)

CLINICAL SUMMARY. Eosinophilic fasciitis (EF) (53) is a scleroderma-like disorder characterized by inflammation and thickening of the deep fascia. It has a rapid onset often after exercise, associated with pain, swelling, and progressive induration of the skin leading to exaggerated deep grooving of the skin around superficial veins. This disorder is often accompanied by peripheral eosinophilia and hypergammaglobulinemia, and has been associated with aplastic anemia. EF often involves one or more extremities. In only a few cases are there lesions on the trunk, and the face is almost invariably spared. In nearly

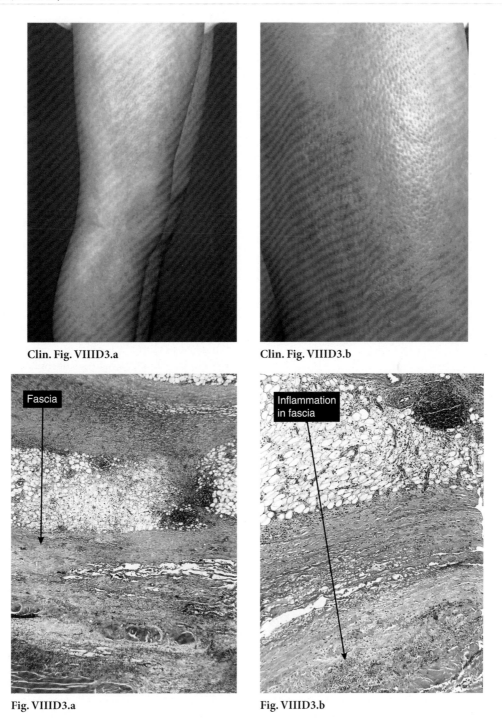

Clin. Fig. VIIID3.a

Clin. Fig. VIIID3.b

Fascia

Inflammation in fascia

Fig. VIIID3.a

Fig. VIIID3.b

Clin. Fig. VIIID3.a. *Eosinophilic fasciitis.* The outer thigh skin is swollen and indurated.

Clin. Fig. VIIID3.b. *Eosinophilic fasciitis.* The skin appears sclerotic with surface dimpling. Morphea is in the differential diagnosis.

Fig. VIIID3.a. *Eosinophilic fasciitis, low power.* This deep biopsy shows subcutaneous fat in the upper portion of the photomicrograph and fascia in the lower half. The subcutaneous septum is markedly thickened and there is an associated predominantly septal inflammatory reaction which focally extends into the lobules.

Fig. VIIID3.b. *Eosinophilic fasciitis, medium power.* The subcutaneous septum shows fibrosis and inflammation with focal extension into the lobules. (*continues*)

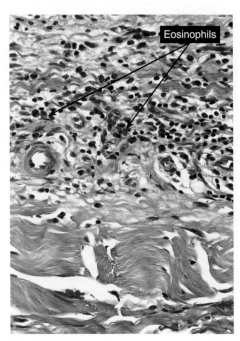

Fig. VIIID3.c

Fig. VIIID3.c. *Eosinophilic fasciitis, high power.* Eosinophils are often not as numerous as in this example, and in some cases may be rare or absent.

all reported cases, Raynaud phenomenon and visceral lesions of scleroderma have been absent. The disorder has a varied course: some patients improve spontaneously, others improve with corticosteroids, while still others may have relapses and remissions. EF shares many features with generalized morphea: they both may have inflammation and fibrosis of the fascia, as well as blood eosinophilia and hypergammaglobulinemia. Also, antinuclear antibodies are present in a significant number of cases. The term morphea profunda ("deep morphea"), analogous to lupus erythematosus profundus (i.e., "deep lupus"), has been applied to this disorder.

HISTOPATHOLOGY. Although an incisional biopsy including fascia been considered the gold standard for diagnosis of EF, radiologic imaging, particularly MRI, is now used for diagnosis and monitoring of cases (54). The fascia is markedly thickened, appears homogeneous, and is permeated by a mononuclear inflammatory infiltrate. In some instances, the infiltrate in the fascia contains an admixture of eosinophils. The underlying skeletal muscle in some cases shows myofiber degeneration, severe inflammation with a component of eosinophils, and focal scarring; in other cases, however, it is not involved. In most cases the fibrous septa separating deeply located fat lobules are thicker, paler staining, and more homogeneous and hyaline than normal subcutaneous connective tissue. In other cases, the collagen in the lower reticular dermis

appears pale and homogeneous, and the entire subcutaneous fat is replaced by horizontally oriented, thick, homogeneous collagen containing only few fibroblasts and merging with the fascia.

Conditions to consider in the differential diagnosis:

> eosinophilic fasciitis
> eosinophilic panniculitis
> arthropod bites
> parasites

VIIID4 With Many Lymphocytes

Lymphocytic infiltrates diffusely involve the subcutis.

Subcutaneous Panniculitis-Like T-Cell Lymphoma

CLINICAL SUMMARY. SPTCL (55) may present with subcutaneous nodules, usually on the extremities. As recently reviewed by Willemze, SPTCL was initially defined as a cytotoxic T-cell lymphoma that preferentially involves the subcutis, with either an α/β or a γ/δ T-cell phenotype. More recent studies showed clinical, histologic, and immunophenotypic differences between SPTCL with an α/β T-cell phenotype and SPTCL with a γ/δ T-cell phenotype, concluding that they represent different entities. Currently the term SPTCL is only used for cases with an α/β T-cell phenotype, while cases expressing the γ/δ T-cell receptor are reclassified as primary cutaneous gamma/delta T-cell lymphoma (PCGD-TCL). SPTCL and PCGD-TCL are the two most common types of cutaneous T-cell lymphoma presenting with panniculitis-like lesions (56). Some patients with this condition have associated hemophagocytic syndrome, which is more common in PCGD-TCL.

HISTOPATHOLOGY. The morphologic pattern overlaps with angiocentric lymphoma, as infiltration of vessel walls often accompanies subcutaneous infiltrates. Histopathologic features include a dense, subcutaneous infiltrate with a mixed septal and lobular distribution. The neoplastic cells have cytologic features similar to those of medium-sized or large-cell pleomorphic T-cell lymphoma, with irregularly shaped, variably sized hyperchromatic nuclei, with small nucleoli; rarely, anaplastic large cells are prominent. In cases with hemophagocytic element, phagocytosis of erythrocytes by nonneoplastic macrophages is present in the subcutaneous infiltrate or the bone marrow. Foci of karyorrhexis and fat necrosis can occur and can be associated with a granulomatous inflammatory reaction. The neoplastic cells express a mature helper T-cell phenotype but can show loss of CD5 and CD7. Subcutaneous T-cell lymphomas resemble panniculitis at scanning magnification, and in the cases in which small pleomorphic T cells predominate, their infiltrates may not be obviously malignant, even under close

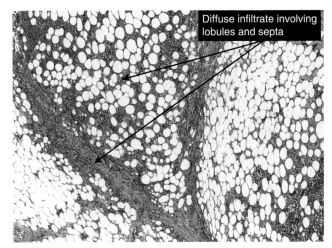

Fig. VIIID4.a

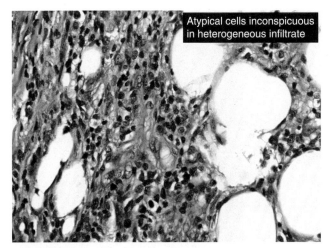

Fig. VIIID4.b

Fig. VIIID4.a. *Subcutaneous T-cell lymphoma, low power.* A septal and lobular infiltrate may mimic an inflammatory panniculus, but the infiltrate is very dense. (P. Leboit and T. McCalmont.)

Fig. VIIID4.b. *Subcutaneous T-cell lymphoma, high power.* Neoplastic lymphocytes are often inconspicuous in a heterogeneous infiltrate of macrophages, lymphocytes of varying sizes, and eosinophils. Genotypic analysis can be useful as an adjunct diagnostic tool in such instances. (P. Leboit and T. McCalmont.)

scrutiny. Atypical lymphocytes can be seen running along the edge of adipocytes, helpful clue to the diagnosis. Subcutaneous lobular lymphoid infiltrates, termed "atypical lymphocytic lobular panniculitis (LLP)," have been characterized as representing a spectrum of histologic, immunophenotypic, and molecular abnormalities which range from the clearly benign to the clearly neoplastic. Lymphoid atypia, erythrophagocytosis, loss of certain pan T-cell markers, a reduced CD4/8 ratio, and TCR rearrangement are attributes that help to define these subcuticular T-cell lymphoid dyscrasias, however some cases continue to defy precise classification (57).

Cutaneous gamma/delta T-cell lymphoma (CGD-TCL) is an aggressive lymphoma that, when involving the subcutaneous fat, can mimic the less aggressive (alpha/beta) subcutaneous panniculitic T-cell lymphoma and also the benign condition lupus erythematosus profundus, and multiple biopsies and perhaps observation over time may be needed to obtain a correct diagnosis (58).

Conditions to consider in the differential diagnosis:

> lupus panniculitis
> chronic lymphocytic leukemia
> subcutaneous T-cell lymphoma
> histiocytic cytophagic panniculitis (early lesion)

VIIID5 With Cytophagic Histiocytes

Histiocytes with phagocytized erythrocytes diffusely infiltrate the subcutis. Rosai–Dorfman disease is a prototypic example (59).

Sinus Histiocytosis With Massive Lymphadenopathy (SHML, Rosai–Dorfman)

CLINICAL SUMMARY. Massive cervical lymphadenopathy, usually bilateral and painless, is the most common manifestation. This is generally a benign disorder in spite of a propensity to form large masses and to disseminate to both nodal and extranodal sites. In most patients the disease resolves spontaneously, others have persistent problems, and very few die. Skin is the most common extranodal site, with over 10% of patients having cutaneous involvement. The lesions are typically papules or nodules. A similar percentage has soft tissue involvement, usually of the subcutaneous tissue. Occasionally the soft tissue lesion may present as a breast mass or panniculitis. Although the disorders are clearly related, the cutaneous form of the disease occurs in an older and ethnically more diverse group and is less likely to be associated with systemic symptoms than the systemic form (60). The IHC profile (S100+, CD68+, CD1a–) is relatively specific (61). Recent studies have identified mutations in the MAK kinase pathway indicating that this is a neoplastic condition at least in these cases (62).

HISTOPATHOLOGY. The skin lesions contain a polymorphous infiltrate in which histiocytes with abundant cytoplasm are the most prominent element. Occasionally they may be multinucleated or have a foamy cytoplasm. However, the hallmark histologic feature is emperipolesis of lymphocytes. On occasion, red cells can also be taken up. In the lymph nodes, the sinuses are greatly dilated and crowded with inflammatory cells, particularly histiocytes. Here they tend to have an abundant foamy cytoplasm and

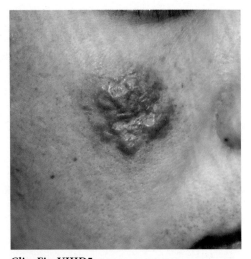

Clin. Fig. VIIID5

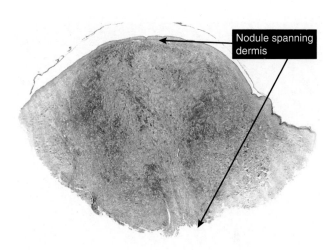

Nodule spanning dermis

Fig. VIIID5.a

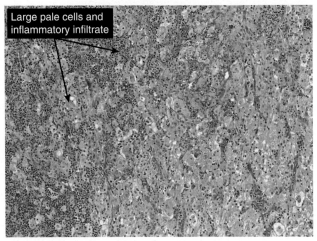

Large pale cells and inflammatory infiltrate

Fig. VIIID5.b

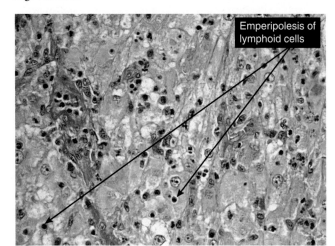

Emperipolesis of lymphoid cells

Fig. VIIID5.c

Clin. Fig. VIIID5. *Rosai–Dorfman disease.* A multinodular tumor in the dermis and subcutis, without epidermal involvement.

Fig. VIIID5.a. *Rosai–Dorfman disease, low power.* A nodular infiltrate spanning the dermis and entering the subcutis, with pale-staining cells centrally. (W. Burgdorf.)

Fig. VIIID5.b. *Rosai–Dorfman disease, medium power.* Typical pattern of strands of pale sinus histiocytes admixed with darker-staining lymphocytes. (W. Burgdorf.)

Fig. VIIID5.c. *Rosai–Dorfman disease, high power.* Numerous large histiocytes, some of which have ingested lymphocytes, demonstrating emperipolesis. (W. Burgdorf.)

also display emperipolesis. The histiocytes are S100+ and CD1a–, and do not contain Birbeck granules. About 50% are CD30 positive. Perivascular plasma cells are frequently seen in the infiltrate.

Conditions to consider in the differential diagnosis:

alpha-1-antitrypsin deficiency (late lesion)
histiocytic cytophagic panniculitis (late lesion)
Rosai–Dorfman disease (SHML)
cutaneous lymphoid hyperplasia

VIIID6 With Granulomas

There is granulomatous inflammation involving the subcutis.

Mycobacterial Panniculitis

Mycobacterial infection of the fat can produce a *mycobacterial panniculitis* that can mimic erythema nodosum as well as erythema induratum. Special stains for acid-fast bacteria and cultures are important for the

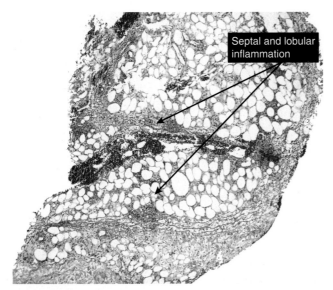

Fig. VIIID6.a

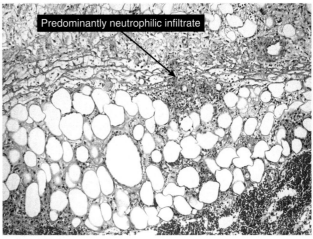

Fig. VIIID6.b

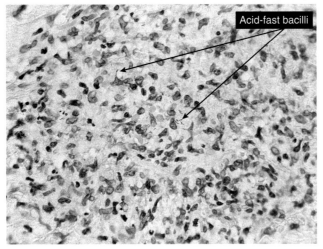

Fig. VIIID6.c

Fig. VIIID6.a. *Mycobacterial panniculitis, low power.* Direct mycobacterial infection of the fat has produced both a septal and lobular panniculitis. (N.S. McNutt, A. Moreno, F. Contreras.)

Fig. VIIID6.b. *Mycobacterial panniculitis, medium power.* The infiltrate is mixed with collections of neutrophils. (N.S. McNutt, A. Moreno, F. Contreras.)

Fig. VIIID6.c. *Mycobacterial panniculitis, high power.* Staining for mycobacteria shows that numerous red, acid-fast bacilli are present in this example. (N.S. McNutt, A. Moreno, F. Contreras.)

identification of the mycobacteria that are responsible. Often nontuberculous mycobacteria are involved in countries with a low incidence of tuberculosis, and in immunodeficient subjects (63). Granulomas may be inconspicuous or absent in many of these situations. A high index of suspicion is important, and modified acid-fast staining may be required to demonstrate the organisms.

Erythema Nodosum Leprosum (Type 2 Leprosy Reaction)

CLINICAL SUMMARY. Erythema nodosum leprosum, or ENL, occurs most commonly in lepromatous leprosy (LL) and less frequently in borderline lepromatous leprosy (BL) (64). Immune complex production and deposition as well as complement activation are regarded as the principal pathogenetic mechanism, while new data

show that cell-mediated immunity is also important. ENL is characterized by an inflammatory infiltrate of neutrophils with vasculitis and/or panniculitis. There is deposition of immune complexes and complement together with Mycobacterium leprae antigens in the skin. The major T-cell subtype in ENL is the CD4 cell, in contrast to LL leprosy where CD8 cells predominate (65). It may be observed in patients under treatment or in untreated patients. Clinically, there is a widespread eruption accompanied by fever, malaise, arthralgia, and leukocytosis. On the skin there are tender, red plaques and nodules together with areas of erythema and occasionally also purpura and vesicles. Ulceration, however, is rare (66).

HISTOPATHOLOGY. The skin and subcutaneous lesions are foci of acute inflammation superimposed on chronic

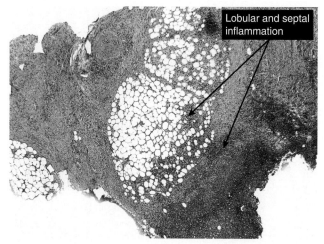

Fig. VIIID6.d

Fig. VIIID6.e

Fig. VIIID6.f

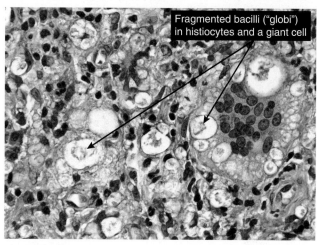

Fig. VIIID6.g

Fig. VIIID6.d. *Erythema nodosum leprosum, low power.* The architecture on scanning magnification may resemble erythema nodosum. Superiorly there is a large vessel within a fat lobule which is occluded and surrounded by a dense infiltrate.

Fig. VIIID6.e. *Erythema nodosum leprosum, low power.* This profile demonstrates dense inflammation within the septa and focally within the lobules. Vascular involvement is also evident.

Fig. VIIID6.f. *Erythema nodosum leprosum, medium power.* A granuloma composed of histiocytes and giant cells is present at the edge of a fat lobule. Clear spaces are identifiable within histiocytes.

Fig. VIIID6.g. *Erythema nodosum leprosum, high power.* Close inspection of the clear spaces within foamy macrophages and giant cells reveals numerous clumps of fragmented bacilli ("globi") within the foamy cells, which are known as "lepra" or "Virchow" cells. Neutrophils are scattered throughout this granuloma.

multibacillary leprosy. Polymorph neutrophils may be scanty or so abundant as to form a dermal abscess with ulceration. Whereas foamy macrophages containing fragmented bacilli are usual, in some patients no bacilli remain and macrophages have a granular pink hue on Wade-Fite staining, indicating mycobacterial debris. A necrotizing vasculitis affecting arterioles, venules, and capillaries occurs in some cases; these patients may have superficial ulceration.

Conditions to consider in the differential diagnosis:

palisaded granulomas
subcutaneous granuloma annulare/pseudorheumatoid nodule
rheumatoid nodules
tuberculosis/mycobacteria
Crohn disease
gummatous tertiary syphilis

erythema nodosum leprosum
chronic erythema nodosum
mycobacterial panniculitis
subcutaneous sarcoidosis
epithelioid sarcoma

VIIIE   SUBCUTANEOUS ABSCESSES

A collection of neutrophils and necrotic material in the subcutis, usually surrounded by granulation tissue and fibrosis.

VIIIE1   With Neutrophils

The center of the abscess contains pus, which is viscous because of the presence of DNA fragments derived from neutrophils and dead organisms. Acute or chronic bacterial abscesses, and deep fungal infections, including "phaeohyphomycotic cyst" are prototypic.

Phaeohyphomycotic Cyst

CLINICAL SUMMARY. Phaeohyphomycosis (67) has been defined as a subcutaneous or systemic infection by dematiaceous, mycelia-forming fungi, that is, those fungi

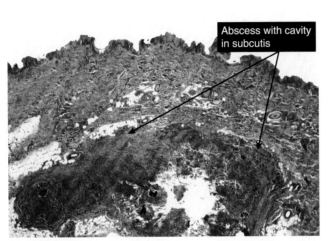

Fig. VIIIE1.a

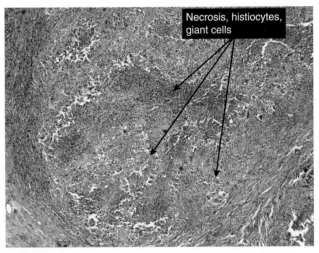

Fig. VIIIE1.b

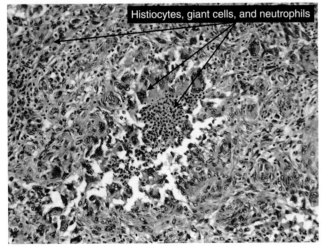

Fig. VIIIE1.c

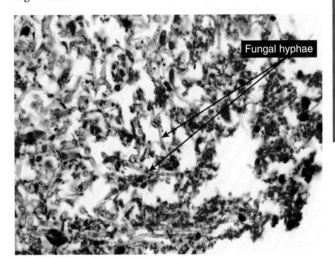

Fig. VIIIE1.d

Fig. VIIIE1.a. *Phaeohyphomycotic "cyst" (abscess).* A subcutaneous nodule was comprised of sheets of neutrophils, with demonstrable fungal hyphae at higher magnification.

Fig. VIIIE1.b. *Phaeohyphomycotic cyst, low power.* There is a dense infiltrate in the dermis with a central collection of neutrophils surrounded by granulomatous inflammation.

Fig. VIIIE1.c. *Phaeohyphomycotic cyst, medium power.* There are alternating zones of neutrophilic abscesses and granulomatous inflammation with histiocytes and multinucleated giant cells.

Fig. VIIIE1.d. *Phaeohyphomycotic cyst, high power.* Fungal forms may be most likely to be found in the areas of neutrophilic inflammation. The fungi may or may not contain brown pigment.

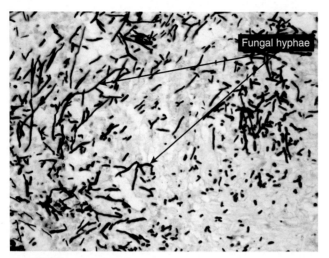

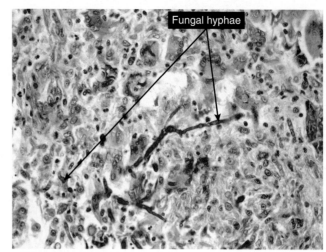

Fig. VIIIE1.e   **Fig. VIIIE1.f**

Fig. VIIIE1.e. *Phaeohyphomycotic cyst, high power, GMS stain.* This silver stain highlights many organisms in this phaeohyphomycotic cyst.

Fig. VIIIE1.f. *Phaeohyphomycotic cyst, high power, PAS stain.* The organisms also stain positively with a periodic acid Schiff stain.

having dark-walled hyphae. This is a histopathologic definition of a disease process that can be caused by many different organisms and that can have multiple different clinical presentations. Subcutaneous phaeohyphomycosis typically presents as a solitary abscess or nodule on the extremity of an adult male. A history of trauma or a splinter can sometimes be elicited. Fungal infection should be suspected in all subcutaneous cystic lesions, especially in endemic areas. Excised tissue should always be sent for culture and histopathology (68).

HISTOPATHOLOGY. Lesions of subcutaneous phaeohyphomycosis start as small, often stellate foci of suppurative granulomatous inflammation. The area of inflammation gradually enlarges and usually forms a single large cavity with a surrounding fibrous capsule, the so-called phaeohyphomycotic cyst. The central space is filled with pus formed of polymorphonuclear leukocytes and fibrin. There is a surrounding granulomatous reaction composed of histiocytes, including epithelioid cells and multinucleated giant cells, lymphocytes, and plasma cells. Diligent search may identify an associated splinter in the tissue or liquid pus. The organisms are found within the cavity and at its edge, often within histiocytes. The hyphae often have irregularly placed branches and show constrictions around their septa. Mycelia, if present, are more loosely arranged than the compact masses of hyphae seen in eumycetoma. Pigment is not always obvious.

Conditions to consider in the differential diagnosis:

deep fungal infections
phaeohyphomycotic cyst

North American blastomycosis
chromoblastomycosis
cutaneous alternariosis
paracoccidioidomycosis
coccidioidomycosis
sporotrichosis
acute or chronic bacterial abscesses
protothecosis
mycobacterial panniculitis

References

1. Wick MR. Panniculitis: a summary. *Semin Diagn Pathol* 2017; 34(3):261–272.
2. Requena L, Yus ES. Panniculitis. Part I. Mostly septal panniculitis. *J Am Acad Dermatol* 2001;45:163–183.
3. Chopra R, Chhabra S, Thami GP, et al. Panniculitis: clinical overlap and the significance of biopsy findings. *J Cutan Pathol* 2010;37(1):49–58.
4. Chen KR, Carlson JA. Clinical approach to cutaneous vasculitis. *Am J Clin Dermatol* 2008;9(2):71–92. Review.
5. Frumholtz L, Laurent-Roussel S, Aumaître O, et al; French Vasculitis Study Group. Clinical and pathological significance of cutaneous manifestations in ANCA-associated vasculitides. *Autoimmun Rev* 2017;16(11):1138–1146.
6. Carlson JA. The histological assessment of cutaneous vasculitis. *Histopathology* 2010;56(1):3–23. Review.
7. Morgan AJ, Schwartz RA. Cutaneous polyarteritis nodosa: a comprehensive review. *Int J Dermatol* 2010;49(7):750–756.
8. Sanchez NP, Van Hale HM, Su WP. Clinical and histopathologic spectrum of necrotizing vasculitis. Report of findings in 101 cases. *Arch Dermatol* 1985;121:220–224.
9. Chen KR. The misdiagnosis of superficial thrombophlebitis as cutaneous polyarteritis nodosa: features of the internal elastic

lamina and the compact concentric muscular layer as diagnostic pitfalls. *Am J Dermatopathol* 2010;32(7):688–693.

10. Kossard S. Defining lymphocytic vasculitis. *Australas J Dermatol* 2000;41:149–155.

11. Carlson JA, Chen KR. Cutaneous vasculitis update: neutrophilic muscular vessel and eosinophilic, granulomatous, and lymphocytic vasculitis syndromes. *Am J Dermatopathol* 2007;29(1):32–43.

12. Rademaker M, Lowe DG, Munro DD. Erythema induratum (Bazin's disease). *J Am Acad Dermatol* 1989;21:740–745.

13. Magalhães TS, Dammert VG, Samorano LP, et al. Erythema induratum of Bazin: epidemiological, clinical and laboratorial profile of 54 patients. *J Dermatol* 2018;45(5):628–629.

14. Bayer-Garner IB, Cox MD, Scott MA, et al. Mycobacteria other than Mycobacterium tuberculosis are not present in erythema induratum/nodular vasculitis: a case series and literature review of the clinical and histologic findings. *J Cutan Pathol* 2005;32:220–222.

15. Chen YH, Yan JJ, Chao SC, et al. Erythema induratum: a clinicopathologic and polymerase chain reaction study. *J Formos Med Assoc* 2001;100:244–249.

16. Segura S, Pujol RM, Trindade F, et al. Vasculitis in erythema induratum of Bazin: a histopathologic study of 101 biopsy specimens from 86 patients. *J Am Acad Dermatol* 2008;59(5):839–851.

17. Requena L, Requena C. Erythema nodosum. *Dermatol Online J* 2002;8:4.

18. Leung AKC, Leong KF, Lam JM. Erythema nodosum. *World J Pediatr* 2018;14(6):548–554.

19. Mössner R, Zimmer L, Berking C, et al. Erythema nodosum-like lesions during BRAF inhibitor therapy: report on 16 new cases and review of the literature. *J Eur Acad Dermatol Venereol* 2015;29(9):1797–1806.

20. Rubin M, Lynch FW. Subcutaneous granuloma annulare. *Arch Dermatol Syphiligr* 1966;93:416.

21. Stefanaki K, Tsivitanidou-Kakourou T, Stefanaki C, et al. Histological and immunohistochemical study of granuloma annulare and subcutaneous granuloma annulare in children. *J Cutan Pathol* 2007;34(5):392–396.

22. Requena L, Fernández-Figueras MT. Subcutaneous granuloma annulare. *Semin Cutan Med Surg* 2007;26(2):96–99. Review.

23. Fett N, Werth VP. Update on morphea: part I. Epidemiology, clinical presentation, and pathogenesis. *J Am Acad Dermatol* 2011;64(2):217–228; quiz 229–230. Review.

24. Knobler R, Moinzadeh P, Hunzelmann N, et al. European Dermatology Forum S1-guideline on the diagnosis and treatment of sclerosing diseases of the skin, Part 1: localized scleroderma, systemic sclerosis and overlap syndromes. *J Eur Acad Dermatol Venereol* 2017;31(9):1401–1424.

25. Tuffanelli DL. Lupus panniculitis. *Sem Dermatol* 1985;4:79.

26. Massone C, Kodama K, Salmhofer W, et al. Lupus erythematosus panniculitis (lupus profundus): clinical, histopathological, and molecular analysis of nine cases. *J Cutan Pathol* 2005;32:396–404.

27. LeBlanc RE, Tavallaee M, Kim YH, et al. Useful parameters for distinguishing subcutaneous panniculitis-like T-Cell lymphoma from lupus erythematosus panniculitis. *Am J Surg Pathol* 2016;40(6):745–754.

28. Park HS, Choi JW, Kim BK, et al. Lupus erythematosus panniculitis: clinicopathological, immunophenotypic, and molecular studies. *Am J Dermatopathol* 2010;32(1):24–30.

29. Chow S, Pasternak S, Green P, et al. Histiocytoid neutrophilic dermatoses and panniculitides: variations on a theme. *Am J Dermatopathol* 2007;29(4):334–341.

30. Hytiroglou P, Phelps RG, Wattenberg DJ, et al. Histiocytic cytophagic panniculitis: molecular evidence for a clonal T-cell disorder. *J Am Acad Dermatol* 1992;27:333.

31. Craig AJ, Cualing H, Thomas G, et al. Cytophagic histiocytic panniculitis—a syndrome associated with benign and malignant panniculitis: case comparison and review of the literature. *J Am Acad Dermatol* 1998;39(5 Pt 1):721–736. Review.

32. Pasqualini C, Jorini M, Carloni I, et al. Cytophagic histiocytic panniculitis, hemophagocytic lymphohistiocytosis and undetermined autoimmune disorder: reconciling the puzzle. *Ital J Pediatr* 2014;40(1):17.

33. Takeshita M, Okamura S, Oshiro Y, et al. Clinicopathologic differences between 22 cases of CD56-negative and CD56-positive subcutaneous panniculitis-like lymphoma in Japan. *Hum Pathol* 2004;35:231–239.

34. Al-Samkari H, Berliner N. Hemophagocytic lymphohistiocytosis. *Annu Rev Pathol* 2018;13:27–49.

35. White JW Jr, Winkelmann RK. Weber-Christian panniculitis: a review of 30 cases with this diagnosis. *J Am Acad Dermatol* 1998;39:56–62.

36. Norwood-Galloway A, Lebwohl M, Phelps RG, et al. Subcutaneous fat necrosis of the newborn with hypercalcemia. *J Am Acad Dermatol* 1987;16:435–439.

37. Burden AD, Krafchik BR. Subcutaneous fat necrosis of the newborn: a review of 11 cases. *Pediatr Dermatol* 1999;16:384–387.

38. Jeong HS, Dominguez AR. Calciphylaxis: controversies in pathogenesis, diagnosis and treatment. *Am J Med Sci* 2016;351(2):217–227.

39. Zembowicz A, Navarro P, Walters S, et al. Subcutaneous thrombotic vasculopathy syndrome: an ominous condition reminiscent of calciphylaxis: calciphylaxis sine calcifications? *Am J Dermatopathol* 2011;33(8):796–802.

40. Essary LR, Wick MR. Cutaneous calciphylaxis. An under recognized clinicopathologic entity. *Am J Clin Pathol* 2000;113:280–287.

41. Hughes PSH, Apisarnthanarax P, Mullins JF. Subcutaneous fat necrosis associated with pancreatic disease. *Arch Dermatol* 1975;111:506–510.

42. Peters MS, Winkelmann RK. The histopathology of localized lipoatrophy. *Br J Dermatol* 1986;114:27–36.

43. Hussain I, Garg A. Lipodystrophy syndromes. *Endocrinol Metab Clin North Am* 2016;45(4):783–797.

44. Snow JL, Su WP. Lipomembranous (membranocystic) fat necrosis. Clinicopathologic correlation of 38 cases. *Am J Dermatopathol* 1996;18:151–155.

45. Alegre VA, Winkelmann RK, Aliaga A. Lipomembranous changes in chronic panniculitis. *J Am Acad Dermatol* 1988;19:39–46.

46. Duncan WC, Freeman RG, Heaton CL. Cold panniculitis. *Arch Dermatol* 1966;94:722–724.

47. Winer LH, Steinberg TH, Lehman R, et al. Tissue reactions to injected silicone liquids. *Arch Dermatol* 1964;90:588–593.

48. Forstrom L, Winkelmann RK. Factitial panniculitis. *Arch Dermatol* 1974;110:747–750.

49. Lancerotto L, Tocco I, Salmaso R, et al. Necrotizing fasciitis: classification, diagnosis, and management. *J Trauma Acute Care Surg* 2012;72(3):560–566.

50. Lee CY, Li YY, Huang TW, et al. Synchronous multifocal necrotizing fasciitis prognostic factors: a retrospective case series study in a single center. *Infection* 2016;44(6):757–763.

51. Wong CH, Wang YS. The diagnosis of necrotizing fasciitis. *Curr Opin Infect Dis* 2005;18:101–106.

VIII Disorders of the Subcutis

52. Johnson EF, Tolkachjov SN, Gibson LE. Alpha-1 antitrypsin deficiency panniculitis: clinical and pathologic characteristics of 10 cases. *Int J Dermatol* 2018;57(8):952–958.

53. Helfman T, Falanga V. Eosinophilic fasciitis. *Clin Dermatol* 1994;12:449–455.

54. Mazori DR, Femia AN, Vleugels RA. Eosinophilic Fasciitis: an updated review on diagnosis and treatment. *Curr Rheumatol Rep* 2017;19(12):74.

55. Perniciaro C, Zalla MJ, White JW Jr, et al. Subcutaneous T-cell lymphoma: report of two additional cases and further observations. *Arch Dermatol* 1993;129:1171–1176.

56. Willemze R. Cutaneous lymphomas with a panniculitic presentation. *Semin Diagn Pathol* 2017;34(1):36–43.

57. Magro CM, Crowson AN, Kovatich AJ, et al. Lupus profundus, indeterminate lymphocytic lobular panniculitis and subcutaneous T-cell lymphoma: a spectrum of subcuticular T-cell lymphoid dyscrasia. *J Cutan Pathol* 2001;28:235–247.

58. Aguilera P, Mascaró JM Jr, Martinez A, et al. Cutaneous gamma/delta T-cell lymphoma: a histopathologic mimicker of lupus erythematosus profundus (lupus panniculitis). *J Am Acad Dermatol* 2007;56(4):643–647.

59. Perrin C, Michiels JF, Lacour JP, et al. Sinus histiocytosis (Rosai-Dorfman disease) clinically limited to the skin: an immunohistochemical and ultrastructural study. *J Cutan Pathol* 1993;20:368–374.

60. Wang KH, Chen WY, Liu HN. Cutaneous Rosai-Dorfman disease: clinicopathological profiles, spectrum and evolution of 21 lesions in six patients. *Br J Dermatol* 2006;154:277–286.

61. Ahmed A, Crowson N, Magro CM. A comprehensive assessment of cutaneous Rosai-Dorfman disease. *Ann Diagn Pathol* 2019;40:166–173.

62. Baraban E, Sadigh S, Rosenbaum J, et al. Cyclin D1 expression and novel mutational findings in Rosai-Dorfman disease. *Br J Haematol* 2019;186(6):837–844.

63. Inwald D, Nelson M, Cramp M, et al. Cutaneous manifestations of mycobacterial infection in patients with AIDS. *Br J Dermatol* 1994;130:111–114.

64. Hussain R, Lucas SB, Kifayet A, et al. Clinical and histological discrepancies in diagnosis of ENL reactions classified by assessment of acute phase proteins SAA and CRP. *Int J Lepr* 1995; 63:222–230.

65. Kahawita IP, Lockwood DN. Towards understanding the pathology of erythema nodosum leprosum. *Trans R Soc Trop Med Hyg* 2008;102(4):329–337.

66. Negera E, Walker SL, Girma S, et al. Clinico-pathological features of erythema nodosum leprosum: a case-control study at ALERT hospital, Ethiopia. *PLoS Negl Trop Dis* 2017;11(10): e0006011.

67. McGinnis MR. Chromoblastomycosis and phaeohyphomycosis: new concepts, diagnosis, and mycology. *J Am Acad Dermatol* 1983;8:1.

68. Priyadharshini G, Varghese RG, Phansalkar M, et al. Subcutaneous fungal cyst masquerading as benign lesions—a series of eight cases. *J Clin Diagn Res* 2015;9(10): EM01-4.

Tumors
  of adipose tissue
    angiolipoma, 451, 453f
    lipoma, 451, 452
    liposarcomas, 454, 454f
    nevus lipomatosus superficialis, 451, 452f
    pleomorphic lipomas, 454, 454f
    spindle cell lipoma, 452, 453f, 454f
  apocrine, 376, 377f, 378f
  of cartilaginous tissue, 455
  eccrine, 366
    circumscribed, symmetrical, 366–373
    infiltrative, asymmetrical, 373–376
  epithelial, 406–408
  fibrohistiocytic spindle cell, 409
  glomus, 447, 450f
  of large hematolymphoid cells, 397–403
  of lymphocytes
    and mixed cell types, 330–332
    or hemopoietic cells, 325–330, 327t
  mast cell, 403–404, 403f, 404f
  melanocytic, 346, 346t
  melanocytic spindle cell, 433–
  of osseous tissue, 455–456
  pilar, 379–387
  and proliferations of angiogenic cells, 435–451
  with prominent necrosis, 404–406
  schwannian/neural spindle cell, 423–428
  sebaceous, 387–391
  of small cells, 332–335
  squamous cell
    inverted follicular keratosis, 337–339
    proliferating trichilemmal cyst, 341
    prurigo nodularis, 342–343, 342f
    pseudoepitheliomatous hyperplasia, 339
    solitary keratoacanthoma, 336–337
    squamous cell carcinoma, 335–336

U

Ulcers, chronic, and sinuses
  chancroid, 290–291, 290f
  chondrodermatitis nodularis helicis, 292f, 293
  pyoderma gangrenosum, 291–293, 291f
Urticaria, 84, 85f, 86f, 223–224, 225f
Urticarial bullous pemphigoid, 86f, 87
Urticaria pigmentosa, 98–99, 99f, 254, 255f, 403–404
  lichenoid examples, 141

V

Vacuolar dermatitis
  apoptotic cells, absent
    dermatomyositis, 156–157, 157f
  apoptotic/necrotic cells prominent
    erythema multiforme, 152–155, 153f
    fixed drug eruption, 154, 155, 155f
    graft-versus-host disease, acute, 155, 155f, 156f
  basement membranes thickened
    discoid lupus erythematosus, 159, 160f, 161f
  variable apoptosis
    subacute cutaneous lupus erythematosus, 157, 158f, 159f
Varicella-zoster virus, 186f, 187
Vasculitis, 95
  granulomatous, 513–515
  leukocytoclastic, 144–145, 144f, 145f, 237, 238f, 239f
  lymphocytes predominant
    cytomegalovirus infection, 235, 235f
    erythema chronicum migrans, 235, 236f
    pernio or chilblains, 232
    pityriasis lichenoides, 232–235, 233f, 234f
  lymphocytic, 513
  mixed cell/granulomas, 146, 147f

  eosinophilic granulomatosis with polyangiitis, 240
  papulonecrotic tuberculid, 240, 241f
  neutrophilic (See Neutrophilic vasculitis)
  neutrophilic, 512–513
  neutrophils prominent
    erythema elevatum diutinum, 239, 240f
    neutrophilic small-vessel vasculitis, 237–239
    polyarteritis nodosa/microscopic polyangiitis, 236, 237f
  septic, 145, 145f, 146f
  true, defined, 231
Vasculopathy, 156
  with lymphocytic inflammation, 147–149, 148f
  with scant inflammation, 149–150, 149f, 150f
Vellus hair cyst, 457, 459f
Venous lake, 447, 449f
Verruca plana, 6, 55, 57, 57f
Verruca vulgaris, 55, 56f
Verruciform xanthoma, 391, 393f
Verrucous melanoma, 64, 130, 131f
Vertical growth phase (VGP), 358
VGP. See Vertical growth phase(VGP)
Viral exanthem, 79–80, 80f
Vitiligo, 14, 15f

W

Warty dyskeratoma, 194–195, 194f
Wells syndrome, 255, 256f
Woringer-Kolopp disease, 55

X

Xanthelasma, 252f, 253, 253f, 391, 392f
Xanthomas/xanthelasma, 391
X-linked ichthyosis, 2t, 3, 3f